CONTEMPORARY HEMATOLOGY

Judith E. Karp, MD, Series Editor

For further volumes:
http://www.springer.com/series/7681

Francine Foss
Editor

T-Cell Lymphomas

Humana Press

Editor
Francine Foss, MD
Department of Medical Oncology/Hematology
Yale University School of Medicine
New Haven, CT, USA

ISBN 978-1-4939-5732-3 ISBN 978-1-62703-170-7 (eBook)
DOI 10.1007/978-1-62703-170-7
Springer New York Heidelberg Dordrecht London

Softcover re-print of the Hardcover 1st edition 2013

Printed on acid-free paper

Humana Press is a brand of Springer
Springer is part of Springer Science+Business Media (www.springer.com)

I would like to dedicate this book to my colleagues internationally who have brought their tremendous expertise and energy to the clinical challenge of diagnosing and treating patients with T-cell malignancies. In particular, two individuals who have been tremendously inspirational to me. Dr. Thomas Waldmann has inspired me from my earliest days at the National Cancer Institute with his tireless and dedicated pursuit of the T-cell in all of its respects and for his seminal contributions to our understanding of T-cell biology and therapeutics. Among his other achievements, Tom defined the Interleukin-2 receptor subunits, developed the first interleukin-2-targeted monoclonal antibody, and was the co-discoverer of interleukin-15. Dr. John Murphy, a world expert in the structural analysis and biology of toxins, developed a novel concept for targeting cytokine receptors and constructed the first fusion toxin (denileukin diftitox) which was FDA-approved for the treatment of T-cell lymphoma.
I had the pleasure of working with Jack's group both at the bench and in the early clinical development of denileukin diftitox and have the greatest admiration for his brilliance and tenacity. Both of these scientists are unsung heroes for many patients suffering from the rare hematologic disorders.

Francine Foss, MD

Preface

The mature T- and NK-cell lymphomas are rare, comprising approximately 10 % of all malignant lymphomas. The incidence of T-cell lymphoma is variable around the world, with a higher incidence compared to B-cell lymphomas in the Asian basin. While the overall incidence of B-cell lymphomas has begun to decline in the United States, the incidence of T-cell lymphomas continues to rise. The evolution of T-cell lymphoma biology and therapy has lagged behind that of B-cell lymphomas, partly due to the fact that in the lymphoproliferative world, T-cell lymphomas have only recently been identified as distinct from their B-cell counterparts. Early lymphoma classification systems made no distinction between B- and T-cell lymphomas. The Working Formulation grouped lymphomas by size and grade and identified them based on clinical behavior (aggressive vs. indolent). In the mid-1990s, the Revised European American Lymphoma Classification attempted to identify distinct clinicopathologic entities based on immunophenotypic and molecular features and included the subset of T-cell lymphomas. More recently, the World Health Organization (WHO) has attempted to further classify lymphomas based on clinical, morphologic, phenotypic, and molecular genetic features to define disease entities and provisional entities. Within the mature T/NK-cell neoplasms, there are 20 entities or provisional entities, with the most common types being the nodal T-cell lymphomas.

The history of T-cell lymphomas is rich and significant advances have been made over the past few years. The identification of thc first human retrovirus HTLV-1 was made in 1980, the setting of a patient with aggressive T-cell leukemia/lymphoma from whom the HUT102 cell line was derived, and the first application of a T-cell-targeted monoclonal antibody, the anti-TAC antibody directed against the CD25 epitope, was conducted by the Waldmann group at the NCI in patients with HTLV-1-associated T-cell leukemia. The propagation of the HTLV-1 retrovirus in vitro was facilitated via a HUT78/H9 cell line representing a mature CD4+ cutaneous T-cell lymphoma. More recently, molecular profiling has identified and distinguished distinct subsets of aggressive nodal T-cell lymphomas within the group of peripheral T-cell lymphomas which are "not otherwise specified" and has led to the identification of a follicular dendritic cell origin for angioimmunoblastic T-cell lymphoma. The importance of the Notch signaling pathway has been shown in T-ALL by the presence of activating NOTCH mutations in over 50 % of patients. Expression of ALK fusion proteins in anaplastic large cell lymphoma has been associated with an adverse outcome and may identify yet another unique subset of T-cell lymphomas. The demonstration of in vitro cytotoxicity of L-asparaginase in NK/T-cell lymphoma cell lines has led to clinical trials using this active agent in refractory NK/T-cell lymphoma patients and has largely changed the therapeutic landscape for these diseases.

From a therapeutic perspective, these and other advances have led to an explosion in the development of novel therapeutic approaches for the T-cell lymphoproliferative disorders. Currently there are a number of FDA-approved therapies for T-cell malignancies, including the IL2 fusion toxin denileukin diftitox, the RXR retinoid bexarotene, the histone deacetylase inhibitors vorinostat, and romidepsin for cutaneous T-cell lymphomas, and pralatrexate, a folate antagonist and romidepsin for peripheral T-cell lymphomas, brentuximab vedotin, a CD30-targeted fusion toxin for anaplastic large cell lymphomas, and the nucleoside analog nelarabine for T-cell ALL. A number of new agents targeting specific receptors and metabolic pathways are currently in clinical trials and are on the horizon.

This book is a comprehensive overview of the T-cell lymphoproliferative disorders both in adults and in children and includes both the cutaneous and the systemic T-cell malignancies. The experts in the field have done an excellent job summarizing the highlights in each disorder with the intent to introduce the reader to the salient clinical and biological features of these diseases as well as future directions for research and novel approaches. I would like to thank all of my collaborators for their insights and ongoing tireless efforts to address the unmet needs within the field of T-cell lymphoproliferative disorders.

New Haven, CT, USA Francine Foss, MD

Acknowledgments

I would like to acknowledge the dedication and persistence of Dotty Saccavino, my administrative assistant, without whom this book would not be possible.

New Haven, CT, USA Francine Foss, MD

Contents

Contributors

Farah Rukhsana Abdulla, MD Department of Dermatology, Southern California Permanente Medical Group, Fontana, CA, USA

Lapo Alinari, MD, PhD Department of Internal Medicine, The Ohio State University, Columbus, OH, USA

Mitchell S. Cairo, MD Pediatric Hematology/Oncology/Stem Cell Transplantation, New York Medical College, NY, USA

Chan Cheah, MBBS (Hons) Division of Cancer Medicine, Peter MacCallum Cancer Centre, Melbourne, VIC, Australia

Bertrand Coiffier, MD, PhD Department of Hematology, Hospices Civils de Lyon and Université Claude Bernard, Lyon, France

Paolo Corradini, MD Division of Hematology, Fondazione IRCCS Istituto Nazionale dei Tumori Milano, Milan, Italy

Claudiu V. Cotta, MD, PhD Department of Pathology and Laboratory Medicine Institute, Cleveland Clinic, Cleveland, OH, USA

Nam H. Dang, MD, PhD Department of Medicine, Division of Hematology and Oncology, University of Florida, Gainesville, FL, USA

Laurence de Leval, MD, PhD Institute of Pathology, CHUV, Lausanne, Switzerland

Claire Dearden, MD Department of Haemato-Oncology, The Royal Marsden Hospital and Institute of Cancer Research, London, UK

Michael Dickinson, MBBS (Hons), FRACP, FRCPA Division of Cancer Medicine, Peter MacCallum Cancer Centre, Melbourne, VIC, Australia

Madeleine Duvic, MD Department of Dermatology, UT-MD Anderson Cancer Center, Houston, TX, USA

Richard L. Edelson, MD Department of Dermatology, Yale University School of Medicine, New Haven, CT, USA

Nader Kim El-Mallawany, MD Departments of Pediatric Hematology, Oncology, Blood and Marrow Transplantation, Columbia University, New York, NY, USA

Adolfo A. Ferrando, MD, PhD Institute for Cancer Genetics, Departments of Pediatrics and Pathology, Columbia University Medical Center, New York, NY, USA

Francine Foss, MD Department of Medical Oncology/Hematology, Yale University School of Medicine, New Haven, CT, USA

Varsha Gandhi, PhD Departments of Experimental Therapeutics and Leukemia, MD Anderson Cancer Center, Houston, TX, USA

Philippe Gaulard, MD Département de Pathologie, Hôpital Henri Mondor, Créteil, France

Michael Girardi, MD, FAAD Department of Dermatology, Yale University School of Medicine, New Haven, CT, USA

Christian Gisselbrecht, MD Department of Hemato-Oncology, Saint Louis, Paris, France

Elisabeth Grey-Davies, MD Department of Haemato-Oncology, The Royal Marsden Hospital and Institute of Cancer Research, Surrey, UK

Eric D. Hsi, MD Pathology and Laboratory Medicine Institute, Cleveland Clinic, Cleveland, OH, USA

S. David Hudnall, MD Department of Pathology, Yale University School of Medicine, New Haven, CT, USA

Marshall E. Kadin, MD Department of Dermatology and Skin Surgery, Boston University of Medicine and Roger Williams Medical Center, Providence, RI, USA

Youn H. Kim, MD Department of Dermatology, Stanford Cancer Center/ Stanford University School of Medicine, Stanford, CA, USA

Frederick Lansigan, MD Department of Hematology and Oncology, Dartmouth-Hitchcock Medical Center, Norris Cotton Cancer Center, Lebanon, NH, USA

Megan S. Lim, MD, PhD Department of Pathology, University of Michigan Medical School, Ann Arbor, MI, USA

Merry Jennifer Markham, MD Department of Medicine, Division of Hematology and Oncology, University of Florida, Gainesville, FL, USA

Badri Modi, MD Department of Dermatology, Yale University School of Medicine, New Haven, CT, USA

Pier Paolo Piccaluga, MD, PhD Department of Hematology and Oncological Sciences "L. and A. Seràgnoli", S. Orsola-Malpighi Hospital, Via Massarenti, Bologna, Italy

Stefano Aldo Pileri, MD Department of Hematology and Oncological Sciences "L. and A. Seràgnoli", S. Orsola-Malpighi Hospital, Via Massarenti, Bologna, Italy

Pierluigi Porcu, MD Department of Hematology, The Ohio State University, Columbus, OH, USA

H. Miles Prince, MBBS (Hons), MD, MRACMA, FRACP, FRCPA Sir Peter MacCallum Department of Oncology, Division of Cancer Medicine, Peter MacCallum Cancer Centre, Melbourne, Parkville, Australia

Christiane Querfeld, MD Section of Dermatology, University of Chicago, Chicago, IL, USA

José Rodríguez, MD, PhD Department of Internal Medicine, Hospital Universitario Severo Ochoa, Leganés, Spain

Steven T. Rosen, MD Department of Medicine, Division of Hematology/Oncology, Robert H. Lurie Comprehensive Cancer Center, Northwestern University, Chicago, IL, USA

David Sibon, MD, PhD Hématologie Adulte, Hôpital Necker, AP-HP, Université Paris Descartes, Sorbonne Paris Cité, Paris, France

Kensei Tobinai, MD, PhD Department of Hematology, National Cancer Center Hospital, Tokyo, Japan

Kunihiro Tsukasaki, MD, PhD Department of Hematology, National Cancer Centre Hospital East, Chiba, Japan

Pieter Van Vlierberghe, PhD Institute for Cancer Genetics, Columbia University Medical Center, New York, NY, USA

Julie M. Vose, MD Section of Hematology/Oncology, Nebraska Medical Center, Omaha, NE, USA

Sophia S. Wang, PhD Department of Population Sciences, City of Hope National Medical Center, Duarte, CA, USA

Motoko Yamaguchi, MD, PhD Department of Hematology and Oncology, Mie University Graduate School of Medicine, Tsu, Japan

Pier Luigi Zinzani, MD, PhD Institute of Hematology "Seràgnoli", University of Bologna, Bologna, Italy

Pierluigi Porcu, MD Department of Hematology, The Ohio [illegible]
Columbus, OH, USA

[illegible]

1 Histopathology and Classification of T-Cell Lymphomas

Claudiu V. Cotta and Eric D. Hsi

Introduction

T and NK cells derive from bone marrow precursor cells that undergo maturation in the central lymphoid organs (bone marrow and thymus) [1]. In the case of T-cells, maturation in the thymus includes T-cell receptor gene rearrangement, expression of T-cell receptor complex, and selection of αβ– or γδ-type T-cells [2–4]. These mature post-thymic T-cells reside in the peripheral lymphoid tissues, and lymphomas of these cells are considered peripheral T-cell lymphomas. NK cells mature in the bone marrow, do not require thymic "education," and circulate in the peripheral lymphoid organs [2–4]. The incidence of peripheral T-cell and NK-cell lymphomas varies across the world [5]. T/NK-cell neoplasms are more common in Asia and Latin America, probably a consequence of host genetic factors as well as environmental factors including infection with human T leukemia virus 1 (HTLV1), Epstein–Barr virus (EBV), and probably other viruses [6, 7]. In Northern Europe, enteropathy-associated T-cell lymphoma (EATCL) is common in Irish and Welsh populations, particularly those with certain HLA haplotypes [8, 9]. In the United States, the mature T/NK-cell neoplasms represent only 10–15% of non-Hodgkin lymphomas with an incidence of approximately 1.79/100,000 person-years [10].

The 2008 (World Health Organization [WHO]) classification of lymphomas applies clinical, morphologic, phenotypic, and molecular genetic features to define disease entities and provisional entities [1]. Some diseases are defined based on the presence of specific genetic abnormalities such as ALK+ anaplastic large cell lymphoma (ALCL), in which *anaplastic lymphoma kinase* (ALK) expression results for translocation of *ALK*. This is a major advance as prior classification systems relied primarily on histopathologic features alone. Within the mature T/NK cell neoplasms, there are 20 entities or provisional entities [5]. Figure 1.1 shows relative frequencies of the T-cell lymphomas other than primary cutaneous T-cell lymphomas. This list of lymphoma/leukemias of peripheral T or NK cells will likely change again as more is learned about the immunology and molecular genetics of these neoplasms.

Because of the heterogeneous composition of the lymphomatous infiltrate in many T/NK-cell lymphomas and the increased reliance on immunophenotypic and genetic features for the diagnosis and subclassification of T-cell lymphomas, procurement of adequate tissue, and proper handling of the fresh tissue is critical. Thus a few words on specimen processing are warranted. Communication among the hematologist, the

C.V. Cotta
Department of Pathology and Laboratory Medicine Institute, Cleveland Clinic, Cleveland, OH, USA

E.D. Hsi (✉)
Pathology and Laboratory Medicine Institute, Cleveland Clinic, 9500 Euclid Avenue, L11, Cleveland, OH 44195, USA
e-mail: hsie@ccf.org

F. Foss (ed.), *T-Cell Lymphomas*, Contemporary Hematology,
DOI 10.1007/978-1-62703-170-7_1, © Springer Science+Business Media New York 2013

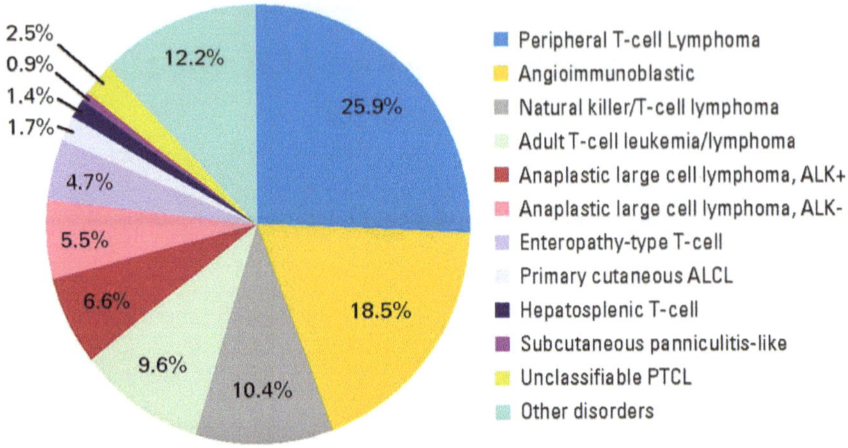

Fig. 1.1 Distribution of 1,314 cases by consensus diagnosis. Relative frequencies of mature T-cell lymphoma subtypes (except primary cutaneous types) in an adult patient population. Significant differences exist in different geographic regions (reprinted from International T-Cell Lymphoma Project [5], with permission from American Society of Clinical Oncology)

surgeon/procedure physician, and the pathologist is critical. In cases suspected of being lymphoma, an established "lymphoma protocol" should exist in which tissue is submitted in the fresh, sterile state to the pathology laboratory. This should be agreed upon by all parties so that clinicians and surgeons know that special handling is required and notify the laboratory at the time of procedure. Upon receipt of the fresh tissue, the pathologist can immediately evaluate the tissue by frozen section or touch imprints to assess specimen adequacy and to appropriately triage specimen for ancillary studies. If lymphoma is suspected, fresh tissue can be sent for cytogenetic studies, flow cytometry, and routine histopathology. Cultures can be sent if infection is suspected. The frozen tissue block can be retained at −20 °C or −70 °C for several days until it is decided whether further molecular genetic studies such as B- or T-cell receptor gene rearrangement studies are required. High-quality nucleic acids can be extracted from frozen tissues as opposed to fixed tissue and are the preferred source. The common practice of thawing the frozen block for permanent section "control" of the frozen is not indicated in lymphoma diagnosis since the morphology of that permanent section is substandard for fine morphologic/cytologic detail. After selecting tissue for these ancillary studies, the bulk of the remaining tissue can then undergo routine fixation and processing for histopathology studies.

With these introductory comments, we now focus on the pathologic features of the common peripheral T/NK-cell lymphomas and their differential diagnostic considerations.

Peripheral T-Cell Lymphoma, Not Otherwise Specified (PTCL, NOS)

PTCL, NOS is the most common type of PTCL, representing approximately 25% of T-cell lymphomas [5, 11] (Fig. 1.1). Rare in children [12], PTCL, NOS is most often diagnosed in older adults [11]. While bone marrow, spleen, skin, and liver can be involved, the most common presentation is nodal [13]. B-Symptoms can accompany the lymphadenopathy, and extensive leukemic involvement is rare. PTCL, NOS has an aggressive clinical course, with a relative low (20–30%) 5 year failure-free survival [13–16].

The morphologic features are somewhat variable (probably a consequence of the fact that PTCL, NOS is not a homogeneous category). There is usually effacement of the normal lymph node architecture (Fig. 1.2a). Partial involvement may occur with the involvement of the paracortical region. A lymphoepithelioid pattern (so-called

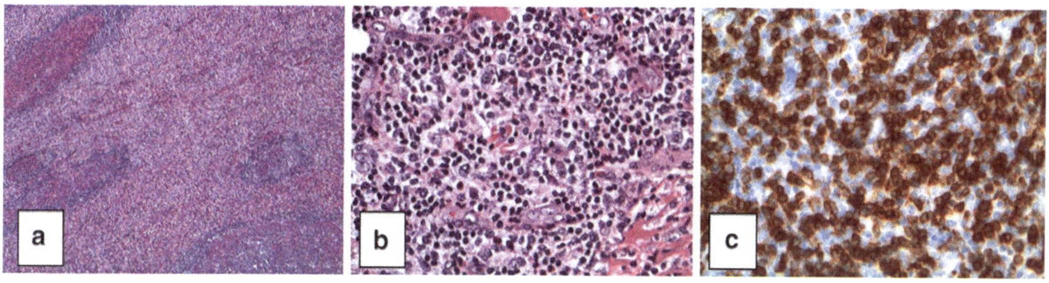

Fig. 1.2 Peripheral T-cell lymphoma, not otherwise specified (PTCL, NOS). (**a**) HE ×40. An interfollicular infiltrate progressively replacing the follicles. (**b**) HE ×400. The abnormal infiltrate comprises atypical lymphocytes with abundant cytoplasm and irregular nuclei, histiocytes, eosinophils, and plasma cells. (**c**) CD3 ×400. The neoplastic cells are positive for CD3

Lennert lymphoma) can sometimes be seen in which the tumor is composed almost exclusively of small to intermediate neoplastic cells and histiocytes that form epithelioid granulomas [1]. Occasional reactive inflammatory cells such as histiocytes, plasma cells, and/or eosinophils are often seen (Fig. 1.2b). In addition, increased vascularity within the infiltrate is characteristic. The lymphoma cells may be monomorphous or quite polymorphous and pleomorphic. In most cases, the lymphoma cells are of intermediate size, have irregular nuclear borders, and have moderate amounts of pale cytoplasm. The presence of small or very large cells does not rule out this diagnosis. Nucleoli range from small and inconspicuous to very large. In some cases, large B-cells with reactive features (immunoblasts) or Reed–Sternberg-like cells can be identified. Rare cases can have follicular patterns similar to B-cell follicular lymphoma and are thought to be derived from follicular T-helper (T_{Fh}) cells [17, 18]. Whether this latter pattern represents a distinct entity is uncertain and awaits further investigation.

Immunophenotypic analysis shows most PTCL, NOS cells to be positive for CD3 (Fig. 1.2c) and CD4, but CD8-positive cases have also been described [19–21]. The cells are most often αβ T-cells and are thus positive for TCRβ (βF1). The most commonly lost "pan" T-cell markers are CD7 and CD5. When expressed, CD30 is detected with variable intensity, at levels significantly lower than those seen in ALCL. CD56 and cytotoxic markers such as granzyme B, perforin, and TIA-1 can be seen mainly in lesions positive for CD8 and are rare in cases positive for CD4. One to two percent of PTCL, NOS are positive for B-cell markers, mainly CD20, but this finding is not associated with positivity for Pax5. The cases with follicular pattern express follicular markers such as BCL-6, CD10, CXCL13, and PD1. The latter are markers expressed in T_{Fh}.

Gene expression profiling studies suggest a relationship with activated T-cells rather than with resting T-cells and suggest dysregulation of important cellular pathways such as proliferation, apoptosis, adhesion, and extracellular matrix remodeling [22]. No characteristic genetic abnormalities have been described in PTCL, NOS. However, gains of chromosomes 3, 5, 7q, 8q, 17q, and 22q have been described. Other abnormalities include loss of genetic material on chromosomes 1, 2, 3, 4q, 5q, 6q, 7, 8, 9p, 10q, 11, 12q, and 13q [23].

Angioimmunoblastic T-Cell Lymphoma

Approximately 15% of total T-cell lymphomas fall into this category [5]. Most patients are adults and present with generalized lymphadenopathy, high-stage disease, and B-symptoms. Involvement of extranodal sites such as skin, liver, spleen, and bone marrow is common [24–26]. Patients appear to have evidence of immune system dysfunction, including recurrent infections, cold agglutinins, polyclonal hypergammaglobulinemia, autoimmune hemolytic anemia, and rheumatoid factor [27]. The immune deficiencies associated with

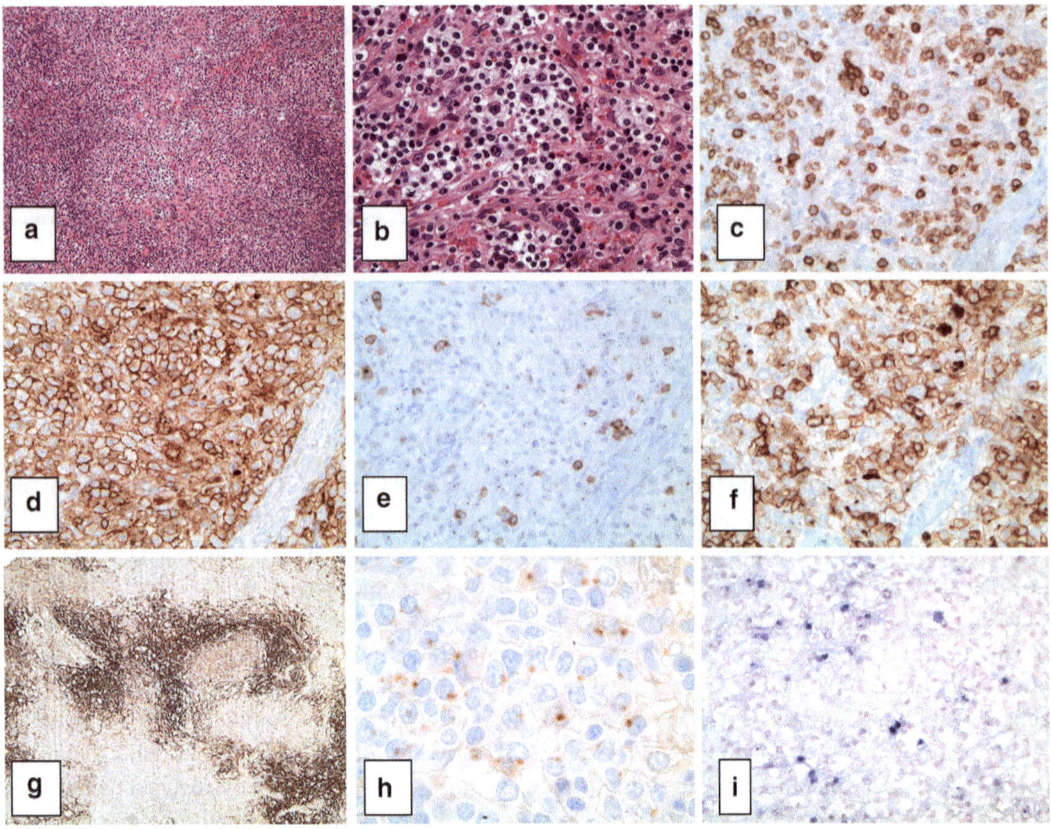

Fig. 1.3 Angioimmunoblastic T-cell lymphoma. (**a**) HE ×100 sheets of intermediate-sized cells completely efface the lymph node architecture. Vascular proliferation noticeable in the background. (**b**) HE ×400. Same features as in (**a**), with a better illustration of the retraction artifact, a consequence of the abundant cytoplasm. (**c**) CD3 ×400. (**d**) CD4 ×400. (**e**) CD7 ×100 (**f**) CD10 ×400. (**g**) CD21 ×100. (**h**) CXCL13 ×400. (**i**) EBER ×100

angioimmunoblastic T-cell lymphoma (AITL) are at least partially responsible for the poor prognosis of AITL (median survival less than 3 years). In up to 25% of cases of AITL, aggressive B-cell lymphomas can develop, further complicating the clinical course of this neoplasm [28].

Histologically, the lymph node is diffusely replaced by a neoplastic infiltrate (Fig. 1.3a). Germinal centers are usually absent or, if present, demonstrate regressive transformation. Presence of germinal centers does not preclude the possibility of AITL, since some cases of early involvement may show this feature. The subcapsular sinuses are usually spared or enlarged, even as the neoplastic infiltrate extends into the pericapsular fibroadipose tissue. Numerous proliferating vessels corresponding to high endothelial venules may form an arborizing vascular network (Fig. 1.3b). The infiltrate is polymorphous, a feature that while characteristic may cause diagnostic difficulty since many of the cells are reactive inflammatory cells such as eosinophils, histiocytes, small lymphocytes, and plasma cells. The neoplastic cells are usually intermediate-sized cells, with abundant cytoplasm, often leading to a "clear cell" or "fried egg" appearance (Fig. 1.3b). Atypia may be mild. The spacing of cells may impart a relatively depleted look at low magnification. Rare large immunoblasts are usually present and Reed–Sternberg-like cells may be seen. While difficult to observe on hematoxylin and eosin stains, follicular dendritic cells proliferate and form distorted networks, usually in paracortical and perivascular areas (Fig. 1.3g).

The immunophenotype of AITL indicates that the cell of origin of this lesion is the CD4-positive follicular T-helper cell [24–26, 29]. The lymphoma cells are positive for CD2, CD3 (Fig. 1.3c), CD4 (Fig. 1.3d), CD5, CD7, CD45, and βF1. Characteristically, they are also positive for T_{FH} markers such as CD10 (Fig. 1.3f), CXCL13 (Fig. 1.3h), PD1, and ICOS [30]. The immunoblasts are positive for EBV in most cases (Fig. 1.3i). The proliferating follicular dendritic cells are positive for CD21, CD23, and CD35, markers that also highlight the abnormal architecture of these proliferations. Occasionally, the lymphoma cells show abnormal loss of T-cell markers (Fig. 1.3f).

The large B-cell component may progress to sheets of monoclonal cells, warranting a diagnosis of EBV+ DLBL that may obscure the underlying AITL [31]. In some cases, a treated AITL may relapse as EBV+ DLBL.

While the above features make AITL recognizable in a lymph node, specific morphologic features may be lacking when involving an extranodal site such as skin or bone marrow. A high index of suspicion is required so that appropriate studies can be performed to confirm lymphomatous involvement.

Molecular genetic testing for T- and B-cell receptor gene rearrangements shows a T-cell clone in >95% of cases. A B-cell clone (EBV-driven) can be detected in half of the cases [32, 33]. Gene expression profiles performed in cases of AITL show similarity between T_{Fh} and AITL cells [34]. Conventional cytogenetic analysis usually does not lead to the identification of characteristic abnormalities. The most often encountered abnormalities are trisomies of chromosomes 3, 5, and X [24].

Anaplastic Large Cell Lymphoma, ALK-Positive

By definition, the neoplasms in this category are positive for translocations involving the *ALK* located at 2p23 [1]. Most patients are young, in the first three decades of life (mean age 21.3 years) [35, 36], with a slight male predominance. Approximately two-thirds of patients present with advanced-stage disease and B-symptoms [36]. Forty-six percent of patients have extranodal involvement with bone, bone marrow, spleen, and subcutaneous tissue being the most common sites. The prognosis of ALK+ ALCL is favorable, as the 5 year survival approaches 80%. Interestingly, patients with different translocations involving *ALK* have similar survival [37]. The adult or older patients with ALCL seem to have a worse prognosis than pediatric patients.

Histologic sections can show one of several morphologic variants. In all the variants, the distribution of the neoplastic cells is predominantly intra-sinusoidal, with the neoplastic cells forming sheets [36, 38]. Perivascular cuffs of malignant cells can be seen in some cases (Fig. 1.4b). In more advanced cases, the lymph node is completely effaced. The neoplastic cells in the common, classical variant (over 60% of cases) are large, with abundant cytoplasm and one or multiple nuclei (Fig. 1.4a). The nuclei are abnormally lobated, often with conspicuous eosinophilic nucleoli. Cells with indented or comma-shaped nuclei and abundant cytoplasm (so-called "hallmark cells") are characteristically seen. In addition to the common type, there are several other morphologic variants: lymphohistiocytic, small cell, Hodgkin-like, sarcomatoid, and giant cell rich. Some cases may demonstrate more than one variant and, upon relapse, transformation to another variant morphology may occur [35].

The immunophenotype of this entity is characterized by strong positivity for CD30 in most large cells, with a membrane and Golgi pattern, similar to that observed in Reed–Sternberg cells [1, 39] (Fig. 1.4b). Many of the T-lineage markers are lost, making lineage determination difficult. The stain for CD3 is negative in many cases (Fig. 1.4d), but expression of CD2, CD4, or CD5 can be preserved. EMA and CD43 can be detected in most cases [35, 40]. A finding limited to ALCL is the concurrent expression of CD4 and of cytotoxic markers such as granzyme B, TIA-1, and perforin [41, 42]. Similar to Reed–Sternberg cells, the neoplastic cells in ALCL can be negative for CD45 (LCA). Clusterin reactivity in a dot-like Golgi pattern may be helpful in identifying cases of ALCL [43]. By definition, ALK expression can be demonstrated (Fig. 1.4c).

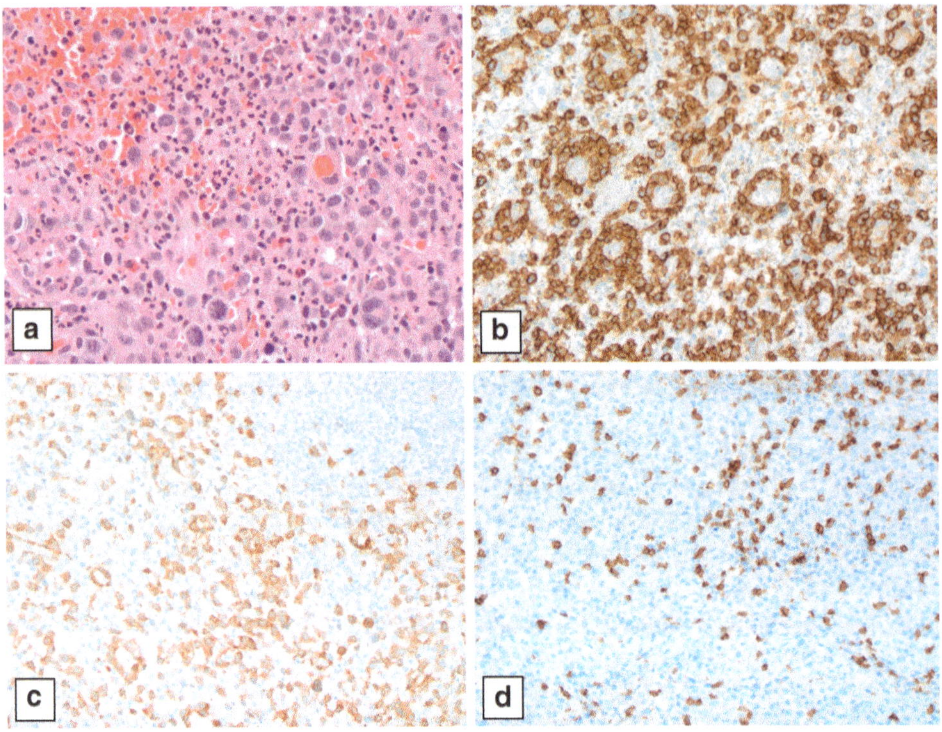

Fig. 1.4 Anaplastic large T-cell lymphoma, ALK positive. (**a**) HE ×400. Sheets of large cells, with one or multiple nuclei with conspicuous nucleoli. (**b**) CD30 ×200. (**c**) ALK1 ×200. Cytoplasmic and nuclear patterns. (**d**) CD3 ×200

The karyotype of ALCL, ALK+ is characterized by translocations involving *ALK*. The consequence of these translocations is abnormal expression of ALK, a protein normally present on the membrane of embryonic and central nervous system cells. Most cases of ALCL, ALK positive harbor the t(2;5)(p23;q35) translocation (*NPM1-ALK*) [44, 45]. The second most common translocation is t(1;2)(q25;p23) (*TPM3-ALK*), the rest of the cases having one of the other abnormalities: Inv(2)(p23q35) (*ATIC-ALK*), t(2;3)(p23;q12) (*TFG-ALK*), t(2;17)(p23;q23) (*CLTC-ALK*), t(X;2)(q11-12;p23)(*MSN-ALK*), t(2;19)(p23;p13.1) (*TPM4-ALK*), t(2;22)(p23;q11.2) (*MYH9-ALK*), t(2;17)(p23;q25) *(ALO17-ALK)* [44, 45]. Additional genetic abnormalities can be identified in ALCL, but their clinical significance is unclear. The intracellular distribution of ALK is determined by the partner of translocation. In the cases with *NPM-ALK* fusion (the majority of ALCL), the staining pattern is cytoplasmic and nuclear (NPM shuttles between the nucleus and the cytoplasm). Cytoplasmic staining with perinuclear intensification characterizes cases with *TPM3-ALK*. Diffuse cytoplasmic staining can be seen in cases with translocations involving *ATIC, TFG, TPM4, MYH9, ALO17*. Exclusive membrane positivity is seen in cases with *MSN*. Granular cytoplasmic stain is the consequence of *CLTC-ALK* translocation.

Most cases of ALCL, ALK+ have clonal rearrangements of the *TCR* gamma locus.

ALCL, ALK negative is a provisional category in the current WHO classification [1]. Unlike the ALK-positive cases, ALCL, ALK-negative patients are older adults (median age 58 years), with a similar slight male preponderance [46]. The prognosis of patients with ALCL, ALK negative is significantly worse than that of patients with ALCL, ALK positive and may be superior to patients with PTCL NOS [36]. The sites of involvement are similar to those for ALK positive ALCL. The diagnosis of cases with primary exclusive skin involvement is difficult, as

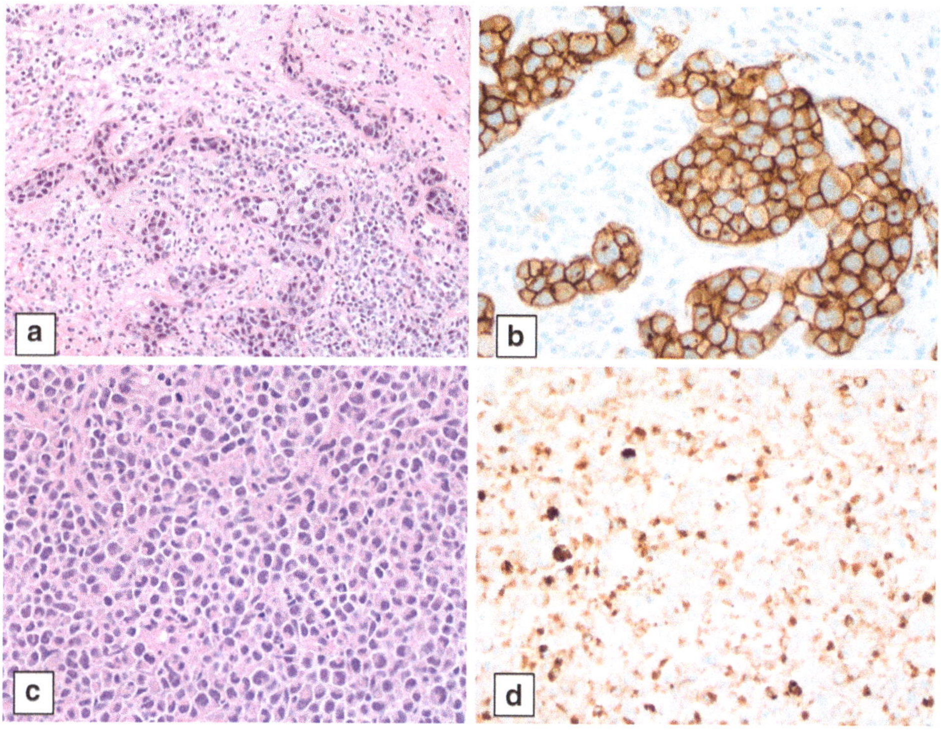

Fig. 1.5 Anaplastic large T-cell lymphoma, ALK negative. (**a**) HE ×200. Large atypical cells with intra-sinusoidal pattern. (**b**) CD30 ×400. (**c**) HE ×400. (**d**) Clusterin ×400. Paranuclear dots

the morphology of these lesions does not allow their differentiation from other CD30-positive primary cutaneous T-cell lymphoproliferative disorders. The histologic characteristics of ALCL, ALK negative are similar to those of ALCL, ALK positive, the common variant, with the exception of negativity for ALK (Fig. 1.5a–d). In cases with a morphology deviating from that of classical ALCL, the diagnosis of PTCL, NOS is preferred. Obviously, no translocations involving ALK can be identified by conventional cytogenetics in ALCL, ALK negative.

Adult T-Cell Leukemia/Lymphoma

Adult T-cell leukemia/lymphoma (ATLL) is a lymphoproliferative disorder associated with HTLV-I infection [1]. This retrovirus is endemic in specific geographic areas such as Southwestern Japan, the Caribbean basin, South American, and Africa. The oncogenic mechanism through which HTLV-1 induces neoplasia is not completely elucidated, but studies suggest that the viral Tax and HBZ gene products are important in the pathogenesis of ATLL [47–49]. It is increasingly clear that genetic and epigenetic changes in host cells are important in transformation and development of this disease [50]. The prognosis of patients with ATLL depends on the form of ATLL (see below), serum calcium, and lactate dehydrogenase [51, 52]. The patients with chronic and smoldering forms have a protracted course, while acute forms result rapidly in death. Suppression of the immune system of ATLL patients can result in lethal infections.

The clinical presentation of ATLL is variable, as there are acute forms, lymphomatous, chronic, and smoldering cases of ATLL [53, 54]. Bone marrow, lymph node, and skin involvement are common. In the acute presentation, there are increased white blood cell counts (with malignant

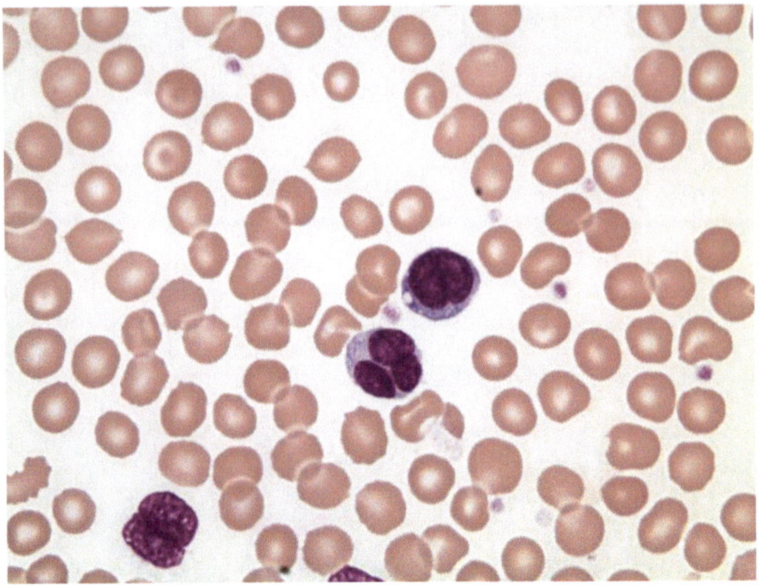

Fig. 1.6 Adult T-cell leukemia/lymphoma. Peripheral blood, ×1,000. Atypical lymphocyte ("flower cell")

cells) and extensive bone marrow involvement. Hypercalcemia can be secondary to bone destruction. Hepatosplenomegaly systemic symptoms and infections are frequent. In the smoldering presentation, the WBC is not significantly increased and malignant cells are less than 5% of the circulating cells. Bone marrow involvement is limited (and there is no hypercalcemia). In lymphomatous cases, there are widespread enlarged lymph nodes, variable blood involvement, and elevated lactate dehydrogenase. Infections are a consequence of immunodeficiencies. In the chronic form, the most common presentation is with a skin rash, which can slowly progress. The acute form can be present at diagnosis, but in a significant number of cases, they arise in patients with the chronic or smoldering forms of ATLL [54].

The morphology of the neoplastic cells is variable, from small to large. Most cells in leukemic cases are of intermediate size, with moderate cytoplasm and irregular nuclei ("flower cells") (Fig. 1.6). The patterns of tissue involvement are also variable, from diffuse sheets of intermediate cells, to patterns reminiscent of AITL or ALCL. Large, Hodgkin-like cells that are positive for EBV are further indication of the immunosuppressed status of the patient. In the skin, the neoplastic cells can form infiltrates similar to MF in tumor or plaque stages.

As the cell of origin is the CD4-positive T-helper cells, the immunophenotype of ATLL is positive for CD2, CD3, CD4, and CD5. CD7 is usually lost, but there is strong positivity for CD25 [55]. Also expressed are CCR4 and FOXP3 [56]. Large, anaplastic cells can be positive for CD30. However, this does not warrant a diagnosis of ALCL.

There are no specific cytogenetic abnormalities in ATLL, but molecular tests can identify clonal rearrangements of the *TCR* genes. Integration of HTLV-I in the host genome differentiates patients with ATLL from healthy carriers [47, 48, 55].

In addition to tests designed to characterize the tumor cells, immunologic and molecular tests designed to identify exposure and infection with HTLV-I should always be integrated in the workup of cases of ATLL.

Extranodal NK/T-Cell Lymphoma, Nasal Type (ENKTL)

This is a neoplasm of cytotoxic cells (NK cell most often) characterized by vascular damage, necrosis, and tissue destruction, usually associated

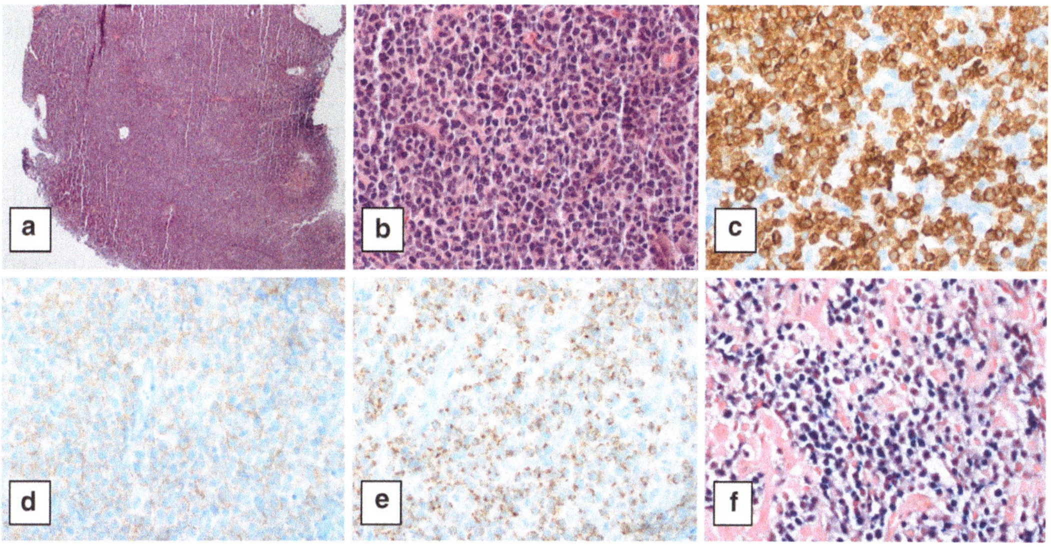

Fig. 1.7 Extranodal NK/T-cell lymphoma, nasal type. (**a**) HE ×20. Focal areas of necrosis. (**b**) HE ×400. Pleomorphic cells with diffuse pattern, with dense chromatin. (**c**) CD3 ×400. The stain for CD3 is positive, as the epitope is detected in the cytoplasm (the cells are negative for surface CD3). (**d**) CD56 ×400. The lymphoma cells are positive for CD56. (**e**) TIA-1 ×400. (**f**) EBER ×400

with EBV [1]. This association suggests that EBV plays an important etiologic role in pathogenesis of this lymphoma.

The increased prevalence of this neoplasm in Asians and Native Americans also points to a component of genetic susceptibility of these populations to this type of neoplasms [57]. Most patients are adult males and cases arising in post-transplant patients have been described. There is involvement of the nasal cavity or other areas of the upper aerodigestive tract. Local extension and destruction of midline facial structures occur, explaining the prior descriptive term for this lymphoma—lethal midline granuloma. Involvement of extranasal sites may also occur as the primary site of disease such as skin, testis, soft tissue, and gastrointestinal tract. Advanced-stage disease may involve bone marrow, and hemophagocytosis may be present. Historically ENKTL was thought to have a poor prognosis [58, 59]. However, due to advances in therapy, the outcome of ENKTL is now variable as a significant subset of patients responds to radiation and chemotherapy [60, 61]. Extranasal presentation is thought to be a poor prognosis feature [62].

Most times, the symptoms at presentation are the result of extensive tissue destruction by neoplastic infiltrate that involve the vasculature. This imparts an angiocentric and angiodestructive pattern. Fibrinoid necrosis may be seen even without neoplastic infiltrate. As a consequence, necrosis is a constant feature (Fig. 1.7a). The cells can infiltrate and fill the nasal cavities or can form tumor nodules at the involved locations. The malignant cells can be small, without conspicuous morphologic abnormalities, intermediate-sized, with irregular nuclear contour and fine or blastoid chromatin, or large, with vesicular chromatin (Fig. 1.7b). Most cases have intermediate-sized cells, and in all cases, a prominent inflammatory infiltrate can be associated with the neoplastic cells, probably a consequence of the necrosis. The cell size has been thought to have prognostic value with small cell cases being thought to have a better prognosis than large cell ones. Blood and bone marrow involvement can occur. On imprints or blood/bone marrow Wright–Giemsa smears, the cells have open chromatin and moderate amounts of cytoplasm with azurophilic granules.

The immunophenotype is that of cytotoxic cells, most often NK cells (positive for CD2, CD56, granzyme B, perforin, and TIA-1 and negative for surface CD3, CD4, CD5, and βF1) [59] (Fig. 1.7c–e). The great majority (if not all) of cases are positive for EBV (Fig. 1.7f). Most tumor cells should be EBV+ [58].

Molecular studies in most cases show no evidence of clonal rearrangement of the TCR receptor genes. The presence of rare cases positive for TCR δ clonal rearrangements has suggested that probably not all these neoplasms are of NK lineage, justifying their naming as NK/T-cell tumors [63]. While not pathognomonic for this entity, abnormalities of chromosome 6 (del(6)(q21q26) and i(6)(p10)) are relatively common. Other cytogenetic abnormalities that can be seen involve the chromosomes 1, 2, 4, 5, 6, 7, 11, and 15 [64, 65].

Aggressive NK-cell leukemia is a neoplasm with leukemic presentation and accelerated, fatal clinical course [1]. The association with EBV, the similar immunophenotype of the malignant cells, as well as the higher incidence in Asians has led to the hypothesis that it may represent the leukemic counterpart of the extranodal NK/T-cell lymphoma, nasal type. However, this idea is not yet fully accepted, as the patients with aggressive NK-cell leukemia tend to be younger than those with ENKTL, the skin is spared, and some genetic abnormalities seem to have preferential association with only one of the two entities [1, 66, 67]. As these cases are relatively rare, the existing data are probably not sufficient for a definitive conclusion.

EBV-Positive T-Cell Lymphoproliferative Disorders of Childhood (EBVTCLD)

EBVTCLD are composed of two main entities [1]: Hydroa vacciniforme-like lymphoma and systemic EBV-positive T-cell lymphoproliferative disease of childhood. This latter entity is rare and is characterized by the proliferation of EBV-infected T-cells with a cytotoxic phenotype. It progresses rapidly usually leading to death. Many of its features overlap with those of aggressive NK-cell leukemia [68–70]. This systemic disease arises in two types of circumstances [71]: shortly after an acute EBV [69, 70, 72] infection and in chronic active EBV infection (CAEBV) [68]. In the former setting, the process has been described to be associated with fulminant hemophagocytic syndrome. The cases of CAEBV that previously have been associated with clonal T-cell populations now are understood to be part of the spectrum of manifestation of the EBV-positive T-cell lymphoproliferative disorders of childhood.

The clinical presentation of EBVTCLD is acute, with fever and constitutional symptoms. The patients develop hepatosplenomegaly and pancytopenia. The EBV titers are high and EBV viral DNA is present in blood. The patients rapidly progresses with the development of coagulopathy, multisystem organ failure, sepsis, and hemophagocytic syndrome.

Morphologically, the pattern of involvement is not characteristic, as malignant cells with no definitive cytologic abnormalities infiltrate organs without forming tumors. Most malignant cells are present in the sinuses of lymph nodes, bone marrow, spleen, liver. Immunophenotyping may be required to see the extent of the lymphomatous infiltrate.

The immunophenotype of the cells is positive for CD2, CD3, TIA-1, and EBV. Cases evolving from CAEBV are positive for CD4 [71, 73], while cases from fulminant mononucleosis are positive for CD8 [72].

There are no pathognomonic conventional cytogenetic abnormalities associated with EBVTCLD, but the tests for *TCR* genes can identify clonal rearrangements.

Hydroa vacciniforme-like lymphoma is a cutaneous T- or NK-cell neoplasm primarily identified in the skin of children from Asia, and South and Central America. It can be precipitated by events such as sun or mosquito bite sensitivity (also, it involves the sun-exposed skin) [74–76].

Morphologically, the lesions are papulovesicular eruptions that progress to ulceration and scarring, becoming associated with lymphadenopathy and hepatosplenomegaly. The neoplastic cells involve all the skin layers and display

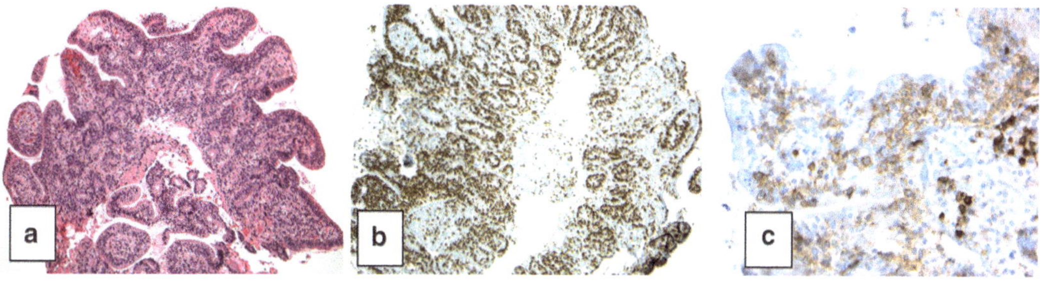

Fig. 1.8 Enteropathy-associated T-cell lymphoma. (**a**) HE ×100. Atypical infiltrate in the lamina propria, invading the crypts. The overall architecture is abnormal, with effacement of the villi. (**b**) CD3 ×100. The cells in the lamina propria and in the surface mucosa are positive. (**c**) CD8 ×400. The lymphoma cells are positive

angiocentricity, leading to necrosis. They are usually small, without overt cytologic atypia.

The immunophenotype is that of cytotoxic T-cells (positive for CD2, CD3, CD5, CD8) or that of NK cells (positive for CD2, CD56) and in most cases are positive for EBV.

The molecular tests show positivity for *TCR* rearrangement of tumors composed of T-cells and negativity for the tumors of NK cells.

Enteropathy-Associated T-Cell Lymphoma (EATCL)

EATCL is a neoplasm thought to be derived from intra-epithelial T-cells. It is most prevalent in areas with high incidence of celiac disease (Northern Europe) [9]. Patients that have EATCL associated with celiac disease usually are positive for HLA DQ2 or DQ8, pointing to host genetic factors being involved in this lymphoma [77]. Patients present with abdominal pain. Many patients do not have a preexisting diagnosis of celiac disease. Patients with established celiac disease may develop EATCL. Such patients may have refractory celiac disease and present with loss of response to therapy and intestinal perforation. Most patients have a poor prognosis and death is often the result of intestinal complications (perforation, obstruction, malabsorption).

Morphologically, the lymphoma forms intestinal masses with superficial mucosal ulceration. The pattern of the neoplastic infiltrate is usually diffuse. A key histologic feature is invasion of the surface and crypt epithelium. The presence of the neoplastic infiltrate is associated with villous atrophy and/or crypt hyperplasia (features of celiac disease) (Fig. 1.8a). When the specimen is small, or the biopsy is obtained at the edge of the lesion, the tumor infiltrate may be sparse, and abnormalities of the mucosal architecture and the lymphoid infiltrate in the epithelium and lamina propria may suggest the correct diagnosis [78]. The morphology of the tumor cells is variable and is the basis for the classification of EATCL in two subcategories. In classical EATCL (type 1), the tumor cells are relatively polymorphous, medium-sized, with irregular nuclei with vesicular chromatin and small nucleoli. There is significant inter-case variability in the morphology of the neoplastic cells, some cases may be quite pleomorphic, having the cytologic appearance suggestive of ALCL. In type II EATCL, the neoplastic cells are relatively monomorphic, small to intermediate sized, with clumped chromatin and pale cytoplasm. This latter type of EATCL is rarer (10–20% of cells) and often is not associated with a history (or evidence) of celiac disease.

The immunophenotype of the two types of EATCL is that of cytotoxic T-cells. They typically express CD3 (Fig. 1.8b), CD7, CD103, and βF1 but are negative for CD5, CD4, CD8, and CD56. Uncommonly, cases may be CD8+. Cases of type II EATCL differ in their phenotype and are more commonly CD8+/CD56+ [78] (Fig. 1.8c). In many cases, a subset of the tumor cells is positive for CD30. EBV is negative.

Molecular tests show that the *TCR* genes are clonally rearranged in both types of EATCL. The association with HLA DR2 or DR8 is stronger for classical EATCL. Both types of EATCL are positive for segmental amplification of 9q31.3-qter or for deletions in 16q12.1 [8]. The classical form can also show gains of 1q and 5q, while amplifications of MYC (8q24) can be seen in the type II (monomorphic) variant.

Hepatosplenic T-Cell Lymphoma (HSTCL)

This is a rare type of lymphoma, mostly diagnosed in young or middle-aged males with a median age of 38 years in a recent series [79]. Most cases are γδ-T-cell lymphomas, although αβ-T-cell types are reported in 20% of cases [80–83]. The lymphoma involves the liver, spleen, and the bone marrow with an intra-sinusoidal pattern. A significant fraction of these lymphomas arise in the context of immunosuppression, often in the post-transplant setting or in the context of inflammatory bowel disease patients treated with immunomodulatory therapy (thiopurines and TNF-α inhibitors) [83, 84]. Patients present with hepatosplenomegaly, altered liver functions, and often with marked thrombocytopenia. It is an aggressive lymphoma with median overall survival of less than 1 year [79, 85].

The morphologic findings consist of an abundant, intra-sinusoidal infiltrate in the liver, spleen, and bone marrow (Fig. 1.9a). This infiltrate is composed of small to intermediate cells with moderate to abundant pale cytoplasm and nuclei without major atypical features.

The immunophenotype is that of γδ T-cells or, less commonly, αβ T-cells. They express CD3 (Fig. 1.9b), TCRδ (if γδ T-cell type), TIA1 (Fig. 1.9c), and granzyme M. These cells are negative for CD7 and for granzyme B or perforin. As on NK cells, the killer inhibitor receptors (KIRs) are expressed, but the cells can be negative for CD94 [83].

Molecular studies have shown that these tumors have clonal rearrangements of the *TCR* γ genes. Only the αβ cases have clones with rearranged *TCR* β genes. Most cases of HSTCL harbor abnormalities of chromosome 7: isochromosome 7q or ring chromosome 7. Other abnormalities may include trisomy 8 and loss of sex chromosomes [83].

Subcutaneous Panniculitis-Like T-Cell Lymphoma

This is a rare type of lymphoma preferentially involving the subcutaneous fibroadipose tissue. The cell of origin is thought to be the mature cytotoxic αβ T-cell [1, 86, 87].

Subcutaneous panniculitis-like T-cell lymphoma (SPTCL) is slightly more common in females than in males, and in early stages, it may show features similar to those of lupus profundus panniculitis (some patients may have a history of systemic lupus erythematosus) [87]. The lesions are most often located on the trunk or on the extremities and can range from small to several centimeters in diameters. The infiltrate lacks epidermotropism, and ulceration is relatively rare. Unlike γδ T-cell lymphomas, SPTCL has a good prognosis (5 year survival of 80%) [88]. In SPTCL cases with poor prognosis,

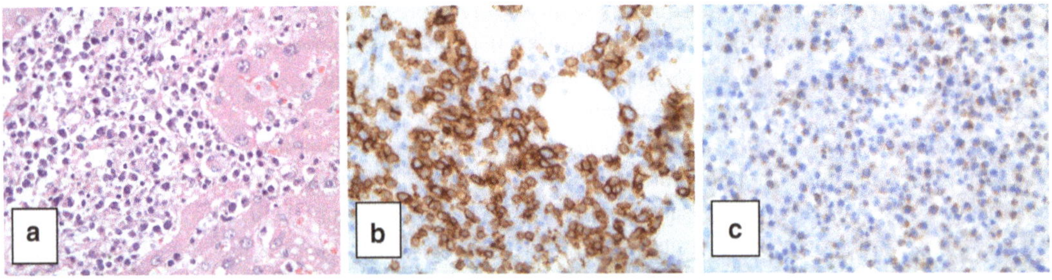

Fig. 1.9 Hepatosplenic T-cell lymphoma. (**a**) HE ×200. Intra-sinusoidal infiltrate. (**b**) CD3 ×200. (**c**) TIA-1 ×200

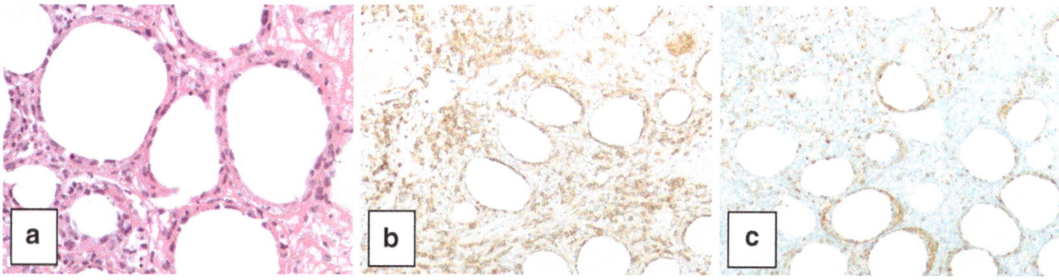

Fig. 1.10 Subcutaneous panniculitis-like T-cell lymphoma. (**a**) HE ×400. Rimming of the adipocytes. (**b**) CD8 ×200. (**c**) Granzyme B ×200

hemophagocytic syndrome has been described as a constant feature [87].

Morphologically, the tumor infiltrate involves the subcutaneous fat lobules and spares the septa. The neoplastic cells are small, with nuclear atypia, and they completely surround or "rim" the adipocytes (Fig. 1.10a). This latter feature is characteristic, albeit not specific [89]. Fat necrosis and increased histiocytes are constant features of most tumors.

The immunophenotype is that of mature cytotoxic αβ T-cells, with random losses of normal surface markers. As such, the cells express T-cell markers such as CD2 and CD3, TCRβ, and are usually CD8+/CD4– (Fig. 1.10b). Cytotoxic molecules are expressed such as granzyme B (Fig. 1.10c), TIA1, and perforin. CD56 is not expressed. Molecular findings confirm the clonal rearrangement of *TCR* γ or β.

Mycosis Fungoides (MFs)

MF is the most common type of cutaneous T-cell lymphoma, with approximately 1,000 new cases diagnosed in the United States each year [11]. The cell of origin is the mature CD4-positive T-cell with propensity for homing in the skin [1]. The median age at diagnosis is 55 years, with a male predominance. It is twice as common in African Americans than in Caucasians [90]. It has an indolent clinical course with slow progression, oftentimes spanning a decade or more [90]. Diagnosis may be delayed due to the indolent course and subtle manifestations. Patients present with erythematous patches with fine scale in non-sun exposed areas and can progress to thickened plaques, and finally to tumors [91]. The prognosis of patients with MF is dependent on the extent of skin involvement and on the clinical stage. Patients with limited skin involvement have an excellent prognosis, while the patients with tumors or increased large cells have a more aggressive course, requiring systemic chemotherapy [91]. Lymph node or leukemic dissemination may occur and portend a poor prognosis. Modern clinical staging systems such as the ISLC/EORTC proposal make use of clinical and pathologic features to stratify patients. The pathologic features now have specific criteria for blood and lymph node involvement. The former requires morphologic, flow cytometric, and molecular genetic assessment of the blood [92].

Clinical variants have been recognized. Folliculotropic MF involves the head and neck and manifests as small folliculotropic papules, sometimes with alopecia [93, 94]. Pagetoid reticulosis is a localized lesion, usually involving the extremities. It may become a solitary plaque that remains localized [95]. Granulomatous slack skin presents with pendulous folds of lax skin involving intertriginous areas [96, 97].

The neoplastic infiltrate of MF can form patches, plaques, or tumors (in order of the progression). At early stages (patch), the malignant cells display remarkable epidermotropism [98] (Fig. 1.11). In the epidermis, most lymphoma cells are seen in the basal layer and are usually surrounded by areas of clearing or halos. Neoplastic cells may cluster within the epidermis to form Pautrier microabscesses (Fig. 1.11b). In the superficial dermis, the infiltrate is mainly in

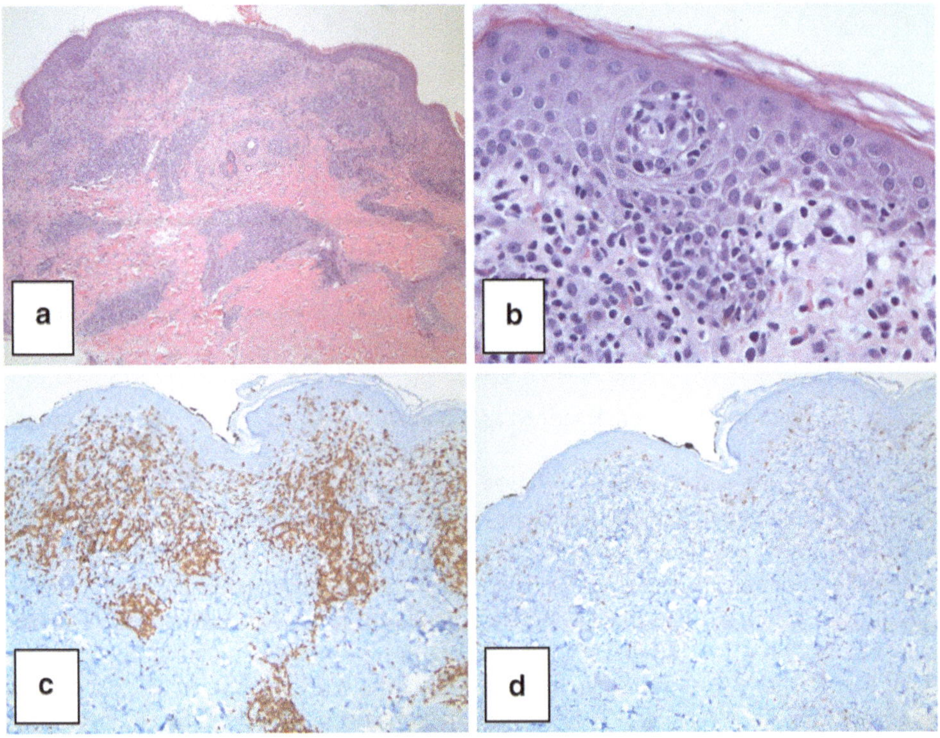

Fig. 1.11 Mycosis fungoides. (**a**) HE ×40. Infiltrate in the superficial dermis, with epidermotropism. (**b**) HE ×400. Pautrier microabscess, in the superficial dermis. The cells in the microabscess are atypical lymphocytes. (**c**) CD3 ×100. Most cells in the infiltrate are T-lymphocytes. (**d**) CD7 ×100. The lymphoma cells show abnormal loss of CD7 expression

a band-like pattern (lichenoid pattern) (Fig. 1.11a). Initially, the MF cells are small or intermediate, with scant-to-moderate cytoplasm and dense, hyperchromatic nuclei with irregular cerebriform contours (Fig. 1.11). Eosinophils and histiocytes are often admixed within the infiltrate. The progression of MF to plaque or tumor stage is generally associated with reduction in epidermotropism. This may be completely lost in the tumor stage, and clinical history may be required to appropriately designate the tumor as MF rather than a non-MF T- cell lymphoma.

Large, transformed cells may be present within the infiltrate. When large cells, with irregular nuclei, vesicular chromatin, and nucleoli, represent more than 25% of total cells, the diagnosis of MF with transformation to large cell lymphoma is recommended [99–101]. Significant diagnostic difficulties are encountered in cases with morphology of MF with large cell transformation at presentation, as the large cells can often be positive for CD30, leading to a morphology and immunophenotype that can overlap that of lymphomatoid papulosis (LyP), primary cutaneous ALCL, and systemic ALCL, ALK negative involving the skin [86]. However, these cases should not be considered ALCL. As the neoplasm progresses, it involves the lymph nodes [102]. Initially, the involved lymph nodes show dermatopathic changes, considered a benign change [103]. Increasing numbers of atypical cells can be recognized either in small clusters or more easily in later stages as overt architectural distortion of the lymph node by clearly neoplastic cells. Proof of involvement in the earliest stages may be found by molecular studies but clinical staging systems do not recommend routine lymph node biopsy (unless pathologically enlarged) or gene rearrangement studies [104, 105]. At advanced stages, the pattern of lymph node involvement may be indistinguishable from that seen in PTCL NOS.

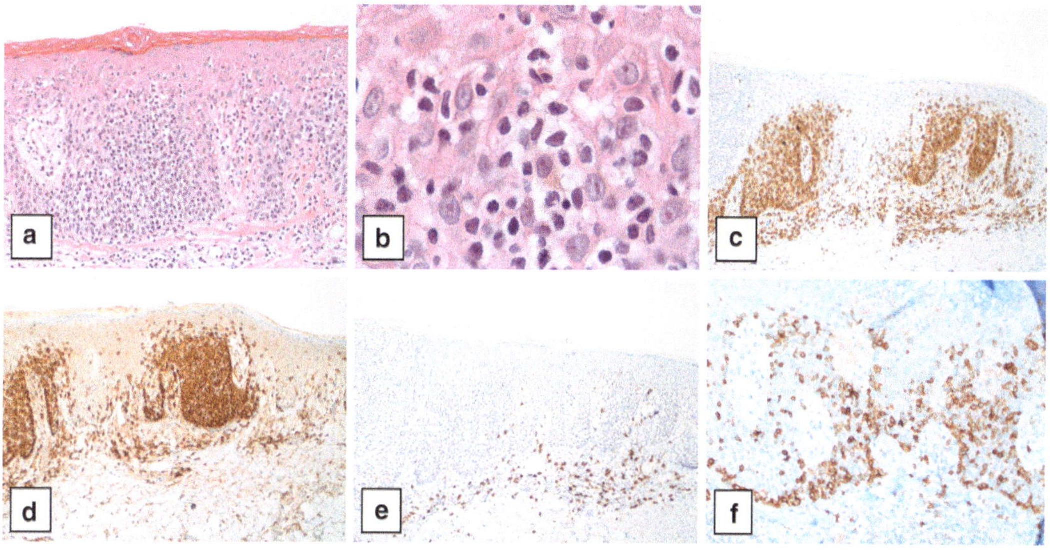

Fig. 1.12 Mycosis fungoides, pagetoid reticulosis. (**a**) HE ×200. Atypical infiltrate with marked epidermotropism and relative sparing of the dermis. (**b**) HE ×1,000. The lymphoma cells are small, with marked nuclear irregularities. (**c**) CD3 ×100. The atypical lymphocytes are CD3+ T-cells. (**d**) CD4 ×100. The lymphoma cells are positive for CD4. (**e**) CD8 ×100. There are very few cytotoxic T-cells in the infiltrate. (**f**) CD30 ×100. Characteristic for this entity, some of the small cells in the infiltrate are positive for CD30

The clinical variants mentioned have morphologic patterns differing from the classical MF (described above). Folliculotropic MF, a variant with a worse prognosis that that of classical MF, is defined by an abundant neoplastic infiltrate in the hair follicles, in the absence of significant involvement of the superficial epidermis [93, 94]. The follicles show mucinous degeneration. In Pagetoid reticulosis (Woringer–Kolopp), the disease is localized and the neoplastic cells infiltrate only the epidermis with sparing of the dermis [95] (Fig 1.12a, b). The rare granulomatous slack skin is characterized by extensive histiocytic and granulomatous proliferation [96, 97].

The immunophenotype of the neoplastic cells is characterized by negativity for CD7 (Fig. 1.11e) in approximately 50% of cases. This feature, however, is not specific as this can occur in some reactive lesions. The MF cells are usually positive for CD2, CD3, CD4, CD5, and CLA (cutaneous lymphocyte antigen). Only rare cases are positive for CD8 [106].

Molecular studies performed on the skin lesions from MF can identify monoclonal T-cell receptor rearrangements. Again, while supportive of lymphoma, uncommon reactive lesions may show monoclonal gene rearrangements. In difficult cases, it may be necessary to study multiple lesions from the same patient over time to demonstrate a persistent malignant clone [107]. There are no characteristic chromosomal abnormalities for MF: in a significant number of cases there are losses of genetic material from 1p, 10q, 17q, 19, gains of 3p25, 8p22, 11q13, 19p13, or numeric abnormalities of 6, 13, 15, 17 [108, 109].

Sezary Syndrome (SS)

Sezary syndrome represents 5% or less of new cases of MF and can be considered the leukemic form of MF. It is clinically aggressive with 5 year survivals in the 10–20% range. The diagnosis of SS implies the triad of erythroderma, generalized lymphadenopathy, and abnormal lymphocytes with characteristic morphology (cerebriform lymphocytes-Sezary cells) in the skin, lymph nodes, and blood [1] (Fig. 1.13). Furthermore, one or more of the following should be present: greater than 1,000 cells/μL Sezary cells, a CD4:CD8 ratio >10 in blood by flow cytometry, loss of pan-T-cell antigens, or demonstration of a

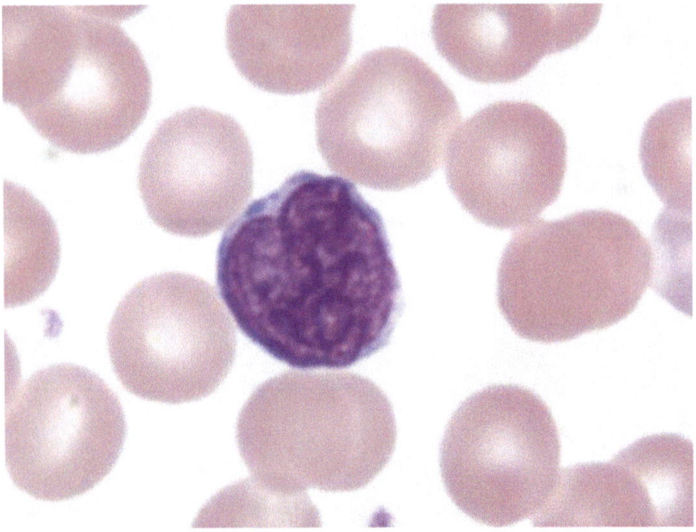

Fig. 1.13 Sezary syndrome. Peripheral blood, Wright–Giemsa ×1,000. The cell has a characteristic "cerebriform" nucleus

T-cell clone by molecular methods [92, 110, 111]. The morphology of the Sezary cells is best appreciated on peripheral blood smears. The cells are usually intermediate sized, with dispersed chromatin and nuclear convolutions; however, small cell variants are described with a more condensed, mature chromatin pattern but retaining the nuclear irregularities.

Primary Cutaneous CD30-Positive T-Cell Lymphoproliferative Disorders

The two entities in this category have significantly overlapping morphologic, immunophenotypic, and molecular features, which make them difficult to differentiate in the absence of an extensive, detailed clinical history [1, 36, 112]. Moreover, advanced stages of MF and cutaneous involvement by systemic ALCL can lead to patterns similar to those in this category.

Primary cutaneous ALCL differs from the nodal ALCL by its initial presentation (exclusively involving the skin) and negativity for ALK [36, 112]. This is a disease of older adults, with male predominance although pediatric cases are described. The cell of origin is not well characterized although it probably is a malignant counterpart of activated T-cells. The clinical course is variable, as spontaneous regression of the lesions can occur. The 5 year survival is over 90% [113].

Grossly, the skin lesions are usually single papules or ulcerated nodules, most >2 cm, but cases with multiple lesions have also been described. Histologically, the malignant infiltrate involves the superficial layers of the skin. The cells are large, with moderate cytoplasm and irregular nuclei, with fine chromatin and conspicuous nucleoli. Variants with smaller cells have been described. In most cases, the neoplastic cells are associated with histiocytes and eosinophils. When associated with ulcerations, the malignant cells can be surrounded by numerous inflammatory cells that can obscure the overall architecture of the infiltrate. A neutrophil-rich variant has been described, and in this variant, the neoplastic cells are a small minority of the lesion [114].

The immunophenotype of c-ALCL is characterized by positivity for CD4, granzyme B, TIA-1, perforin, and CD30. Clusterin is also expressed, with a Golgi dot-like pattern but is not specific as it can be seen in LyP, transformed MF, and some reactive conditions [115]. T-cell markers such as CD2, CD5, or CD3 can be lost. The neoplastic cells are negative for EMA, ALK, or CD15.

Molecular studies show clonal rearrangements of TCR genes. Rearrangements of

BUSP22 occur in up to 57% of cases and may be diagnostically useful [116].

LyP is a self-healing cutaneous lesion. It occurs mainly on the trunk and extremities of adults (median age of 45 years), with a male predominance [113]. The prognosis of these patients is excellent, as most lesions spontaneously regress. However, as there are no reliable prognostic indicators, close clinical follow-up is recommended.

Grossly, the lesions are multiple, small (<2 cm) papules with waxing and waning course, usually at different stages of development [113]. In a small minority of the patients, the lesions are preceded by MF. There are three histologic patterns of LyP [86]: type A with small clusters of pleomorphic, CD30 positive cells on a background of benign reactive cells, type C with sheets of anaplastic CD30 positive cells and limited mixed inflammatory infiltrate, and type B, with an epidermotropic infiltrate of small atypical cells, often negative for CD30.

The immunophenotype of the atypical cells in LyP is similar to those of the cells in c-ALCL, and molecular studies can identify clonal rearrangements of *TCR* genes [117]. *BUSP22* rearrangements are generally absent from LyP lesions [116].

Primary Cutaneous γδ T-Cell Lymphoma

This is a rare neoplasm of gamma-delta cytotoxic T-cells usually confined to the skin (mainly of extremities) and mucosa, mainly diagnosed in adults [118, 119]. A subset of cases can be associated with hemophagocytic syndrome [120]. The cell of origin is considered to be the activated cytotoxic γδ T-cells. This is an aggressive type of lymphoma, with a relatively short median survival (15 months) [120].

Gross examination can show several types of lesions: subcutaneous tumors, patches or plaques, ulcerations [120]. Histologic examination can divide the lesions in epidermotropic, dermal, and subcutaneous tumors. Overall, the pattern of involvement is similar to that seen in SPTCL, with the difference that usually there is significant involvement of dermis in primary cutaneous γδ T-cell lymphoma (PCGDTCL). Epidermis is often also involved and ulceration can be present. The malignant cells are intermediate to large, with dense chromatin. In the subcutaneous fibroadipose tissue, these cells can display adipocyte rimming. Necrosis and apoptosis are often prominent features of these tumors.

The immunophenotype of PCGDTCL is CD2+, CD3+, CD56+, TCRδ+. The cells are negative for CD4, CD5, CD8, βF1 [120].

Molecular studies have shown most of the cases to have clonal *TCR* γ rearrangements [121]. There is very little information on the cytogenetics of these lesions.

Primary Cutaneous CD8-Positive Aggressive Epidermotropic Cytotoxic T-Cell Lymphoma

A provisional entity in the WHO 2008 classification of tumors of hematopoietic and lymphoid tissue, primary cutaneous CD8-positive aggressive epidermotropic cytotoxic T-cell lymphoma, is a rare entity occurring mainly in adults [1, 86]. The cell of origin is the cytotoxic αβ T-cell with skin homing abilities. In contrast with CD4-positive primary cutaneous T-cell lymphoma, as its name suggests, this neoplasm has an aggressive clinical course [122].

Clinical examination shows the patients to have disseminated papules, nodules or tumors, with central necrosis, ulceration and hyperkeratotic plaques. In advanced stages, the tumor shows extensive visceral dissemination [86, 122]. Microscopic examination shows a malignant process with lichenoid pattern and marked epidermotropism. Overall, the pattern can be reminiscent of that of pagetoid reticulosis, with the difference that the lesions are widespread. The epidermis can show reactive changes, such as acanthosis, atrophy, necrosis, spongiosis. As the tumor invades deeper structures, it can display angiocentricity and angioinvasion, sometimes resulting in necrosis. The tumor cells are of variable size, most often small, with irregular nuclei, often with dense chromatin, sometimes with blastic chromatin [86, 122].

The immunophenotype of the lymphoma cells is positive for CD3, CD8, βF1, granzyme B, perforin, TIA-1. These cells are negative for CD4, CD5, and CD7. In most cases, they are also negative for CD2 [123].

While there are no conventional cytogenetic abnormalities identified to date, molecular studies almost always show clonal rearrangements of the *TCR* genes.

Primary Cutaneous CD4-Positive Small/Medium T-Cell Lymphoma

This is another provisional entity in the WHO 2008 classification [1]. It is a rare tumor defined as a (most often solitary) tumor mass with the appearance of the tumor stage of MF, in a patient without a history of MF, or without patches or plaques [124]. The tumor cells are thought to be malignant counterparts of skin-homing CD4-positive T-cells. This is considered an indolent lymphoma with prognosis of the patients with this type of lymphoma is relatively similar to that of patients with MF.

Gross examination shows usually a single skin nodule. Histologic examination shows a dense infiltrate mainly in the dermis, but also expanding in the subcutaneous tissue and displaying moderate epidermotropism (significantly less than MF). The lymphoma cells are small/intermediate T-cells, with abnormal nuclei, similar to those seen in MF.

The immunophenotype of the malignant cells is positive for CD3, CD4 and is negative for CD8 or CD30.

There are no data on the cytogenetics of this lesion. Molecular studies for clonal *TCR* rearrangements are positive.

T-Cell Prolymphocytic Leukemia

T-cell prolymphocytic leukemia (T-PLL) is an aggressive T-cell neoplasm involving the peripheral blood, lymph nodes, bone marrow, liver, spleen, and skin [1]. The cell of origin is a post-thymic (non-lymphoblastic) T-cell. This neoplasm is most often detected in adult males and has an aggressive course, with a median survival of less than 1 year [125–127]. An early indolent phase has been described, but most patients then enter an aggressive terminal phase [128].

The clinical presentation of T-PLL patients is generalized lymphadenopathy, rapidly increasing lymphocyte counts, hepatosplenomegaly. Cytopenias can be a consequence of bone marrow involvement. In a significant number of cases, the skin is extensively involved [129] (Fig. 1.14b, c).

Histologic examination of the involved tissues does not show a pathognomonic pattern, although sometimes it involves paracortical zones and spares normal structures such as lymphoid follicles in lymph nodes. Usually, the neoplastic infiltrate is composed of small cells, with dense chromatin (Fig. 1.14). Since the morphologic features are not entirely specific, clinical history is important at arriving at the correct diagnosis. On bone marrow or peripheral blood smears, the

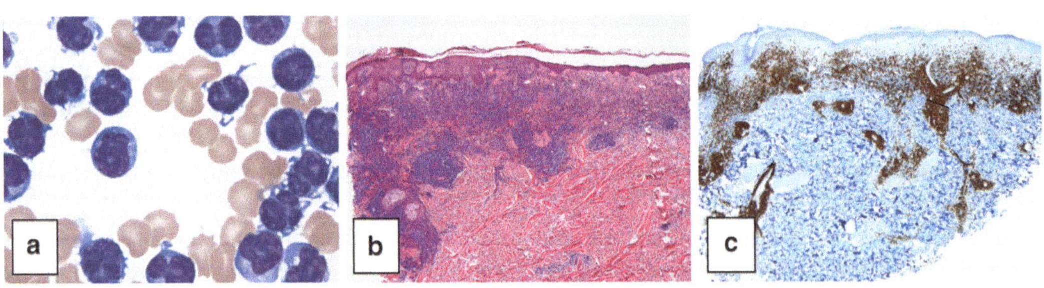

Fig. 1.14 T-cell prolymphocytic leukemia. (**a**) Peripheral blood, Wright–Giemsa ×1,000. Lymphocytosis with small lymphocytes. The nuclei are irregular, with knobs and notches, smudged chromatin, and small nucleoli. Cytoplasmic blebs are visible on the surface. (**b**) Skin, HE ×40. Dense small lymphocytic infiltrate, with limited epidermotropism. (**c**) TCL1 ×40. The lymphoma cells are positive

lymphoma cells are small to intermediate, with light basophilic cytoplasm without granules. The cell surface can show membrane blebbing. The nuclei are irregular, with notches or knobs, relatively dense chromatin, and usually central nucleoli [130] (Fig. 1.14a).

The immunophenotype of T-PLL cells is CD2+, CD3+, CD7+. Most cases (60%) are positive for CD4, 25% of cases are positive for both CD4 and CD8, while rare cases (15%) are positive for CD8 [130]. Another immunophenotypic feature characteristic of T-PLL (in addition to positivity for both CD4 and CD8) is positivity for TCL1, a protein normally expressed in B-cells [131] (Fig. 1.14c).

Molecular studies identify clonal rearrangements of *TCR* γ or β genes. Genetic abnormalities include inv(14)(q11q32) or t(14;14)(q11;q32) [125, 132]. The results of these abnormalities is the transposition of *TCL1A* and *TCL1B* in the *TCR* α gene locus (and hence their overexpression). A variant translocation is t(X;14)(q28;q11), resulting in the translocation of *MTCL1*. Other abnormalities described in T-PLL are idic(8p11), t(8;8)(p11-12;q12) and trisomy 8q. The observation that T-PLL is more frequent in patients with ataxia-telangiectasia has let to the identification of missense mutations of ATM (at 11q23). A minority of cases has mutations on chromosomes 6 or 17 [133].

T-Cell Large Granular Lymphocytic Leukemia

T-cell large granular lymphocytic leukemia (T-LGLL) is defined as an increase in circulating large granular lymphocytes lasting usually over 6 months and in most cases reaching levels of $2–20 \times 10^9$/L [1]. Most patients are adults, with no sex predilection. The disease is most often indolent with a prolonged course, characterized by cytopenias, splenomegaly. Many patients also have rheumatoid arthritis, circulating immune complexes, or other abnormalities of the immune system. Recent studies have shown a propensity for coexistence of B-cell dyscrasias including monoclonal gammopathy of undetermined significance, monoclonal B-cell lymphocytosis, and overt B-cell lymphoma/leukemia [134, 135]. Clones of cytotoxic T-cells have also been described in post-transplant patients. The cells of origin are cytotoxic T-cells, either CD8 positive or $\gamma\delta$. With the exception of rare cases with an aggressive course, T-LGLL is an indolent disease, with a protracted clinical course [136–139].

In the peripheral blood, the abnormal T-LGLs have features relatively similar to those of normal T-LGLs, but the granules can be more coarse or less numerous. The bone marrow can be normocellular (in most cases) or hypocellular. The T-LGLs can form aggregates, but most often are diffusely distributed, mainly with an intra-sinusoidal pattern. Benign lymphoid aggregates can also be present and could signal abnormal immune processes [140].

The cytotoxic cells are positive for CD2, CD3, CD5, CD7, CD8, CD16, CD57. Rarely CD5 or CD7 can be lost. Cytotoxic molecules such as granzyme B, perforin, TIA-1 are a constant feature. Very few cases are positive for CD4 (but not for co-expression of CD4 and CD8). TCR-Vbeta analysis shows restricted Vbeta family usage, and KIR analysis shows restricted KIR patterns [141]. Electron-microscopy shows the granules to be tubular array filled with proteins, probably cytotoxic.

Conventional cytogenetic analysis of T-LGLL is usually noncontributory, but when abnormalities are identified they are nonspecific. Molecular studies show *TCR* γ chain rearrangements [137]. Recently, somatic mutations in STAT3 have been found in 30- 40 % of T-LGLL cases [142].

References

1. Swerdlow SH, Campo E, Harris NL, Jaffe ES, Pileri SA, Stein H, et al., editors. WHO classification of tumours of haematopoietic and lymphoid tissues. Lyon: IARC; 2008.
2. Cotta CV, Hsi ED. Pathobiology of mature T-cell lymphomas. Clin Lymphoma Myeloma. 2008;8 Suppl 5:S168–79.
3. Delves PJ, Roitt IM. The immune system. Second of two parts. N Engl J Med. 2000;343:108–17.

4. Delves PJ, Roitt IM. The immune system. First of two parts. N Engl J Med. 2000;343:37–49.
5. Vose J, Armitage J, Weisenburger D. International peripheral T-cell and natural killer/T-cell lymphoma study: pathology findings and clinical outcomes. J Clin Oncol. 2008;26:4124–30.
6. Au WY, Weisenburger DD, Intragumtornchai T, et al. Clinical differences between nasal and extranasal natural killer/T-cell lymphoma: a study of 136 cases from the International Peripheral T-Cell Lymphoma Project. Blood. 2009;113:3931–7.
7. Oshimi K, Kawa K, Nakamura S, et al. NK-cell neoplasms in Japan. Hematology. 2005;10:237–45.
8. Deleeuw RJ, Zettl A, Klinker E, et al. Whole-genome analysis and HLA genotyping of enteropathy-type T-cell lymphoma reveals 2 distinct lymphoma subtypes. Gastroenterology. 2007;132:1902–11.
9. Zettl A, deLeeuw R, Haralambieva E, Mueller-Hermelink HK. Enteropathy-type T-cell lymphoma. Am J Clin Pathol. 2007;127:701–6.
10. O'Leary HM, Savage KJ. Update on the World Health Organization classification of peripheral T-cell lymphomas. Curr Hematol Malig Rep. 2009;4:227–35.
11. Morton LM, Wang SS, Devesa SS, Hartge P, Weisenburger DD, Linet MS. Lymphoma incidence patterns by WHO subtype in the United States, 1992–2001. Blood. 2006;107:265–76.
12. Hutchison RE, Laver JH, Chang M, et al. Non-anaplastic peripheral t-cell lymphoma in childhood and adolescence: a Children's Oncology Group study. Pediatr Blood Cancer. 2008;51:29–33.
13. Rizvi MA, Evens AM, Tallman MS, Nelson BP, Rosen ST. T-cell non-Hodgkin lymphoma. Blood. 2006;107:1255–64.
14. Campo E, Gaulard P, Zucca E, et al. Report of the European Task Force on Lymphomas: workshop on peripheral T-cell lymphomas. Ann Oncol. 1998; 9:835–43.
15. Lopez-Guillermo A, Cid J, Salar A, et al. Peripheral T-cell lymphomas: initial features, natural history, and prognostic factors in a series of 174 patients diagnosed according to the R.E.A.L. classification. Ann Oncol. 1998;9:849–55.
16. Han X, Kilfoy B, Zheng T, et al. Lymphoma survival patterns by WHO subtype in the United States, 1973–2003. Cancer Causes Control. 2008; 19:841–58.
17. de Leval L, Savilo E, Longtine J, Ferry JA, Harris NL. Peripheral T-cell lymphoma with follicular involvement and a CD4+/bcl-6+ phenotype. Am J Surg Pathol. 2001;25:395–400.
18. Rudiger T, Ichinohasama R, Ott MM, et al. Peripheral T-cell lymphoma with distinct perifollicular growth pattern: a distinct subtype of T-cell lymphoma? Am J Surg Pathol. 2000;24:117–22.
19. Beck RC, Stahl S, O'Keefe CL, Maciejewski JP, Theil KS, Hsi ED. Detection of mature T-cell leukemias by flow cytometry using anti-T-cell receptor V beta antibodies. Am J Clin Pathol. 2003;120:785–94.
20. Warnke RA, Jones D, Hsi ED. Morphologic and immunophenotypic variants of nodal T-cell lymphomas and T-cell lymphoma mimics. Am J Clin Pathol. 2007;127:511–27.
21. Went P, Agostinelli C, Gallamini A, et al. Marker expression in peripheral T-cell lymphoma: a proposed clinical-pathologic prognostic score. J Clin Oncol. 2006;24:2472–9.
22. Piccaluga PP, Agostinelli C, Califano A, et al. Gene expression analysis of peripheral T cell lymphoma, unspecified, reveals distinct profiles and new potential therapeutic targets. J Clin Invest. 2007;117: 823–34.
23. Zettl A, Rudiger T, Konrad MA, et al. Genomic profiling of peripheral T-cell lymphoma, unspecified, and anaplastic large T-cell lymphoma delineates novel recurrent chromosomal alterations. Am J Pathol. 2004;164:1837–48.
24. Dogan A, Attygalle AD, Kyriakou C. Angioimmunoblastic T-cell lymphoma. Br J Haematol. 2003;121:681–91.
25. Dunleavy K, Wilson WH, Jaffe ES. Angioimmunoblastic T cell lymphoma: pathobiological insights and clinical implications. Curr Opin Hematol. 2007;14:348–53.
26. Grogg KL, Attygalle AD, Macon WR, Remstein ED, Kurtin PJ, Dogan A. Angioimmunoblastic T-cell lymphoma: a neoplasm of germinal-center T-helper cells? Blood. 2005;106:1501–2.
27. Lachenal F, Berger F, Ghesquieres H, et al. Angioimmunoblastic T-cell lymphoma: clinical and laboratory features at diagnosis in 77 patients. Medicine (Baltimore). 2007;86:282–92.
28. Attygalle AD, Kyriakou C, Dupuis J, et al. Histologic evolution of angioimmunoblastic T-cell lymphoma in consecutive biopsies: clinical correlation and insights into natural history and disease progression. Am J Surg Pathol. 2007;31:1077–88.
29. Grogg KL, Attygalle AD, Macon WR, Remstein ED, Kurtin PJ, Dogan A. Expression of CXCL13, a chemokine highly upregulated in germinal center T-helper cells, distinguishes angioimmunoblastic T-cell lymphoma from peripheral T-cell lymphoma, unspecified. Mod Pathol. 2006;19:1101–7.
30. Marafioti T, Paterson JC, Ballabio E, et al. The inducible T-cell co-stimulator molecule is expressed on subsets of T cells and is a new marker of lymphomas of T follicular helper cell-derivation. Haematologica. 2010;95:432–9.
31. Willenbrock K, Brauninger A, Hansmann ML. Frequent occurrence of B-cell lymphomas in angioimmunoblastic T-cell lymphoma and proliferation of Epstein-Barr virus-infected cells in early cases. Br J Haematol. 2007;138:733–9.
32. Tan BT, Seo K, Warnke RA, Arber DA. The frequency of immunoglobulin heavy chain gene and T-cell receptor gamma-chain gene rearrangements and Epstein-Barr virus in ALK+ and ALK- anaplastic large cell lymphoma and other peripheral T-cell lymphomas. J Mol Diagn. 2008;10:502–12.

33. Tan BT, Warnke RA, Arber DA. The frequency of B- and T-cell gene rearrangements and Epstein-Barr virus in T-cell lymphomas: a comparison between angioimmunoblastic T-cell lymphoma and peripheral T-cell lymphoma, unspecified with and without associated B-cell proliferations. J Mol Diagn 2006;8:466–75; quiz 527.
34. Piccaluga PP, Agostinelli C, Califano A, et al. Gene expression analysis of angioimmunoblastic lymphoma indicates derivation from T follicular helper cells and vascular endothelial growth factor deregulation. Cancer Res. 2007;67:10703–10.
35. Benharroch D, Meguerian-Bedoyan Z, Lamant L, et al. ALK-positive lymphoma: a single disease with a broad spectrum of morphology. Blood. 1998;91:2076–84.
36. Savage KJ, Harris NL, Vose JM, et al. ALK- anaplastic large-cell lymphoma is clinically and immunophenotypically different from both ALK+ ALCL and peripheral T-cell lymphoma, not otherwise specified: report from the International Peripheral T-Cell Lymphoma Project. Blood. 2008;111:5496–504.
37. Falini B, Pulford K, Pucciarini A, et al. Lymphomas expressing ALK fusion protein(s) other than NPM-ALK. Blood. 1999;94:3509–15.
38. Klapper W, Bohm M, Siebert R, Lennert K. Morphological variability of lymphohistiocytic variant of anaplastic large cell lymphoma (former lymphohistiocytic lymphoma according to the Kiel classification). Virchows Arch. 2008;452:599–605.
39. Stein H, Mason DY, Gerdes J, et al. The expression of the Hodgkin's disease associated antigen Ki-1 in reactive and neoplastic lymphoid tissue: evidence that Reed-Sternberg cells and histiocytic malignancies are derived from activated lymphoid cells. Blood. 1985;66:848–58.
40. Bonzheim I, Geissinger E, Roth S, et al. Anaplastic large cell lymphomas lack the expression of T-cell receptor molecules or molecules of proximal T-cell receptor signaling. Blood. 2004;104:3358–60.
41. Foss HD, Anagnostopoulos I, Araujo I, et al. Anaplastic large-cell lymphomas of T-cell and null-cell phenotype express cytotoxic molecules. Blood. 1996;88:4005–11.
42. Krenacs L, Wellmann A, Sorbara L, et al. Cytotoxic cell antigen expression in anaplastic large cell lymphomas of T- and null-cell type and Hodgkin's disease: evidence for distinct cellular origin. Blood. 1997;89:980–9.
43. Wellmann A, Thieblemont C, Pittaluga S, et al. Detection of differentially expressed genes in lymphomas using cDNA arrays: identification of clusterin as a new diagnostic marker for anaplastic large-cell lymphomas. Blood. 2000;96:398–404.
44. Chiarle R, Voena C, Ambrogio C, Piva R, Inghirami G. The anaplastic lymphoma kinase in the pathogenesis of cancer. Nat Rev Cancer. 2008;8:11–23.
45. Drexler HG, Gignac SM, von Wasielewski R, Werner M, Dirks WG. Pathobiology of NPM-ALK and variant fusion genes in anaplastic large cell lymphoma and other lymphomas. Leukemia. 2000;14:1533–59.
46. Stein H, Foss HD, Durkop H, et al. CD30(+) anaplastic large cell lymphoma: a review of its histopathologic, genetic, and clinical features. Blood. 2000;96:3681–95.
47. Nicot C. Current views in HTLV-I-associated adult T-cell leukemia/lymphoma. Am J Hematol. 2005; 78:232–9.
48. Nicot C, Harrod RL, Ciminale V, Franchini G. Human T-cell leukemia/lymphoma virus type 1 nonstructural genes and their functions. Oncogene. 2005;24:6026–34.
49. Satou Y, Yasunaga J, Yoshida M, Matsuoka M. HTLV-I basic leucine zipper factor gene mRNA supports proliferation of adult T cell leukemia cells. Proc Natl Acad Sci U S A. 2006;103:720–5.
50. Yasunaga J, Taniguchi Y, Nosaka K, et al. Identification of aberrantly methylated genes in association with adult T-cell leukemia. Cancer Res. 2004;64:6002–9.
51. Ohshima K, Suzumiya J, Kato A, Tashiro K, Kikuchi M. Clonal HTLV-I-infected CD4+ T-lymphocytes and non-clonal non-HTLV-I-infected giant cells in incipient ATLL with Hodgkin-like histologic features. Int J Cancer. 1997;72:592–8.
52. Yamamura M, Honda M, Yamada Y, et al. Increased levels of interleukin-6 (IL-6) in serum and spontaneous in vitro production of IL-6 by lymph node mononuclear cells of patients with angio-immunoblastic lymphadenopathy with dysproteinemia (AILD), and clinical effectiveness of cyclosporin A. Leukemia. 1996;10:1504–8.
53. Ohshima K. Pathological features of diseases associated with human T-cell leukemia virus type I. Cancer Sci. 2007;98:772–8.
54. Shimoyama M. Diagnostic criteria and classification of clinical subtypes of adult T-cell leukaemia-lymphoma. A report from the Lymphoma Study Group (1984–87). Br J Haematol. 1991;79:428–37.
55. Matutes E. Adult T-cell leukaemia/lymphoma. J Clin Pathol. 2007;60:1373–7.
56. Karube K, Ohshima K, Tsuchiya T, et al. Expression of FoxP3, a key molecule in CD4CD25 regulatory T cells, in adult T-cell leukaemia/lymphoma cells. Br J Haematol. 2004;126:81–4.
57. Liang X, Graham DK. Natural killer cell neoplasms. Cancer. 2008;112:1425–36.
58. Hasserjian RP, Harris NL. NK-cell lymphomas and leukemias: a spectrum of tumors with variable manifestations and immunophenotype. Am J Clin Pathol. 2007;127:860–8.
59. Jaffe ES, Krenacs L, Kumar S, Kingma DW, Raffeld M. Extranodal peripheral T-cell and NK-cell neoplasms. Am J Clin Pathol. 1999;111:S46–55.
60. Kwong YL, Chan AC, Liang RH. Natural killer cell lymphoma/leukemia: pathology and treatment. Hematol Oncol. 1997;15:71–9.
61. Liang R, Todd D, Chan TK, et al. Treatment outcome and prognostic factors for primary nasal lymphoma. J Clin Oncol. 1995;13:666–70.
62. Au WY. Current management of nasal NK/T-cell lymphoma. Oncology (Williston Park). 2010;24:352–8.

63. Ng SB, Lai KW, Murugaya S, et al. Nasal-type extranodal natural killer/T-cell lymphomas: a clinicopathologic and genotypic study of 42 cases in Singapore. Mod Pathol. 2004;17:1097–107.
64. Siu LL, Chan V, Chan JK, Wong KF, Liang R, Kwong YL. Consistent patterns of allelic loss in natural killer cell lymphoma. Am J Pathol. 2000;157:1803–9.
65. Zhang Y, Wong KF, Siebert R, et al. Chromosome aberrations are restricted to the CD56+, CD3- tumour cell population in natural killer cell lymphomas: a combined immunophenotyping and FISH study. Br J Haematol. 1999;105:737–42.
66. Song SY, Kim WS, Ko YH, Kim K, Lee MH, Park K. Aggressive natural killer cell leukemia: clinical features and treatment outcome. Haematologica. 2002;87:1343–5.
67. Suzuki R, Suzumiya J, Nakamura S, et al. Aggressive natural killer-cell leukemia revisited: large granular lymphocyte leukemia of cytotoxic NK cells. Leukemia. 2004;18:763–70.
68. Kimura H, Hoshino Y, Kanegane H, et al. Clinical and virologic characteristics of chronic active Epstein-Barr virus infection. Blood. 2001;98:280–6.
69. Su IJ, Chen RL, Lin DT, Lin KS, Chen CC. Epstein-Barr virus (EBV) infects T lymphocytes in childhood EBV-associated hemophagocytic syndrome in Taiwan. Am J Pathol. 1994;144:1219–25.
70. Suzuki K, Ohshima K, Karube K, et al. Clinicopathological states of Epstein-Barr virus-associated T/NK-cell lymphoproliferative disorders (severe chronic active EBV infection) of children and young adults. Int J Oncol. 2004;24:1165–74.
71. Kasahara Y, Yachie A, Takei K, et al. Differential cellular targets of Epstein-Barr virus (EBV) infection between acute EBV-associated hemophagocytic lymphohistiocytosis and chronic active EBV infection. Blood. 2001;98:1882–8.
72. Quintanilla-Martinez L, Kumar S, Fend F, et al. Fulminant EBV(+) T-cell lymphoproliferative disorder following acute/chronic EBV infection: a distinct clinicopathologic syndrome. Blood. 2000;96:443–51.
73. Jones JF, Shurin S, Abramowsky C, et al. T-cell lymphomas containing Epstein-Barr viral DNA in patients with chronic Epstein-Barr virus infections. N Engl J Med. 1988;318:733–41.
74. Barrionuevo C, Anderson VM, Zevallos-Giampietri E, et al. Hydroa-like cutaneous T-cell lymphoma: a clinicopathologic and molecular genetic study of 16 pediatric cases from Peru. Appl Immunohistochem Mol Morphol. 2002;10:7–14.
75. Iwatsuki K, Satoh M, Yamamoto T, et al. Pathogenic link between hydroa vacciniforme and Epstein-Barr virus-associated hematologic disorders. Arch Dermatol. 2006;142:587–95.
76. Zhang Y, Nagata H, Ikeuchi T, et al. Common cytological and cytogenetic features of Epstein-Barr virus (EBV)-positive natural killer (NK) cells and cell lines derived from patients with nasal T/NK-cell lymphomas, chronic active EBV infection and hydroa vacciniforme-like eruptions. Br J Haematol. 2003;121:805–14.
77. Howell WM, Leung ST, Jones DB, et al. HLA-DRB, -DQA, and -DQB polymorphism in celiac disease and enteropathy-associated T-cell lymphoma. Common features and additional risk factors for malignancy. Hum Immunol. 1995;43:29–37.
78. Chott A, Haedicke W, Mosberger I, et al. Most CD56+ intestinal lymphomas are CD8+ CD5-T-cell lymphomas of monomorphic small to medium size histology. Am J Pathol. 1998;153:1483–90.
79. Falchook GS, Vega F, Dang NH, et al. Hepatosplenic gamma-delta T-cell lymphoma: clinicopathological features and treatment. Ann Oncol. 2009;20:1080–5.
80. Lai R, Larratt LM, Etches W, et al. Hepatosplenic T-cell lymphoma of alphabeta lineage in a 16-year-old boy presenting with hemolytic anemia and thrombocytopenia. Am J Surg Pathol. 2000;24:459–63.
81. Macon WR, Levy NB, Kurtin PJ, et al. Hepatosplenic alphabeta T-cell lymphomas: a report of 14 cases and comparison with hepatosplenic gammadelta T-cell lymphomas. Am J Surg Pathol. 2001;25:285–96.
82. Suarez F, Wlodarska I, Rigal-Huguet F, et al. Hepatosplenic alphabeta T-cell lymphoma: an unusual case with clinical, histologic, and cytogenetic features of gammadelta hepatosplenic T-cell lymphoma. Am J Surg Pathol. 2000;24:1027–32.
83. Vega F, Medeiros LJ, Gaulard P. Hepatosplenic and other gammadelta T-cell lymphomas. Am J Clin Pathol. 2007;127:869–80.
84. Gaulard P, Belhadj K, Reyes F. Gammadelta T-cell lymphomas. Semin Hematol. 2003;40:233–43.
85. Belhadj K, Reyes F, Farcet JP, et al. Hepatosplenic gammadelta T-cell lymphoma is a rare clinicopathologic entity with poor outcome: report on a series of 21 patients. Blood. 2003;102:4261–9.
86. Willemze R, Jaffe ES, Burg G, et al. WHO-EORTC classification for cutaneous lymphomas. Blood. 2005;105:3768–85.
87. Willemze R, Jansen PM, Cerroni L, et al. Subcutaneous panniculitis-like T-cell lymphoma: definition, classification, and prognostic factors: an EORTC Cutaneous Lymphoma Group Study of 83 cases. Blood. 2008;111:838–45.
88. Massone C, Lozzi GP, Egberts F, et al. The protean spectrum of non-Hodgkin lymphomas with prominent involvement of subcutaneous fat. J Cutan Pathol. 2006;33:418–25.
89. Lozzi GP, Massone C, Citarella L, Kerl H, Cerroni L. Rimming of adipocytes by neoplastic lymphocytes: a histopathologic feature not restricted to subcutaneous T-cell lymphoma. Am J Dermatopathol. 2006;28:9–12.
90. Keehn CA, Belongie IP, Shistik G, Fenske NA, Glass LF. The diagnosis, staging, and treatment options for mycosis fungoides. Cancer Control. 2007;14:102–11.
91. van Doorn R, Van Haselen CW, van Voorst Vader PC, et al. Mycosis fungoides: disease evolution and

prognosis of 309 Dutch patients. Arch Dermatol. 2000;136:504–10.
92. Olsen E, Vonderheid E, Pimpinelli N, et al. Revisions to the staging and classification of mycosis fungoides and Sezary syndrome: a proposal of the International Society for Cutaneous Lymphomas (ISCL) and the cutaneous lymphoma task force of the European Organization of Research and Treatment of Cancer (EORTC). Blood. 2007;110:1713–22.
93. Gibson LE, Muller SA, Leiferman KM, Peters MS. Follicular mucinosis: clinical and histopathologic study. J Am Acad Dermatol. 1989;20:441–6.
94. van Doorn R, Scheffer E, Willemze R. Follicular mycosis fungoides, a distinct disease entity with or without associated follicular mucinosis: a clinicopathologic and follow-up study of 51 patients. Arch Dermatol. 2002;138:191–8.
95. Haghighi B, Smoller BR, LeBoit PE, Warnke RA, Sander CA, Kohler S. Pagetoid reticulosis (Woringer-Kolopp disease): an immunophenotypic, molecular, and clinicopathologic study. Mod Pathol. 2000;13:502–10.
96. LeBoit PE. Granulomatous slack skin. Dermatol Clin. 1994;12:375–89.
97. van Haselen CW, Toonstra J, van der Putte SJ, van Dongen JJ, van Hees CL, van Vloten WA. Granulomatous slack skin. Report of three patients with an updated review of the literature. Dermatology. 1998;196:382–91.
98. Massone C, Kodama K, Kerl H, Cerroni L. Histopathologic features of early (patch) lesions of mycosis fungoides: a morphologic study on 745 biopsy specimens from 427 patients. Am J Surg Pathol. 2005;29:550–60.
99. Cerroni L, Rieger E, Hodl S, Kerl H. Clinicopathologic and immunologic features associated with transformation of mycosis fungoides to large-cell lymphoma. Am J Surg Pathol. 1992;16:543–52.
100. Diamandidou E, Colome-Grimmer M, Fayad L, Duvic M, Kurzrock R. Transformation of mycosis fungoides/Sezary syndrome: clinical characteristics and prognosis. Blood. 1998;92:1150–9.
101. Vergier B, de Muret A, Beylot-Barry M, et al. Transformation of mycosis fungoides: clinicopathological and prognostic features of 45 cases. French Study Group of Cutaneous Lymphomas. Blood. 2000;95:2212–8.
102. Sausville EA, Worsham GF, Matthews MJ, et al. Histologic assessment of lymph nodes in mycosis fungoides/Sezary syndrome (cutaneous T-cell lymphoma): clinical correlations and prognostic import of a new classification system. Hum Pathol. 1985;16:1098–109.
103. Scheffer E, Meijer CJ, Van Vloten WA. Dermatopathic lymphadenopathy and lymph node involvement in mycosis fungoides. Cancer. 1980;45:137–48.
104. Sausville EA, Eddy JL, Makuch RW, et al. Histopathologic staging at initial diagnosis of mycosis fungoides and the Sezary syndrome. Definition of three distinctive prognostic groups. Ann Intern Med. 1988;109:372–82.
105. Zackheim HS, Amin S, Kashani-Sabet M, McMillan A. Prognosis in cutaneous T-cell lymphoma by skin stage: long-term survival in 489 patients. J Am Acad Dermatol. 1999;40:418–25.
106. Ralfkiaer E. Immunohistological markers for the diagnosis of cutaneous lymphomas. Semin Diagn Pathol. 1991;8:62–72.
107. Vega F, Luthra R, Medeiros LJ, et al. Clonal heterogeneity in mycosis fungoides and its relationship to clinical course. Blood. 2002;100:3369–73.
108. Mao X, Lillington D, Scarisbrick JJ, et al. Molecular cytogenetic analysis of cutaneous T-cell lymphomas: identification of common genetic alterations in Sezary syndrome and mycosis fungoides. Br J Dermatol. 2002;147:464–75.
109. Mao X, Lillington DM, Czepulkowski B, Russell-Jones R, Young BD, Whittaker S. Molecular cytogenetic characterization of Sezary syndrome. Genes Chromosomes Cancer. 2003;36:250–60.
110. Vonderheid EC, Bernengo MG, Burg G, et al. Update on erythrodermic cutaneous T-cell lymphoma: report of the International Society for Cutaneous Lymphomas. J Am Acad Dermatol. 2002;46:95–106.
111. Wieselthier JS, Koh HK. Sezary syndrome: diagnosis, prognosis, and critical review of treatment options. J Am Acad Dermatol. 1990;22:381–401.
112. Kempf W, Kutzner H, Cozzio A, et al. MUM1 expression in cutaneous CD30+ lymphoproliferative disorders: a valuable tool for the distinction between lymphomatoid papulosis and primary cutaneous anaplastic large-cell lymphoma. Br J Dermatol. 2008;158:1280–7.
113. Bekkenk MW, Geelen FA, van Voorst Vader PC, et al. Primary and secondary cutaneous CD30(+) lymphoproliferative disorders: a report from the Dutch Cutaneous Lymphoma Group on the long-term follow-up data of 219 patients and guidelines for diagnosis and treatment. Blood. 2000;95:3653–61.
114. Burg G, Kempf W, Kazakov DV, et al. Pyogenic lymphoma of the skin: a peculiar variant of primary cutaneous neutrophil-rich CD30+ anaplastic large-cell lymphoma. Clinicopathological study of four cases and review of the literature. Br J Dermatol. 2003;148:580–6.
115. Olsen SH, Ma L, Schnitzer B, Fullen DR. Clusterin expression in cutaneous CD30-positive lymphoproliferative disorders and their histologic simulants. J Cutan Pathol. 2009;36:302–7.
116. Feldman AL, Law M, Remstein ED, et al. Recurrent translocations involving the IRF4 oncogene locus in peripheral T-cell lymphomas. Leukemia. 2009;23:574–80.
117. Weiss LM, Wood GS, Trela M, Warnke RA, Sklar J. Clonal T-cell populations in lymphomatoid papulosis. Evidence of a lymphoproliferative origin for a clinically benign disease. N Engl J Med. 1986;315:475–9.
118. Burg G, Kempf W, Cozzio A, et al. WHO/EORTC classification of cutaneous lymphomas 2005: histological and molecular aspects. J Cutan Pathol. 2005;32:647–74.

119. Jaffe ES, Krenacs L, Raffeld M. Classification of cytotoxic T-cell and natural killer cell lymphomas. Semin Hematol. 2003;40:175–84.
120. Toro JR, Liewehr DJ, Pabby N, et al. Gamma-delta T-cell phenotype is associated with significantly decreased survival in cutaneous T-cell lymphoma. Blood. 2003;101:3407–12.
121. Przybylski GK, Wu H, Macon WR, et al. Hepatosplenic and subcutaneous panniculitis-like gamma/delta T cell lymphomas are derived from different Vdelta subsets of gamma/delta T lymphocytes. J Mol Diagn. 2000;2:11–9.
122. Berti E, Cerri A, Cavicchini S, et al. Primary cutaneous gamma/delta T-cell lymphoma presenting as disseminated pagetoid reticulosis. J Invest Dermatol. 1991;96:718–23.
123. Massone C, Chott A, Metze D, et al. Subcutaneous, blastic natural killer (NK), NK/T-cell, and other cytotoxic lymphomas of the skin: a morphologic, immunophenotypic, and molecular study of 50 patients. Am J Surg Pathol. 2004;28:719–35.
124. Garcia-Herrera A, Colomo L, Camos M, et al. Primary cutaneous small/medium CD4+ T-cell lymphomas: a heterogeneous group of tumors with different clinicopathologic features and outcome. J Clin Oncol. 2008;26:3364–71.
125. Dearden CE. T-cell prolymphocytic leukemia. Med Oncol. 2006;23:17–22.
126. Dungarwalla M, Matutes E, Dearden CE. Prolymphocytic leukaemia of B- and T-cell subtype: a state-of-the-art paper. Eur J Haematol. 2008;80: 469–76.
127. Krishnan B, Matutes E, Dearden C. Prolymphocytic leukemias. Semin Oncol. 2006;33:257–63.
128. Cavazzini F, Cuneo A, Bardi A, Castoldi G. Indolent T-cell prolymphocytic leukemia: a case report and a review of the literature. Am J Hematol. 2003; 74:145–7.
129. Magro CM, Morrison CD, Heerema N, Porcu P, Sroa N, Deng AC. T-cell prolymphocytic leukemia: an aggressive T cell malignancy with frequent cutaneous tropism. J Am Acad Dermatol. 2006;55:467–77.
130. Foucar K. Mature T-cell leukemias including T-prolymphocytic leukemia, adult T-cell leukemia/lymphoma, and Sezary syndrome. Am J Clin Pathol. 2007;127:496–510.
131. Herling M, Patel KA, Teitell MA, et al. High TCL1 expression and intact T-cell receptor signaling define a hyperproliferative subset of T-cell prolymphocytic leukemia. Blood. 2008;111:328–37.
132. Pekarsky Y, Hallas C, Isobe M, Russo G, Croce CM. Abnormalities at 14q32.1 in T cell malignancies involve two oncogenes. Proc Natl Acad Sci U S A. 1999;96:2949–51.
133. Costa D, Queralt R, Aymerich M, et al. High levels of chromosomal imbalances in typical and small-cell variants of T-cell prolymphocytic leukemia. Cancer Genet Cytogenet. 2003;147:36–43.
134. Howard MT, Bejanyan N, Maciejewski JP, Hsi ED. T/NK large granular lymphocyte leukemia and coexisting monoclonal B-cell lymphocytosis-like proliferations. An unrecognized and frequent association. Am J Clin Pathol. 2010;133:936–41.
135. Viny AD, Lichtin A, Pohlman B, Loughran T, Maciejewski J. Chronic B-cell dyscrasias are an important clinical feature of T-LGL leukemia. Leuk Lymphoma. 2008;49:932–8.
136. Alekshun TJ, Sokol L. Diseases of large granular lymphocytes. Cancer Control. 2007;14:141–50.
137. O'Malley DP. T-cell large granular leukemia and related proliferations. Am J Clin Pathol. 2007;127:850–9.
138. Rose MG, Berliner N. T-cell large granular lymphocyte leukemia and related disorders. Oncologist. 2004;9:247–58.
139. Sokol L, Loughran Jr TP. Large granular lymphocyte leukemia. Oncologist. 2006;11:263–73.
140. Morice WG, Kurtin PJ, Tefferi A, Hanson CA. Distinct bone marrow findings in T-cell granular lymphocytic leukemia revealed by paraffin section immunoperoxidase stains for CD8, TIA-1, and granzyme B. Blood. 2002;99:268–74.
141. Morice WG, Kurtin PJ, Myers JL. Expression of cytolytic lymphocyte-associated antigens in pulmonary lymphomatoid granulomatosis. Am J Clin Pathol. 2002;118:391–8.
142. Koskela HL, EIUFISS S, Ellonen P, et. al. Somatic mutations in large granular lymphocytic leukemia, NENS J Meu 2012; 366: 1905–13.

2 Epidemiology and Prognosis of T-Cell Lymphoma

Sophia S. Wang and Julie M. Vose

Introduction

NHL incidence rates rose steadily in the second half of the twentieth century. This observation motivated the conduct of numerous large-scale population-based epidemiologic studies of NHL in the last decade whose goals were to understand the rising rates and to uncover the etiology of NHL and its heterogeneous subtypes. In these studies, however, T-cell lymphomas and its subtypes are underrepresented due to the low incidence of disease and the relatively small proportion of NHL cases that are considered T-cell lymphomas. Like B-cell lymphomas, T-cell lymphomas comprise multiple subtypes with different incidence rates and patterns that likely reflect their distinct etiologies (e.g., mycosis fungoides and adult T-cell leukemia/lymphoma (ATL)). In recent years, the incidence rates of many B-cell lymphomas have begun to decline in the United States (US). In contrast, incidence rates for T-cell lymphomas have continued to rise. With consortial efforts and multidisciplinary approaches to epidemiologic research, the major hurdles for uncovering T-cell lymphoma risk factors may finally be surmountable.

Patterns of Occurrence

T/NK-cell lymphoid neoplasms account for approximately 6% of all lymphoid neoplasms. B-cell lymphoid neoplasms account for 80% of all lymphoid neoplasms and Hodgkin lymphomas account for 7%. During the 10-year period from 1997 to 2006 as recorded in the US Surveillance, Epidemiology and End Results (SEER) cancer registries, incidence rates for B-cell lymphoid neoplasms (27.96 per 100,000 persons) was greatly elevated above T/NK-cell lymphoid neoplasms (2.09) and Hodgkin lymphoma (2.71) (Table 2.1). Within T/NK-cell lymphoid neoplasms, incidence rates were highest for peripheral T-cell lymphoma (PTCL) (0.78) followed by mycosis fungoides/Sezary syndrome (0.54) and T/NK-cell lymphoid neoplasms, not otherwise specified (NOS) (0.49). Incidence of ATL was rare in the US (0.04). The most common PTCL subtype was PTCL-NOS (0.41) followed by anaplastic large cell lymphoma (ALCL) (0.28), cutaneous T-cell lymphoma (0.25), and angioimmunoblastic lymphoma (0.10). The remaining PTCL subtypes (subcutaneous panniculitis-like T-cell lymphoma, hepatosplenic T-cell lymphoma, enteropathy type T-cell lymphoma) were rare and had incidence rates of 0.01 per 100,000 persons.

S.S. Wang
Department of Population Sciences, City of Hope National Medical Center, Duarte, CA, USA

J.M. Vose (✉)
Section of Hematology/Oncology, 987680 Nebraska Medical Center, Omaha, NE 68198-7680, USA
e-mail: jmvose@unmc.edu

F. Foss (ed.), *T-Cell Lymphomas*, Contemporary Hematology,
DOI 10.1007/978-1-62703-170-7_2,

Table 2.1 Incidence of hematopoietic neoplasms by subtype and ICD-O-3 codes, 13 SEER registries, 1997–2006

Hematopoietic neoplasm subtype	ICD-O-3 codes[a, b]	No.	Rate[c]
Lymphoid neoplasms, total	–	127,234	34.55
B-cell lymphoid neoplasms, total	9590–9591(B), 9596(B), 9670–9671, 9673, 9675(B), 9678–9680, 9684, 9687, 9689–9691, 9695, 9698–9699, 9727(B), 9728, 9731–9734, 9761, 9764, 9820(B), 9823, 9826, 9832(B), 9833, 9835(B), 9836, 9940, 9970(B)	102,100	27.96
T/NK-cell lymphoid neoplasms, total	9590–9591(T/NK), 9596(T/NK), 9675(T/NK), 9700–9702, 9705, 9708–9709, 9714, 9716–9719, 9727(T/NK), 9729, 9820(T/NK), 9827, 9831, 9832(T/NK), 9834, 9835(T/NK), 9837, 9948, 9970(T/NK)	7,868	2.09
Mycosis fungoides/Sézary syndrome	9700–9701	2,037	0.54
Peripheral T-cell lymphoma	9675(T/NK), 9702, 9705, 9708, 9714, 9716, 9827	2,921	0.78
Angioimmunoblastic lymphoma	9705	368	0.10
Anaplastic large cell lymphoma	9714	1,051	0.28
Peripheral T-cell lymphoma, NOS	9675(T/NK), 9702, 9708, 9716, 9827	1,502	0.41
Adult T-cell leukemia/lymphoma	9827	146	0.04
T/NK-cell lymphoid neoplasms, NOS	9590–9591(T/NK), 9596(T/NK), 9709, 9717–9719, 9820(T/NK), 9831, 9948, 9970 (T/NK)	1,812	0.49
Lymphoblastic leukemia/lymphoma[d]	9727–9729, 9835–9837	6,591	1.67
B-cell lymphoblastic leukemia/lymphoma	9727(B), 9728, 9835(B), 9836	4,012	1.02
T-cell lymphoblastic leukemia/lymphoma	9727(T/NK), 9729, 9835(T/NK), 9837	1,001	0.25
Unknown type lymphoblastic leukemia/lymphoma	9727, 9835(unknown)	1,578	0.40
Prolymphocytic leukemia	9832–9834	281	0.08
Hodgkin lymphoma	9650–9655, 9659, 9661–9665, 9667	10,644	2.71
Unknown type lymphoid neoplasms	9590–9591(unknown), 9596(unknown), 9675(unknown), 9820(unknown), 9970(unknown)	4,971	1.36

ICD-O International classification of diseases for oncology; *NK* natural killer cell; NOS not otherwise specified; *SEER* Surveillance, Epidemiology, and End Results

[b]Codes followed by parentheses indicate that immunophenotyping data (B-cell, T/NK-cell, or unknown) were used to assign cases to that lymphoid neoplasm subtype

[c]All incidence rates are age-adjusted to the 2000 US population and expressed per 100,000 person-years

[d]Also known as acute lymphoblastic leukemia (ALL)

In general, lymphoid neoplasm incidence increases monotonically with age and is higher in males than females. This pattern is similarly reflected in total T/NK cell lymphoid neoplasms (Fig. 2.1). However, differences emerge between individual subtypes. For example, T-cell lymphoblastic leukemia has a bimodal distribution where children (<15 years) and older adults (≥65 years) have higher incidence. Mycosis fungoides/Sezary syndrome incidence begins in teenagers and T/NK cell-NOS incidence is limited to adults 45 years and above. PTCL incidence rates are higher among Black males and females and angioimmunoblastic lymphoma incidence rates are highest in Black males.

Further differences in risk patterns emerge by demographic groups. Like B-cell lymphoid neoplasms, incidence of T/NK-cell lymphoid neoplasms in all categories of race are higher in men than women (Tables 2.2 and 2.3). However, unlike B-cell lymphoid neoplasms which predominantly develop in white populations, T-cell

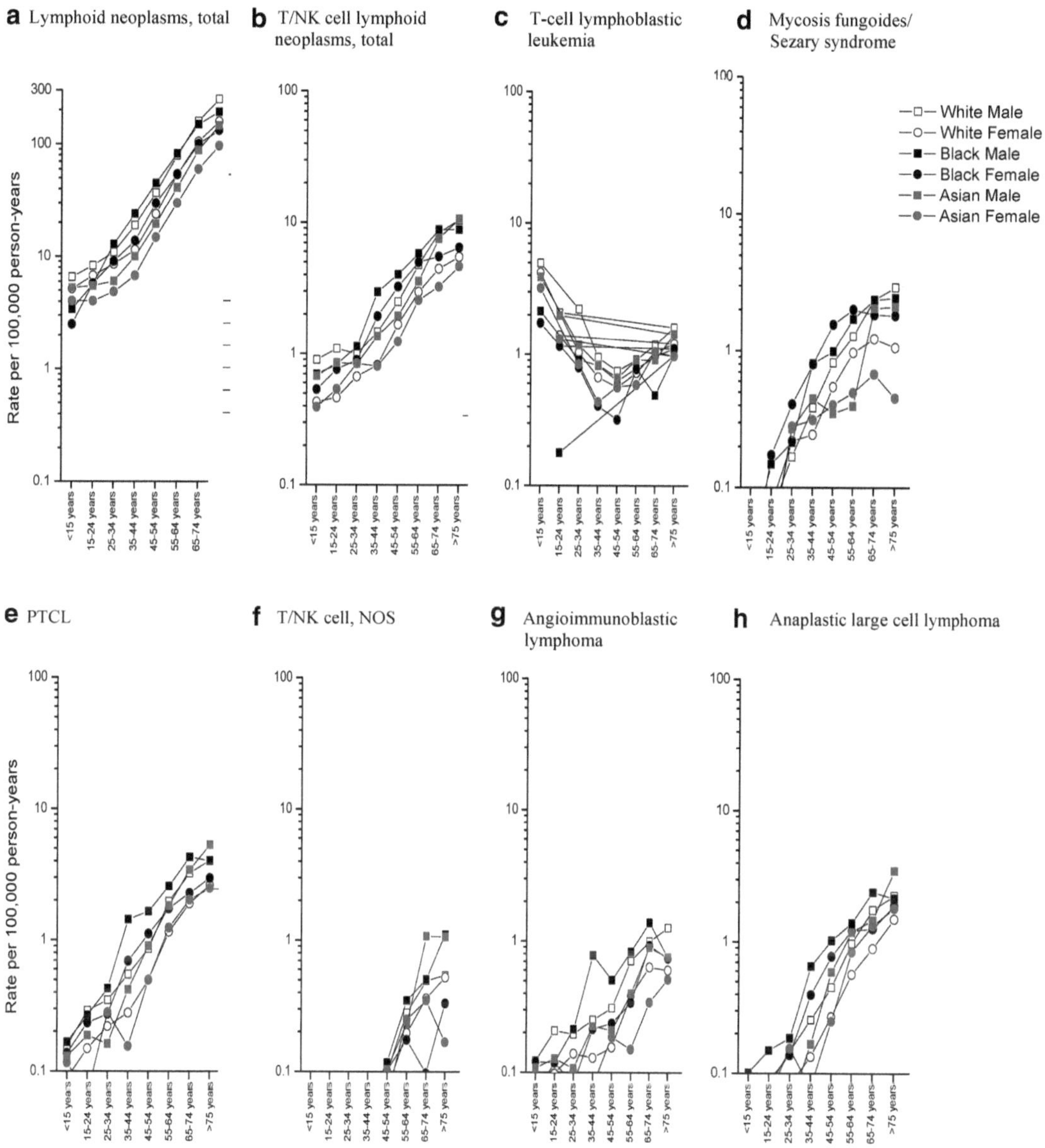

Fig. 2.1 Incidence of lymphoid neoplasms by subtype, race, sex, and age, 13 SEER registries, 1997–2006. *All incidence rates are age-adjusted to the 2000 United States population within age groups

lymphoid neoplasms appear to occur similarly in black and white populations. For the 1997–2006 time period within the US SEER cancer registry, incidence rates of T-cell lymphoid neoplasms among black men were 3.06 per 100,000, followed by white men (2.65), and Asian men (2.31) (Table 2.2). Among women, incidence rates were highest among black women (2.28) followed by white (1.49), and Asian women (1.29). This pattern is generally consistent across the T/NK-cell lymphoid neoplasm subtypes except the PTCL subtype angioimmunoblastic lymphoma where rates are higher among Asian males (0.17) than black (0.15) or white (0.11) males (Tables 2.2 and 2.3).

Incidence rates of all lymphoid neoplasms appear to have plateaued in the US (Fig. 2.2). However, while the incidence of B-cell lymphoid neoplasms has slowed particularly among white men, rates for T/NK-cell lymphoid neoplasms

Table 2.2 Incidence of lymphoid neoplasms by subtype, race, and sex, 13 SEER registries, 1997–2006

	Male								Female							
	White		Black		Asian		AI/AN		White		Black		Asian		AI/AN	
Lymphoid neoplasm subtype	No.	Rate[a]	No.	Rate[a]	No.	Rate[a]	No.	Rate[a]	No.	Rate[a]	No.	Rate[a]	No.	Rate[a]	No.	Rate[a]
Lymphoid neoplasms, total	58,204	44.64	6,072	41.96	4,449	25.16	354	18.77	47,150	29.42	5,352	28.10	3,812	17.55	333	15.93
B-cell lymphoid neoplasms, total	46,885	36.46	4,642	33.89	3,514	20.27	261	14.57	38,213	23.70	4,079	22.19	3,092	14.36	286	13.89
T/NK-cell lymphoid neoplasms, total	3,597	2.65	505	3.06	429	2.31	45	2.10	2,334	1.49	467	2.28	290	1.29	16	0.72
Mycosis fungoides/Sézary syndrome	872	0.65	120	0.77	85	0.46	8	0.45	601	0.39	170	0.83	66	0.28	2	0.07
Peripheral T-cell lymphoma	1,286	0.96	215	1.33	173	0.97	17	0.83	900	0.57	168	0.84	123	0.56	8	0.40
Angioimmunoblastic lymphoma	146	0.11	19	0.15	29	0.17	0	0.00	139	0.09	16	0.08	15	0.07	0	0.00
Anaplastic large cell lymphoma	506	0.37	81	0.46	50	0.26	10	0.49	310	0.20	52	0.26	31	0.14	4	0.17
Peripheral T-cell lymphoma, NOS	634	0.48	115	0.72	94	0.54	7	0.33	451	0.28	100	0.51	77	0.35	4	0.23
Adult T-cell leukemia/lymphoma	36	0.03	18	0.11	12	0.07	2	0.10	39	0.02	26	0.13	10	0.05	0	0.00
T/NK-cell lymphoid neoplasms, NOS	867	0.65	88	0.59	101	0.56	12	0.60	567	0.36	74	0.38	63	0.28	4	0.20
Lymphoblastic leukemia/lymphoma	3,071	2.08	242	1.02	346	1.63	43	1.22	2,327	1.58	217	0.92	274	1.27	35	1.12
B-cell lymphoblastic leukemia/lymphoma	1,828	1.23	123	0.52	206	0.97	24	0.67	1,490	1.01	105	0.45	191	0.89	25	0.76
T-cell lymphoblastic leukemia/lymphoma	527	0.35	71	0.30	68	0.31	7	0.18	236	0.16	52	0.22	35	0.15	2	0.05
Unknown type lymphoblastic leukemia/lymphoma	716	0.49	48	0.21	72	0.35	12	0.37	601	0.40	60	0.25	48	0.23	8	0.31
Prolymphocytic leukemia	148	0.12	20	0.13	6	0.03	1	0.04	88	0.05	10	0.05	5	0.02	0	0.00
Hodgkin lymphoma	4,818	3.29	586	2.95	293	1.38	20	0.85	4,035	2.68	527	2.24	254	1.07	15	0.57
Unknown type lymphoid neoplasms	2,148	1.71	287	1.82	140	0.85	16	0.89	1,942	1.14	216	1.12	128	0.60	8	0.44

AI/AN American Indian or Alaska Native; *CLL/SLL* Chronic lymphocytic leukemia/small lymphocytic lymphoma; *DLBCL* diffuse large B-cell lymphoma; *NK* natural killer cell; *NOS* not otherwise specified; *SEER* surveillance, epidemiology, and end results

[a]All incidence rates are age-adjusted to the 2000 US population and expressed per 100,000 person-years

Surveillance, epidemiology, and end results (SEER) Program (www.seer.cancer.gov) SEER*Stat Database: Incidence—SEER 13 Regs Limited-Use, Nov 2008 Sub (1992–2006) <Katrina/Rita Population Adjustment>—Linked To County Attributes—Total US, 1969–2006 Counties, National Cancer Institute, DCCPS, Surveillance Research Program, Cancer Statistics Branch, released April 2009, based on the November 2008 submission

Table 2.3 Incidence rate[a] ratios for lymphoid neoplasms by subtype, race, and sex, 13 SEER registries, 1997–2006

	Male:Female IRR			White:Black IRR		White:Asian IRR	
Lymphoid neoplasm subtype	White	Black	Asian	Males	Females	Males	Females
Lymphoid neoplasms, total	1.5	1.5	1.4	1.1	1.0	1.8	1.7
B-cell lymphoid neoplasms, total	1.5	1.5	1.4	1.1	1.1	1.8	1.6
T/NK-cell lymphoid neoplasms, total	1.8	1.3	1.8	0.9	0.7	1.1	1.2
Mycosis fungoides/Sézary syndrome	1.7	0.9	1.6	0.8	0.5	1.4	1.4
Peripheral T-cell lymphoma	1.7	1.6	1.7	0.7	0.7	1.0	1.0
Angioimmunoblastic lymphoma	1.3	1.9	2.6	0.7	1.1	0.6	1.3
Anaplastic large cell lymphoma	1.8	1.8	1.9	0.8	0.8	1.4	1.4
Peripheral T-cell lymphoma, NOS	1.7	1.4	1.5	0.7	0.6	0.9	0.8
Adult T-cell leukemia/lymphoma	1.2	0.8	1.5	0.3	0.2	0.4	0.5
T/NK-cell lymphoid neoplasms, NOS	1.8	1.6	2.0	1.1	1.0	1.2	1.3
Lymphoblastic leukemia/lymphoma	1.3	1.1	1.3	2.0	1.7	1.3	1.2
B-cell lymphoblastic leukemia/lymphoma	1.2	1.2	1.1	2.4	2.3	1.3	1.1
T-cell lymphoblastic leukemia/lymphoma	2.2	1.3	2.0	1.2	0.7	1.1	1.0
Unknown type lymphoblastic leukemia/lymphoma	1.2	0.8	1.5	2.4	1.6	1.4	1.8
Prolymphocytic leukemia	2.3	2.3	1.5	0.9	0.9	3.6	2.3
Hodgkin lymphoma	1.2	1.3	1.3	1.1	1.2	2.4	2.5
Unknown type lymphoid neoplasms	1.5	1.6	1.4	0.9	1.0	2.0	1.9

CLL/SLL Chronic lymphocytic leukemia/small lymphocytic lymphoma; *DLBCL* diffuse large B-cell lymphoma; *IRR* Incidence rate ratio; *NK* natural killer cell; *NOS* not otherwise specified; *SEER* surveillance, epidemiology, and end results

~=Calculation of the IRR was precluded by zero cases diagnosed among Asian males

Bolded IRRs were not statistically significant at $P<0.05$ (95% CI included 1.0)

95% CIs available from the author

[a]All incidence rates are age-adjusted to the 2000 US population

Surveillance, epidemiology, and end results (SEER) Program (www.seer.cancer.gov) SEER*Stat Database: Incidence—SEER 13 Regs Limited-Use, Nov 2008 Sub (1992–2006) <Katrina/Rita Population Adjustment>—Linked To County Attributes—Total US, 1969–2006 Counties, National Cancer Institute, DCCPS, Surveillance Research Program, Cancer Statistics Branch, released April 2009, based on the November 2008 submission

continue to rise for men and women of all race groups. Specifically, from 1997 to 2006, incidence rates of T/NK-cell lymphoid neoplasms in the US have risen with an annual percent change of 1.17 (Table 2.4). The annual increase in incidence was highest for Black males (2.2) and Asian females (2.3). Only among Asian males did rates appear to decline during this time period (−0.45). By subtype, rates declined for mycosis fungoides/Sezary syndrome within all race groups (Fig. 2.2 and Table 2.4). Incidence rates for PTCL increased (3.78) and strikingly so for the PTCL subtype, angioimmunoblastic lymphoma (14). Incidence also increased strikingly for PTCL-NOS (5.5) but declined for ALCL (−2.0) (Table 2.4 and Fig. 2.2). That anaplastic large cell lymphoma declined during the same period that angioimmunoblastic lymphomas increased raises some question regarding potential coding changes within the cancer registry for these two subtypes.

Incidence rates for lymphoid neoplasms also vary by geography and there are some particular differences by subtypes. For example, the human T-cell lymphotropic virus I (HTLV-1) is endemic to Japan and the Caribbean, resulting in elevated rates of ATLs in these regions. In general, the occurrence of lymphoid neoplasms is higher in developed countries. In these countries which are largely of Caucasian descent such as the US, T/NK-cell lymphoid neoplasms comprise less than 10% of all lymphoid neoplasms. There is some evidence, however, that the proportion of T-cell lymphoid neoplasms in Asian countries is higher (15–25%, excluding ATL) [1–3] and that rates of nasal type NK/T-cell lymphoma in

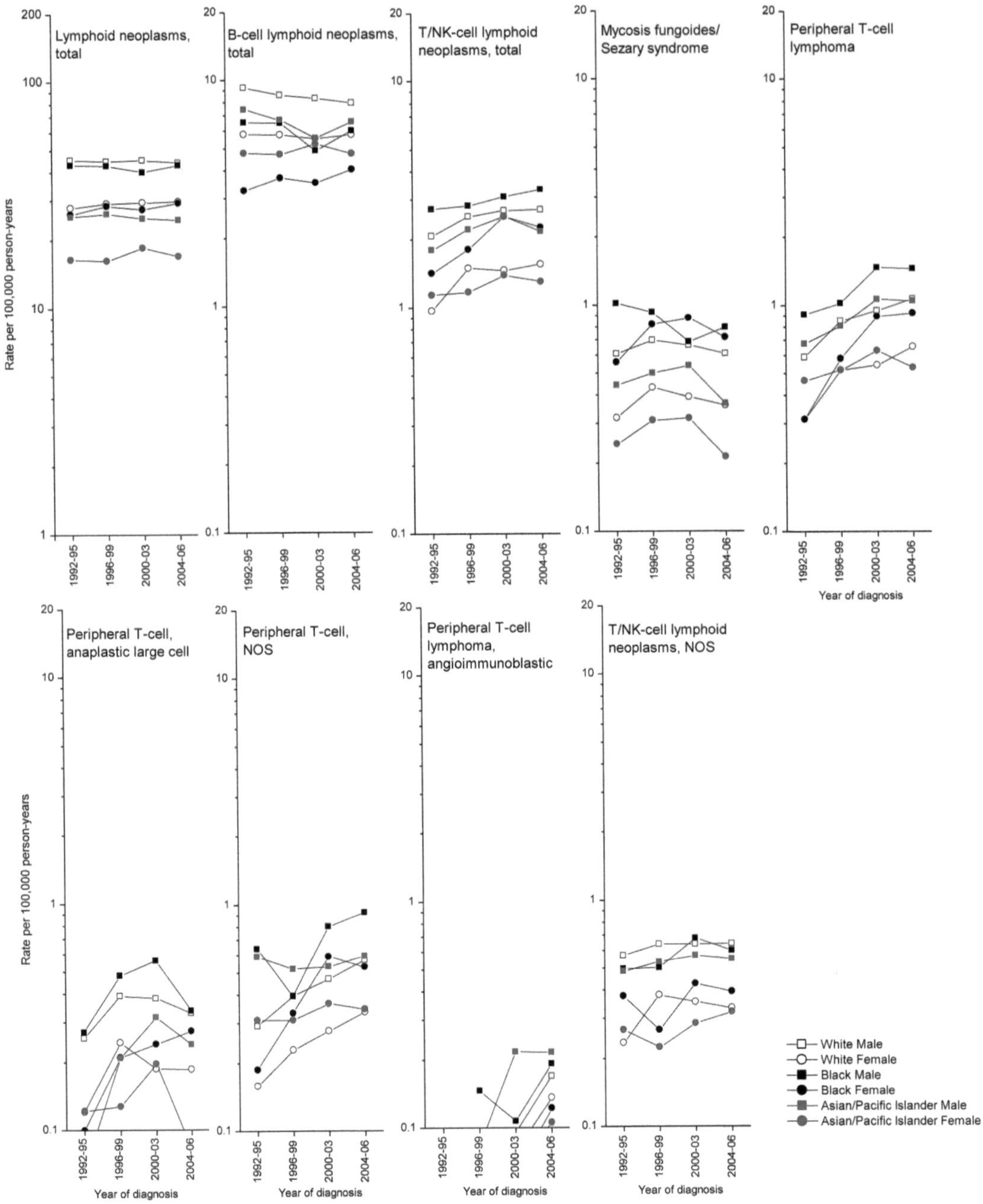

Fig. 2.2 Trends in incidence of lymphoid neoplasms by subtype, race, and sex, 13 SEER registries, 1992–1995 to 2004–2006. *All incidence rates are age-adjusted to the 2000 United States population and presented for four fixed time periods (1992–1995, 1996–1999, 2000–2003, 2004–2006). ^Presentation of trends for certain populations was precluded by at least one annual rate of zero

particular are higher in Asians than Caucasians [4]. Within the US, Asians also have varying rates; among US Asians in four SEER registries (1996–2004), incidence rates are highest among Filipino (1.1), Asian Indian/Pakistani (0.8), and Japanese (0.8) populations; rates are lower than Whites in Korean (0.6), Vietnamese (0.6), and Chinese (0.4) populations [5].

Table 2.4 Annual percent changes in lymphoid neoplasm incidence rates* by subtype, race, and sex, 13 SEER registries, 1997–2006

	Males				Females		
	Total†	White	Black	Asian	White	Black	Asian
Lymphoid neoplasms, total	−0.0427	−0.0962	0.0928	−0.7623	0.2345	0.3877	−0.0268
B-cell lymphoid neoplasms, total	0.4161	0.3813	0.3388	−0.4618	0.8241*	0.5558	−0.2574
T/NK-cell lymphoid neoplasms, total	1.1691	0.8756	2.2072	−0.4532	1.3093	0.8126	2.3118
Mycosis fungoides/Sézary syndrome	−1.9107*	−2.0273	−2.6149	−3.0275	−1.5175	−3.0766	−3.0828
Peripheral T-cell lymphoma	3.7821*	3.1657*	4.8475	3.7147	4.5589*	2.4256	−0.0645
Peripheral T—angioimmunoblastic	14.1737*	13.2487*	~	~	16.0677*	14.9347	~
Peripheral T—anaplastic large cell	−2.0075	−2.3261	−3.6173	3.5916	−1.7437	−1.1701	~
Peripheral T—NOS*	5.5460*	5.4049*	9.7284	2.0159	6.0618*	3.575	0.0936
T/NK-cell lymphoid neoplasms, NOS	−0.2212	−0.1506	2.0884	−2.0632	−1.8366	4.9163	5.956
Lymphoblastic leukemia/lymphoma	1.034	1.6265	−0.4829	−0.2968	0.1719	3.6541	3.6677
Prolymphocytic leukemia	−1.9903	−2.6652	7.7941	~	−0.0031	~	~
Hodgkin lymphoma	0.3216	−0.0205	1.899	2.9156	0.0263	2.2964	5.9063*
Unknown type lymphoid neoplasms	−8.4295*	−8.5848*	−9.4694*	−9.6691*s	−8.0173*	−6.2642	−6.6906*

CLL/SLL chronic lymphocytic leukemia/small lymphocytic lymphoma; *DLBCL* diffuse large B-cell lymphoma; *NK* natural killer cell; *NOS* not otherwise specified; *SEER* Surveillance, Epidemiology, and End Results
~ = Calculation of the annual percent change was precluded by at least one annual rate of zero
Surveillance, epidemiology, and end results (SEER) Program (www.seer.cancer.gov) SEER*Stat Database: Incidence—SEER 13 Regs Limited-Use, Nov 2008 Sub (1992–2006) <Katrina/Rita Population Adjustment>—Linked To County Attributes—Total US, 1969–2006 Counties, National Cancer Institute, DCCPS, Surveillance Research Program, Cancer Statistics Branch, released April 2009, based on the November 2008 submission

Risk Factors for T-Cell Lymphomas

Few risk factors for T-cell lymphomas are known. Although numerous studies of NHL were conducted worldwide in the last decade, the low incidence of T-cell lymphomas and the low proportion of NHLs that T-cell lymphomas comprise provided individual studies with few cases and virtually no statistical power to evaluate modest risk factors for T-cell lymphomas or its subtypes. The formation of consortia in the last decade for epidemiologic studies where case-control and/or cohort studies conduct pooled analyses to increase sample sizes to evaluate modest risk factors for tumors and their major subtypes has contributed to the understanding of NHL etiology. Specifically, the International Epidemiology Lymphoma Consortium (InterLymph) has allowed evaluation of over 10,000 NHL cases and a comparable number of controls. The numbers of T-cell lymphomas within the InterLymph Consortium now approaches a thousand. To date, a number of risk factors have been linked to NHL and some of the major NHL subtypes, including: family history of hematopoietic malignancies, medical conditions and viral infections, occupational and environmental exposures, behavioral factors such as dietary intake, and personal exposures such as use of hair dyes. These risk factors and others are summarized with regard to their potential relevance for T-cell lymphomas (Table 2.5).

Family and Personal History

A number of studies including registry databases from Sweden and Denmark [6, 7] have linked increased NHL risk among those with a first-degree relative with NHL. No individual study has had sufficient power to evaluate T-cell lymphoma risk with family history. A recent pooled analysis from the InterLymph Consortium of 10,211 NHL cases and 11,905 controls included 447 T-cell lymphoma cases. In addition to confirming a 50% increase in risk for NHL with family history of NHL, the pooled analysis

Table 2.5 Summary status of potential risk factors for T-cell lymphomas

Risk factors	Status	Risk association	Subtype specificity
Family and personal history			
Family history	Hypothesized	Increased risk	
Personal history	Hypothesized	Increased risk for NHL (numbers too small to delineate T-cell lymphomas)	
Autoimmune disorders			
Celiac disease	Established	Increased risk	Extranodal
Psoriasis	Hypothesized	Increased risk	
Immunosuppressive therapies and organ transplants	Established	Increased risk for all NHL (including T-cell lymphomas)	
Atopy			
Eczema	Hypothesized	Increased risk	
Infections			
HTLV-1	Established	Increased risk	ATLL
HIV, HCV, *Helicobacter pylori*	Hypothesized	Increased risk for NHL (numbers too small to delineate T-cell lymphomas)	
Occupational/pesticide exposures	Hypothesized	Increased risk for NHL (numbers too small to delineate T-cell lymphomas)	
Behavioral risk factors			
Smoking	Hypothesized	No association	Mycosis fungoides,
Alcohol	Hypothesized	Decreased risk	PTCL
Height/weight	Hypothesized	Increased risk for NHL (numbers too small to delineate T-cell lymphomas)	
Sun exposure	Hypothesized	Decreased risk for NHL (numbers too small to delineate T-cell lymphomas)	
Diet/hair dye use	Hypothesized	Increased risk for NHL (numbers too small to delineate T-cell lymphomas)	
Genetic susceptibility			
TNF G-308A	Hypothesized	Increased risk	Mycosis fungoides

reported increased T-cell lymphoma risks among those reporting a first-degree male relative with multiple myeloma (OR = 5.8, 95% CI = 1.5–21.4). T-cell lymphoma risk was also elevated among individuals 50 years or younger and who reported a family history of leukemia (OR = 2.3, 95% CI = 1.0–5.6), compared with individuals who were older than 50 years [8]. There was no elevation in T-cell lymphoma risk among those reporting a family history of NHL or Hodgkin lymphoma.

Based on a US childhood cancer survivor study, children with mycosis fungoides and Sezary syndrome have elevated NHL risks [9]. Risks for lymphoma (NHL standard incidence ratio = 5.08, 95% CI = 3.34–7.38) were also found elevated in a study that followed patients with mycosis fungoides and Sezary syndrome [10]. Whether these subsequent risks for NHL were more likely to be T-cell lymphomas is unclear.

Autoimmune Disorders

Autoimmune conditions are an established risk factor for NHL specific conditions implicated in NHL risk include Sjogren's syndrome, systemic lupus erythematosus, and Celiac disease [11]. Of these, it is well established that Celiac disease patients possess elevated NHL risk that is predominant for T-cell lymphomas. High risk for NHL mortality and risk has been reported in an Italian [12], US [13] and Swedish cohort studies [14], and in a Swedish registry-based study [15]. Results from the pooled InterLymph Consortium analysis of autoimmune conditions and NHL which included 766 T-cell lymphomas risk further support an association between Celiac disease and extranodal T-cell lymphoma (OR = 6.21, 95% CI = 2.82–13.6) [16]. The study also implicates psoriasis with increased T-cell lymphoma risk (OR = 1.63, 95% CI = 1.03–2.57).

Primary Immunodeficiencies and Organ Transplants

Individuals who are recipients of organ transplants and immunosuppressive therapy also have elevated NHL risks. Although B-cell lymphomas are more common, T-cell lymphomas also develop post-transplantation.

Atopy

Atopic conditions such as asthma, allergies and eczema are hypothesized to induce mild immune deficiencies that would prefer a Th2 immune response and result in decreased NHL risk. Contrary to this hypothesis, a recent pooled analysis of various atopic conditions within the InterLymph Consortium did not report an association with asthma and allergy but did observe increased risk for T-cell lymphoma among those who reported having eczema (OR = 1.92, 95% CI = 1.43–2.58). Further data from cohort studies are needed to confirm these associations in analyses not potentially biased by disease status [17].

Infections

A number of infectious agents are linked to NHL etiology, either by directly causing lymphomagenesis or providing a cellular milieu that depresses immune function or induces chronic inflammation. The association between HTLV-1 and ATL is well established and HTLV-1 was the first retrovirus established as causal for lymphoma [18, 19]. In southern Japan and the Caribbean, HTLV-1 infection is endemic and is attributable to 56 and 78% of ATL cases, respectively [19]. Further increased ATL risks are reported among those infected with both HTLV-1 and the gastrointestinal parasite also endemic in the same regions, Strongyloides stercoralis [20]. Other infections associated with NHL include the human immunodeficiency virus, hepatitis C virus, and *Helicobacter pylori*, but none affect T-cell lymphomas preferentially.

Occupational Exposures

Occupations linked with elevated NHL risks include: farmers, livestock workers, printers, teachers, wood workers, dry cleaners, barbers, and hairdressers [21, 22]. NHL is one of the malignancies caused by exposure to non-arsenical insecticides; tetrachloroethylene and trichloroethylene; benzene, 2,3,7,8-Tetrachlorodibenzo-*para*-dioxin; and 1,3-Butadiene [23]. Persistent organochlorine exposure including polychlorinated biphenyls, dioxins, furans [24], and pesticide exposure such as DDE [25] and alpha-chlordane [26] have also been associated with increased NHL risk. At present, no preferential risk for T-cell lymphomas has been reported.

Behavioral Risk Factors

Unlike most other cancers, smoking does not appear to be a strong risk factor for developing NHL. By subtypes, however, a pooled analysis from nine case-control studies within the InterLymph Consortium of 6,594 cases reported elevated risks for follicular lymphoma among smokers but not other subtypes [27]. Null associations were reported for T-cell lymphoma and its subtypes, mycosis fungoides, and PTCL. Similar results were reported in a pooled analysis of six European case-control studies of 1,742 cases [28].

Reduced NHL risks have been reported with alcohol consumption. A large pooled analysis of nine case-control studies reported risks of 0.73 for current drinkers [29] and are also supported by cohort studies [30–32]. No differential effect of the association was observed by subtype;

among T-cell lymphomas, decreased risks were observed for mycosis fungoides and PTCL.

Taller individuals and excess weight are also implicated in NHL risk though no preference for T-cell lymphomas has been demonstrated [33]. No preference for T-cell lymphomas has also been demonstrated for sunlight exposure, which is implicated in reducing NHL risk [34]. Other hypothesized NHL risk factors include dietary intake and hair dye use, but to date no associations with T-cell lymphomas have been shown [35].

Genetic Susceptibility

The most consistently demonstrated genetic variants associated with NHL risk are a polymorphism in the promoter region of the tumor necrosis factor (*TNF*) gene (–308G->A) and the interleukin 10 –3575T->A polymorphism, both of which are preferentially associated with DLBCL [36]. Analyses of all NHL subtypes within the InterLymph Consortium for these genetic variants comprising approximately 6,500 NHL cases and 6,700 controls and included over 300 T-cell lymphomas found no association with either proinflammatory cytokine with overall T-cell lymphoma risk. However, increased risk for mycosis fungoides was reported with the *TNF* G-308A variant allele (OR for AG/AA compared to GG genotype = 1.53, 95% CI = 1.02, 2.28; p-trend = 0.03 for each additional variant allele), albeit with just over 100 cases [37]. No other genetic variants have been implicated specifically for T-cell lymphoma risk or that of its subtypes.

Future Directions in Epidemiologic Research

The majority of T-cell lymphomas remain unexplained. As our understanding of NHL epidemiology has moved from studying NHL as a single entity to evaluating individual NHL subtypes with the recognition that the descriptive epidemiology of NHL subtypes are distinct, a similar approach for understanding T-cell lymphomas is clearly needed. To date, most epidemiologic studies have combined the heterogeneous T-cell lymphoma subtypes into a single entity to increase sample size and power for association studies. However, not only do T-cell lymphoma subtypes have differential treatment, survival and prognosis, but their distinct descriptive epidemiology clearly suggest differences in their etiology and thus also require evaluation as individual entities.

Based on descriptive epidemiology, we know that there are striking differences between T-cell lymphoma subtypes, by age, over time and by race/ethnicity. Based on epidemiologic research and consortia-based pooling efforts of NHL to date, potential risk factors for T-cell lymphoma and some subtypes include Celiac disease for extranodal T-cell lymphomas and a genetic variant in *TNF* for mycosis fungoides. Risk factors that are inversely associated with T-cell lymphomas include alcohol consumption and exposure to sunlight. Although a growing number of viral and bacterial infections are associated with NHL, their specific role in T-cell lymphomas remains unclear, with the exception of HTLV-1 and acute T-cell leukemia/lymphoma (ATLL). Translating clues from case reports to epidemiologic associations will also remain an important avenue of research, such as research on the reported links between breast implants and ALCLs of the breast. Research in understanding the role of genetic variants in T-cell lymphoma etiology is still in its infancy as most studies have been underpowered to adequately evaluate genetic associations. We thus encourage the inclusion of T-cell lymphomas from consortial efforts in ongoing genome-wide association studies to further our understanding of genes and pathways that may play important roles in T-cell lymphoma etiology.

Risk factors for T-cell lymphomas identified from case-control studies will require further confirmation from cohort studies where survival bias is minimized. For some exposures, cohort studies will be needed to establish temporality, particularly where prediagnostic specimens are optimal for evaluation. For example, some biomarker-based exposures such as persistent organochlorine exposure that can be measured in serial prediagnostic serum are optimally measured prospectively. Combining data from epidemiologic case-control and cohort studies with large clinical series may also prove fruitful for overcoming the rarity of the tumor for identifying additional T-cell lymphoma risk factors. In addition, the ability to incorporate detailed clinical data to epidemiologic analyses may further our understanding of T-cell lymphoma etiology. Within clinical case series, case–case comparisons may also be beneficial for identifying similar or distinct etiologies across subtypes. Finally, continued attention to striking individual case reports will be instrumental for generating new hypotheses and providing new clues with regard to the etiology of T-cell lymphomas and their subtypes.

Prognosis of T-Cell Lymphoma

Peripheral T-Cell Lymphoma-Not Otherwise Specified

This is the most common type of peripheral T-cell NHL and is a heterogeneous mix of different types of PTCL. PTCL-NOS is the "diffuse large cell" equivalent of B-cell NHL. There are two morphologic variants recognized, the T-zone lymphoma variant and the lymphoepithelioid cell variant. Patients with PTCL-NOS have predominantly nodal lymphoma that presents in adults (median age 61 years), with a male: female ratio of 1.5:1.0 [38]. Patients typically have advanced stage disease with 60% having stage IV disease and many patients having unfavorable characteristics such as B-symptoms, elevated lactic dehydrogenase (LDH), bulky disease, poor performance status, and extranodal disease so that >50% of patients fall into the unfavorable International Prognostic Index (IPI) category 3–5 [37]. Another prognostic model for PTCL-NOS has been utilized by Gallamini et al. [39] which uses the characteristics of age >60, LDH>normal, performance status≥2, and bone marrow involvement to predict outcome and was found to be more discriminatory that the standard IPI for this group of patients.

Angioimmunoblastic Lymphoma

Angioimmunoblastic T-cell lymphoma (AITL), previously known as angioimmunoblastic lymphadenopathy with dysproteinemia, was the second most common PTCL in the International T-Cell Lymphoma Classification Project [40]. This type accounts for 18.5% of the PTCL's. The median age at diagnosis is 64 years, with a male predominance and the majority of patients present with advanced stage disease. Other features include a high percentage of patients with B-symptoms, skin rash, effusions, hypergammaglobulinemia, and other immunologic or rheumatologic abnormalities [41]. The prognosis of AITL is similar to PTCL-NOS with only about 10% of patients alive 10 years after their diagnosis (Fig. 2.3) [40].

Anaplastic Large Cell Lymphoma (Primary Systemic Type)

ALCL, primary systemic type accounts for 2–3% of all NHLs [1] and 10.2% of all T/NK-cell lymphomas [40]. This NHL is usually nodal, although extranodal sites can certainly be involved as well. There are two major subtypes of systemic ALCL, anaplastic lymphoma kinase (ALK)-positive and ALK-negative. ALK-positive systemic ALCL is typically diagnosed in younger patients (median age 34 years, with a male predominance) and ALK-negative in older ones (median age 58 years), although this is not an exclusive cutoff [40]. The ALK status of patients with systemic ALCL is very important as patients with ALK-positive ALCL have a 5-year OS of 70% compared to a 5-year OS of 49% for ALK-negative ALCL [40]. The chromosomal translocation t(2;5)(p23;q35) is associated with this type of lymphoma and results in the fusion protein NPM–ALK [42] (Fig. 2.3).

ALCL, Primary Cutaneous

This is a rare type of NK/T-cell lymphoma, occurring in 1.7% of the T-cell lymphomas [40]. It typically presents in one or more areas in the skin, often in the same region of the body. It is most frequently ALK-negative, but has in general a fairly good prognosis with 5-year OS of 90% and 5-year progression-free survival of 55% [40]. This pattern indicates an indolent type of lymphoma with relapses and the ability to treat the patient repeatedly with either chemotherapy and/or radiotherapy.

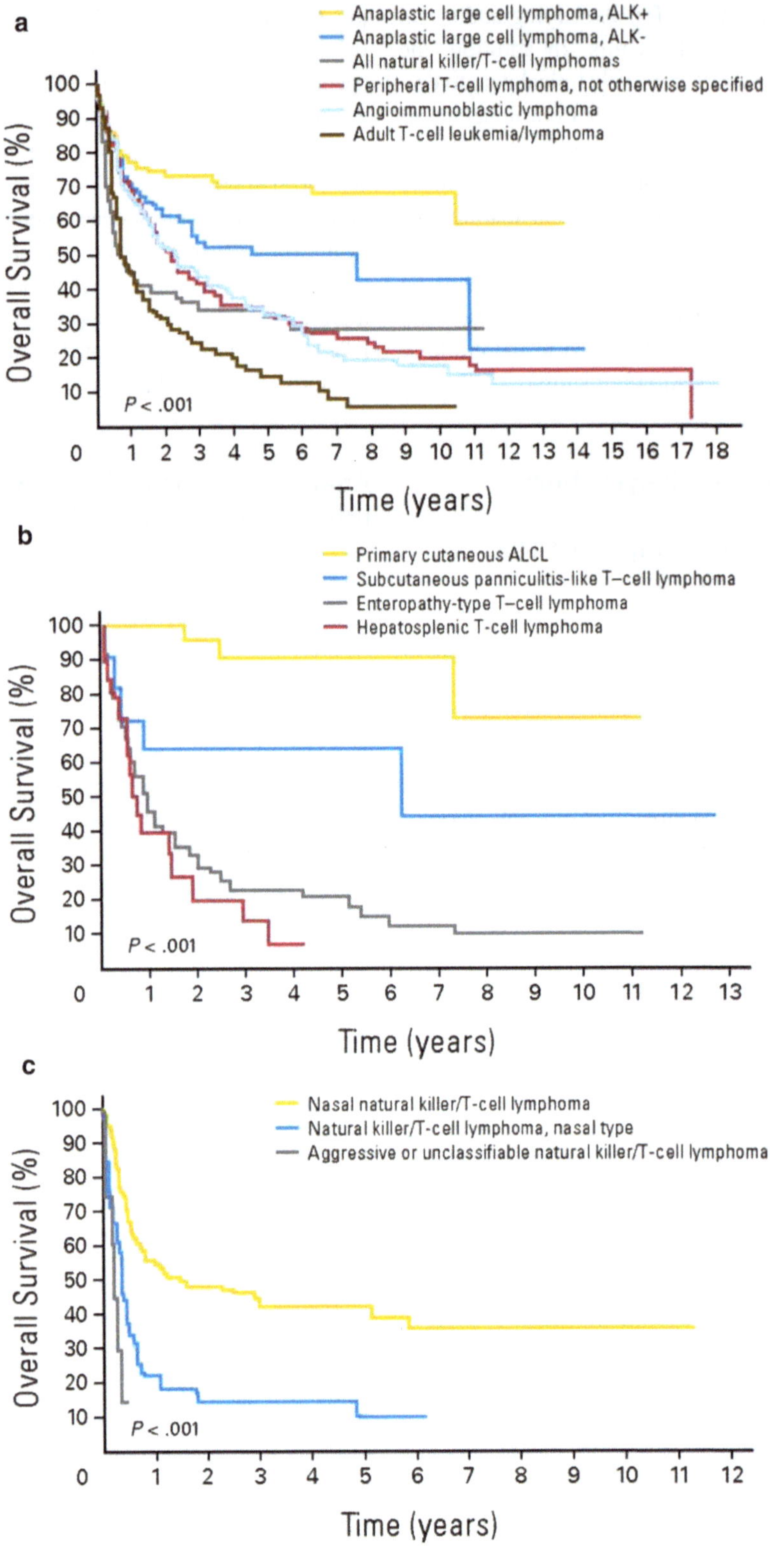

Fig. 2.3 Overall survival of various subtypes of PTCL (Reprinted from Vose et al. [40], With permission from American Society of Clinical Oncology)

Extranodal NK/T-Cell Lymphoma, Nasal and Extranasal (Nasal Type)

These lymphomas were previously called angiocentric lymphomas and are found mostly in Asia, South, and Central America [43]. Nasal NK/T-cell lymphoma is typically seen in the nasal and paranasal sinus areas and is associated with EBV infection [44]. These patients often have localized stage I/II disease but an aggressive clinical course. Patients with extranasal NK/T-cell lymphoma (nasal type) typically present with other extranodal sites of disease (skin, respiratory tract, gastrointestinal, and genitourinary). The 5-year OS with this type of lymphoma is 42% from the International T-cell Study [40] (Fig. 2.3).

Acute T-Cell Leukemia/Lymphoma

ATLL has four subtypes based on clinicopathologic features and prognosis: acute, lymphoma, chronic, and smoldering. Patients with the acute type present with Hypercalcemia, leukemic manifestations, bone and tumor lesions and have a very poor prognosis with a median survival time of 6 months [45]. Patients with the lymphomatous type typically have nodal, hepatosplenic, bone, and gastrointestinal involvement and a median survival of 10 months. Patients with the chronic and smoldering type have a more indolent course. The retrovirus HTLV-1 is critical to the development of ATLL [46]. In endemic areas such as southern Japan, up to 40% of the population is infected with the virus. However, ATLL develops in only 2–3% of the patients who are carriers of the HTLV-1 virus.

Other rare subtypes of PTCL such as hepatosplenic T-cell lymphoma, enteropathy type T-cell lymphoma, and subcutaneous panniculitis type T-cell lymphoma (gamma-delta subtype) have a very poor prognosis with standard therapy.

Summary

Despite the overall decline observed for non-Hodgkin lymphoma incidence, the incidence of T-cell lymphomas continues to rise. The distinct incidence patterns by T-cell lymphoma subtypes suggests that risk factors may also be specific to each T-cell lymphoma subtype as reflected in two of the established risk factors (e.g., celiac disease and extranodal T-cell lymphomas; HTLV-1 and ATLL). This is consistent with the distinct clinical characteristics and prognosis that is observed for each T-cell lymphoma subtype. A predominance of some T-cell lymphoma subtypes by geographic locale (e.g., ATLL and extranodal NK/T-cell lymphoma) further supports the hypothesis of distinct etiologies and need for treatment by subtype. The rarity of T-cell lymphomas has historically posed challenges for furthering our understanding of these tumors. However, we expect important clues to emerge as on-going large international consortium efforts aim to accrue sufficient sample sizes of T-cell lymphomas and its subtypes for both etiological and prognostic studies.

Acknowledgements We thank J. Daniel Carreon for guidance on descriptive statistics and graphical presentation.

References

1. Au WY, Lo J. HTLV-1-related lymphoma in Hong Kong Chinese. Am J Hematol. 2005;78:80–1.
2. Naresh KN, Srinivas V, Soman CS. Distribution of various subtypes of non-Hodgkin's lymphoma in India: a study of 2773 lymphomas using R.E.A.L. and WHO Classifications. Ann Oncol. 2000;11:63–7.
3. Ng CS, Chan J, Lo S, Poon Y. Immunophenotypic analysis of non-Hodgkin's lymphomas in Chinese. A study of 75 cases in Hong Kong. Pathology. 1986; 18:419–25.
4. Kadin ME, Berard CW, Nanba K, Wakasa H. Lymphoproliferative diseases in Japan and Western countries: Proceedings of the United States—Japan Seminar, September 6 and 7, 1982, in Seattle, Washington. Hum Pathol. 1983;14:745–72.
5. Carreon JD, Morton LM, Devesa SS, Clarke CA, Gomez SL, Glaser SL, et al. Incidence of lymphoid neoplasms by subtype among six Asian ethnic groups in the United States, 1996–2004. Cancer Causes Control. 2008;19:1171–81.
6. Goldin LR, Landgren O, McMaster ML, Gridley G, Hemminki K, Li X, et al. Familial aggregation and heterogeneity of non-Hodgkin lymphoma in population-based samples. Cancer Epidemiol Biomarkers Prev. 2005;14:2402–6.
7. Goldgar DE, Easton DF, Cannon-Albright LA, Skolnick MH. Systematic population-based assessment

of cancer risk in first-degree relatives of cancer probands. J Natl Cancer Inst. 1994;86:1600–8.
8. Wang SS, Slager SL, Brennan P, Holly EA, De SS, Bernstein L, et al. Family history of hematopoietic malignancies and risk of non-Hodgkin lymphoma (NHL): a pooled analysis of 10 211 cases and 11 905 controls from the International Lymphoma Epidemiology Consortium (InterLymph). Blood. 2007;109:3479–88.
9. Friedman DL, Kadan-Lottick NS, Whitton J, Mertens AC, Yasui Y, Liu Y, et al. Increased risk of cancer among siblings of long-term childhood cancer survivors: a report from the childhood cancer survivor study. Cancer Epidemiol Biomarkers Prev. 2005;14:1922–7.
10. Huang KP, Weinstock MA, Clarke CA, McMillan A, Hoppe RT, Kim YH. Second lymphomas and other malignant neoplasms in patients with mycosis fungoides and Sezary syndrome: evidence from population-based and clinical cohorts. Arch Dermatol. 2007;143:45–50.
11. Ehrenfeld M, Abu-Shakra M, Buskila D, Shoenfeld Y. The dual association between lymphoma and autoimmunity. Blood Cells Mol Dis. 2001;27:750–6.
12. Corrao G, Corazza GR, Bagnardi V, Brusco G, Ciacci C, Cottone M, et al. Mortality in patients with coeliac disease and their relatives: a cohort study. Lancet. 2001;358:356–61.
13. Green PH, Fleischauer AT, Bhagat G, Goyal R, Jabri B, Neugut AI. Risk of malignancy in patients with celiac disease. Am J Med. 2003;115:191–5.
14. Peters U, Askling J, Gridley G, Ekbom A, Linet M. Causes of death in patients with celiac disease in a population-based Swedish cohort. Arch Intern Med. 2003;163:1566–72.
15. Askling J, Linet M, Gridley G, Halstensen TS, Ekstrom K, Ekbom A. Cancer incidence in a population-based cohort of individuals hospitalized with celiac disease or dermatitis herpetiformis. Gastroenterology. 2002;123:1428–35.
16. Ekstrom SK, Vajdic CM, Falster M, Engels EA, Martinez-Maza O, Turner J, et al. Autoimmune disorders and risk of non-Hodgkin lymphoma subtypes: a pooled analysis within the InterLymph Consortium. Blood. 2008;111:4029–38.
17. Vajdic CM, Falster MO, de Sanjose S, Martinez-Maza O, Becker N, Bracci PM, et al. Atopic disease and risk of non-Hodgkin lymphoma: an InterLymph pooled analysis. Cancer Res. 2009;69:6482–9.
18. Mueller N. Overview of the epidemiology of malignancy in immune deficiency. J Acquir Immune Defic Syndr. 1999;21:S5–10.
19. Manns A, Cleghorn FR, Falk RT, Hanchard B, Jaffe ES, Bartholomew C, et al. Role of HTLV-I in development of non-Hodgkin lymphoma in Jamaica and Trinidad and Tobago. The HTLV Lymphoma Study Group. Lancet. 1993;342:1447–50.
20. Mortreux F, Gabet AS, Wattel E. Molecular and cellular aspects of HTLV-1 associated leukemogenesis in vivo. Leukemia. 2003;17:26–38.
21. Siemiatycki J, Richardson L, Boffetta P. Occupation. In: Schottenfeld D, Fraumeni JF, editors. Cancer Epidemiology and Prevention. New York: Oxford University Press; 2006. p. 322–54.
22. Boffetta P, de Vocht F. Occupation and the risk of non-Hodgkin lymphoma. Cancer Epidemiol Biomarkers Prev. 2007;16:369–72.
23. International Agency for Research on Cancer. IARC Monographs on the evaluation of carcinogenic risks to humans: Dry cleaning, some chlorinated solvents and other industrial chemicals. Lyon, France: International Agency for Research on Cancer;1995.
24. Engel LS, Lan Q, Rothman N. Polychlorinated biphenyls and non-Hodgkin lymphoma. Cancer Epidemiol Biomarkers Prev. 2007;16:373–6.
25. Colt JS, Severson RK, Lubin J, Rothman N, Camann D, Davis S, et al. Organochlorines in carpet dust and non-Hodgkin lymphoma. Epidemiology. 2005;16:516–25.
26. Colt JS, Davis S, Severson RK, Lynch CF, Cozen W, Camann D, et al. Residential insecticide use and risk of non-Hodgkin's lymphoma. Cancer Epidemiol Biomarkers Prev. 2006;15:251–7.
27. Morton LM, Hartge P, Holford TR, Holly EA, Chiu BC, Vineis P, et al. Cigarette smoking and risk of non-Hodgkin lymphoma: a pooled analysis from the International Lymphoma Epidemiology Consortium (interlymph). Cancer Epidemiol Biomarkers Prev. 2005;14:925–33.
28. Besson H, Brennan P, Becker N, Nieters A, De SS, Font R, et al. Tobacco smoking, alcohol drinking and non-Hodgkin's lymphoma: European multicenter casecontrol study (Epilymph). Int J Cancer. 2006;119:901–8.
29. Morton LM, Zheng T, Holford TR, Holly EA, Chiu BC, Costantini AS, et al. Alcohol consumption and risk of non-Hodgkin lymphoma: a pooled analysis. Lancet Oncol. 2005;6:469–76.
30. Gaziano JM, Gaziano TA, Glynn RJ, Sesso HD, Ajani UA, Stampfer MJ, et al. Light-to-moderate alcohol consumption and mortality in the Physicians' Health Study enrollment cohort. J Am Coll Cardiol. 2000;35:96–105.
31. Chiu BC, Cerhan JR, Gapstur SM, Sellers TA, Zheng W, Lutz CT, et al. Alcohol consumption and non-Hodgkin lymphoma in a cohort of older women. Br J Cancer. 1999;80:1476–82.
32. Lim U, Morton LM, Subar AF, Baris D, Stolzenberg-Solomon R, Leitzmann M, et al. Alcohol, smoking, and body size in relation to incident Hodgkin's and non-Hodgkin's lymphoma risk. Am J Epidemiol. 2007;166:697–708.
33. Willett EV, Morton LM, Hartge P, Becker N, Bernstein L, Boffetta P, et al. Non-Hodgkin lymphoma and obesity: a pooled analysis from the InterLymph Consortium. Int J Cancer. 2008;122:2062–70.
34. Kricker A, Armstrong BK, Hughes AM, Goumas C, Smedby KE, Zheng T, et al. Personal sun exposure and risk of non Hodgkin lymphoma: a pooled analysis from the Interlymph Consortium. Int J Cancer 2008;122:144–54.

35. Zhang Y, Sanjose SD, Bracci PM, Morton LM, Wang R, Brennan P, et al. Personal use of hair dye and the risk of certain subtypes of non-Hodgkin lymphoma. Am J Epidemiol. 2008;167:1321–31.
36. Rothman N, Skibola CF, Wang SS, Morgan G, Lan Q, Smith MT, et al. Genetic variation in TNF and IL10 and risk of non-Hodgkin lymphoma: a report from the InterLymph Consortium. Lancet Oncol. 2006; 7:27–38.
37. Skibola CF, Bracci PM, Nieters A, Brooks-Wilson A, de Sanjosé S, Hughes AM, et al. Tumor necrosis factor (TNF) and lymphotoxin-alpha (LTA) polymorphisms and risk of non-Hodgkin lymphoma in the InterLymph Consortium. Am J Epidemiol. 2010;71(3):267–76.
38. Rudiger T, Weisenburger DD, Anderson JR, et al. Peripheral T-cell lymphoma (excluding anaplastic large-cell lymphoma): results from the Non-Hodgkin's Lymphoma Classification Project. Ann Oncol. 2002;13:140–9.
39. Gallamini A, Stelitano C, Calvi R, et al. Peripheral T-cell lymphoma unspecified (PTCL-U): a new prognostic model from a retrospective multicenter clinical study. Blood. 2004;103:2474–9.
40. Vose JM, Armitage JO, Weisenburger DD. International peripheral T-cell lymphoma study: pathology findings and clinical outcomes. J Clin Oncol. 2008;26:4124–30.
41. Siegert W, Nerl C, Agthe A, et al. Angioimmunoblastic lymphadenopathy (AILD)-type T-cell lymphoma: prognostic impact of clinical observations and laboratory findings at presentation: the Kiel Lymphoma Study Group. Ann Oncol. 1995;6:659–64.
42. Weisenburger DD, Gordon BG, Vose JM, et al. Occurrence of the t(2;5)(p23p35) in non-Hodgkin's lymphoma. Blood. 1996;87:3860–8.
43. Jaffe ES, Chan JK, Su IJ, et al. Report of the Workshop on Nasal and Related Extranodal Angiocentric T/Natural Killer Cell Lymphomas: definitions, differential diagnosis, and epidemiology. Am J Surg Pathol. 1996;20:103–11.
44. Cheung MM, Chan JK, Lau WH, et al. Primary non-Hodgkin's lymphoma of the nose and nasopharynx: clinical features, tumor immunphenotype, and treatment outcome of 113 patients. J Clin Oncol. 1998; 16:70–7.
45. Shimoyama M. Diagnostic criteria and classification of clinical subtypes of adult T-cell leukaemia-lymphoma: a report from the Lymphoma Study Group (1984–1987). Br J Haematol. 1991;79:428–37.
46. Chen YC, Wang CH, Su IJ, et al. Infection of human T-cell leukemia virus type I and development of human T-cell leukemia lymphoma in patients with hematologic neoplasms: a possible linkage to blood transfusion. Blood. 1989;74:388–94.

Molecular Profiling and Prognosis in T-Cell Lymphomas

3

Pier Paolo Piccaluga and Stefano Aldo Pileri

Background

In 1994, the Revised European–American Lymphoma (REAL) Classification introduced new standards in the lymphoma field [1]. In particular, it stated for the first time that a classification of lymphoid tumors should consist in a list of "real" entities, each defined by the amalgamation of cell morphology, phenotype, molecular genetics, clinical data, and identification of a normal counterpart, if possible [1]. After a validation trial [2], the REAL Classification was adopted by the World Health Organization (WHO) as guideline for lymphoma diagnosis and therapy [3]. On such occasion, its methodology was extended to all tumors of the haematopoietic system [3]. According to patients' survival without any treatment, non-Hodgkin lymphomas (NHLs) are classified as indolent (survival measurable in years) and aggressive (survival measurable in months).

Peripheral T-cell lymphomas (PTCLs) belong to the aggressive lymphoma group [4]. They represent approximately 12% of all lymphoid neoplasms [4, 5]. Their incidence varies in different countries and races, being higher in HTLV-1 endemic areas (Asia, Caribbean basin, and some parts of the United States) [4, 5]. PTCLs are a heterogeneous group of tumors that can be roughly subdivided into specified and not otherwise specified (NOS) forms [5, 6]. In particular, the latter—corresponding to about 35% of T-cell lymphomas—cannot be further classified on the basis of morphology, phenotype, and conventional molecular studies [4]. Usually, they occur in the fifth–sixth decade of life, without sex predilection [7–10]. Although PTCLs/NOS can present as isolated disease, they more often have a widespread dissemination (stage III–IV) with nodal, skin, liver, spleen, bone-marrow, and peripheral blood involvement [7–10]. B-symptoms are recorded in about 45% of cases at diagnosis. A haemophagocytic syndrome may also be encountered [7–10].

The tumor morphology is highly variable, comprising cells of different size and shape [4]. PTCLs/NOS may contain prominent reactive components, including small lymphocytes, eosinophils, plasma cells, histiocytes, and epithelioid elements [4].

Immunohistochemistry does generally show T-cell associated molecule expression, although the phenotypic profile is aberrant in about 80% of cases [11].

Clonal rearrangements of T-cell receptor encoding genes are generally detected [12]. The karyotype is aberrant in more than 80% of cases and often characterized by complex abnormalities. However, specific alterations have not been identified [13]. Recently, some recurrent lesions have been documented by comparative genomic hybridization and SNPs analysis [14, 15].

P.P. Piccaluga • S.A. Pileri (✉)
Haematopathology Section, Department of Hematology and Oncological Sciences "L. and A. Seràgnoli", S. Orsola-Malpighi Hospital, Pavillon 8, Via Massarenti 9, 40138 Bologna, Italy
e-mail: stefano.pileri@unibo.it

F. Foss (ed.), *T-Cell Lymphomas*, Contemporary Hematology,
DOI 10.1007/978-1-62703-170-7_3, © Springer Science+Business Media New York 2013

On clinical grounds, PTCLs/NOS are among the most aggressive NHLs. In the majority of cases, the response to conventional chemotherapy is indeed frustrating, with relapse free and overall survival (OS) rates at 5 years below 30% [5].

Besides the PTCL/NOS category, histological classification remains anyway a basic prognostic indicator in the PTCL setting [5, 6, 8, 16]. First, nodal and extranodal entities are clinically well distinct, as extranodal tumors, and specially the cutaneous forms, often display a relatively good outcome [5]. In addition, among nodal PTCLs, the distinction between anaplastic large cell lymphoma (ALCL) and other entities as well as the distinction of ALK$^+$ and ALK$^-$ cases among ALCLs retain a significant prognostic impact [5, 6, 8, 16]. In fact, ALK$^+$ ALCL, particularly when occurring in children and young adults, have a significantly better clinical outcome if compared with all other forms [5, 6]. Importantly, it was recently suggested to include ALK$^-$ ALCL within the PTCLs/NOS basing on the lack of evidences of clear biological differences between them. However, new clinical and molecular findings demonstrated that ALK$^-$ ALCL and PTCL/NOS are distinct entities, also presenting with different clinical outcome [6, 17, 18].

In addition to the basic distinction of the different entities, in that last years several attempts have been made in order to further characterize the molecular pathology of PTCLs and identify reliable prognostic indicators to be offered to clinicians. Indeed, novel insights have been provided by gene expression profile (GEP) studies, specially as far as tumor histogenesis, molecular pathogenesis, and possibly new targeted therapies are concerned. On the other hand, novel and more refined prognostic scores have been proposed, which will be also discussed in this chapter.

Gene Expression Profiling of Peripheral T-Cell Pymphoma

The pathobiology of PTCLs has been neglected for a long time. The main reasons for that probably relied on the relative rarity of the disease, as well as the extreme difficulty to culture these neoplastic cells ex vivo. However, in the last few years, a new interest on PTCLs did emerge. Specially, these lymphomas have been then the object of different studies based on the application of high throughput technologies and several reports dealt with the GEP of the different subtypes [17–32] (Table 3.1). In particular, on one hand, some authors focused on specific topics: that is, the GEP of mycosis fungoides, ALK$^+$ and ALK$^-$ ALCLs, angioimmunoblastic lymphomas (AITL), γδ-T-cell lymphomas, adult T-cell lymphoma/leukemia (ATLL), and extranodal NK/T lymphoma nasal-type, respectively [19, 25, 26, 28–31]. On the other hand, others analyzed larger collections of PTCLs of the NOS, AITL, and ALCL types [17, 18, 20, 23, 24, 32]. However, some of these studies suffer of limitations that vary from the usage of chips with a restricted number of genes [20, 23, 24] to the lack of a reliable normal counterpart for comparison [20, 24]. Specifically, Martinez-Delgado et al. reported that PTCL/NOS corresponds to a heterogeneous group of tumors, whose GEP is difficult to interpret due to the significant amount of infiltrating reactive cells. According to these authors, the only clinically relevant information provided by GEP pertains the expression level of genes belonging to the NFκB pathway (see below) [20]. Ballester et al. [23] found that the GEP could discriminate among PTCLs of the NOS, AITL, and ALCL types, although the former did not share a single profile. Using a multi-class predictor, the authors separated their cases into three molecular subgroups called U1, U2, and U3. The U1 gene expression signature included genes known to be associated with poor outcome in other tumors, such as *CCND2*. The U2 subgroup was associated with over-expression of genes involved in T-cell activation, including *NFKB1* and *BCL2*. The third group was mainly defined by the over-expression of genes involved in the IFN/JAK/STAT pathway and comprised most histiocyte-rich tumors. This finding suggests that the signatures recorded by Ballester et al. might be at least in part influenced by reactive components. Nevertheless, at present, it is not defined yet whether the presence of specific reactive components may significantly affect the tumor behavior

Table 3.1 Summary of the main gene expression profile studies dealing with peripheral T-cell lymphomas

Reference	Disease(s) explored	Comments
Tracey et al. [19]	MF	The manuscript explored GEP of MF and showed concurrent deregulation of multiple genes involved in the TNF signaling pathway
Martinez-Delgado et al. [20]	PTCL/NOS	The authors found significant differences between the peripheral and lymphoblastic T-cell lymphomas, which include a deregulation of nuclear factor-κB signaling pathway
Martinez-Delgado et al. [21]	PTCL/NOS	The Authors found two different subgroups of PTCL based on the expression of NFκB-related genes. One-third of PTCL showed clearly reduced expression of NFκB genes, while the other group was characterized by high expression of these genes. Of interest, the expression profile associated to reduced expression of NFκB genes was significantly associated with shorter survival of patients
Ballester et al. [23]	PTCL/NOS, AILT, ALCL	According to this study, PTCL/NOS could be divided into three molecular subgroups called U1, U2, and U3. The U1 gene expression signature included genes known to be associated with poor outcome in other tumors, such as *CCND2*. The U2 subgroup was associated with over-expression of genes involved in T-cell activation and apoptosis, including NFKB1 and BCL2. The U3 subgroup was mainly defined by over-expression of genes involved in the IFN/JAK/STAT pathway. Notably, such distinction possibly reflected, at least in part, the presence of reactive components in the PTCL samples
De Leval et al. [26]	AILT	The molecular profile of AITL was characterized by a strong microenvironment and over-expression of several genes characteristic of normal follicular helper T (TFH) cells (*CXCL13, BCL6, PDCD1, CD40L, NFATC1*). Such finding was reinforced by gene set enrichment analysis, which demonstrated that the AITL molecular signature was significantly enriched in TFH-specific genes
Piccaluga et al. [17]	PTCL/NOS	The Authors showed that PTCLs/NOS are most closely related to activated peripheral T-lymphocytes, either CD4+ or CD8+, basing on the GEP. In addition, PTCLs/NOS displayed deregulation of relevant functional cell programs. In particular, among others, *PDGFRA*, a gene encoding for a tyrosine–kinase receptor, turned out to be aberrantly expressed by PTCL/NOS. Notably, both phosphorylation of PDGFRA and sensitivity of cultured PTCL cells to imatinib were demonstrated
Piccaluga et al. [81]	PTCL/NOS	In this study, the Authors found that CD52 is expressed in approximately 40% of PTCLs/NOS at the same level as in normal T-lymphocytes, being aberrantly down-regulated in the remaining cases. Notably, they concluded that the estimation of CD52 expression may provide a rationale for the selection of patients with a higher probability of response to the anti-CD52 antibody, alemtuzumab
Piccaluga et al. [28]	AILT	In this manuscript, the Authors reported that AILT and other PTCLs have rather similar GEP, possibly sharing common oncogenic pathways. In addition, they found that the molecular signature of follicular T-helper cells was significantly over-expressed in AILT. Finally, several genes deregulated in AILT, representing potential therapeutic targets such as *PDGFRA* and *VEGF*, were identified
Lamant et al. [25]	ALCL	This study focused, for the first time, on ALCLs. Unsupervised analysis classified ALCL in 2 clusters, corresponding essentially to morphologic subgroups and clinical variables. Supervised analysis showed that ALK+ALCL and ALK−ALCL have different GEPs, further confirming that they are different entities

(continued)

Table 3.1 (continued)

Reference	Disease(s) explored	Comments
Cuadros et al. [27]	PTCL/NOS	In this study, the Authors identified five clusters of genes, the expression of which varied significantly among the samples. Genes in these clusters were functionally related to different cellular processes such as proliferation, inflammatory response, and T-cell or B-cell lineages. Notably, over-expression of genes in the proliferation signature was associated significantly with shorter survival of patients
Miyazaki [29]	γδ-TCL	This study focused on the GEP of 7 γδ-TCL cases Notably, hepatosplenic γδ-TCLs were clustered together, while the other γδ-TCLs were scattered within the αβ-TCLs In addition, a classifier based on GEP was developed, able to distinguish γδTCL
Pise-Masison [30]	ATLL	This study focused on ATLL and provided evidence that BIRC5 plays an important role in ATL cell viability as well as other important insights into ATLL pathogenesis and potential targeted therapies
Huang et al. [31]	NKTCL	This study highlighted emerging oncogenic pathways in NKTCL and identified novel diagnostic and therapeutic targets. In particular, deregulation of the AKT, JAKSTAT, and NFκB pathways was documented. In addition, aberrant expression of *PDGFRA*, and sensitivity to imatinib were demonstrated
Iqbal et al. [32]	PTCL/NOS, AILT, ALCL, ATLL	This study collected a large panel of PTCLs within the ITCLP and provided important information. First, confirmed the existence of at least 2 PTCL/NOS subtypes, based on the cellular derivation, the helper and cytotoxic ones. Second, the author suggested that the latter are provided with a worse prognosis. Finally, a molecular classificatory was built for AITL, ATLL, and ALK^+ ALCL
Piva et al. [18]	PTCL/NOS, AILT, ALCL	This study specially focused on ALCLs. It was shown that the molecular signature of ALK^+ cases largely relies on STAT3 signaling. In addition, it was shown that ALCLs are distinct from other PTCLs and selected genes can discriminate ALK^+ vs. ALK^- or ALK^- vs. PTCL/NOS

MF mycosis fungoides, *PTCL/NOS* peripheral T-cell lymphoma, not otherwise specified, *AILT* peripheral T-cell lymphoma, angioimmunoblastic type, *ALCL* anaplastic large cell lymphoma, *ATLL* Adult T-cell leukemia/lymphoma, *γδ-TCL* γδ T-cell lymphoma, *NKTCL* NK/T-cell lymphoma, nasal-type, *ITCLP* International T-cell lymphoma project, *GEP* gene expression profile

in the field of PTCL/NOS, as it appeared in the case of some B-cell derived lymphomas (namely, follicular and Hodgkin lymphomas) [33, 34], and possibly AITL (see below) [32].

Subsequently, Piccaluga et al. [17] have published a GEP study based on the analysis of 28 PTCLs/NOS, all corresponding to lymph node biopsies and containing an amount of neoplastic cells that exceeded the 70% value of the whole examined population. The mRNA extracted from these cases was hybridized on the HG U133 2.0 *Plus* gene chip. The obtained results were compared with those of six AITLs, six ALCLs (two ALK^+ and four ALK^-), and 20 samples of normal T-lymphocytes, purified from the peripheral blood and tonsil and corresponding to the main T-cell subsets ($CD4^+$, $CD8^+$, resting, and activated). Thus, the study of Piccaluga et al. significantly differs from most previous reports [20, 23, 24] in terms of methodology and selection criteria. In addition, it provides for the first time the rationale for possible targeted therapies in PTCL/NOS by offering clear evidence of their effectiveness ex vivo. In particular, the GEP detected by Piccaluga et al. [17] indicates that PTCLs/NOS are distinct from the other lymphoid malignancies and normal T-lymphocytes, establishing a clear relationship between PTCL/NOS and normal cellular counterparts and providing the basis for a better understanding of their pathogenesis.

More recently, Iqbal and Colleagues analyzed a large series of PTCLs, collected within the International T-cell lymphoma Project (ITCLP) [32]. Importantly, they could build a robust molecular classifier for ATLL, AITL and ALK^{+} ALCL. On the other hand, PTCLs/NOS were confirmed to have a more heterogeneous profile possibly related to those of the normal counterparts. In addition, importantly, this study provided novel evidences on AITL and PTCL/NOS prognostication (see below). Additional, important, information have been then offered by Piva et al. [18]. In their study, the authors mainly focused on the molecular pathogenesis of ALCLs but also established the relationship between ALCL and PTCL/NOS. Importantly, they showed that ALCLs are molecularly distinct from PTCL/NOS, thus flattening the diffuse, though not biologically based, proposal of including ALK^{-} ALCL within the group of PTCL/NOS. Consistently, in the course of their analysis, Piccaluga et al. [17] already found that all ALCLs tended to cluster together, irrespectively of their ALK positivity or negativity, though in a more limited number of cases. In all, this suggests that—besides the occurrence or not of a translocation involving the ALK gene at 2p23—these tumors share a set of deregulated pathways. On the other hand, it is possible to clearly differentiate ALK^{+} and ALK^{-} cases basing on GEP, as shown by different authors [18, 25, 32]. To this regard, in particular, it was demonstrated the strong biological relevance of the ALK/STAT3 signaling in characterizing the global molecular profile of ALK+ALCL [18].

Histogenesis of PTCLs

In the REAL and subsequent WHO classifications of lymphomas, the recognition of the non-neoplastic cellular counterpart is regarded as a main factor contributing to the definition of the single disease entity. However, differently from the field of B-NHLs, the vast majority of PTCLs have not yet definitely associated to a normal counterpart, mainly due to the complexity of T-cell compartment, as well as the bizarre morphology and largely aberrant phenotype of the neoplastic elements. Nevertheless, the recent GEP studies provided evidences which may be the basis for a future classification of these tumors. First, robust data were generated supporting the concept that AITL cells correspond to follicular T-helper (F_{TH}) cells [26, 28]. Specifically, De Leval and Colleagues studied 18 AITL cases and by gene set enrichment analysis [35] found that AITL signature is significantly enriched in molecules characteristic of normal T_{FH}, including *CXCL13, BCL6, PDCD1, CD40L*, and *NFATC1* [26]. At the same time, Piccaluga et al., by using a different algorithm, also showed that the GEP of AITL is definitely related to that of T_{FH} lymphocytes [28]. Noteworthy, both the studies proved that such feature is restricted to AITL cases [26, 28], though a small fraction of PTCLs/NOS, more often characterized by clear cell cytology, presence of blastic EBV^{+} B-cells, and sometimes, follicular architecture [4] also presents with T_{FH} molecular pattern [26]. Importantly, GEP results were validated by the immunohistochemical demonstration of F_{TH} markers, such as CD10, BCL6, CXCL13, PD1, CCR5, SAP, and ICOS, in AITL [26, 28, 36–40], and were largely in keeping with the observations previously made by Rüdiger et al. [41]. Subsequently, the expression of the same molecules was confirmed in follicular PTCL/NOS [42].

As far as PTCLs/NOS are concerned, interestingly, GEP results suggested that these tumors are more closely related to activated rather than resting T-cells [17]. As in normal mature T-lymphocytes, it was possible to identify two main subgroups of PTCL/NOS, with GEPs related to either CD4 or CD8 elements [17]. Notably, this characteristic did not correspond to the immunophenotype with regards to the expression of the single CD4 and CD8 molecules [17], reflecting the aberrancy in tumor phenotypes [11]. Importantly, the existence of these two molecularly distinct subgroups of PTCL/NOS was later confirmed by the ITCLP study [32]. Remarkably, the latter, also suggested that cases with cytotoxic molecular profile may be provided with a worse prognosis (see below). Finally, ALCLs, according to GEP, appeared to be related to either T_{H17} [32] (Piccaluga, unpublished) or T_{H1} lymphocytes (Piccaluga, unpublished).

Overall, the recognition of normal counterparts for different PTCLs has both biological and practical relevance. On one hand, in fact, it provides the basis for the recognition of cellular abnormalities and comprehension of the interaction with the microenvironment (i.e., the relationship of TFH-derived neoplastic cells and follicular dendritic cells, mast cells etc. in AITL). On the other, it can be used in clinics for easier differential diagnosis, by applying new cell specific markers (i.e., a panel of F_{TH}-associated markers for the distinction of AITL and PTCL/NOS) [40].

Molecular Pathogenesis of PTCL

Besides histogenetic information, different GEP studies provided relevant insights into the functional alterations of PTCLs. First, a careful comparison of PTCL/NOS with the closest normal cellular counterparts revealed, in fact, the extensive deregulation of genes, which control functions that are typically damaged in malignant cells, such as matrix remodeling, cell adhesion, transcription regulation, proliferation, and apoptosis. In particular, the analysis of Piccaluga et al. [17] might explain the dissemination pattern of PTCL/NOS, with frequent extranodal and bone-marrow involvement and spread to peripheral blood [4], by showing the up-regulation of *FN1*, *LAMB1*, *COL1A2*, *COL3A1*, *COL4A1*, *COL4A2*, and *COL12A1*, that is, of genes which promote local invasion and metastasis in different types of human cancers [43–45]. In addition, it revealed the deregulation of genes involved in apoptosis (e.g., *MOAP1*, *ING3*, *GADD45A*, and *GADD45B*) [46–52] and chemo-resistance (such as *CYR61* and *NNMT*) [43–45, 53–64], which may be responsible for the poor response to conventional chemotherapy. Secondly, a couple of GEP studies suggested the possible deregulation of NFκB pathway in a certain number of PTCL/NOS cases [20, 21, 23]. Indeed, it was shown that around 30–40% of cases present with nuclear localization (i.e., activation) of NFκB elements and peculiar GEP [65]. Noteworthy, it was then demonstrated that a fraction of PTCL/NOS presents with REL locus abnormalities, including amplifications and translocations, finally leading to NFκB constitutive activation [15]. Interestingly, on the other hand, down-regulation of *BCL10* (an upstream activator of NFκB in human lymphocytes) was reported to occur in PTCL/NOS [17, 66] with consequent NFκB shut off. However, it is still debated whether (1) such cases NFκB negative cases have a worse clinical outcome and (2) whether anti-NFκB approaches can be eventually effective.

Finally, different studies characterized an aberrant tyrosine–kinase (TK) signaling in PTCLs [17, 18, 22, 31]. In particular, Piccaluga et al. showed that PTCLs/NOS constantly express the *PDGRA* gene and present with consistent phosphorylation (i.e., activation) of the encoded protein [17, 22]. Intriguingly, the same authors also found PDGF ligands to be produced by PTCL/NOS cells, proposing the intriguing hypothesis of an autocrine/paracrine loop activating this signaling [67]. Noteworthy, it was later on showed that also other T/NK-derived tumors present with such phenomenon with relevant therapeutic implications (see below) [31]. Moreover, Piva et al. demonstrated that STAT3 activation induced by ALK is a major contributor to ALK^+ ALCL molecular signature [18].

Importantly, immunohistochemistry was largely adopted in order to provide in situ validation of the genomic data by showing correspondence between mRNA and protein expression, as seen, for example, with *PDGFRA* [17, 22] and *BCL10* [17, 66]. In addition, by comparison with normal tissues, immunohistochemistry allowed the identification of staining patterns corresponding to the synthesis of ectopic or paraphysiologic products by neoplastic cells. On the other hand, the phenotypic test highlighted the possibility that some of the results obtained by gene expression profiling may depend on non-neoplastic cellular components present in the analyzed sample, as seen for caldesmon [17].

Identifying Novel Targeted Therapies for PTCL

Tyrosine–Kinase Inhibitors

Basing on the evidence of TK deregulation in different subtypes of PTCLs, the application of TK inhibitors (TKI) has been tested ex vivo [17, 31]. In particular, Piccaluga et al. [17] designed experiments aiming to test the sensitivity of PTCL/NOS cells to different TKI, including imatinib mesylate. The results obtained were of interest, with about 50% cytotoxic effect seen at 48 h with a 1 μmol concentration. Notably, imatinib exerted a limited effect on the viability of normal lymphocytes. On the other hand, Huang et al. treated with imatinib T/NK-tumor-derived cell lines, and obtained analog results [31]. Finally, as far as ALCL are concerned, consistently with GEP data, Chiarle et al. clearly showed that targeting ALK+ and its downstream STAT3 is an effective strategy in ALK+ ALCL [68, 69].

Histone–Deacetylase Inhibitors

Interestingly, GEP analyses provided evidence for the silencing of genes, possibly regulated by epigenetic mechanisms such as acetylation (e.g., *GADD45A* and *GADD45B*), and suggested to test histone–deacetylase inhibitors (HDACi) against PTCL/NOS primary cells and cell lines [17]. Notably, these compounds induced a dramatic reduction in cell viability, with G0–G1 cell cycle arrest and apoptosis at therapeutic concentrations, suggesting a possible role for this class of drugs in PTCL/NOS therapy. Noteworthy, this idea was also supported by some clinical preliminary observations [70]. Interestingly, the association of HDACi and daunorubicin apparently had a slight additive effect, as already observed in other settings [71]. Notably, the triple combination of TKI, HDACi, and anthracyclines produced a remarkable effect on cell viability: it might represent a promising option for future therapeutic applications.

Anti-angiogenetic Therapy

Increased angiogenesis is a major characteristic of AITL. However, its molecular basis has been unknown for a long time. Recently, a couple of studies documented the up-regulation of the *VEGF* gene in this tumor [26, 28]. Importantly, immunohistochemistry, extensively applied to a large series of cases on tissue microarrays, demonstrated that VEGF is mainly expressed by the neoplastic elements [28] and not only by the abundant vascular component, as initially proposed [26]. Remarkably, it was further shown that AITL cells do also express a VEGF-receptor±±±, VEGFR2/KDR [28], suggesting the hypothesis of an autocrine/paracrine stimulation also in this setting. In addition, it suggested the possible AITL sensitivity to anti-angiogenetic drugs, such as thalidomide and bevacizumab. Indeed, several reports have then documented their positive activity in AITL cases [72–77]

Monoclonal Antibodies

During the last few years, therapeutic monoclonal antibodies (MoAb) have become a major component of anti-lymphoma approaches. However, as far as PTCLs are concerned, a significant limitation emerged, differently from what seen in B-NHL. In particular, PTCLs were demonstrated to extensively present with the aberrant expression of T-cell-associated molecules [11, 17]. This phenomenon is indeed relevant in the clinical practice. In fact, some antigens against which, MoAb have been designed, such as CD4 [78] and, specially, CD52 [79, 80], are frequently down-regulated in T-cell tumors [11, 17, 81–83]. Based on these findings, different authors agreed that the estimation of CD52 expression may provide a rationale for the selection of patients with higher probability of responding to alemtuzumab, by avoiding the risk of unwanted toxicity [81]. Similar consideration will have to be applied to other antigens/MoAbs available in the future.

Prognostication of Peripheral T-Cell Lymphomas

Several prognostic indicators (summarised in Table 3.2) have been proposed that will be detailedly discussed in the following.

International Prognostic Index

The international prognostic index (IPI) was first introduced in 1993 with the intent of identifying patients with aggressive NHL and different risk of treatment failure, relapse, and death [84]. It is based on clinical parameters, such as tumor stage, presence of extranodal localizations, age, lactate dehydrogenase (LDH) level, and performance status (PS). Notably, it was built up on B-NHL rather than T-NHL cases, and, specially, diffuses large B-cell lymphomas (DLBCL). However, its ability to stratify PTCL patients was reported in the following years. In particular, the International Lymphoma Study Group showed that overall and relapse free survival were significantly different in patients with low (0/1) vs. high (4/5) IPI, in patients with all PTCL type but ALCL (5-year OS, 36 vs. 15%; 5-year failure free survival, FFS, 27 vs. 10%) [2]. On the other hand, subsequent studies showed that IPI was particularly effective for prognostication of both ALK^+ and ALK^- ALCL [6, 85]. In particular, in ALK^+ ALCL, the 5-year OS was 94 ± 5% for the low/low intermediate risk group vs. 41 ± 12% for the high/high intermediate group ($p < 0.0001$) [85]. Noteworthy, the IPI was more relevant than ALK expression in stratifying patients with ALCL (relative risk, 3.50 vs. 0.29, respectively), though both were significant prognostic factors [85]. In addition, in a large study within the ITCLP, the IPI effectively identified risk groups with different prognoses within both ALK^+ and ALK^- ALCL, although those with an IPI score of 3 or more fell into the poor-risk category regardless of ALK status [6].

Furthermore, Suzumiya et al. recently reported on a large series of patients with aggressive adult T-cell leukemia/lymphoma (ATLL), providing evidence that IPI, platelet count, and B-symptoms were significant prognostic factors [86]. Interestingly, multivariate analysis indicated that only the IPI was an independent predictor of OS in this series, though the IPI significantly predicted for OS only in the lymphoma type of ATLL ($p = 0.04$), but not in the acute one ($p = 0.24$) [86].

Overall, IPI identifies patients at higher risk, being the expression of disease extension on one hand, and patient's frailty on the other. Indeed, it does offer neither specific biological hints nor potential target for overcoming drug resistance. In addition, it was soon clear that IPI was not as effective in PTCLs/NOS and AITLs (the two commonest PTCL types) as in the original series of DLBCLs, probably reflecting, at least in part, the fact that PTCL therapy is basically derived from B-NHLs and specific trials have been lacking for a long time. In particular, the extensive use of anthracyclines did not appear to provide significant benefits in PTCL patients [5]. Thus, novel scores have been investigated in this setting in the last few years (see below).

Prognostic Index for PTCL/NOS

In 2004, an Italian group (*Intergruppo Italiano Linfomi, IIL*) proposed a novel prognostic model based on a retrospective multi-centric clinical analysis of 385 patients [87]. Specifically, the new model, named *Prognostic Index for PTCL-U* (PIT), included bone-marrow involvement, age, PS, and LDH. When these four variables were combined in four groups, the PIT could identify patient subgroups with different outcomes. Noteworthy, the PIT turned out to be slightly more effective than IPI in stratifying PTCL patients (log-rank 66.79 vs. 55.94) and was then proposed as reference tool. In addition a simplified, two-classes PIT appeared to be superior to a simplified two-classes IPI (log-rank 49.36 vs. 30.23) [87]. However, PIT was based on a series lacking systematic histological review and though its value was confirmed within the ITCLP, it did not resulted superior to IPI. In particular, the PIT was also applied to ALK^+ and ALK^- ALCL and was similarly predictive of FFS and OS in both groups [6]. However, given that the distribution of patients across the risk groups was very similar with the two prognostic models and that bone-marrow involvement is rarely observed in ALCL, the PIT actually seems to mirror the IPI in this setting [6].

In addition, as it does not include tumor-specific biologic factors, cannot be intended for the future application of targeted therapies.

Clinical-Pathologic Prognostic Score (Bologna Score)

Immunohistochemical markers have been largely proposed for prognostication of malignant

Table 3.2 Summary of prognostic markers and scores in peripheral T-cell lymphomas

Prognostic indicator	PTCL subtype	Reference
Histotype	All	The Non-Hodgkin's Lymphoma Classification Project [2]
		Vose et al. [5]
		Savage et al. [6]
		Lopez-Guillermo et al. [8]
		Ascani et al. [16]
IPI	All	The Non-Hodgkin's Lymphoma Classification Project [2]
	ALCL	Savage et al. [6]
		Falini et al. [85]
	ATLL	Suzumiya et al. [86]
	NK/TCL	Au et al. [108]
PIT	PTCL/NOS	Gallamini et al. [87]
		Savage et al. [6]
Bologna score	PTCL/NOS	Went et al. [11]
	AITL	Briones et al. [66]
Korean prgnostic index	NKTCL	Lee et al. [105]
NK prognostic index	NKTCL	Suzuki et al. [118]
EBV integration	PTCL/NOS	Went et al. [11]
	AITL	Kluin et al. [89]
		Dupuis et al. [90]
	NKTCL	Au et al. [108]Cheung et al. [60]
		Chim et al. [115]
		Huang et al. [116]
		Lee et al. [117]
		Ng et al. [114]
Proliferation (evaluated by)	PTCL/NOS	Went et al. [11]
Ki-67		Cuadros et al. [27]
Molecular signature		
Cellular derivation	PTCL/NOS	Went et al. [11]
		Bekkenk et al. [91]
		Kojima et al. [92]
		Iqbal et al. [32]
NFκB activation	PTCL/NOS	Martinez-Delgado et al. [21]
		Ballester et al. [23]
		Briones et al. [66]
CYP3A	PTCL/NOS	Rodriguez-Antona et al. [100]

PTCL/NOS peripheral T-cell lymphoma, not otherwise specified, *AILT* peripheral T-cell lymphoma, angioimmunoblastic type, ALCL anaplastic large cell lymphoma, *ATLL* Adult T-cell leukemia/lymphoma, *NKTCL* NK/T-cell lymphoma, nasal-type

lymphomas. As far as PTCLs are concerned, in a large collection of Italian cases, Went et al. recently found that high Ki-67 expression, Epstein–Barr virus (EBV) status, and CD15 staining were associated with the worst outcome in PTCL/NOS [11]. Interestingly, EBV has repeatedly been proposed as a negative prognosticator in PTCLs [88], both among Asian and European patients [89, 90]. Specifically, Went et al. found EBV-positivity in 5 and 3% of PTCLs, NOS, and AITL respectively: this value is definitely lower than the one recorded by Dupuis et al. in a

French cohort. Such discrepancies might reflect geographic or racial differences. No other immunohistochemical marker alone or in combination was associated with a poor outcome, although patients with tumors expressing CD57 or $CD4^+/CD8^-$ phenotype showed a tendency for a better outcome, the possible prognostic relevance of the latter having also been proposed by others [91, 92].

Furthermore, based on their collective largely provided with follow-up data and previous experience in the literature [87, 93–98], Went et al. developed a new score integrating both patient- and tumor-specific characteristics (age >60 years, PS, LDH, and Ki-67 marking ≥80%) and identifying three clear-cut groups of patients with different responses to therapy and life-expectancy. Such score seemed to show an improved ability to predict patient-outcome compared to previous indices, including IPI ($p<0.001$ vs. 0.1) and PIT ($p<0.001$ vs. 0.0043) [11]. In particular, according to the Bologna score, patients were clustered into three groups, which showed significantly different clinical outcome (median OS 37 vs. 23 vs. 6 months, respectively; $p<0.001$) [11].

Interestingly, the ability of the Bologna score was recently validated by a Spanish group [66].

Remarkably, all the factors contributing to the scoring system proposed by Went et al. [11] are part of the routine workup, making their integration simple and cost-effective, and incorporate both patient- and tumor-specific characteristics.

Gene Expression Profiling

In the last few years, several studies dealt with the gene expression profiling (GEP) of nodal PTCLs [17, 18, 20–23, 25–32, 81, 99], possibly providing novel insight into PTCL prognostication. First, a few reports suggested that PTCLs/NOS may present with up- or down-regulation of NFκB molecules [20, 21, 23], with possible prognostic relevance [21, 23]. In particular, cases with higher levels of NFκB-related molecules or other evidence of NFκB activation showed a better median OS (25 months, range 0–124 months, vs. 12 months, range 0–19 months; $p=0.032$) [21, 23]. This observation was then confirmed by another Spanish group, the 5-year OS being 45% vs. 0%, in $NF\kappa B^+$ and $NF\kappa B^-$ cases, respectively ($p=0.04$) [66]. However, all these studies included a relatively limited number of cases, by mixing different histotypes [21, 66], or cases with prominent non-neoplastic components [23], which might have influenced, at least in part the results.

In addition, basing on GEP obtained from 35 nodal PTCL cases (23 PTCLs/NOS and 12 AITLs), it was suggested that over-expression of genes involved in a so-called "proliferation signature" was associated significantly with shorter survival of patients [27]. This proliferation signature included genes commonly associated with the cell cycle, such as *CCNA*, *CCNB*, *TOP2A*, and *PCNA* [27]. Notably, this evidence of high proliferation as a possible adverse prognostic factor was definitely in line with what reported by Went et al. [11] and what observed within the ITCLP (unpublished), highlighting the importance of such parameter.

Finally, our Group, basing on GEP analyses, indicated that PTCLs/NOS can be subclassified according to their histogenesis. In particular, at least two subgroups were described, derived from activated helper and cytotoxic elements, respectively [17]. Importantly, such finding was recently confirmed by Iqbal et al. [32]. Intriguingly, in this report, it was also suggested that the cytotoxic profile may be associated with unfavorable outcome, though this evidence was based on a limited series and warrants further validation. On the other hand, a possible more favorable outcome for PTCL cases with helper phenotype had been also previously suggested by others [11, 91, 92].

Overall, GEP studies provided evidences that molecular features may be useful in defining the prognosis of PTCL patients. However, no complete explanation has been offered as far as the molecular bases of drug resistance are concerned. Notably, our group described for the first time the expression of molecules associated to drug resistance in solid tumors such as *CYR61* and *NNMT* in PTCL/NOS [17]. Furthermore, Rodríguez-Antona et al. recently found that a high expression of cytochrome P450 3A (CYP3A), an enzyme involved in the inactivation of chemotherapy drugs, was associated to poor response to the standard PTCL chemotherapy, suggesting that CYP3A could be useful as a predictor of response [100]. Indeed, the molecular classification of PTCLs and the identification of key events in their molecular pathology will be probably the basis for future prognostication and targeted treatment in this field as in the case of DLBCL [101, 102].

Prognostication of NK/T-Cell Lymphoma, Nasal-Type

Extranodal natural killer/T-cell lymphoma, nasal-type is a distinct entity in the WHO classification of lymphoid tumors, more frequent in Asia and Central–South America than in Western countries [103–108]. Morphologically, tissue invasion, vascular destruction, and necrosis are the most prominent features; EBV is always integrated in the genome of neoplastic cells [107]. Most of the cases derive from natural killer (NK) cells and are characterized by a typical NK phenotype and T-cell receptor genes in germ-line configuration; however, in some instances a cytotoxic T lymphocyte origin was recognized [107]. The nasal cavity and the upper aerodigestive tract (nasal NK/T-cell lymphoma) are the most commonly involved sites, but skin, gastrointestinal tract, lung, testis, and soft-tissues (extra-nasal NK/T-cell lymphoma) can be also affected [103, 104, 107, 109].

The prognosis of extranodal natural killer/T-cell lymphoma is poor, being the worst among the PTCL categories [108]: survival rate is 30–40%, anyway some differences exist between nasal and non-nasal disease as the latter is more aggressive [107, 108, 110], therefore the inclusion of radiotherapy in treatment protocols improved outcome of nasal natural killer/T-cell lymphoma in stage I or II [106–108, 111, 112]. Among nasal forms, adverse prognostic factors are unfavorable IPI, advanced stage disease (stage III or IV), high circulating EBV DNA levels, and detection of EBV in bone-marrow cells by in situ hybridization [107, 108, 111, 113–117]. Some studies suggest that high proportion of large/transformed cells in tumoral population have a negative impact on survival: anyway the significance of cytological features as prognostic indicator is still uncertain [106–109]. The primary extra-nasal cases are highly aggressive with poor response to therapy even in patients with localized disease [107, 108].

Importantly, a new prognostic index, proposed by a Korean group, specifically developed for NK/T-cell tumors and based on four parameters, ("B" symptoms, LDH levels, stage and regional lymph node involvement) demonstrated a better prognostic stratification of NK/T-cell lymphomas as compared with IPI [105].

In addition, recently, another study showed that four factors (non-nasal-type, stage, performance status and numbers of extranodal involvement) were significant prognostic factors in NK/T-cell lymphomas [118]. Using these four variables, a NK prognostic index was successfully constructed, the 4-year OS of patients with zero, one, two and three or four adverse factors being 55, 33, 15, and 6%, respectively [118].

Conclusion

PTCLs have represented for a long time an orphan pathology. This can be explained by their relatively low incidence (that is anyway higher that of a "common" tumor, such as Hodgkin's lymphoma), the difficulties encountered in their analysis, and their dismal prognosis. During the last few years, however, a great deal of interest has developed shedding new light on the pathobiology of these tumors and leading to the proposal of more effective prognosticators. In particular, though IPI is somehow effective for PTCL prognostication, novel more refined and possibly disease specific scores have been explored, and several models including clinical–pathological and molecular features have been proposed, their validation process being now ongoing. In addition, innovative therapeutic schedules have been recently proposed, based on the application of the newly developed micro-array techniques. The morning of a new era seems quite close that will actually dissipate the shadows which have wrapped PTCLs for several decades.

References

1. Harris NL, Jaffe ES, Stein H, et al. A revised European–American classification of lymphoid neoplasms: a proposal from the International Lymphoma Study Group. Blood. 1994;84(5):1361–92.
2. The Non-Hodgkin's Lymphoma Classification Project. A clinical evaluation of the International Lymphoma Study Group classification of non-Hodgkin's lymphoma. Blood. 1997;89(11):3909–18.
3. WHO. Classification of tumors of hematopoietic and lymphoid tissues. IVth ed. Lyon: IARC; 2008.
4. Pileri S, Ralfkiaer E, Weisenburger D, et al. Peripheral T-cell lymphoma, not otherwise specified. In: Swerdlow S, Campo E, Harris NL, et al., editors. WHO Classification of tumors of hematopoietic and lymphoid tissues. IVth ed. Lyon: IARC; 2008. p. 429.
5. Vose J, Armitage J, Weisenburger D. International peripheral T-cell and natural killer/T-cell lymphoma study: pathology findings and clinical outcomes. J Clin Oncol. 2008;26(25):4124–30.
6. Savage KJ, Harris NL, Vose JM, et al. ALK-anaplastic large-cell lymphoma is clinically and immunophenotypically different from both ALK+ALCL and peripheral T-cell lymphoma, not otherwise specified: report from the International Peripheral T-Cell Lymphoma Project. Blood. 2008;111(12):5496–504.
7. Evens AM, Gartenhaus RB. Treatment of T-cell non-Hodgkin's lymphoma. Curr Treat Options Oncol. 2004;5(4):289–303.
8. Lopez-Guillermo A, Cid J, Salar A, et al. Peripheral T-cell lymphomas: initial features, natural history, and prognostic factors in a series of 174 patients diagnosed according to the R.E.A.L. Classification. Ann Oncol. 1998;9(8):849–55.
9. Gisselbrecht C, Gaulard P, Lepage E, et al. Prognostic significance of T-cell phenotype in aggressive non-Hodgkin's lymphomas. Groupe d'Etudes des Lymphomes de l'Adulte (GELA). Blood. 1998;92(1):76–82.
10. Effect of age on the characteristics and clinical behavior of non-Hodgkin's lymphoma patients. The Non-Hodgkin's Lymphoma Classification Project. Ann Oncol. 1997;8(10):973–8.
11. Went P, Agostinelli C, Gallamini A, et al. Marker expression in peripheral T-cell lymphoma: a proposed clinical-pathologic prognostic score. J Clin Oncol. 2006;24(16):2472–9.
12. Rudiger T, Weisenburger DD, Anderson JR, et al. Peripheral T-cell lymphoma (excluding anaplastic large-cell lymphoma): results from the Non-Hodgkin's Lymphoma Classification Project. Ann Oncol. 2002;13(1):140–9.
13. Zettl A, Rudiger T, Konrad MA, et al. Genomic profiling of peripheral T-cell lymphoma, unspecified, and anaplastic large T-cell lymphoma delineates novel recurrent chromosomal alterations. Am J Pathol. 2004;164(5):1837–48.
14. Oshiro A, Tagawa H, Ohshima K, et al. Identification of subtype-specific genomic alterations in aggressive adult T-cell leukemia/lymphoma. Blood. 2006;107(11):4500–7.
15. Hartmann S, Gesk S, Scholtysik R, et al. High resolution SNP array genomic profiling of peripheral T cell lymphomas, not otherwise specified, identifies a subgroup with chromosomal aberrations affecting the REL locus. Br J Haematol. 2010;148(3):402–12.
16. Ascani S, Zinzani PL, Gherlinzoni F, et al. Peripheral T-cell lymphomas. Clinico-pathologic study of 168 cases diagnosed according to the R.E.A.L. Classification. Ann Oncol. 1997;8(6):583–92.
17. Piccaluga PP, Agostinelli C, Califano A, et al. Gene expression analysis of peripheral T cell lymphoma, unspecified, reveals distinct profiles and new potential therapeutic targets. J Clin Invest. 2007;117(3):823–34.
18. Piva R, Agnelli L, Pellegrino E, et al. Gene expression profiling uncovers molecular classifiers for the recognition of anaplastic large-cell lymphoma within peripheral T-cell neoplasms. J Clin Oncol. 2010;28(9):1583–90.
19. Tracey L, Villuendas R, Dotor AM, et al. Mycosis fungoides shows concurrent deregulation of multiple genes involved in the TNF signaling pathway: an expression profile study. Blood. 2003;102(3):1042–50.
20. Martinez-Delgado B, Melendez B, Cuadros M, et al. Expression profiling of T-cell lymphomas differentiates peripheral and lymphoblastic lymphomas and defines survival related genes. Clin Cancer Res. 2004;10(15):4971–82.
21. Martinez-Delgado B, Cuadros M, Honrado E, et al. Differential expression of NF-kappaB pathway genes among peripheral T-cell lymphomas. Leukemia. 2005;19(12):2254–63.
22. Piccaluga PP, Agostinelli C, Zinzani PL, Baccarani M, Dalla Favera R, Pileri SA. Expression of platelet-derived growth factor receptor alpha in peripheral T-cell lymphoma not otherwise specified. Lancet Oncol. 2005;6(6):440.
23. Ballester B, Ramuz O, Gisselbrecht C, et al. Gene expression profiling identifies molecular subgroups among nodal peripheral T-cell lymphomas. Oncogene. 2006;25(10):1560–70.
24. Mahadevan D, Spier C, Della Croce K, et al. Transcript profiling in peripheral T-cell lymphoma, not otherwise specified, and diffuse large B-cell lymphoma identifies distinct tumor profile signatures. Mol Cancer Ther. 2005;4(12):1867–79.
25. Lamant L, de Reynies A, Duplantier MM, et al. Gene-expression profiling of systemic anaplastic large-cell lymphoma reveals differences based on ALK status and two distinct morphologic ALK+ subtypes. Blood. 2007;109(5):2156–64.
26. de Leval L, Rickman DS, Thielen C, et al. The gene expression profile of nodal peripheral T-cell lymphoma demonstrates a molecular link between angioimmunoblastic T-cell lymphoma (AITL) and

follicular helper T (TFH) cells. Blood. 2007; 109(11):4952–63.
27. Cuadros M, Dave SS, Jaffe ES, et al. Identification of a proliferation signature related to survival in nodal peripheral T-cell lymphomas. J Clin Oncol. 2007;25(22):3321–9.
28. Piccaluga PP, Agostinelli C, Califano A, et al. Gene expression analysis of angioimmunoblastic lymphoma indicates derivation from T follicular helper cells and vascular endothelial growth factor deregulation. Cancer Res. 2007;67(22):10703–10.
29. Miyazaki K, Yamaguchi M, Imai H, et al. Gene expression profiling of peripheral T-cell lymphoma including gammadelta T-cell lymphoma. Blood. 2009;113(5):1071–4.
30. Pise-Masison CA, Radonovich M, Dohoney K, et al. Gene expression profiling of ATL patients: compilation of disease-related genes and evidence for TCF4 involvement in BIRC5 gene expression and cell viability. Blood. 2009;113(17):4016–26.
31. Huang Y, de Reynies A, de Leval L, et al. Gene expression profiling identifies emerging oncogenic pathways operating in extranodal NK/T-cell lymphoma, nasal-type. Blood. 2010;115(6):1226–37.
32. Iqbal J, Weisenburger DD, Greiner TC, et al. Molecular signatures to improve diagnosis in peripheral T-cell lymphoma and prognostication in angioimmunoblastic T-cell lymphoma. Blood. 2010;115(5): 1026–36.
33. Dave SS, Wright G, Tan B, et al. Prediction of survival in follicular lymphoma based on molecular features of tumor-infiltrating immune cells. N Engl J Med. 2004;351(21):2159–69.
34. Steidl C, Lee T, Shah SP, et al. Tumor-associated macrophages and survival in classic Hodgkin's lymphoma. N Engl J Med. 2010;362(10):875–85.
35. Watson A, Mazumder A, Stewart M, Balasubramanian S. Technology for microarray analysis of gene expression. Curr Opin Biotechnol. 1998;9(6): 609–14.
36. Dupuis J, Boye K, Martin N, et al. Expression of CXCL13 by neoplastic cells in angioimmunoblastic T-cell lymphoma (AITL): a new diagnostic marker providing evidence that AITL derives from follicular helper T cells. Am J Surg Pathol. 2006;30(4):490–4.
37. Grogg KL, Attygale AD, Macon WR, Remstein ED, Kurtin PJ, Dogan A. Expression of CXCL13, a chemokine highly upregulated in germinal center T-helper cells, distinguishes angioimmunoblastic T-cell lymphoma from peripheral T-cell lymphoma, unspecified. Mod Pathol. 2006;19(8):1101–7.
38. Roncador G, Garcia Verdes-Montenegro JF, Tedoldi S, et al. Expression of two markers of germinal center T cells (SAP and PD-1) in angioimmunoblastic T-cell lymphoma. Haematologica. 2007;92(8):1059–66.
39. Marafioti T, Paterson JC, Ballabio E, et al. The inducible T-cell co-stimulator molecule is expressed on subsets of T cells and is a new marker of lymphomas of T follicular helper cell-derivation. Haematologica. 2010;95(3):432–9.
40. Laurent C, Fazilleau N, Brousset P. A novel subset of T-helper cells: follicular T-helper cells and their markers. Haematologica. 2010;95(3):356–8.
41. Rudiger T, Geissinger E, Muller-Hermelink HK. 'Normal counterparts' of nodal peripheral T-cell lymphoma. Hematol Oncol. 2006;24(4):175–80.
42. Huang Y, Moreau A, Dupuis J, et al. Peripheral T-cell lymphomas with a follicular growth pattern are derived from follicular helper T cells (TFH) and may show overlapping features with angioimmunoblastic T-cell lymphomas. Am J Surg Pathol. 2009;33(5):682–90.
43. Tapper J, Kettunen E, El-Rifai W, Seppala M, Andersson LC, Knuutila S. Changes in gene expression during progression of ovarian carcinoma. Cancer Genet Cytogenet. 2001;128(1):1–6.
44. Sado Y, Kagawa M, Naito I, et al. Organization and expression of basement membrane collagen IV genes and their roles in human disorders. J Biochem (Tokyo). 1998;123(5):767–76.
45. van den Boom J, Wolter M, Kuick R, et al. Characterization of gene expression profiles associated with glioma progression using oligonucleotide-based microarray analysis and real-time reverse transcription-polymerase chain reaction. Am J Pathol. 2003;163(3):1033–43.
46. Jin S, Tong T, Fan W, et al. GADD45-induced cell cycle G2-M arrest associates with altered subcellular distribution of cyclin B1 and is independent of p38 kinase activity. Oncogene. 2002;21(57):8696–704.
47. Papa S, Zazzeroni F, Bubici C, et al. Gadd45 beta mediates the NF-kappa B suppression of JNK signalling by targeting MKK7/JNKK2. Nat Cell Biol. 2004;6(2):146–53.
48. Chen F, Lu Y, Zhang Z, et al. Opposite effect of NF-kappa B and c-Jun N-terminal kinase on p53-independent GADD45 induction by arsenite. J Biol Chem. 2001;276(14):11414–9.
49. Hirose T, Sowa Y, Takahashi S, et al. p53-independent induction of Gadd45 by histone deacetylase inhibitor: coordinate regulation by transcription factors Oct-1 and NF-Y. Oncogene. 2003;22(49):7762–73.
50. Tan KO, Tan KM, Chan SL, et al. MAP-1, a novel proapoptotic protein containing a BH3-like motif that associates with Bax through its Bcl-2 homology domains. J Biol Chem. 2001;276(4):2802–7.
51. Nagashima M, Shiseki M, Pedeux RM, et al. A novel PHD-finger motif protein, p47ING3, modulates p53-mediated transcription, cell cycle control, and apoptosis. Oncogene. 2003;22(3):343–50.
52. Gunduz M, Ouchida M, Fukushima K, et al. Allelic loss and reduced expression of the ING3, a candidate tumor suppressor gene at 7q31, in human head and neck cancers. Oncogene. 2002;21(28):4462–70.
53. Lee MS, Hanspers K, Barker CS, Korn AP, McCune JM. Gene expression profiles during human CD4+ T cell differentiation. Int Immunol. 2004;16(8): 1109–24.
54. Chtanova T, Newton R, Liu SM, et al. Identification of T cell-restricted genes, and signatures for different T cell responses, using a comprehensive

collection of microarray datasets. J Immunol. 2005; 175(12):7837–47.
55. Chtanova T, Tangye SG, Newton R, et al. T follicular helper cells express a distinctive transcriptional profile, reflecting their role as non-Th1/Th2 effector cells that provide help for B cells. J Immunol. 2004;173(1):68–78.
56. Hosack DA, Dennis Jr G, Sherman BT, Lane HC, Lempicki RA. Identifying biological themes within lists of genes with EASE. Genome Biol. 2003; 4(10):R70.
57. Han JS, Macarak E, Rosenbloom J, Chung KC, Chaqour B. Regulation of Cyr61/CCN1 gene expression through RhoA GTPase and p38MAPK signaling pathways. Eur J Biochem. 2003;270(16):3408–21.
58. Leu SJ, Liu Y, Chen N, Chen CC, Lam SC, Lau LF. Identification of a novel integrin alpha 6 beta 1 binding site in the angiogenic inducer CCN1 (CYR61). J Biol Chem. 2003;278(36):33801–8.
59. Schober JM, Lau LF, Ugarova TP, Lam SC. Identification of a novel integrin alphaMbeta2 binding site in CCN1 (CYR61), a matricellular protein expressed in healing wounds and atherosclerotic lesions. J Biol Chem. 2003;278(28):25808–15.
60. Tsai MS, Bogart DF, Castaneda JM, Li P, Lupu R. Cyr61 promotes breast tumorigenesis and cancer progression. Oncogene. 2002;21(53):8178–85.
61. Tsai MS, Hornby AE, Lakins J, Lupu R. Expression and function of CYR61, an angiogenic factor, in breast cancer cell lines and tumor biopsies. Cancer Res. 2000;60(20):5603–7.
62. Lin MT, Chang CC, Chen ST, et al. Cyr61 expression confers resistance to apoptosis in breast cancer MCF-7 cells by a mechanism of NF-kappaB-dependent XIAP up-regulation. J Biol Chem. 2004;279(23):24015–23.
63. Kassem H, Sangar V, Cowan R, Clarke N, Margison GP. A potential role of heat shock proteins and nicotinamide N-methyl transferase in predicting response to radiation in bladder cancer. Int J Cancer. 2002;101(5):454–60.
64. Xu J, Capezzone M, Xu X, Hershman JM. Activation of nicotinamide N-methyltransferase gene promoter by hepatocyte nuclear factor-1{beta} in human papillary thyroid cancer cells. Mol Endocrinol. 2005;19(2):527–39.
65. Piccaluga P, Agostinelli C, Righi S, et al. Expression of classical NF-kappa B pathway molecules in peripheral t-cell lymphoma not otherwise specified. In: 10th International Conference on Malignant Lymphoma; 2008 June, 4–6; 2008; Lugano, CH; 2008. p. #231.
66. Briones J, Moga E, Espinosa I, et al. Bcl-10 protein highly correlates with the expression of phosphorylated p65 NF-kappaB in peripheral T-cell lymphomas and is associated with clinical outcome. Histopathology. 2009;54(4):478–85.
67. Piccaluga P, Rossi M, De Falco G, et al. PDGFRA activity deregulation in PTCL/NOS is a consequence of miRNA deregulation and autocrine loop sustainment. In: American Association for Cancer Research Annual Meeting; 2009 April 18–22; Denver Philadelphia (PA): AACR; 2009.
68. Chiarle R, Simmons WJ, Cai H, et al. Stat3 is required for ALK-mediated lymphomagenesis and provides a possible therapeutic target. Nat Med. 2005;11(6):623–9.
69. Chiarle R, Martinengo C, Mastini C, et al. The anaplastic lymphoma kinase is an effective oncoantigen for lymphoma vaccination. Nat Med. 2008;14(6): 676–80.
70. Duvic M, Talpur R, Ni X, et al. Phase 2 trial of oral vorinostat (suberoylanilide hydroxamic acid, SAHA) for refractory cutaneous T-cell lymphoma (CTCL). Blood. 2007;109(1):31–9.
71. Sanchez-Gonzalez B, Yang H, Bueso-Ramos C, et al. Antileukemia activity of the combination of an anthracycline with a histone deacetylase inhibitor. Blood. 2006;108(4):1174–82.
72. Strupp C, Aivado M, Germing U, Gattermann N, Haas R. Angioimmunoblastic lymphadenopathy (AILD) may respond to thalidomide treatment: two case reports. Leuk Lymphoma. 2002;43(1):133–7.
73. Bruns I, Fox F, Reinecke P, et al. Complete remission in a patient with relapsed angioimmunoblastic T-cell lymphoma following treatment with bevacizumab. Leukemia. 2005;19(11):1993–5.
74. Dogan A, Ngu LS, Ng SH, Cervi PL. Pathology and clinical features of angioimmunoblastic T-cell lymphoma after successful treatment with thalidomide. Leukemia. 2005;19(5):873–5.
75. Ramasamy K, Lim Z, Pagliuca A, Salisbury JR, Mufti GJ, Devereux S. Successful treatment of refractory angioimmunoblastic T-cell lymphoma with thalidomide and dexamethasone. Haematologica 2006;91(8 Suppl): ECR44.
76. Aguiar Bujanda D. Complete response of relapsed angioimmunoblastic T-cell lymphoma following therapy with bevacizumab. Ann Oncol. 2008;19(2): 396–7.
77. Gottardi M, Danesin C, Canal F, et al. Complete remission induced by thalidomide in a case of angioimmunoblastic T-cell lymphoma refractory to autologous stem cell transplantation. Leuk Lymphoma. 2008;49(9):1836–8.
78. Kim YH, Duvic M, Obitz E, et al. Clinical efficacy of zanolimumab (HuMax-CD4): two phase 2 studies in refractory cutaneous T-cell lymphoma. Blood. 2007;109(11):4655–62.
79. Enblad G, Hagberg H, Erlanson M, et al. A pilot study of alemtuzumab (anti-CD52 monoclonal antibody) therapy for patients with relapsed or chemotherapy-refractory peripheral T-cell lymphomas. Blood. 2004;103(8):2920–4.
80. Gallamini A, Zaja F, Patti C, et al. Alemtuzumab (Campath-1 H) and CHOP chemotherapy as first-line treatment of peripheral T-cell lymphoma: results of a GITIL (Gruppo Italiano Terapie Innovative nei Linfomi) prospective multicenter trial. Blood. 2007; 110(7):2316–23.

81. Piccaluga PP, Agostinelli C, Righi S, Zinzani PL, Pileri SA. Expression of CD52 in peripheral T-cell lymphoma. Haematologica. 2007;92(4):566–7.
82. Rodig SJ, Abramson JS, Pinkus GS, et al. Heterogeneous CD52 expression among hematologic neoplasms: implications for the use of alemtuzumab (CAMPATH-1 H). Clin Cancer Res. 2006; 12(23):7174–9.
83. Chang ST, Lu CL, Chuang SS. CD52 expression in non-mycotic T- and NK/T-cell lymphomas. Leuk Lymphoma. 2007;48(1):117–21.
84. A predictive model for aggressive non-Hodgkin's lymphoma. The International Non-Hodgkin's Lymphoma Prognostic Factors Project. N Engl J Med. 1993;329(14):987–94.
85. Falini B, Pileri S, Zinzani PL, et al. ALK+lymphoma: clinico-pathological findings and outcome. Blood. 1999;93(8):2697–706.
86. Suzumiya J, Ohshima K, Tamura K, et al. The International Prognostic Index predicts outcome in aggressive adult T-cell leukemia/lymphoma: analysis of 126 patients from the International Peripheral T-Cell Lymphoma Project. Ann Oncol. 2009;20(4): 715–21.
87. Gallamini A, Stelitano C, Calvi R, et al. Peripheral T-cell lymphoma unspecified (PTCL-U): a new prognostic model from a retrospective multicentric clinical study. Blood. 2004;103(7):2474–9.
88. Cheng AL, Su IJ, Chen YC, Uen WC, Wang CH. Characteristic clinicopathologic features of Epstein-Barr virus-associated peripheral T-cell lymphoma. Cancer. 1993;72(3):909–16.
89. Kluin PM, Feller A, Gaulard P, et al. Peripheral T/NK-cell lymphoma: a report of the IXth Workshop of the European Association for Haematopathology. Histopathology. 2001;38(3):250–70.
90. Dupuis J, Emile JF, Mounier N, et al. Prognostic significance of Epstein-Barr virus in nodal peripheral T-cell lymphoma, unspecified: A Groupe d'Etude des Lymphomes de l'Adulte (GELA) study. Blood. 2006;108(13):4163–9.
91. Bekkenk MW, Vermeer MH, Jansen PM, et al. Peripheral T-cell lymphomas unspecified presenting in the skin: analysis of prognostic factors in a group of 82 patients. Blood. 2003;102(6):2213–9.
92. Kojima H, Hasegawa Y, Suzukawa K, et al. Clinicopathological features and prognostic factors of Japanese patients with "peripheral T-cell lymphoma, unspecified" diagnosed according to the WHO classification. Leuk Res. 2004;28(12):1287–92.
93. Caulet-Maugendre S, Patey M, Granier E, Joundi A, Gentile A, Caulet T. Quantitative analysis of cellular proliferative activity in 35 T-cell non-Hodgkin's lymphomas. Use of proliferating cell nuclear antigen and Ki-67 (MIB-1) antibodies and nucleolar organizer regions. Anal Quant Cytol Histol. 1996;18(5): 337–44.
94. Miller TP, Grogan TM, Dahlberg S, et al. Prognostic significance of the Ki-67-associated proliferative antigen in aggressive non-Hodgkin's lymphomas: a prospective Southwest Oncology Group trial. Blood. 1994;83(6):1460–6.
95. Mochen C, Giardini R, Costa A, Silvestrini R. MIB-1 and S-phase cell fraction predict survival in non-Hodgkin's lymphomas. Cell Prolif. 1997;30(1): 37–47.
96. Montalban C, Obeso G, Gallego A, Castrillo JM, Bellas C, Rivas C. Peripheral T-cell lymphoma: a clinicopathological study of 41 cases and evaluation of the prognostic significance of the updated Kiel classification. Histopathology. 1993;22(4):303–10.
97. Sheval EV, Churakova JV, Dudnik OA, Vorobjev IA. Examination of the proliferative activity of tumor cells in human lymphoid neoplasms using a morphometric approach. Cancer. 2004;102(3):174–85.
98. Tiemann M, Schrader C, Klapper W, et al. Histopathology, cell proliferation indices and clinical outcome in 304 patients with mantle cell lymphoma (MCL): a clinicopathological study from the European MCL Network. Br J Haematol. 2005; 131(1):29–38.
99. Gazzola A, Bertuzzi C, Agostinelli C, Righi S, Pileri SA, Piccaluga PP. Physiological PTEN expression in peripheral T-cell lymphoma not otherwise specified. Haematologica. 2009;94(7):1036–7.
100. Rodriguez-Antona C, Leskela S, Zajac M, et al. Expression of CYP3A4 as a predictor of response to chemotherapy in peripheral T-cell lymphomas. Blood. 2007;110(9):3345–51.
101. Agostinelli C, Piccaluga PP, Went P, et al. Peripheral T cell lymphoma, not otherwise specified: the stuff of genes, dreams and therapies. J Clin Pathol. 2008; 61(11):1160–7.
102. Lenz G, Staudt LM. Aggressive lymphomas. N Engl J Med. 2010;362(15):1417–29.
103. Quintanilla-Martinez L, Franklin JL, Guerrero I, et al. Histological and immunophenotypic profile of nasal NK/T cell lymphomas from Peru: high prevalence of p53 overexpression. Hum Pathol. 1999;30(7):849–55.
104. Oshimi K, Kawa K, Nakamura S, et al. NK-cell neoplasms in Japan. Hematology. 2005;10(3):237–45 (Amsterdam, Netherlands).
105. Lee J, Suh C, Park YH, et al. Extranodal natural killer T-cell lymphoma, nasal-type: a prognostic model from a retrospective multicenter study. J Clin Oncol. 2006;24(4):612–8.
106. Barrionuevo C, Zaharia M, Martinez MT, et al. Extranodal NK/T-cell lymphoma, nasal type: study of clinicopathologic and prognosis factors in a series of 78 cases from Peru. Appl Immunohistochem Mol Morphol. 2007;15(1):38–44.
107. Chan J, Quintanilla-Martinez L, Ferry J, Peh S-C. Extranodal NK/T-cell lymphoma, nasal-type. In: Swerdlow S, Campo E, Harris NL, et al., editors. WHO Classification of tumors of hematopoietic and lymphoid tissues. IVth ed. Lyon: IARC; 2008. p. 285.
108. Au WY, Weisenburger DD, Intragumtornchai T, et al. Clinical differences between nasal and

extranasal natural killer/T-cell lymphoma: a study of 136 cases from the International Peripheral T-Cell Lymphoma Project. Blood. 2009;113(17):3931–7.
109. Kwong YL, Chan AC, Liang R, et al. CD56+ NK lymphomas: clinicopathological features and prognosis. Br J Haematol. 1997;97(4):821–9.
110. Chan JK. Natural killer cell neoplasms. Anat Pathol. 1998;3:77–145.
111. Cheung MM, Chan JK, Lau WH, Ngan RK, Foo WW. Early stage nasal NK/T-cell lymphoma: clinical outcome, prognostic factors, and the effect of treatment modality. Int J Radiat Oncol Biol Phys. 2002;54(1):182–90.
112. Kuo TT, Shih LY, Tsang NM. Nasal NK/T cell lymphoma in Taiwan: a clinicopathologic study of 22 cases, with analysis of histologic subtypes, Epstein-Barr virus LMP-1 gene association, and treatment modalities. Int J Surg Pathol. 2004;12(4):375–87.
113. Au WY, Pang A, Choy C, Chim CS, Kwong YL. Quantification of circulating Epstein-Barr virus (EBV) DNA in the diagnosis and monitoring of natural killer cell and EBV-positive lymphomas in immunocompetent patients. Blood. 2004;104(1): 243–9.
114. Ng SB, Lai KW, Murugaya S, et al. Nasal-type extranodal natural killer/T-cell lymphomas: a clinicopathologic and genotypic study of 42 cases in Singapore. Mod Pathol. 2004;17(9):1097–107.
115. Chim CS, Ma SY, Au WY, et al. Primary nasal natural killer cell lymphoma: long-term treatment outcome and relationship with the International Prognostic Index. Blood. 2004;103(1):216–21.
116. Huang WT, Chang KC, Huang GC, et al. Bone marrow that is positive for Epstein-Barr virus encoded RNA-1 by in situ hybridization is related with a poor prognosis in patients with extranodal natural killer/T-cell lymphoma, nasal type. Haematologica. 2005; 90(8):1063–9.
117. Lee J, Suh C, Huh J, et al. Effect of positive bone marrow EBV in situ hybridization in staging and survival of localized extranodal natural killer/T-cell lymphoma, nasal-type. Clin Cancer Res. 2007; 13(11):3250–4.
118. Suzuki R, Suzumiya J, Yamaguchi M, et al. Prognostic factors for mature natural killer (NK) cell neoplasms: aggressive NK cell leukemia and extranodal NK cell lymphoma, nasal type. Ann Oncol. 2010;21(5):1032–40.

Molecular and Clinical Aspects of Angioimmunoblastic T-Cell Lymphoma

4

Laurence de Leval, Francine Foss, and Philippe Gaulard

Introduction: Historical Perspective

Angioimmunoblastic T-cell lymphoma (AITL) was originally described in the 1970s as "angioimmunoblastic lymphadenopathy (AILD) with dysproteinemia" by Frizzera et al. [1] and subsequently as "immunoblastic lymphadenopathy" [2] or "lymphogranulomatosis X" [3]. The disease was initially reported as a non-neoplastic lymphoproliferative disorder and believed to represent an abnormal "hyperimmune" reaction of the B-cell system or an atypical lymphoid process, despite a clinical course characterized by multiple relapses, the development of malignant lymphoma in some cases, and a fatal outcome in the majority of patients [2]. Subsequently, Shimoyama and colleagues reported morphologic features of malignancy in cases with clinical and histological features otherwise similar to those of AILD, for which they proposed the designation of "immunoblastic T-cell lymphoma," and that they suggested to consider as a variant of PTCL [4]. In addition, later in the 1980s, the identification of clonal cytogenetic abnormalities and the demonstration of clonal T-cell receptor (TCR) gene rearrangements definitively established the neoplastic nature of the disease [5–8].

Thereafter, AITL was recognized as one of the most common forms of PTCL in the REAL and subsequent WHO classifications of hematologic malignancies [9, 10]. According to a recent international survey, AITL represents the second most common form of mature T/NK-cell malignancies, accounting for 18.5% of the cases worldwide [11]. Interestingly, there are important geographic variations, and the disease is more common in Europe (representing 29% of the cases) than in North America or Asia, where its prevalence is estimated to 16% and 18% of the cases, respectively [12]. The reasons for this heterogeneous distribution across different countries are not known. Part of it might be explained by the overall low prevalence of T-cell neoplasms in Western countries and a relative overrepresentation of other NK/T-cell lymphoma types in Asia, but true differences might exist. Yet no risk factors or etiologic agent(s) have been identified, and no racial predisposition is recognized.

L. de Leval
Institute of Pathology, CHUV, Lausanne, Switzerland

F. Foss
Department of Medical Oncology/Hematology, Yale University School of Medicine, New Haven, CT, USA

P. Gaulard (✉)
Département de Pathologie, Hôpital Henri Mondor, 51 Avenue du Maréchal de Lattre de Tassigny, 94010 Créteil, France
e-mail: philippe.gaulard@hmn.aphp.fr

F. Foss (ed.), *T-Cell Lymphomas*, Contemporary Hematology,
DOI 10.1007/978-1-62703-170-7_4,

Pathological Spectrum of Angioimmunoblastic T-Cell Lymphoma

Architectural Patterns

Lymph nodes almost constantly involved in AITL represent the tissue most frequently harvested for pathologic analysis and diagnosis (Table 4.1). AITL displays distinctive pathological features. According to Attygalle and colleagues, lymph node involvement in AITL can be classified according to three overlapping architectural patterns [13–16]. In pattern I (AITL with hyperplastic follicles) seen least frequently, the lymph node has a partially preserved architecture and contains hyperplastic follicles with numerous tingible body macrophages, poorly developed mantles, and ill-defined borders, merging into the paracortex expanded by a polymorphous infiltrate comprising often inconspicuous neoplastic cells, which tend to distribute in the vicinity of the hyperplastic follicles. In pattern II (AITL with depleted follicles), occasional depleted follicles are present. The pattern III (AITL without follicles), by far the most frequent, is characterized by complete loss of architecture, absence of residual B-cell follicles, and prominent irregular proliferation of FDCs. Conversely, FDCs are normal or minimally increased in patterns I and II. These three patterns, reported to comprise increasing numbers of neoplastic cells and to evolve toward a more diffuse distribution, are thought to reflect morphologic evolution of the disease rather than clinical progression [13–16].

Usual Morphologic Features

In pattern III most commonly encountered, the architecture of the lymph node is effaced, often with capsular and perinodal infiltration sparing the peripheral cortical sinus. The lymph node is occupied by a diffuse polymorphous infiltrate including variable proportions of medium-sized neoplastic T cells, admixed with small lymphocytes, histiocytes or epithelioid cells, immunoblasts, eosinophils, and plasma cells, and associated with prominent arborizing blood vessels and a perivascular proliferation of FDCs (Fig. 4.1a, b). Typically, the lymphoma cells are medium-sized cells with round or slightly irregular nuclei and abundant clear cytoplasm and distinct cell membranes (Fig. 4.1c). They are often less abundant than the reactive background and may even comprise only a minority of the T-cell compartment [17, 18]. This neoplastic component,

Table 4.1 Major pathological features of angioimmunoblastic T-cell lymphoma

Criteria	Characteristic features
Pattern of lymphoproliferation	Diffuse nodal involvement (pattern III)
	Less common: with hyperplastic follicles (pattern I) or with regressed follicles (pattern II)
	Increased density of high-endothelial venules
Cytologic features	Polymorphic infiltrate: neoplastic and reactive cells
	Neoplastic cells: small to medium-sized, clear cytoplasm
	Reactive cells: B-cell blasts, plasma cells, eosinophils, histiocytes
	FDC expansion
Immunophenotype	CD2+, CD3+/dim, CD4+/dim, CD5+, CD7−/+, CD8−, CD10+, CD10+/-
	Positivity for Tfh markers (BCL-6, CXCL13, PD1, ICOS, SAP, c-MAF)
Molecular genetics	Monoclonal *TCR* gene rearrangement in up to 95% of the cases
	Monoclonal or oligoclonal *IGH* and/or *IGK* and/or *IGL* gene rearrangement in up to 33% of the cases
Cytogenetics	Trisomies of chromosomes 3, 5, and 21, gain of X, and loss of 6q
EBV	Detected in the majority of cases, in B cells

EBV Epstein–Barr virus; *FDC* follicular dendritic cell; *Tfh* follicular helper T cell

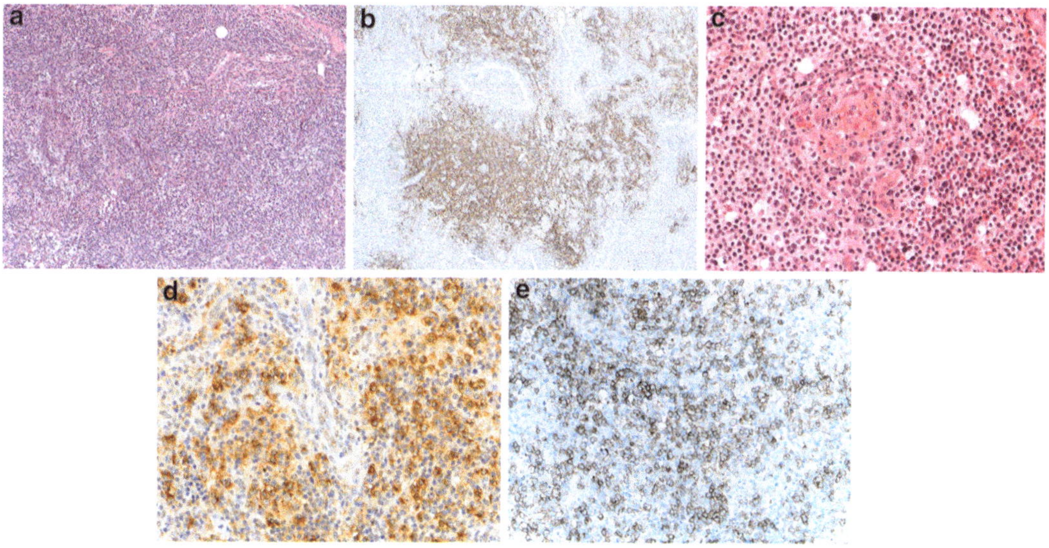

Fig. 4.1 Typical histopathologic features of angioimmunoblastic T-cell lymphoma. (**a**) Lymph node involvement characterized by a diffuse lymphoproliferation associated with arborizing blood vessels (×100); (**b**) follicular dendritic cell (FDC) proliferation in angioimmunoblastic T-cell lymphoma highlighted by CD21 immunostaining (×25); (**c**) high magnification showing medium-sized neoplastic lymphoid cells with clear cytoplasm (×200); (**d**) CXCL13 usually produces intense cytoplasmic staining of most tumor cells (×200); (**e**) PD1 is positive in most neoplastic cells (×200)

which may be difficult to readily identify by morphology alone and is better highlighted by immunohistochemistry for T-cell markers, tends to form small clusters around high endothelial venules. In a subset of cases, the neoplastic cells are smaller with only slight pleomorphism and atypia, and without striking clear cell component. The disease is accompanied by a variable number of scattered large B-blasts often infected by the EBV, which may morphologically mimic Reed–Sternberg cells.

Morphologic Variants According to Cell Content

A subset of cases contain a high proportion of large B-cell blasts (>25%) (*B-cell-rich AITL*), which are usually but not always infected by EBV; the importance of the large B-cell component does not seem to impact the clinical outcome [18, 19]. Although the neoplastic infiltrate in disease tissues is often subtle, a subset of AITL cases (less than 10%) comprise an overt lymphomatous proliferation of sheets of "clear" neoplastic cells [20]. Such cases, referred to as "clear cell-rich AITL," do not appear to differ from usual cases in terms of clinical outcome [18]. The *epithelioid variant* of AITL, characterized by a high content of epithelioid cells, raises differential diagnosis issues as it can suggest a granulomatous disease or be mistaken for other histiocyte-rich lymphomas such as the lymphoepithelioid variant of PTCL, NOS (Lennert's lymphoma), mixed cellularity Hodgkin lymphoma, or even with B-cell lymphomas (lymphoplasmacytic lymphoma or T-cell/histiocyte-rich large B-cell lymphoma in cases rich in large B cells) [21].

Immunophenotype

In involved tissues, the majority of infiltrating lymphocytes are T cells comprising an admixture of CD4+ and CD8+ cells, among which the tumor cell population may be difficult to identify [22, 23]. Nevertheless, it is established that in the majority of cases, the neoplastic cells of AITL consist of mature αβ CD4+ CD8− T cells [17, 23–25]. Aberrancies in the pattern of expression of pan-T-cell antigens are frequently observed—although this may be difficult to assess due to the low content in neoplastic cells—most commonly loss or reduced expression of CD7 or surface CD3, sometimes low or heterogeneous CD4 expression. Conversely, the expression of CD2 and CD5 is usually intact. Partial expression of CD30 by the neoplastic cells has been documented in up to one-third of the cases [23].

Aberrant CD10 antigen expression first reported in 2002 [13] is now validated by immunohistochemistry and/or flow cytometry as a sensitive marker for AITL, observed in around 80% of the cases [14, 18, 23, 26–28]. In many cases, the expression of CD10 is heterogeneous (detected on an often minor subset of the tumor cells and of variable intensity). Since aberrant CD10 expression is maintained in most involved extranodal sites, it is a useful marker for identification of AITL dissemination [26]. As detailed below, it has been recently shown that neoplastic T cells can be recognized by the expression of several markers of the follicular helper T cells (T_{FH}), such as CXCL13, PD1, inducible costimulator (ICOS), CD200 [29], or BCL6 or c-MAF (Fig. 4.1d, e). Immunohistochemical criteria also include the demonstration of a variable proportion of scattered CD20+ B blasts, often expressing CD30 and EBV-infected, and of a proliferation of FDCs—highlighted by using classical FDC markers CD21, CD23, CNA.42, and/or CD35—typically in association with expanded high endothelial venules.

Extranodal Organs

Extranodal sites, especially bone marrow and skin, are also frequently involved in AITL patients. Bone marrow involvement has been reported to occur in up to 70% of the cases [30]. In the bone marrow, AITL infiltrates are often subtle, appearing as often small single or multiple nodular or interstitial foci of infiltration in a paratrabecular or non-paratrabecular distribution, which are often difficult to distinguish from reactive lymphocytic infiltrates. Accordingly, despite the absence of peripheral blood leukocytosis with lymphocytosis in most patients, low numbers of circulating tumor cells may be demonstrated due to an aberrant immunophenotype (most commonly CD10+ and/or sCD3− or dim) and/or clonal TCR gene rearrangement [30–32].

Exceptionally, AITL may lead to complete replacement of hematopoietic tissues [33]. In addition, secondary changes of the hematopoietic tissue are frequently observed, including bone marrow hypercellularity, eosinophilia, myelofibrosis, hematophagocytosis, or reactive polyclonal plasmacytosis, which may obscure the lymphoma infiltrate [30, 34].

Different histopathologic aspects can be seen in skin biopsies, ranging from subtle nonspecific mild perivascular lymphocytic infiltrate to, more rarely, an overtly lymphomatous diffuse infiltration containing numerous atypical T cells [35, 36]. The distribution of the atypical lymphoid infiltrates in other organs is less well characterized. Splenomegaly and tonsillar swelling are common in AITL, but spleen and Waldeyer's ring are rarely the site of diagnosis [37]. The multiple extranodal sites of involvement can be paralleled with the common detection of tumoral cells in peripheral blood in AITL patients at diagnosis.

Clonality Analysis in AITL

Several large studies have reported clonality analysis of the *TCR* and immunoglobulin *(IG)* genes in AITL [8, 14, 17, 38–42]. In the most recent publications using sensitive PCR techniques, the detection of monoclonal or oligoclonal rearrangement of the *TCR* is found in the majority of cases—although not all—(up to 95% in the series reported by the Biomed-2 consortium when multiplex strategies targeting the β, γ, and δ *TCR* loci). In one recent study, sequence analysis of the rearranged *TCRB* genes showed overrepresentation of the BV17S1 family compared to the use of other Vβ segments [43].

In addition to *TCR* rearrangement, a clonal or oligoclonal rearrangement of the *IG* gene(s) is also found in up to one-third of patients. B-cell clonality tends to be evidenced in cases comprising an increased number of B-cell blasts, which may or may not be associated with EBV infection [41, 44]. Most EBV-infected B cells show ongoing mutational activity and carry hypermutated *IG* genes with destructive mutations, suggesting that in AITL alternative pathways operate to allow the survival of these mutating "forbidden" (Ig-deficient) B cells [44].

Genetic Alterations in AITL

By conventional cytogenetic analysis, clonal aberrations are detected in up to 90% of the cases (reviewed in ref. [45]). The most common recurrent abnormalities are trisomies of chromosomes 3, 5, and 21, gain of X, and loss of 6q [6, 46, 47]. Specific chromosomal abnormalities do not seem to be associated with survival, but complex karyotypes adversely impact the clinical outcome [46, 48]. Genetic heterogeneity manifested by unrelated clonal and non-clonal abnormalities in the same patient has been mentioned in cytogenetic reports, possibly reflective of genetic instability [48], and also perhaps linked to genetic alterations in the EBV-positive B-cell blasts [47]. Intriguingly, whereas a high frequency of chromosomal imbalances was confirmed by matrix-based CGH in a series of 39 AITL, with gains identified more commonly than losses, there was little overlap with classical cytogenetic data: tri somies 3 and 5 were infrequent and the most frequent gains were of 22q, 19, and 11p11-q14, and losses of 13q [49].

Chromosomal breakpoints affecting the *TCR* gene loci appear to be extremely rare: only one of 54 AITLs analyzed in two recent FISH-based studies was found to have a break, involving the *TCR A/B* locus [50, 51]. The molecular alterations underlying the neoplastic transformation remain unknown. Mutations of *p53* are infrequent, and mutations in the 5′ region of *BCL6* have not been detected [52]. A role for the c-MAF transcription factor has been suggested, because its overexpression in transgenic mice induces the development of T-cell lymphomas, and high levels of c-MAF have been detected in human AITL tissues [53]. However, *c-MAF* rearrangements are not evidenced in AITL, and hence the presence of c-MAF protein in AITL neoplastic cells represents an additional witness of their ontogenic derivation from T_{FH} cells rather than the reflection of an oncogenic event [54]. Recently, novel recurrent mutations have been reported in AITL, involving the Ten Eleven Ten 2 (*TET2*) and isocitrate dehydrogenase 2 (*IDH2*) genes in approximately 35% and 20% of the cases, respectively [55, 56].

Molecular Signature Provides Further Evidence That AITL Derives from Follicular Helper T Cells

Critical insights into the understanding of AITL have been gained from molecular profiling analyses. In our study, we firstly defined the global molecular signature of 18 AITL cases in comparison to that of 16 PTCL, NOS samples, and subsequently, given the availability of sorted tumor cell suspensions for profiling, distinguished the respective contributions of the tumor cells and the nontumor cells to the AITL signature [57]. Somewhat in accordance with the known pathological features and diagnostic criteria, the AITL molecular profile was dominated by a strong microenvironment imprint, including overexpression of B-cell- and FDC-related genes, chemokines, and chemokine receptors, and genes related to extracellular matrix and vascular biology. Interestingly, the signature contributed by the neoplastic cells, albeit quantitatively minor, was enriched in genes normally expressed by T_{FH} cells (Fig. 4.2). T_{FH} cells constitute a minor subset of effector T cells with a specific microanatomic distribution in the apical zone of reactive germinal centers, and distinct gene signature and functions separable from the other known Th1, Th2, Th17 effector subsets [58, 59]. The demonstration of molecular similarities between AITL tumor cells and T_{FH} cells at a genome-wide level definitively established the cellular derivation of AITL from T_{FH} cells, initially suspected on the basis of the expression of single T_{FH} markers in

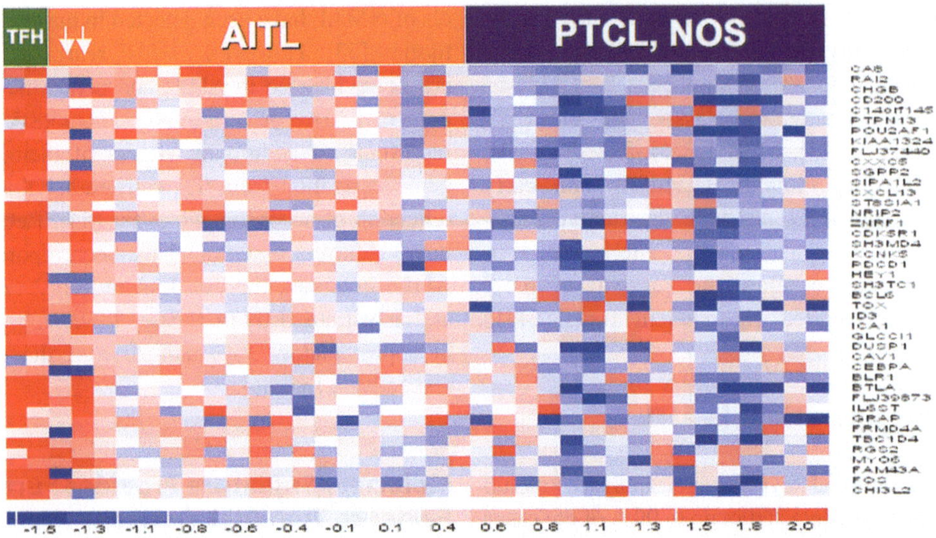

Fig. 4.2 Molecular signatures of AITL and PTCL, NOS by gene expression profiling analysis. Expression data from two normal T_{FH} cell populations, 2 AITL tumor cell suspension samples (*arrows*), 17 AITL tissue samples, and 16 PTCL, NOS samples are shown. The genes represented in this heatmap include a set of 42 core genes representative of normal T_{FH} cells, overexpressed in AITL (by comparison to PTCL, NOS) and overrepresented in sorted AITL tumor cells (*arrows*) in comparison to AITL tissues (as demonstrated by gene set enrichment analyses). Standardized expression ranges from −2.0 (*blue*) to 2.0 (*red*) (adapted from de Leval et al. [57], with permission from John Wiley & Sons, Inc.)

AITL tumor cells, in particular the CXCL13 chemokine [62]. The molecular link between T_{FH} cells and AITL has been confirmed in other gene expression profiling datasets by independent investigators [60, 61].

This peculiar gene expression signature translates into the expression of T_{FH} markers that represent novel diagnostic markers of the disease. Strikingly, cytoplasmic expression of the CXCL13 chemokine is found in the neoplastic cells in most AITL cases [62, 63]. Additional markers of normal T_{FH} cells, including the cell surface molecules CXCR5, CD154, programmed death-1 (PD-1) (a member of the CD28 costimulatory receptor family resulting in negative regulation of T-cell activity), and ICOS (a CD28 homologue with costimulatory function in T-cell activation and expansion), have been demonstrated in AITL by immunohistochemistry [16, 27, 64–68]. Another cytoplasmic protein, SAP (SLAM-associated protein), has been recently validated as a novel marker of both normal germinal center T cells and AITL [66]. Nuclear expressions of the BCL6 and c-MAF transcription factors, which are characteristic of the T_{FH} subset of CD4+ cells, represent other phenotypic traits of AITL tumor cells [15, 28, 54]. On tissue sections, the distribution and the intensity of the immunostainings observed for the different T_{FH} markers tend to correlate and, similar to CD10, to show a relationship to the FDC meshwork. For diagnostic purposes, CXCL13, PD1, and BCL6 currently represent the most useful and robust T_{FH} markers amenable to routine paraffin section immunohistochemistry. In terms of specificity, CXCL13 is probably superior to PD1, ICOS, and BCL6, which can also be expressed in a subset of extrafollicular T cells. It has also been reported that CXCL13 is a more helpful marker than CD10 to recognize the neoplastic nature of subtle infiltrates in extranodal sites, for example, the skin [36].

The cellular derivation of AITL from T_{FH} cells provides a rational model to explain several of the peculiar pathological and biological features inherent to this disease, i.e., the expansion of B cells, the intimate association with germinal centers in early disease stages, and the striking proliferation of FDCs. Among the molecular mediators of T_{FH}

cells, CXCL13 likely plays a key role. New future insights in the precise functions of the network of mediators involved in the generation of T_{FH} cells and their role in the immune system will certainly contribute to the better understanding of the pathogenesis of AITL. The reason why this peculiarly small subset of T cells gives rise to one of the most frequent T-cell lymphoma entity is unexplained and the molecular alterations targeting neoplastic T_{FH} cells and their role in lymphomagenesis remain to be deciphered. Moreover, these recently accumulated data suggest that the morphological spectrum of AITL may be larger than previously defined. Indeed, a T_{FH} imprint has been demonstrated in a subset of cases morphologically classified as PTCL, NOS that may represent evolution from AITL, and in rare forms of PTCL with a follicular growth pattern [57, 69, 70].

Role of the Tumor Microenvironment

Non-neoplastic cells typically represent a quantitatively major component of AITL and, clinically, the manifestations of the disease mostly reflect a deregulated immune and/or inflammatory response rather than direct complications of tumor growth [18] supporting the concept of a paraneoplastic immunological dysfunction (Fig. 4.3). Moreover, AITL patients have defective T-cell responses, linked to both quantitative and qualitative perturbations of T-cell subsets [32, 71]. A depletion in T_{reg} cells and an accumulation of Th_{17} cells have been recently reported in AITL tissues [72, 73]. Interestingly, normal T_{FH} cells suppress T-cell responses by inhibiting the proliferation and function of conventional CD4 T cells,

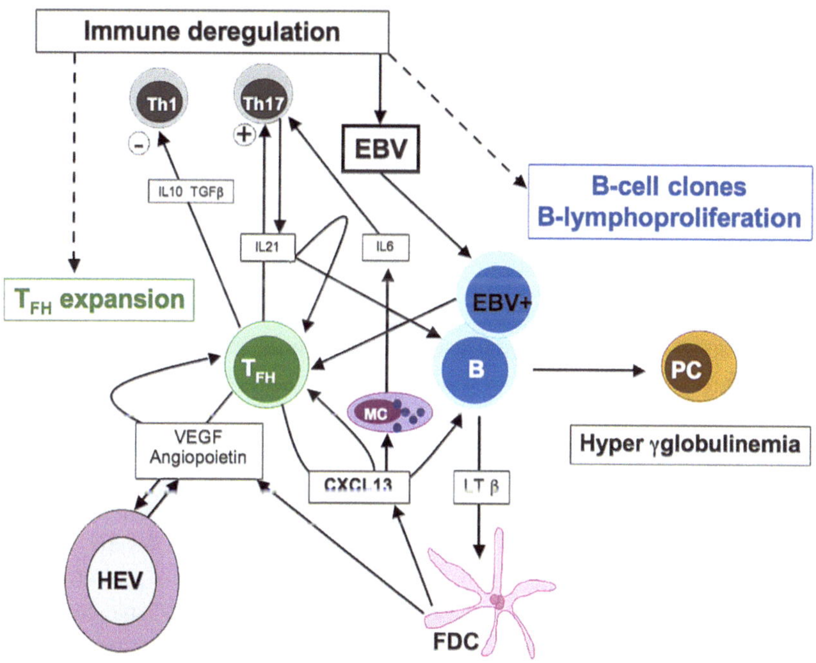

Fig. 4.3 Pathogenetic model of angioimmunoblastic T-cell lymphoma. In AITL, a complex network of interactions take place between the tumor cells and the various cellular components of the reactive microenvironment, the molecular mediators of which are partly deciphered. Different factors released by T_{FH} cells are involved in B-cell recruitment, activation, and differentiation (CXCL13), in the modulation of other T-cell subsets (IL21, IL10, TFGβ), or in promoting vascular proliferation (VEGF, angiopoietin), and may also act as autocrine factors. CXCL13 may also attract mast cells (MC), which are a source of IL6 promoting Th17 differentiation. EBV reactivation occurs in the context of a deregulated immune response, which also favors the expansion of both T_{FH} cells and B cells. TGFβ is a mediator of FDC differentiation and proliferation, and FDC in turn are a source of CXCL13 and VEGF. *B* B-cell; *FDC* FDC; *HEV* high endothelial venule; *MC* mast cell; *PC* plasma cell

especially through TGF-β and IL-10 production [74]. The complex pathways and networks and the mediators linking the various cellular non-neoplastic and neoplastic components are only partly deciphered. Lymphotoxin beta demonstrated in AITL tumor cells [75] and potentially released by B cells under CXCL13 stimulation might be involved in inducing FDC proliferation.

Upregulation of several angiogenic mediators has been demonstrated in AITL. Vascular endothelial growth factor (VEGF) is overexpressed in AITL and probably acts as a key mediator of the prominent vascularization observed in the disease [61, 69]. By immunostaining, neoplastic cells and endothelial cells are positive for both VEGF and its receptor, suggesting the possibility of some paracrine and/or autocrine loop [61, 76]. Moreover, FDCs represent another source of VEGF. The angiopoietin system may also play an important role as angiopoietin 1, which is expressed by AITL neoplastic cells and FDCs [61, 76].

Overall, the importance of the microenvironment and its potential role in tumor growth may have clinical implications for the use of novel targeted therapies.

Infectious Agents in AITL

The etiology of AITL remains unknown, and there are no consistent risk factors for the disease. The original descriptions of AILD emphasized that in many patients the disease was preceded by allergic reactions, infections, and/or administration of drugs, especially antibiotics, which led to the speculation that AITL occurred as a result of abnormal immune reaction. Several reports also mentioned an association with various bacterial or fungal infections. It is now believed that these associations likely reflect the consequences of immune deregulation in AITL patients and do not bear a causal relationship.

EBV-positive cells are detected in most cases of AITL, and it is now established that these EBV-infected cells are B cells, indicating that the virus is unlikely to play a primary role in lymphomagenesis. Zhou et al. recently found that higher EBV viral loads in biopsies correlated with progression of histological patterns and with B-cell clonality [77]. In the latter study, PCR showed the presence of HHV6B in almost half of the cases. The involvement of other herpesviruses, in particular HHV8, appears very unlikely [77]. Although viral infection/reactivation likely occurs as a consequence of the underlying immune dysfunction, EBV and potentially also HHV6B may, through the modulation of cytokines, chemokines, and membrane receptors, play a role in the development of the tumor microenvironment, ultimately favoring disease progression. Interestingly, HHV6B also has immunosuppressive properties.

Clinical Features and Treatment

The median age of presentation for AITL is 59–65 years. A slight or marked male predominance is repeatedly reported. AITL may present as a subacute or acute systemic illness and may be associated with infections or other disorder of immune deregulation. Generalized lymphadenopathy and constitutional symptoms such as fever and weight loss are common features. A high proportion of patients have hepatomegaly and/or splenomegaly. Bone marrow involvement has been reported in up to 70% of the cases and tends to correlate with a higher frequency of B symptoms, hepatosplenomegaly, laboratory abnormalities, and the presence of circulating tumor cells [30]. Up to half of the patients have skin rash—either generalized or a predominantly truncal maculopapular eruption mimicking an inflammatory dermatosis—and/or pruritus, prior to or concurrent with the diagnosis of lymphoma, or at relapse. Nodular lesions, plaques, purpura, and urticarial lesions can also be seen [78]. Overall, most patients have concomitant extranodal disease, and the disease is stage III or IV in more than 80% of cases.

Laboratory tests often disclose a variety of hematological, biochemical, and/or immunological abnormalities. Anemia, polyclonal hypergammaglobulinemia, and hypereosinophilia are the most common alterations seen at diagnosis. Other common findings include lymphopenia, thrombocytopenia, and the presence of various autoantibodies (rheumatoid factor, antinuclear factor, anti-smooth muscle), cryoglobulins, or cold agglutinins.

The prognostic significance of various other clinicobiological and pathological features was evaluated in a retrospective series of 157 AITL patients retrieved from the Goupe d' Etude des Lymphomes de l'Adulte (GELA) LNH87-LNH93 randomized trials [18]. In multivariate analysis, only male sex, mediastinal lymphadenopathy, and anemia adversely affected overall survival.

Clinical Approaches for AITL

The optimal therapeutic approach for AITL has not been determined. Steroids have been used as a single-agent approach, especially in elderly patients. Most patients receive combination chemotherapeutic regimens, such as cyclophosphamide, doxorubicin, vincristine, prednisone (CHOP); and cyclophosphamide, vincristine, prednisolone, bleomycin, doxorubicin, procarbazine, ifosfamide, methotrexate, and etoposide (COPBLAM/IMVP-16), but none of these has increased the long-term survival rate to more than 30%. A number of single-agent therapies have also been used, including methotrexate together with steroids, fludarabine or 2-chlorodeoxyadenosine, and cyclosporine A [79–84]. These reports are often anecdotal or correspond to limited phase II trials with response rates averaging 30%, and there is no consensus whether any of these agents improve outcomes more than conventional treatment, even in combination.

Is More Intensive Treatment with Transplantation Better?

The possible benefit of high-dose chemotherapy with ASCT (HDT-ASCT) for AITL patients was demonstrated in a retrospective multicenter study of the European Group for Blood and Marrow Transplantation, which reported 146 AITL patients who received ASCT in different situations (relapse, refractory, first complete remission) [85]. After a median follow-up of 31 months, the actuarial overall survival (OS) was 67% at 24 months and 59% at 48 months. The estimated progression-free survival (PFS) rates were 70% and 56% at 24 and 48 months, respectively, for patients who received their transplants in CR; 42% and 30% for patients with chemotherapy-sensitive disease; and 23% at both time points for patients with chemotherapy-refractory disease.

There are now emerging data on allogeneic transplantation in small cohorts of patients with PFS and OS rates of 66% and 64% at 3 years, respectively, with a relapse rate at 3 years estimated at 20%. However, whether allogeneic transplantation offers additional benefit over autologous transplantation to young patients remains to be determined.

Newer Agents for AITL

The most commonly used treatment for PTCL is CHOP or variant regimens. However, the results with CHOP are inadequate, and new approaches are needed. The activities of new drugs are being described in studies designed for PTCL patients, and attempts at novel combinations are emerging. Alemtuzumab, a monoclonal anti-CD52 antibody, has recently been added to CHOP for the treatment of PTCL. Twenty-four consecutive patients with newly diagnosed PTCL, including six AITL, enrolled in a prospective multicenter trial received a combination of alemtuzumab with CHOP [86]. There was CR in 17 of 24 (71%) patients. At a median follow-up of 16 months, 13/24 patients (54%) were disease-free with an estimated 2-year OS and failure-free survival of 53% and 48% respectively. Several Phase II trials with alemtuzumab alone or combined with chemotherapy gave encouraging results for first-line treatment, with manageable toxicities. A phase II study of CHOP with denileukin diftitox for 37 untreated PTCL, including 10 AITL, showed clinical activity with an 86% response rate (76% CR) and a 2-year PFS estimate of 41%, and only little added toxicity over CHOP [87]. The addition of rituximab to target CD20-positive B-cells along with CHOP was explored as first-line therapy for AITL, but results were similar to CHOP alone.

Therapies targeting VEGF mediators have been proposed in relation to the expression of both VEGF and its receptor by neoplastic cells of AITL. Bevacizumab has shown anecdotal activity in PTCL, particularly AITL, and has been added to CHOP in an ongoing Eastern Cooperative Oncology Group trial for newly diagnosed patients with PTCL. This study has been associated with enhanced cardiac toxicity [88].

Pralatrexate, a novel antifolic drug, demonstrated activity in PTCL in a study of 111 patients with relapsed and refractory PTCL including 13 AITL [89]. The overall response rate was 27, including 11 CR. Median duration of response was 9 months, and the dose-limiting toxicities were thrombocytopenia and stomatitis. Romidepsin, a novel histone deacetylase inhibitor (HDACi), showed a 35% response rate in relapsed/refractory PTCL, including in several patients with AITL [90].

In summary, despite the use of aggressive regimens with anthracycline-based chemotherapy, AITL is largely incurable without a stem cell transplant. Prognostic factors associated with response to various modalities have not been elucidated. Novel agents are being explored with promising results in small numbers of patients.

Acknowledgments This study was supported in part by grants from FRM (Fondation pour la Recherche Médicale, équipe labellisée) and the Cancer Plan research Programme (Belgium, LdL).

References

1. Frizzera G, Moran E, Rappaport H. Angio-immunoblastic lymphadenopathy with dysproteinemia. Lancet. 1974;1:1070–3.
2. Lukes RJ, Tindle BH. Immunoblastic lymphadenopathy. A hyperimmune entity resembling Hodgkin's disease. N Engl J Med. 1975;292:1–8.
3. Lennert K. [Nature, prognosis and nomenclature of angioimmunoblastic lymphadenopathy (lymphogranulomatosis X or T-zone lymphoma)]. Dtsch Med Wochenschr. 1979;104:1246–7.
4. Shimoyama M, Minato K. [Clinical, cytological and immunological analysis of T-cell type lymphoid malignancies: a classification of T-cell type lymphoid malignancy (author's transl)]. Rinsho Ketsueki. 1979;20:1056–69.
5. Feller AC, Griesser H, Schilling CV, et al. Clonal gene rearrangement patterns correlate with immunophenotype and clinical parameters in patients with angioimmunoblastic lymphadenopathy. Am J Pathol. 1988;133:549–56.
6. Kaneko Y, Maseki N, Homma C, et al. Chromosome translocations involving band 7q35 or 7p15 in childhood T-cell leukemia/lymphoma. Blood. 1988;72:534–8.
7. Tobinai K, Minato K, Ohtsu T, et al. Clinicopathologic, immunophenotypic, and immunogenotypic analyses of immunoblastic lymphadenopathy-like T-cell lymphoma. Blood. 1988;72:1000–6.
8. Weiss LM, Strickler JG, Dorfman RF, Horning SJ, Warnke RA, Sklar J. Clonal T-cell populations in angioimmunoblastic lymphadenopathy and angioimmunoblastic lymphadenopathy-like lymphoma. Am J Pathol. 1986;122:392–7.
9. Harris NL, Jaffe ES, Stein H, et al. A revised European-American classification of lymphoid neoplasms: a proposal from the International Lymphoma Study Group. Blood. 1994;84:1361–92.
10. Jaffe ES, Krenacs L, Raffeld M. Classification of cytotoxic T-cell and natural killer cell lymphomas. Semin Hematol. 2003;40:175–84.
11. Vose J, Armitage J, Weisenburger D. International peripheral T-cell and natural killer/T-cell lymphoma study: pathology findings and clinical outcomes. J Clin Oncol. 2008;26:4124–30.
12. Rudiger T, Weisenburger DD, Anderson JR, et al. Peripheral T-cell lymphoma (excluding anaplastic large-cell lymphoma): results from the Non-Hodgkin's Lymphoma Classification Project. Ann Oncol. 2002;13:140–9.
13. Attygalle A, Al-Jehani R, Diss TC, et al. Neoplastic T cells in angioimmunoblastic T-cell lymphoma express CD10. Blood. 2002;99:627–33.
14. Attygalle AD, Kyriakou C, Dupuis J, et al. Histologic evolution of angioimmunoblastic T-cell lymphoma in consecutive biopsies: clinical correlation and insights into natural history and disease progression. Am J Surg Pathol. 2007;31:1077–88.
15. Ree HJ, Kadin ME, Kikuchi M, et al. Angioimmunoblastic lymphoma (AILD-type T-cell lymphoma) with hyperplastic germinal centers. Am J Surg Pathol. 1998;22:643–55.
16. Rodriguez-Justo M, Attygalle AD, Munson P, Roncador G, Marafioti T, Piris MA. Angioimmunoblastic T-cell lymphoma with hyperplastic germinal centres: a neoplasia with origin in the outer zone of the germinal centre? Clinicopathological and immunohistochemical study of 10 cases with follicular T-cell markers. Mod Pathol. 2009;22:753–61.
17. Willenbrock K, Renne C, Gaulard P, Hansmann ML. In angioimmunoblastic T-cell lymphoma, neoplastic T cells may be a minor cell population. A molecular single-cell and immunohistochemical study. Virchows Arch. 2005;446:15–20.
18. Mourad N, Mounier N, Briere J, et al. Clinical, biologic, and pathologic features in 157 patients with

angioimmunoblastic T-cell lymphoma treated within the Groupe d'Etude des Lymphomes de l'Adulte (GELA) trials. Blood. 2008;111:4463–70.
19. Lome-Maldonado C, Canioni D, Hermine O, et al. Angio-immunoblastic T cell lymphoma (AILD-TL) rich in large B cells and associated with Epstein-Barr virus infection. A different subtype of AILD-TL? Leukemia. 2002;16:2134–41.
20. Merchant SH, Amin MB, Viswanatha DS. Morphologic and immunophenotypic analysis of angioimmunoblastic T-cell lymphoma: emphasis on phenotypic aberrancies for early diagnosis. Am J Clin Pathol. 2006;126:29–38.
21. Patsouris E, Noel H, Lennert K. Angioimmunoblastic lymphadenopathy—type of T-cell lymphoma with a high content of epithelioid cells. Histopathology and comparison with lymphoepithelioid cell lymphoma. Am J Surg Pathol. 1989;13:262–75.
22. Chen W, Kesler MV, Karandikar NJ, McKenna RW, Kroft SH. Flow cytometric features of angioimmunoblastic T-cell lymphoma. Cytometry B Clin Cytom. 2006;70:142–8.
23. Karube K, Aoki R, Nomura Y, et al. Usefulness of flow cytometry for differential diagnosis of precursor and peripheral T-cell and NK-cell lymphomas: analysis of 490 cases. Pathol Int. 2008;58:89–97.
24. Lee PS, Lin CN, Chuang SS. Immunophenotyping of angioimmunoblastic T-cell lymphomas by multiparameter flow cytometry. Pathol Res Pract. 2003;199: 539–45.
25. Stacchini A, Demurtas A, Aliberti S, et al. The usefulness of flow cytometric CD10 detection in the differential diagnosis of peripheral T-cell lymphomas. Am J Clin Pathol. 2007;128:854–64.
26. Attygalle AD, Diss TC, Munson P, Isaacson PG, Du MQ, Dogan A. CD10 expression in extranodal dissemination of angioimmunoblastic T-cell lymphoma. Am J Surg Pathol. 2004;28:54–61.
27. Dorfman DM, Brown JA, Shahsafaei A, Freeman GJ. Programmed death-1 (PD-1) is a marker of germinal center-associated T cells and angioimmunoblastic T-cell lymphoma. Am J Surg Pathol. 2006;30:802–10.
28. Yuan CM, Vergilio JA, Zhao XF, Smith TK, Harris NL, Bagg A. CD10 and BCL6 expression in the diagnosis of angioimmunoblastic T-cell lymphoma: utility of detecting CD10+ T cells by flow cytometry. Hum Pathol. 2005;36:784–91.
29. Dorfman D, Shahsafaei A. CD200 (OX-2 membrane glycoprotein) is expressed by follicular helper T cells and in angioimmunoblastic T-cell lymphoma. Am J Surg Pathol. 2011;35(1):76–83.
30. Cho YU, Chi HS, Park CJ, Jang S, Seo EJ, Huh J. Distinct features of angioimmunoblastic T-cell lymphoma with bone marrow involvement. Am J Clin Pathol. 2009;131:640–6.
31. Baseggio L, Berger F, Morel D, et al. Identification of circulating CD10 positive T cells in angioimmunoblastic T-cell lymphoma. Leukemia. 2006;20:296–303.
32. Delfau-Larue MH, de Leval L, Joly B, et al. Targeting intratumoral B-cells with Rituximab in addition to CHOP in angioimmunoblastic T-cell lymphoma.A clinicobiological study of the GELA. Haematologica. 2012 Feb 27. [Epub ahead of print]
33. Sakai H, Tanaka H, Katsurada T, Yoshida Y, Okamoto E, Ohno H. Angioimmunoblastic T-cell lymphoma initially presenting with replacement of bone marrow and peripheral plasmacytosis. Intern Med. 2007; 46:419–24.
34. Grogg KL, Morice WG, Macon WR. Spectrum of bone marrow findings in patients with angioimmunoblastic T-cell lymphoma. Br J Haematol. 2007;137:416–22.
35. Martel P, Laroche L, Courville P, et al. Cutaneous involvement in patients with angioimmunoblastic lymphadenopathy with dysproteinemia: a clinical, immunohistological, and molecular analysis. Arch Dermatol. 2000;136:881–6.
36. Ortonne N, Dupuis J, Plonquet A, et al. Characterization of CXCL13+ neoplastic t cells in cutaneous lesions of angioimmunoblastic T-cell lymphoma (AITL). Am J Surg Pathol. 2007;31:1068–76.
37. Frizzera G, Moran EM, Rappaport H. Angio-immunoblastic lymphadenopathy. Diagnosis and clinical course. Am J Med. 1975;59:803–18.
38. Attygalle AD, Chuang SS, Diss TC, Du MQ, Isaacson PG, Dogan A. Distinguishing angioimmunoblastic T-cell lymphoma from peripheral T-cell lymphoma, unspecified, using morphology, immunophenotype and molecular genetics. Histopathology. 2007;50:498–508.
39. Bruggemann M, White H, Gaulard P, et al. Powerful strategy for polymerase chain reaction-based clonality assessment in T-cell malignancies. Report of the BIOMED-2 Concerted Action BHM4 CT98-3936. Leukemia. 2007;21:215–21.
40. Kawano R, Ohshima K, Wakamatsu S, Suzumiya J, Kikuchi M, Tamura K. Epstein-Barr virus genome level, T-cell clonality and the prognosis of angioimmunoblastic T-cell lymphoma. Haematologica. 2005;90:1192–6.
41. Tan BT, Warnke RA, Arber DA. The frequency of B- and T-cell gene rearrangements and Epstein-Barr virus in T-cell lymphomas: a comparison between angioimmunoblastic T-cell lymphoma and peripheral T-cell lymphoma, unspecified with and without associated B-cell proliferations. J Mol Diagn. 2006;8:466–75; quiz 527.
42. Vrsalovic MM, Korac P, Dominis M, Ostojic S, Mannhalter C, Kusec R. T- and B-cell clonality and frequency of human herpes viruses-6, -8 and Epstein Barr virus in angioimmunoblastic T-cell lymphoma. Hematol Oncol. 2004;22:169–77.
43. Shah ZH, Harris S, Smith JL, Hodges E. Monoclonality and oligoclonality of T cell receptor beta gene in angioimmunoblastic T cell lymphoma. J Clin Pathol. 2009;62:177–81.
44. Brauninger A, Spieker T, Willenbrock K, et al. Survival and clonal expansion of mutating "forbidden" (immunoglobulin receptor-deficient) Epstein-Barr virus-infected b cells in angioimmunoblastic t cell lymphoma. J Exp Med. 2001;194:927–40.
45. de Leval L, Bisig B, Thielen C, Boniver J, Gaulard P. Molecular classification of T-cell lymphomas. Crit Rev Oncol Hematol. 2009;72(2):125–43.

46. Nelson M, Horsman DE, Weisenburger DD, et al. Cytogenetic abnormalities and clinical correlations in peripheral T-cell lymphoma. Br J Haematol. 2008;141:461–9.
47. Dogan A, Attygalle AD, Kyriakou C. Angioimmunoblastic T-cell lymphoma. Br J Haematol. 2003;121:681–91.
48. Schlegelberger B, Feller A, Godde W, Lennert K. Stepwise development of chromosomal abnormalities in angioimmunoblastic lymphadenopathy. Cancer Genet Cytogenet. 1990;50:15.
49. Thorns C, Bastian B, Pinkel D, et al. Chromosomal aberrations in angioimmunoblastic T-cell lymphoma and peripheral T-cell lymphoma unspecified: a matrix-based CGH approach. Genes Chromosomes Cancer. 2007;46:37–44.
50. Gesk S, Martin-Subero JI, Harder L, et al. Molecular cytogenetic detection of chromosomal breakpoints in T-cell receptor gene loci. Leukemia. 2003;17:738–45.
51. Leich E, Haralambieva E, Zettl A, et al. Tissue microarray-based screening for chromosomal breakpoints affecting the T-cell receptor gene loci in mature T-cell lymphomas. J Pathol. 2007;213:99–105.
52. Kerl K, Vonlanthen R, Nagy M, et al. Alterations on the 5′ noncoding region of the BCL-6 gene are not correlated with BCL-6 protein expression in T cell non-Hodgkin lymphomas. Lab Invest. 2001;81:1693–702.
53. Murakami YI, Yatabe Y, Sakaguchi T, et al. c-Maf expression in angioimmunoblastic T-cell lymphoma. Am J Surg Pathol. 2007;31:1695–702.
54. Bisig B, et al. c-Maf expression in angioimmunoblastic T-cell lymphoma reflects follicular helper T-cell derivation rather than oncogenesis. Histopathology. 2012;60:371–6.
55. Quivoron C, et al. TET2 inactivation results in pleiotropic hematopoietic abnormalities in mouse and is a recurrent event during human lymphomagenesis. Cancer Cell. 2011;20:25–38.
56. Cairns RA, et al. IDH2 mutations are frequent in angioimmunoblastic T-cell lymphoma. Blood. 2012; 119:1901–3.
57. De Leval L, Gisselbrecht C, Gaulard P. Advances in the understanding and management of angioimmunoblastic T-cell lymphoma. Br J Haematol. 2010;148(5):673–89.
58. Fazilleau N, Mark L, McHeyzer-Williams LJ, McHeyzer-Williams MG. Follicular helper T cells: lineage and location. Immunity. 2009;30:324–35.
59. Vinuesa CG, Tangye SG, Moser B, Mackay CR. Follicular B helper T cells in antibody responses and autoimmunity. Nat Rev Immunol. 2005;5:853–65.
60. Iqbal J, Weisenburger DD, Greiner TC, et al. Molecular signatures to improve diagnosis in peripheral T-cell lymphoma and prognostication in angioimmunoblastic T-cell lymphoma. Blood. 2010;115:1026–36.
61. Piccaluga PP, Agostinelli C, Califano A, et al. Gene expression analysis of angioimmunoblastic lymphoma indicates derivation from T follicular helper cells and vascular endothelial growth factor deregulation. Cancer Res. 2007;67:10703–10.
62. Dupuis J, Boye K, Martin N, et al. Expression of CXCL13 by neoplastic cells in angioimmunoblastic T-cell lymphoma (AITL): a new diagnostic marker providing evidence that AITL derives from follicular helper T cells. Am J Surg Pathol. 2006;30:490–4.
63. Grogg KL, Attygalle AD, Macon WR, Remstein ED, Kurtin PJ, Dogan A. Angioimmunoblastic T-cell lymphoma: a neoplasm of germinal-center T-helper cells? Blood. 2005;106:1501–2.
64. Krenacs L, Schaerli P, Kis G, Bagdi E. Phenotype of neoplastic cells in angioimmunoblastic T-cell lymphoma is consistent with activated follicular B helper T cells. Blood. 2006;108:1110–1.
65. Marafioti T, Paterson JC, Ballabio E, et al. The inducible T-cell co-stimulator molecule is expressed on subsets of T cells and is a new marker of lymphomas of T follicular helper cell-derivation. Haematologica. 2010;95:432–9.
66. Roncador G, Garcia Verdes-Montenegro JF, Tedoldi S, et al. Expression of two markers of germinal center T cells (SAP and PD-1) in angioimmunoblastic T-cell lymphoma. Haematologica. 2007;92:1059–66.
67. Xerri L, Chetaille B, Serriari N, et al. Programmed death 1 is a marker of angioimmunoblastic T-cell lymphoma and B-cell small lymphocytic lymphoma/chronic lymphocytic leukemia. Hum Pathol. 2008;39:1050–8.
68. Yu H, Shahsafaei A, Dorfman DM. Germinal-center T-helper-cell markers PD-1 and CXCL13 are both expressed by neoplastic cells in angioimmunoblastic T-cell lymphoma. Am J Clin Pathol. 2009;131:33–41.
69. de Leval L, Rickman DS, Thielen C, et al. The gene expression profile of nodal peripheral T-cell lymphoma demonstrates a molecular link between angioimmunoblastic T-cell lymphoma (AITL) and follicular helper T (TFH) cells. Blood. 2007;109:4952–63.
70. Huang Y, Moreau A, Dupuis J, et al. Peripheral T-cell lymphomas with a follicular growth pattern are derived from follicular helper T cells (TFH) and may show overlapping features with angioimmunoblastic T-cell lymphomas. Am J Surg Pathol. 2009;33:682–90.
71. Pizzolo G, Vinante F, Agostini C, et al. Immunologic abnormalities in angioimmunoblastic lymphadenopathy. Cancer. 1987;60:2412–8.
72. Bruneau J, Canioni D, Renand A, et al. Regulatory T-cell depletion in angioimmunoblastic T-cell lymphoma. Am J Pathol. 2010;177:570–4.
73. Tripodo C, Gri G, Piccaluga PP, et al. Mast cells and Th17 cells contribute to the lymphoma-associated proinflammatory microenvironment of angioimmunoblastic T-cell lymphoma. Am J Pathol. 2010;177:792–802.
74. Marinova E, Han S, Zheng B. Germinal center helper T cells are dual functional regulatory cells with suppressive activity to conventional CD4+ T cells. J Immunol. 2007;178:5010–7.
75. Foss HD, Anagnostopoulos I, Herbst H, et al. Patterns of cytokine gene expression in peripheral T-cell lymphoma of angioimmunoblastic lymphadenopathy type. Blood. 1995;85:2862–9.

76. Zhao WL, Mourah S, Mounier N, et al. Vascular endothelial growth factor-A is expressed both on lymphoma cells and endothelial cells in angioimmunoblastic T-cell lymphoma and related to lymphoma progression. Lab Invest. 2004;84:1512–9.
77. Zhou Y, Attygalle AD, Chuang SS, et al. Angioimmunoblastic T-cell lymphoma: histological progression associates with EBV and HHV6B viral load. Br J Haematol. 2007;138:44–53.
78. Yoon GS, Choi YK, Bak H, et al. Angioimmunoblastic T cell lymphomas: frequent cutaneous skin lesions and absence of human herpes viruses. Ann Dermatol. 2009;21:1–5.
79. Advani R, Warnke R, Sikic BI, Horning S. Treatment of angioimmunoblastic T-cell lymphoma with cyclosporine. Ann Oncol. 1997;8:601–3.
80. Bourgeois E, Auxenfants E, Jouffrey C, Dubest C, Mahieu M, Rose C. [Efficacy of fludarabine in the treatment of angioimmunoblastic lymphoma (AIL)]. Ann Med Interne (Paris). 2000;151:230–1.
81. Gerlando Q, Barbera V, Ammatuna E, Franco V, Florena AM, Mariani G. Successful treatment of angioimmunoblastic lymphadenopathy with dysproteinemia-type T-cell lymphoma by combined methotrexate and prednisone. Haematologica. 2000;85:880–1.
82. Murayama T, Imoto S, Takahashi T, Ito M, Matozaki S, Nakagawa T. Successful treatment of angioimmunoblastic lymphadenopathy with dysproteinemia with cyclosporin A. Cancer. 1992;69:2567–70.
83. Quintini G, Iannitto E, Barbera V, et al. Response to low-dose oral methotrexate and prednisone in two patients with angio-immunoblastic lymphadenopathy-type T-cell lymphoma. Hematol J. 2001;2:393–5.
84. Sallah AS, Bernard S. Treatment of angioimmunoblastic lymphadenopathy with dysproteinemia using 2-chlorodeoxyadenosine. Ann Hematol. 1996;73:295–6.
85. Kyriakou C, Canals C, Goldstone A, et al. High-dose therapy and autologous stem-cell transplantation in angioimmunoblastic lymphoma: complete remission at transplantation is the major determinant of Outcome-Lymphoma Working Party of the European Group for Blood and Marrow Transplantation. J Clin Oncol. 2008;26:218–24.
86. Gallamini A, Zaja F, Patti C, et al. Alemtuzumab (Campath-1 H) and CHOP chemotherapy as first-line treatment of peripheral T-cell lymphoma: results of a GITIL (Gruppo Italiano Terapie Innovative nei Linfomi) prospective multicenter trial. Blood. 2007; 110:2316–23.
87. Foss FM, Sjak-Shie NN, Goy A, Advani R, Jacobsen ED. Phase II study of denileukin diftitox with CHOP chemotherapy in newly-diagnosed PTCL: CONCEPT trial [ASCO meeting abstracts]. J Clin Oncol. 2010; 28:8045.
88. Advani RH, Hong F, Ganjoo KN, et al. Cardiac toxicity associated with the anti-VEGF monoclonal antibody bevacizumab (avastin) in combination with CHOP (A-CHOP) chemotherapy for peripheral T cell lymphoma (PTCL): the ECOG 2404 trial [ASH annual meeting abstracts]. Blood. 2009; 114:1671.
89. O'Connor O, Pro B, Pinter-Brown L, et al. PROPEL: results of the pivotal, multicenter, phase II study of pralatrexate in patients with relapsed or refractory peripheral T-cell lymphoma (PTCL) [ASCO meeting abstracts]. J Clin Oncol. 2009;27:8561.
90. Coiffier B, Pro B, Prince HM, et al. Final results from a pivotal, multicenter, international, open-label, phase 2 Study of romidepsin in progressive or relapsed peripheral T-cell lymphoma (PTCL) following prior systemic therapy [ASH annual meeting abstracts]. Blood. 2010;116:114.

Primary Cutaneous and Systemic CD30+ T-cell Lymphoproliferative Disorders

5

Marshall E. Kadin and Francine Foss

Historical Perspective and Overview

CD30+ lymphoproliferative diseases are a recently recognized group of diseases whose identification was made possible by reaction of the tumor cells with an antibody raised against a Hodgkin lymphoma cell line, L428 [1]. In screening reactivity of the antibody, Stein and coworkers discovered a subset of large-cell lymphomas which also expressed the Hodgkin-associated antigen [2]. The antibody was called Ki-1 after the location of investigators in Kiel, Germany, but later was given the cluster designation CD30. CD30 was found to be a member of the TNF receptor superfamily [3]. Mir and coworkers showed a dual effect of CD30 signaling, causing proliferation of Hodgkin cells but apoptosis of anaplastic large-cell lymphoma (ALCL) cells [4]. In 1985, Kadin and coworkers observed that the atypical Reed–Sternberg-like cells in lymphomatoid papulosis (LyP), a recurrent cutaneous eruption, express CD30 as well as T-cell antigens [5]. This led to clarification of the histogenesis of a spectrum of cutaneous papules, nodules, and tumors, initially thought to be regressing atypical histiocytosis, and later to become known as CD30+ cutaneous lymphoproliferative disorders. This spectrum includes LyP, cutaneous ALCL, and borderline lesions which are not readily be distinguished clinically or histologically from LyP or ALCL. In 1986, Kadin and coworkers described a series of children and adolescents with skin lesions and peripheral lymphadenopathy [6]. Unlike patients with CD30+ cutaneous lymphoproliferative disorders who lack lymphadenopathy, these children with lymphadenopathy at presentation had an aggressive disease requiring multiagent chemotherapy. This clinicopathologic entity became known as systemic ALCL. Rimokh et al. found that cell line Karpas 299 derived from a pleural effusion of a patient with systemic ALCL contained a reciprocal translocation t(2;5)(p23;q35) [7]. Further studies revealed this is a recurrent translocation characteristic of 80% of systemic ALCL [8]. In 1994, Morris et al. cloned the t(2;5) breakpoint and discovered a novel oncogenic protein derived from fusion of nuclear chaperone protein, nucleophosmin (NPM) at chr. 5p35, and a newly recognized tyrosine kinase designated as ALK after Anaplastic Lymphoma Kinase, at 2p23 [9]. Japanese investigators raised a polyclonal antibody against the p80 component of ALK which revealed that ALK positive (ALK+) ALCL has a better prognosis than ALK(−) ALCL [10]. Pulford et al. found ALK to be immunogenic and

M.E. Kadin
Department of Dermatology and Skin Surgery, Boston University of Medicine and Roger Williams Medical Center, Providence, RI, USA

F. Foss (✉)
Department of Medical Oncology/Hematology, Yale University School of Medicine, 333 Cedar Street, FMP 130, PO Box 208032, New Haven, CT 06520, USA
e-mail: Francine.foss@yale.edu

F. Foss (ed.), *T-Cell Lymphomas*, Contemporary Hematology,
DOI 10.1007/978-1-62703-170-7_5, © Springer Science+Business Media New York 2013

raised a monoclonal antibody (ALK-1) which now is used clinically to aid identification and diagnosis of systemic ALCL [11]. Clinical studies later confirmed that ALK+ systemic ALCL is a clinicopathologic entity occurring mainly in children and adolescents with a significantly better prognosis than ALK(−) systemic ALCL or peripheral T-cell lymphoma, not otherwise specified [12].

Cutaneous CD30+ Lymphoproliferative Disorders

Primary cutaneous CD30+ T-cell lymphoproliferative disorders are the second most common type of cutaneous T-cell lymphomas (CTCL). These disorders comprise a spectrum of clinically benign LyP and primary cutaneous anaplastic large-cell lymphoma (PCALCL). The peak incidence is in the fifth decade for LyP and sixth decade for PCACL, but children are also affected. Both LyP and PCALCL have an excellent prognosis. However, LyP is associated with development of malignant lymphoma (mycosis fungoides, Hodgkin lymphoma, or ALCL) in 20% of cases, and also with an increased risk of non-lymphoid cancers. The diagnosis of LyP is difficult and often delayed. PCALCL must be distinguished from secondary skin lesions in systemic ALCL which confer a poor prognosis. Correlation of clinical findings with histopathology and immunopathology (stains for ALK kinase, epithelial membrane antigen (EMA), and cutaneous lymphocyte antigen (CLA)) is important to achieve a correct diagnosis. When a diagnosis of CD30+ PCLPD is established, minimal clinical staging is required. Bone marrow involvement is rare and thus bone marrow biopsy is not indicated. Lymph node involvement is uncommon and when it occurs does not appear to portend a poor prognosis. Low-dose methotrexate (10–25 mg weekly) is the most effective therapy for primary cutaneous lymphoproliferative disorders but is usually reserved only for aggressive cases of LyP and multifocal lesions of cutaneous ALCL. Many patients with LyP can be followed expectantly with special attention to change in character of skin lesions or development of lymphadenopathy. Patients with localized cutaneous ALCL can be treated with irradiation. Extracutaneous spread of disease is an indication for multiagent chemotherapy. Other treatment alternatives are discussed.

Cutaneous CD30+ Lymphoproliferative Disorders

The primary cutaneous CD30-positive (CD30+) T-cell lymphoproliferative disorders are a group of largely indolent diseases that manifest as nodules or tumors of the skin. The European Organization for Research and Treatment of Cancer has developed a modification of the World Health Organization lymphoma classification system that specifically categorizes these entities. According to Willemze et al., the CD30+ diseases include primary ALCL, primary CD30+ lymphoproliferative disorder, and LyP [13]. These comprise about 25% of the CTCL. Often confused with more aggressive T-cell lymphomas with similar histopathologic features, these diseases are difficult to diagnose and poorly understood (Fig. 5.1). LyP patients have clinically benign self-healing skin papules and/or nodules which have the unexpected histopathology of a high-grade malignant lymphoma [14]. Primary cutaneous ALCL also have the histology of a high-grade lymphoma but only 25% of lesions regress spontaneously. Because of their histologic appearance and frequent recurrence, patients with CD30+ PCLPD may be treated unnecessarily with multiagent chemotherapy. However, the prognosis is excellent. Disease-specific survival of LyP patients at 5 years is 100% and overall survival at 5 years is 92% [15, 16]. Disease-specific survival of PCALCL is 85–90% [15, 16].

Diagnosis

LyP often is not diagnosed correctly upon presentation; it is common for symptoms to persist for 1–3 years before a correct diagnosis is established. A variety of diagnoses are entertained but most commonly insect, spider, or mosquito bite.

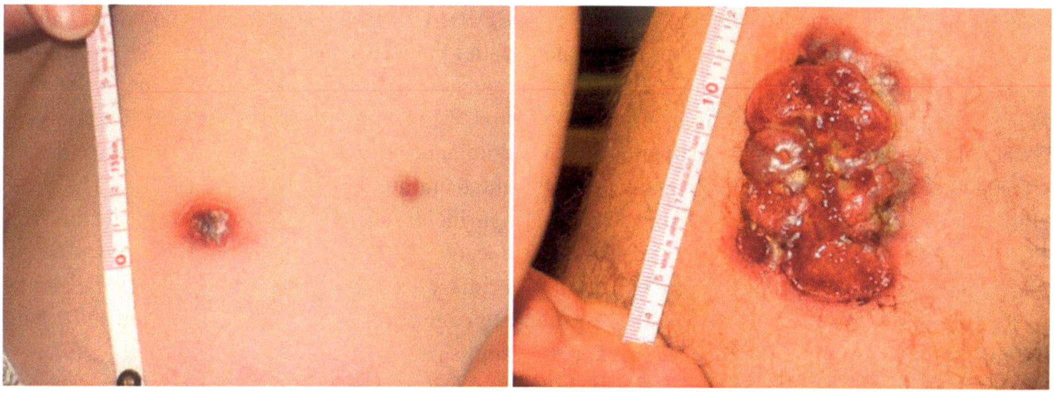

Fig. 5.1 Spectrum of LyP and Cutaneous ALCL in an individual patient. *Left*: Two LyP lesions are seen with erythema and central necrosis in the larger lesion. *Right*: The cutaneous ALCL is larger and elevated without signs of regression

This is likely due to the common occurrence of bites with associated erythema and central necrosis, whereas most patients and many clinicians are unfamiliar with LyP.

Tumor cells in both LyP and PCALCL are derived from activated T-cells which express CD30 antigen. The CD30+ cells are larger than normal lymphocytes and have basophilic cytoplasm and large nuclei with a prominent nucleolus resembling immunoblasts. These cells often are bi- or multinucleated giving the appearance of Reed–Sternberg cells. Mitoses are frequent and often atypical. In LyP, tumor cells are scattered throughout the upper dermis and surrounded by small lymphocytes, neutrophils, and eosinophils. In PCALCL, tumor cells form large clusters or sheets that generally extend from the dermal–epidermal junction down into the subcutaneous fatty tissue. Thus the distinction of LyP from ALCL largely depends on the density of CD30+ tumor cells and the extent of dermal and subcutaneous involvement.

Differential Diagnosis

The frequency of LyP in male children poses an interesting differential diagnosis with pityriasis lichenoides et varioliformis acuta (PLEVA). PLEVA can present with similar cutaneous lesions but has a different prognostic significance. In particular, there is no increased risk to develop lymphoma among patients with PLEVA while the risk of lymphoma in LyP patients approaches 20% [15, 17]. PLEVA is more common in children and young adults than in older patients so the most difficult differential diagnosis is in the age group under 30 years. Skin lesions in PLEVA tend to be hemorrhagic papules whereas LyP lesions vary from papules to small nodules often with central whitening and ulceration due to accumulation of neutrophils in the epidermis. LyP shows more frequent large bizarre cells including bi- or multinucleated cells with basophilic cytoplasm; these cells are CD30+. Such cells are infrequent or absent in PLEVA. Necrosis of individual keratinocytes (Civatte and colloid bodies) is usual in PLEVA but absent in LyP. Further, immunopathology reveals a predominance of CD4+ lymphocytes in LyP but mostly CD8+ lymphocytes in PLEVA. Nodular scabies is also in the differential diagnosis of LyP, particularly in children. Scabies also includes CD30+ cells. It is found in the inguinal and genital areas which can be affected in LyP. In scabies, the CD30+ cells co-express B-cell antigens whereas CD30+ cells in LyP express T-cell antigens.

Distinction from Systemic ALCL

Oncologists need to be aware of the distinction of CD30+ PCLPD from secondary skin lesions in patients with nodal/systemic ALCL. Skin is the most common extranodal site of disease in nodal/systemic ALCL and skin lesions confer an increased risk of failure in childhood ALCL [18, 19]. When skin lesions are a presenting manifestation of nodal/systemic ALCL, the distinction from CD30+ PCLPC is imperative. The distinction of skin lesions in systemic ALCL from CD30+ PCLPC can be difficult on purely clinical grounds and may be difficult as well to achieve by routine histopathology. One of the most helpful approaches is to test the tumor cells for expression of the ALK protein. This is expressed in skin lesions of most patients with nodal/systemic ALCL but not in the large majority of patients with CD30+ PCLPD. Rare exceptions occur and in such cases, therefore a panel of immunologic markers is recommended. EMA is expressed on tumor cells in 82% of nodal/systemic ALCL but <5% of CD30+ PCLPD [20]. CLA also is more frequently expressed in CD30+ PCLPD (44%) than on tumor cells in nodal/systemic ALCL (18%). Thus, a successful immunopathologic distinction of CD30+ PCLPD from nodal/systemic ALCL can be made in most cases.

Staging of Cutaneous CD30+ Lymphoproliferative Disorders

When a diagnosis of CD30+ PCLPD is established, minimal clinical staging is required. Bone marrow involvement is rare and thus bone marrow biopsy is not indicated. Lymph node involvement is uncommon and when it occurs does not appear to portend a poor prognosis [15]. In the case of systemic involvement, regional lymph nodes are the most common sites of involvement. Often this is minimal microscopic involvement with tumor cells confined to lymph node sinuses and not effacing lymph node architecture. This may be detected by immunohistochemical staining for CD30, which in combination with morphology, can reveal microscopic disease.

Etiology

Although CD30+ PCLPD are rare, all races, ages, and both genders are affected. The prevalence of CD30+ CLPD in the USA is unknown but an LyP patient support group includes 850 members indicating a prevalence approaching 3 per million. Most European studies show a male predominance whereas our US registry has a nearly equal number of males and females. The peak age incidence of LyP appears to be in the fifth decade. However, children are also affected. Primary cutaneous ALCL has a peak incidence after age 50 but can also affect children and young adults.

CD30 signaling is known to have an effect on the growth and survival of lymphoid cells. CD30 transcription is under control of a genetically determined polymorphic promoter. Franchina et al. analyzed CD30 promoter microsatellite alleles in 32 unrelated Caucasian patients diagnosed with LyP alone or LyP plus lymphoma, as well as 8 unrelated Caucasian patients with CD30+ primary cutaneous ALCL [21]. Controls were 57 Caucasian healthy volunteers and patients with non-lymphoid malignancies. Patients and controls were gender-matched. We determined that two allelic forms of the CD30 promoter microsatellite repressive element, designated 30M377 and 30M362, are associated with the development of LyP and CD30+ lymphomas in LyP patients, respectively. These findings suggest that allele-specific differences in the control of CD30 transcription may determine the pathogenesis of the spectrum of CD30+ cutaneous lymphoproliferative disorders.

Njisten et al. reported 35 cases of LyP beginning in childhood [22]. These patients had a significantly higher prevalence of atopy (RR3.1, 95%CI). Compared with the general population, patients with childhood-onset LyP had a significantly increased risk of developing non-Hodgkin lymphoma (relative risk, 226.2; 95% confidence interval, 73.4–697.0). Fletcher also reported an association of CD30+ CLPD with atopic eczema beginning in childhood [23]. Three patients had primary cutaneous ALCL, of whom two developed systemic disease and one died. The fourth patient developed LyP type A which resolved after withdrawal of cyclosporine therapy. We concluded that LyP presents similarly in children and adults, including the risk to develop lymphoma, and patients should be closely monitored for development of lymphoma throughout their lives.

A major concern of LyP patients, and parents of children with LyP, is whether the affected individual will develop a malignant lymphoma. There are many reported individual or small series of cases, but few reports of large numbers of affected patients. In one series, including a review of the literature, 50 patients with LyP-associated lymphomas were evaluated [24]. Three main types of LyP-associated lymphomas were distinguished: cases associated with mycosis fungoides (19/50), Hodgkin's disease (12/50), and CD30+ large-cell lymphoma (16/50). Mycosis fungoides and Hodgkin's disease could develop before, after, or concurrent with LyP, but CD30+ large-cell lymphoma always developed in patients with existing LyP, often showing a slow progression from regressing LyP lesions to persistent skin tumors. Patients with mycosis fungoides, Hodgkin's disease, and CD30+ large-cell lymphoma limited to the skin generally had a favorable prognosis. The prognosis of patients developing a systemic CD30+ large-cell lymphoma was generally poor. Some LyP patients develop Hodgkin's disease followed by a systemic CD30+ large-cell lymphoma which also is associated with a poor prognosis. In a subsequent review of 118 LyP patients in the Netherlands, 23 (19%) developed malignant lymphoma, 11 developed mycosis fungoides, 10 CD30+ LCL, and 2 Hodgkin lymphoma [15].

The relationship between LyP, a T-cell disorder, and Hodgkin's disease, primarily a B-cell disorder, is poorly understood. I am aware of patients who had LyP lesions before or after Hodgkin's disease. When the Hodgkin's disease was treated with chemotherapy, the LyP lesions often disappeared but temporarily only to reappear shortly thereafter. In rare cases, a clonal relationship between the CD30+ cells in LyP and Hodgkin's disease was shown by DNA sequencing. A clonal relationship between LyP and mycosis fungoides, and ALCL is firmly established [25, 26].

In a case–control study of 57 patients with biopsy-proven LyP and 67 individually matched controls, there was a significant increased frequency of prior or coexisting lymphoproliferative disorders, an increased frequency of non-lymphoid malignancies, and exposure to radiation therapy [27]. Among patients with LyP, three had a history of Hodgkins disease, three had NHL, and ten had mycosis fungoides; none of the control subjects reported such histories. Prospective study of this group of patients over an 8-year period (1988–1996) revealed that six LyP patients (10.5%) and one control (1.5%) developed non-lymphoid malignancies. Two patients and one controls developed lymphoid malignancies. The expected numbers of non-lymphoid and lymphoid malignancies in the LyP group based on SEER data were 1.93 and 0.15 respectively, yielding a relative risk (with 95% CI) of 3.11 (1.26–6.47) for non-lymphoid malignancies and 13.33 (2.44–44.05) for malignant lymphoma in LyP patients. There was no significant difference between observed and expected numbers of malignancies in the control group. These results confirm that LyP patients are at increased risk to develop lymphoid malignancies but for the first time revealed that they also have an increased risk of non-lymphoid malignancies [27].

The prognosis of LyP patients developing a systemic CD30+ large-cell lymphoma is generally poor. In two such cases, progression of LyP to systemic ALCL was associated with mutations of receptors for the lymphocyte growth inhibitor, transforming growth-factor beta, allowing unregulated growth of the CD30+ cells [28].

Treatment

Control of LyP lesions does not appear to affect the risk to develop lymphoma. Most patients with few or infrequent papules do not require therapy. For patients with extensive papules, nodules, and/or scarring lesions, particularly on the face or hands, or legs, which appear cosmetically disturbing, the most effective therapies are low-dose oral methotrexate or PUVA/UVB. Methotrexate is effective in controlling lesions in approximately 90% of patients and it induces a permanent remission in up to 20% of patients [29]. Vonderheid treated 45 patients with relatively severe LyP, CD30+ CALCL, and interface/borderline lesions with oral methotrexate. During induction, patients received 10–60 mg/week (median 20 mg/week). Clinical improvement usually occurred quickly, typically at doses of 15–20 mg weekly, and satisfactory long-term control was achieved in 39 patients (87%) with maintenance doses given at 10–14-day intervals (range 7–28 days). Responding patients were usually free of active lesions within 4 weeks of receiving the first dose. After methotrexate was discontinued, ten patients remain free of CD30+ lesions for more than 24 months to more than 227 months (median, more than 127 months). The median total duration of methotrexate therapy for all patients exceeded 39 months (range 2–205 months). Adverse effects were generally mild and transient, and included fatigue (47%), nausea (22%), weight loss (13%), diarrhea, or gastrointestinal cramping (10%), increased serum hepatic transaminase levels (27%), anemia (11%), or leukopenia (9%). Early hepatic fibrosis was found in five of ten patients, all of whom had been treated for more than 3 years (range 38–111 months).

The mechanisms of effectiveness of methotrexate in controlling CD30+ CLPD appear to be its inhibitory effect on DNA synthesis, its anti-inflammatory effects, or both. Because the atypical lymphocytes of LyP and related CD30+ CLPD are characterized by high mitotic activity, it is likely that methotrexate inhibits cell proliferation, particularly in the early phase of lesion development. The observation that long-lasting complete remissions occur after relatively short courses (2–5 months) of methotrexate in some patients raises the possibility that high-dose methotrexate therapy, possibly combined with leucovorin (folinic acid) rescue, might provide more than suppressive therapy for some patients. Moreover, low doses of methotrexate appear to have anti-inflammatory effects separate from its anti-proliferative effect. This may explain why LyP may improve with other drugs that have anti-inflammatory effects, including corticosteroids, tetracycline, and retinoids.

In patients who do not respond to MTX, photo(chemo)-therapy should be considered. Although conventional ultraviolet phototherapy (UVB) may be effective, PUVA administered at dosages ranging from 50–480 J/cm twice weekly result in complete clearing or improvement of lesions in most patients.

Alternative Therapies

Although topically administered steroids may be useful in controlling symptoms of LyP (e.g., pruritus), steroid therapy has not been proven to control disease progression or induce remission. Similarly, antibiotic therapy has not been shown to alter the course of LyP, although anecdotally tetracycline has benefited few patients. In such patients, the role of tetracycline may be related to its anti-inflammatory effect rather its antimicrobial effects. In children with symptomatic LyP, a prolonged trial of tetracycline therapy may be used initially, particularly if there are concerns regarding side effects from MTX, photo(chemo) therapy, or other therapies. Nevertheless, neither steroid nor antibiotic therapy can be recommended as routine LyP management.

Interferon α and interferon γ therapy has been used successfully to treat LyP in few patients. The rationale for the use of interferon was provided by Japanese investigators who showed that CD30+ cells in LyP and cutaneous lymphoma have features of Th2 cells, and that skin lesions could be suppressed by local and intravenous injection of IFNα a Th1 cytokine [30]. Austrian dermatologists treated five patients with Interferon alpha subcutaneously three times per week and compared them with a group of six patients receiving photochemotherapy, antibiotics, topical corticosteroids, or surgery in an open trial. Four patients in the IFN group showed a complete remission and one a partial remission within 6 weeks. Two patients developed recurrent disease after discontinuation of short-term IFN therapy (5–7 months), and one patient remained in partial remission. In the control group, one patient went into spontaneous remission, two patients had partial remission of which one developed progressive disease; three patients had recurrent disease despite treatment. Although IFNα can alter the clinical course, it does not induce stable remissions after short-term treatment [31].

Retinoids can induce apoptosis of T-cells. M.D. Anderson investigators reported the use of bexarotene, (Targretin), a rexinoid with selectivity for intracellular retinoid X receptors in treating LyP. Ten patients with chronic and symptomatic LyP were treated prospectively with bexarotene, three orally, and seven with topical gel formulations. A favorable response with decreased numbers or duration of lesions was seen in all patients with objective responses in eight patients [32]. In patients with localized skin disease, oral bexarotene had a 54% overall response rate at an optimal dose of 300 mg/m^2/day (approximately 10 mg/kg). Topical bexarotene 1.0% gel was effective in producing remissions of individual lesions with an overall response rate of 68%.

Other topical agents that have been used historically for treatment of LyP include mechlorethamine or carmustine. There is no role for multiagent systemic chemotherapies in LyP because LyP recurs quickly and predictably in affected patients who have received such treatments [33].

Primary Cutaneous Anaplastic Large-Cell Lymphoma

While spontaneous regression is characteristic of LyP, 25% of primary cutaneous ALCL lesions will regress [26]. This number is sufficiently high to warrant as initial management expectant follow-up for a period of 4–6 weeks. If spontaneous regression occurs, therapy is not indicated, and such patients should be observed from possible disease recurrence. A small number of patients whose disease spontaneously regresses will not have recurrence of their disease. Therefore, observation for spontaneous regression is an appropriate first step in managing this disease [34].

Unfortunately, most patients with primary cutaneous ALCL have disease that does not regress spontaneously [35]. For these patients, choice of therapy depends on disease distribution and whether the lesions are singular or multiple. An exception to this approach may arise when other associated lymphoproliferative disorders such as mycosis fungoides or symptomatic LyP are simultaneously encountered, in which cases the therapeutic approach should be directed against both diseases [25].

Solitary lesions respond to local radiotherapy [34, 36]. Although surgical excision represents an alternative approach, excision specimens may contain margins involved by disease. For this reason, radiotherapy is the preferred treatment for solitary lesions. Radiotherapy consists of electron beam irradiation (4–10 million eV) with a total radiation dose of 40 Gy. Because electron beam therapy penetrates only to the dermis, there are no systemic effects, although side effects include alopecia, atrophy of sweat glands and skin, radio-dermatitis, and edema.

In general, radiotherapy is impractical for patients with multiple non-regressing lesions, although total skin electron beam therapy may be a consideration if other diseases, like mycosis fungoides, are present. For this reason, systemic therapy is the treatment of choice for this group of patients [37]. Because long-term remissions are generally not achieved with multiagent chemotherapy, less toxic, single-agent therapies are preferred. As in LyP, methotrexate can be effective in inducing remissions, but higher weekly doses of methotrexate may be necessary [29]. In affected patients whose disease is refractory or progressive on methotrexate, oral etoposide has been shown to be safe and effective therapy for primary cutaneous ALCL [38]. Other potential therapies are purine nucleoside analogs (e.g., Pentostatin), retinoids, interferon-α, and interleukin-12 [33]. Recently, studies with humanized anti-CD30 antibody have demonstrated efficacy in patients with cutaneous and systemic ALCL.

Finally, it is important to monitor patients for potential dissemination of primary cutaneous ALCL to lymph nodes and systemic organs, as well as development of associated malignancies, particularly mycosis fungoides, Hodgkin lymphoma, and B-cell non-Hodgkin lymphoma. Patients who develop systemic ALCL should be considered for multiagent systemic chemotherapies similar to those used in treatment of systemic ALCL, e.g., cyclophosphamide, doxorubicin, vincristine, and prednisone (CHOP) or CHOP-like regimens [34, 36]. High-dose chemotherapy followed by stem cell rescue may be indicated in affected patients who are at high risk [34, 36]. Determination of high risk may be based on prognostic factors for survival in the international prognostic index (IPI).

Approach to Patients with CD30+ PCLPD

Patients are often frustrated because of the delay in establishing the correct diagnosis. They are also fearful of their prognosis because of the association of LyP with development of other lymphomas and the high-grade histology of their lesions. The first goal is to reassure the patient about his/her favorable prognosis and to answer their questions about their disease. If the lesions scar or interfere with normal activity, therapies such as low-dose methotrexate may be effective but are not indicated for women of child-bearing age who expect to become pregnant, people with a history of liver disease, or blood dyscrasias. Other options include PUVA/UVB and topical treatments. Careful monitoring is necessary due to the increased risk of mycosis fungoides and ALCL in these patients. For patients with suspected PCALCL, clinical evaluation and pathologic studies should be done to exclude nodal/systemic ALCL. Local irradiation of skin tumors is effective, and use of methotrexate for multifocal cutaneous lesions is often successful. Follow-up of skin lesions should be carried out by a dermatologist and consultation by an oncologist when additional irradiation or multiagent chemotherapy is needed.

Systemic Anaplastic Large-Cell Lymphoma

Systemic ALCL comprises 2–3% of all NHLs [39]. The median age for ALK+ ALCL is 35 (male to female ratio: 3.0), while ALK-negative (ALK−) ALCL is 58–61 years with a male to female ratio of 0.9 [40]. Most patients (60%) have extensive disease at presentation [12, 40]. Extranodal sites in ALK− ALCL include bone, subcutaneous tissue, bone marrow, and spleen, while in ALK+ patients, the most common sites are skin, lung, liver, bone, and bone marrow. Blood involvement is rare except in children. More recently, there has been an association between ALCL and breast implants. A number of cases have reported serosal involvement in the implant pocket. De Jong et al. reported an odds ratio of 18.2 (95% confidence interval, 2.1–156.8) for ALCL associated with breast prostheses [41].

NPM-ALK expression in ALCL has been shown to be a significant prognostic factor [10], with 5-year OS of 93% vs. 37% ($P<0.00001$) and 5-year FFS of 88% vs. 37% ($P<0.0001$) [42]. A retrospective review by Savage et al. confirmed the superior survival of systemic ALK+ ALCL compared with ALK− cases (5-year FFS 60% vs. 36%; $P=0.015$; and 5-year OS 70% vs. 49%; $P=0.016$); however as previously discussed, ALK-positive patients were significantly younger than ALK− patients. When they controlled for age, there were no differences in FFS or OS [12]. Table 5.1 reviews the clinical features and outcomes for both ALK+ and ALK− patients. Both the IPI and the prognosis in T-cell lymphoma' scoring system are predictive of progression-free survival (PFS) and OS survival in ALCL [12]. In addition, expression of CD56, a neural cell adhesion molecule, was shown in a series of 143 patients with ALCL to be a predictor of poor survival (approximately 5-year OS: 28% vs. 65%, $P=0.002$) [43]. The inferior outcome associated with CD56 was seen with ALK+ and ALK− patients.

Immunophenotype

ALCL frequently do not stain with T-cell markers. Up to 75% are CD3 negative, and staining is variable with CD2, CD5, CD4, and CD8 [12, 44]. Virtually all ALCL are positive for CD30 [45]. The small cell variant of ALCL may display positive staining only on the less numerous larger cells and not on the smaller lymphocytes. ALCL may express cytotoxic T-cell markers, including

Table 5.1 Clinical Features and outcomes of ALCL based on ALK status

Clinical feature	ALK+	ALK–	P^a	PTCL-NOS	P^b
Total no. patients (%)	87 (55)	72 (45)		331	
Median age, year	34	58	<0.001	57	0.30
Age less than 60 years, no (%)	74 (86)	42 (58)	<0.001	170 (50)	0.21
Male–female ratio	1.7:1	1.5:1	0.74	1.01	0.41
Stage no. (%)					
II	30 (35)	30 (42)	0.38	102 (31)	18
III	25 (29)	15 (21)		87 (20)	
IV	31 (30)	27 (37)		145 (43)	
Elevated LDH, no. (%)	31 (37)	31 (46)	0.28	158 (49)	0.62
Performance status >2, no. (%)	30 (35)	21 (30)	0.56	60 (18)	0.02
Nodal only disease, no. (%)	39 (54)	38 (49)	0.52	124 (42)	0.07
Extranodal sites >1, no. (%)	17 (19.5)	15 (21)	0.84	99 (29)	0.15
Bulky disease >10 cm, no. (%)	17 (21)	6 (11)	0.17	19 (7)	0.25
B Symptoms, no. (%)	52 (60)	41 (57)	0.72	118 (35)	<0.001
Hemoglobin less than 110 g/L, no. (%)	17 (27)	18 (32)	0.54	61 (22)	0.11
Platelets less than 150×10^8/L, no. (%)	6 (10)	6 (11)	0.83	64 (24)	0.03
IPI score, no. (%)					
0, 1	40 (49)	27 (41)	0.50	88 (28)	0.066
2	18 (22)	13 (20)		111 (35)	
3	12 (15)	16 (24)		71 (22)	
4, 5	12 (14)	10 (15)		48 (15)	
5-year FFS (%)	60	36	0.015	20	0.012
5-year OS (%)	70	49	0.016	32	0.032
5-year FFS by IPI, (%)					
0, 1	80	62		35	
2	61	44	0.022	16	
3	23	15		13	
4,5	25	13		8	
5-year OS by IPI %					
0, 1	90	74		52	
2	68 (*P*<0.001)[c]	62	<001[c]	33	<0.001[c]
3	23	31		16	
4, 5	33	13		13	

Reprinted from [12], with permission from the American Society of Hematology
[a] is statistical comparison between Alk+ and ALK-
[b] is statistical comparison between Alk- and PTCL

perforin, granzyme-B, and TIA-1 [46]. EMA may also be expressed in some cases.

ALK positivity in ALCL is due to rearrangement of the ALK gene located at chromosome 2p23. The most common partner is the NPM gene located at chromosome 5q35 resulting in the (2;5)(p23;q35) translocation [47] followed by the non-muscle tropomyosin gene 3 located at chromosome 1q25 resulting in the (1;2)(q25;p23) translocation [46]. Inversion of the ALK gene, Inv(2)(p23q35), also is seen in a small number of cases, and other fusion partners have also been identified [46]. The NPM/ALK fusion protein constitutively activates a number of intracellular pathways, including phosphatidylinositol 3-kinase-AKT, JAK/STAT, and RAS/MEK/ERK.

Treatment of Systemic ALCL

Chemotherapy

The standard treatment for most patients with systemic ALCL has been CHOP-based chemotherapy. Outcomes using CHOP and related aggressive lymphoma regimens can be derived from large intergroup studies. The GELA has reported results from their trials in which systemic ALCL patients were treated with combination chemotherapy regimens including ACVBP (doxorubicin, cyclophosphamide, vindesine, bleomycin, prednisone) followed by a consolidation phase with high-dose methotrexate, ifosfamide, etoposide, asparaginase, and cytosine-arabinoside or m-BACOD (methotrexate, bleomycin, cyclophosphamide, vincristine, dexamethasone), VIMMM (VM26, ifosfamide, mitoxantrone, methyl-gag, methotrexate)/ACVBP, and CHOP [48]. In those studies, the ALCL patients, not stratified for ALK expression, had a CR rate of 69% and OS of 63% at 5 years. In a retrospective report, Falini et al. examined the outcomes according to ALK expression in 78 patients [40]. Overall survival was better for ALK+ patients when compared to ALK− (71% vs. 15%), and 10-year DFS was 28% for ALK− vs. 82% for ALK+ patients. ALK+ patients with intermediate or high IPI had a worse outcome compared to low IPI ALK+ patients (OS 94% vs. 41%).

Addition of etoposide to CHOP has been explored in a number of trials for patients with aggressive T- and B-cell NHL. In the NHL-B1 trial added etoposide to CHOP in younger patients improved overall survival and disease-free survival in T-cell patients, but results were not significant for ALCL patients due to small numbers [49]. The NHL-B2 explored a more aggressive regimen (CHOP-14 vs. CHOP 21) in older patients (>age 61) and favored the more aggressive regimen, but only 3.5% of patients in this trial had ALCL [50]. In a more recent study from the German High Grade Lymphoma Group in which 78 ALK+ and 113 ALK− patients were randomized to CHOP or CHOEP, the 3-year EFS and OS were 75 and 89% for ALK+ and 45% and 62% for ALK− patients respectively [51]. There was an overall improvement in outcome in OS for the ALK+ patients with the addition of etoposide (3-year EFS 91% vs. 57%, $P=0.12$). However, there was no improvement for patients treated with dose-escalated therapy (Mega CHOEP), and in fact, younger patients who received MegaCHOEP had a worse outcome than those receiving CHOEP-14. In this trial, ALK− patients had a similar outcome to patients with other aggressive nodal PTCL subtypes (PTCLu and AITL). There was a difference in outcome for ALK− patients based on IPI in that the low IPI patients had a favorable outcome, as shown in Fig. 5.2.

Transplantation for ALCL

Autologous Stem Cell Transplant

Autologous stem cell transplant (ASCT) has been a standard treatment for patients in first remission with ALK− ALCL and in first relapse for ALK+ ALCL. Retrospective reviews of autologous transplant data have shown that ALCL patients had the best outcome, with a 3-year DFS of 67% when compared with other T-cell subtypes [52]. The European Group for Blood and Marrow Transplantation reported that patients who were in CR or PR at the time of transplant had better outcomes than those who had chemorefractory disease [53]. The GEL-TAMO experience with 123 patients with relapsed/refractory T-cell NHL, of which 25% cases were ALCL, demonstrated that intermediate or high IPI, extranodal disease, and elevated β2-microglobulin at time of transplant were associated with inferior survival [54]. No significant survival differences were noted for ALCL compared with other T-cell subtypes, and ALK status was not available. Nickelsen et al. reported results from ASCT in first remission [55]. The most common subtype in this study was ALK− ALCL (39%). Patients were treated with 4–6 courses of dose-escalated CHOP plus etoposide and then ASCT. Sixty-seven percent of the T-cell NHL patients were able to complete therapy without progression.

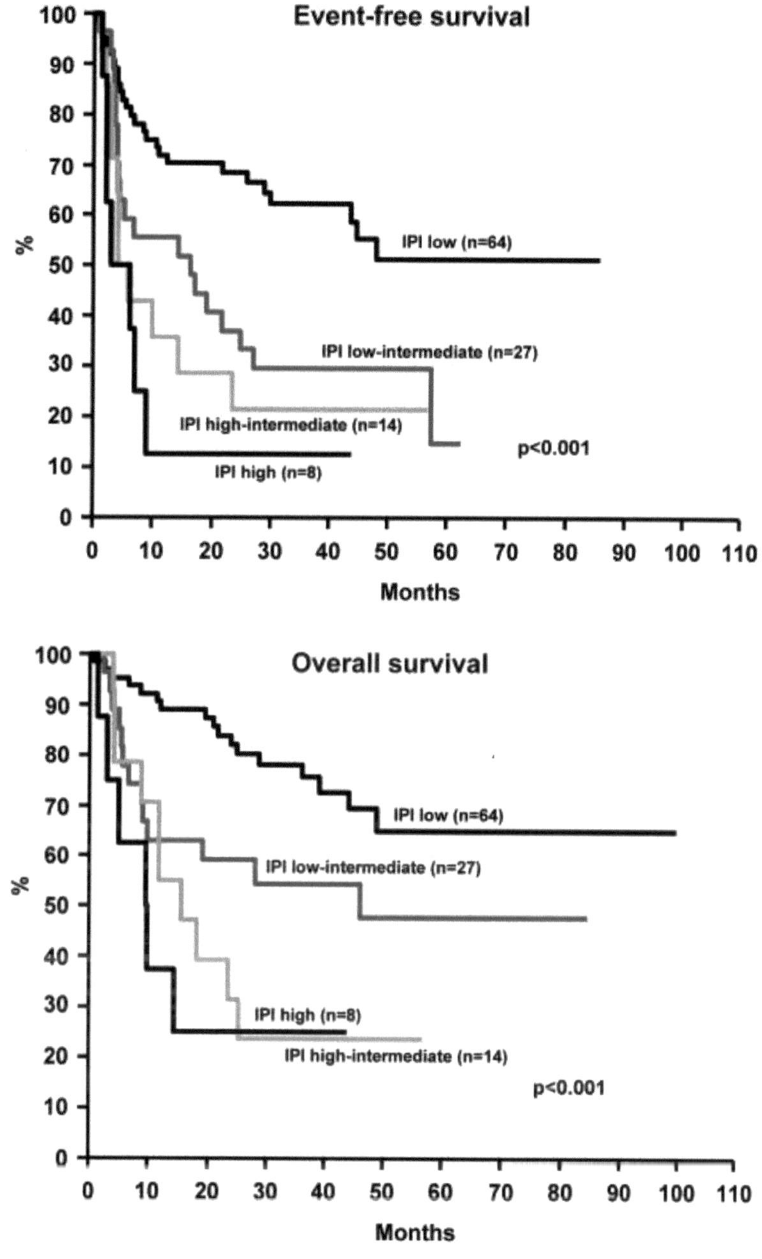

Fig. 5.2 Outcomes based on IPI status for 113 ALK negative ALCL patients after chemotherapy with CHOP or CHOEP in the German High Grade Non-Hodgkins Lymphoma Study Group trials (reprinted from [51], with permission from the American Society of Hematology)

Allogeneic Stem Cell Transplant

Allogeneic stem cell transplantation has been used as a treatment modality in patients with relapsed or refractory ALCL, in many cases after ASCT. A French study reported retrospective results for 77 T-cell lymphomas, 35% of which were ALCL [50]. Fifty-seven patients received myeloablative conditioning; 5-year toxicity-related mortality was 33%. The 5-year EFS and OS for the ALCL patients were 48% and 55%

respectively. ALK status did not impact survival. Of note, chemotherapy-resistant patients also appeared to benefit from allo-SCT with 5-year OS of 29% and successful use of donor lymphocyte infusions (DLI) suggested a graft-versus-lymphoma effect. Corradini et al. reported a small series of 17 patients (four ALCL) with relapsed T-cell NHL who received salvage chemotherapy followed by allo-SCT with reduced intensity conditioning and planned DLI [56, 57]. All patients had sustained engraftment; the estimated 3-year PFS and OS rates were 64 and 81%. All four ALCL patients were event-free at 10, 12, 17, and 36 months.

Novel Therapeutics

There are several FDA-approved agents that are clinically active as single agents for relapsed or refractory ALCL. Pralatrexate is a 10-deaza-aminopterin-analog of methotrexate and a novel targeted antifolate that has shown higher affinity to the reduced folate carrier type 1, increased accumulation and polyglutamylation in tumor cells compared to methotrexate. In a phase I/II study of relapsed/refractory lymphoma, the pralatrexate MTD was 30 mg/m^2 weekly for 6 weeks every 7 weeks [58, 59]. Among 26 evaluable relapsed/refractory T-cell NHL patients, the ORR was 54% (47% by intent-to-treat). Two of the eight CRs seen were systemic ALCL patients (one ALK− and one ALK+) lasting 2 and 22+ months. Denileukin diftitox is a fusion protein which targets the high-affinity interleukin-2 receptor. In a Phase II study of denileukin diftitox in relapsed and refractory T-cell lymphoma patients, two of three patients with ALCL responded (both were ALK-) [60].

Histone deacetylases (HDACs) are a novel class of epigenetic agents which modulate gene expression and regulate acetylation of cellular proteins. The mechanism of HDAC inhibitors in T-cell lymphomas is unknown but may be related to pleotrophic effects on multiple intracellular pathways. Both vorinostat (Zolinza) and romidepsin (Istodax) are FDA-approved: vorinostat for the treatment of CTCL and romidepsin for both cutaneous and aggressive peripheral T-cell lymphomas [59, 61]. Piekarz et al. first reported activity for romidepsin in aggressive T-cell lymphomas, with an ORR of 31% with single-agent romidepsin in 48 relapsed/refractory T-cell NHL patients (4 CR and 11 PR) [62]. The median DOR was 9 months (range 2–61+ months). In a pivotal multicenter trial of 131 patients with aggressive T-cell lymphomas, the objective response rate was 25% (33/130), including 15% (19/130) with CR/CRu. The median duration of response was 17 months, with the longest response ongoing at 34+ months. Of 21 ALK− ALCL patients in the trial, five responded (four CR, one PR) [54].

Immunomodulatory drugs (IMiD drugs) such as lenalidomide have been shown to have a number of biological effects, including modulation of cytokine expression and enhancement of antitumor immunity. Activity of thalidomide had been demonstrated in T-cell lymphoma in one report [63]. A trial exploring the activity of single-agent lenalidomide in relapsed/refractory T-cell NHL has reported an ORR of 30% [64]. Clinical trials examining lenalidomide in combination with other agents in T-cell NHL are being initiated.

Targeted agents

CD30 has been a promising therapeutic target in ALCL. Several anti-CD30 antibodies have been developed and have demonstrated limited clinical activity. MDX-060 (Medarex), a fully human anti-CD30 IgG1k monoclonal antibody, was shown to inhibit growth of CD-30 positive tumor cells in vitro and tumor xenograft models [65]. However, clinical activity was modest with an 8% response rate (6/72) [66]. MDX-1401, a second-generation antibody with improved effector function, has been in Phase I trials which are ongoing. SGN-30 (Seattle Genetics), a chimeric anti-CD30 monoclonal antibody, demonstrated a response rate of 17% in patients with systemic ALCL with median response durations ranging from 27 to 1,460 days [67, 68]. In patients with primary cutaneous ALCL, the ORR was 70% [69]. Figure 5.3 demonstrates a complete clinical response in a patient with refractory ALCL.

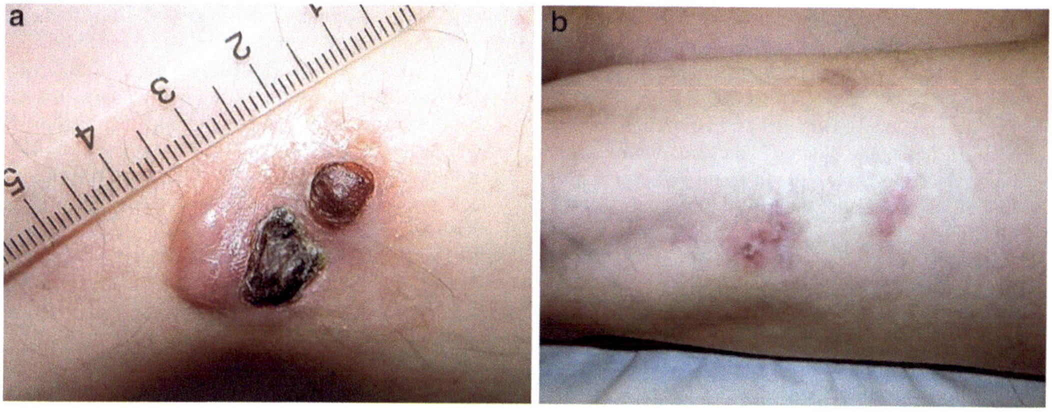

Fig. 5.3 Cutaneous ALCL patient treated with humanized SGN-30 antibody demonstrates complete regression of tumor. (**a**) Pretreatment, (**b**) After six doses of antibody

SGN-35 (brentuximab vedotin) is an antibody-drug conjugate, which was formed by coupling the anti-CD-30 antibody, cAC10, to monomethyl auristatin E (MMAE), an antitubulin agent [68]. In preclinical mouse xenograft models, SGN-35 also induced durable dose-dependent tumor regression compared to either untreated mice or another control group receiving IgG-vcMMAE [68]. In two phase I studies, SGN-35 demonstrated significant clinical activity in relapsed/refractory systemic ALCL [70, 71]. In these trials, 86% of patients (6/7) had documented CR. Subsequently, a phase II multicenter registration trial of brentuximab vedotin was conducted in patients with relapsed or refractory ALCL [72]. The overall response rate was 86% (50 of 58 patients), with CR in 53%. Patients received brentuximab vedotin 1.8 mg/kg q3 weeks for up to 16 cycles. Pts had received a median of 2 (range 1–6) prior systemic therapies, 62% of pts had primary refractory disease, 50% were refractory to their most recent prior therapy, and 22% had never responded to any prior therapy. Median duration of objective response had not been reached but ranged from 0.3 to 45.3 weeks. Fourteen patients moved on to stem cell transplant in remission (seven allogeneic, seven autologous). Peripheral sensory neuropathy was the most frequent side effect and occurred in 36% of patients. The use of brentuximab along with chemotherapy as firstline treatment for systemic anaplastic large-cell lymphomas is under investigation.

Conclusions

The CD30 positive malignancies comprise a spectrum of diseases which include benign cutaneous as well as malignant systemic entities. Cutaneous manifestations are common with systemic anaplastic large-cell lymphomas, which must be clearly distinguished from their more benign cutaneous restricted counterparts. Novel therapeutic approaches for this broad group of diseases target the CD30 antigen and have led to high response rates in relapsed and refractory patients. The appearance of CD30+ lymphomas in the setting of breast implants has recently been observed and these patients may have regression of disease with removal of the implants.

References

1. Schwab U, Stein H, Gerdes J, et al. Production of a monoclonal antibody specific for Hodgkin and Sternberg-Reed cells of Hodgkin's disease and a subset of normal lymphoid cells. Nature. 1982;299:65–7.
2. Stein H, Mason DY, Gerdes J, et al. The expression of the Hodgkin's disease associated antigen Ki-1 in

reactive and neoplastic lymphoid tissue: evidence that Reed-Sternberg cells and histiocytic malignancies are derived from activated lymphoid cells. Blood. 1985;66:848–58.
3. Durkop H, Latza U, Hummel M, Eitelbach F, Seed B, Stein H. Molecular cloning and expression of a new member of the nerve growth factor receptor family that is characteristic for Hodgkin's disease. Cell. 1992;68:421–7.
4. Mir SS, Richter BW, Duckett CS. Differential effects of CD30 activation in anaplastic large cell lymphoma and Hodgkin disease cells. Blood. 2000;96:4307–12.
5. Kadin ME. Common activated helper-T-cell origin for lymphomatoid papulosis, mycosis fungoides, and some types of Hodgkin's disease. Lancet. 1985;2:864–5.
6. Kadin ME, Sako D, Berliner N, et al. Childhood Ki-1 lymphoma presenting with skin lesions and peripheral lymphadenopathy. Blood. 1986;68:1042–9.
7. Rimokh R, Magaud JP, Berger F, et al. A translocation involving a specific breakpoint (q35) on chromosome 5 is characteristic of anaplastic large cell lymphoma ('Ki-1 lymphoma'). Br J Haematol. 1989;71:31–6.
8. Le Beau MM, Bitter MA, Larson RA, et al. The t(2;5)(p23;q35): a recurring chromosomal abnormality in Ki-1-positive anaplastic large cell lymphoma. Leukemia. 1989;3:866–70.
9. Morris SW, Kirstein MN, Valentine MB, et al. Fusion of a kinase gene, ALK, to a nucleolar protein gene, NPM, in non-Hodgkin's lymphoma. Science. 1994; 263:1281–4.
10. Shiota M, Nakamura S, Ichinohasama R, et al. Anaplastic large cell lymphomas expressing the novel chimeric protein p80NPM/ALK: a distinct clinicopathologic entity. Blood. 1995;86:1954–60.
11. Pulford K, Lamant L, Morris SW, et al. Detection of anaplastic lymphoma kinase (ALK) and nucleolar protein nucleophosmin (NPM)-ALK proteins in normal and neoplastic cells with the monoclonal antibody ALK1. Blood. 1997;89:1394–404.
12. Savage KJ, Harris NL, Vose JM, et al. ALK- anaplastic large-cell lymphoma is clinically and immunophenotypically different from both ALK+ ALCL and peripheral T-cell lymphoma, not otherwise specified: report from the International Peripheral T-Cell Lymphoma Project. Blood. 2008;111:5496–504.
13. Willemze R, Jaffe ES, Burg G, et al. WHO-EORTC classification for cutaneous lymphomas. Blood. 2005;105:3768–85.
14. Macaulay WL. Lymphomatoid papulosis. A continuing self-healing eruption, clinically benign–histologically malignant. Arch Dermatol. 1968;97:23–30.
15. Bekkenk MW, Geelen FA, van Voorst Vader PC, et al. Primary and secondary cutaneous CD30(+) lymphoproliferative disorders: a report from the Dutch Cutaneous Lymphoma Group on the long-term follow-up data of 219 patients and guidelines for diagnosis and treatment. Blood. 2000;95:3653–61.
16. Liu HL, Hoppe RT, Kohler S, Harvell JD, Reddy S, Kim YH. CD30+ cutaneous lymphoproliferative disorders: the Stanford experience in lymphomatoid papulosis and primary cutaneous anaplastic large cell lymphoma. J Am Acad Dermatol. 2003;49:1049–58.
17. Wang HH, Myers T, Lach LJ, Hsieh CC, Kadin ME. Increased risk of lymphoid and nonlymphoid malignancies in patients with lymphomatoid papulosis. Cancer. 1999;86:1240–5.
18. Kadin ME. Primary Ki-1-positive anaplastic large-cell lymphoma: a distinct clinicopathologic entity. Ann Oncol. 1994;5 Suppl 1:25–30.
19. Le Deley MC, Reiter A, Williams D, et al. Prognostic factors in childhood anaplastic large cell lymphoma: results of a large European intergroup study. Blood. 2008;111:1560–6.
20. de Bruin PC, Beljaards RC, van Heerde P, et al. Differences in clinical behaviour and immunophenotype between primary cutaneous and primary nodal anaplastic large cell lymphoma of T-cell or null cell phenotype. Histopathology. 1993;23:127–35.
21. Franchina M, Kadin ME, Abraham LJ. Polymorphism of the CD30 promoter microsatellite repressive element is associated with development of primary cutaneous lymphoproliferative disorders. Cancer Epidemiol Biomarkers Prev. 2005;14:1322–5.
22. Nijsten T, Curiel-Lewandrowski C, Kadin ME. Lymphomatoid papulosis in children: a retrospective cohort study of 35 cases. Arch Dermatol. 2004; 140:306–12.
23. Fletcher CL, Orchard GE, Hubbard V, Whittaker SJ, Edelson RL, Russell-Jones R. CD30(+) cutaneous lymphoma in association with atopic eczema. Arch Dermatol. 2004;140:449–54.
24. Beljaards RC, Willemze R. The prognosis of patients with lymphomatoid papulosis associated with malignant lymphomas. Br J Dermatol. 1992;126:596–602.
25. Basarab T, Fraser-Andrews EA, Orchard G, Whittaker S, Russel-Jones R. Lymphomatoid papulosis in association with mycosis fungoides: a study of 15 cases. Br J Dermatol. 1998;139:630–8.
26. Chott A, Vonderheid EC, Olbricht S, Miao NN, Balk SP, Kadin ME. The dominant T cell clone is present in multiple regressing skin lesions and associated T cell lymphomas of patients with lymphomatoid papulosis. J Invest Dermatol. 1996;106:696–700.
27. Wang HH, Lach L, Kadin ME. Epidemiology of lymphomatoid papulosis. Cancer. 1992;70:2951–7.
28. Schiemann WP, Pfeifer WM, Levi E, Kadin ME, Lodish HF. A deletion in the gene for transforming growth factor beta type I receptor abolishes growth regulation by transforming growth factor beta in a cutaneous T-cell lymphoma. Blood. 1999;94:2854–61.
29. Vonderheid EC, Sajjadian A, Kadin ME. Methotrexate is effective therapy for lymphomatoid papulosis and other primary cutaneous CD30-positive lymphoproliferative disorders. J Am Acad Dermatol. 1996; 34:470–81.
30. Yagi H, Tokura Y, Furukawa F, Takigawa M. Th2 cytokine mRNA expression in primary cutaneous CD30 positive lymphoproliferative disorders: successful treatment with recombinant interferon-gamma. J Invest Dermatol. 1996;107:827–32.

31. Schmuth M, Topar G, Illersperger B, Kowald E, Fritsch PO, Sepp NT. Therapeutic use of interferon-alpha for lymphomatoid papulosis. Cancer. 2000;89:1603–10.
32. Krathen RA, Ward S, Duvic M. Bexarotene is a new treatment option for lymphomatoid papulosis. Dermatology. 2003;206:142–7.
33. Drews R, Samel A, Kadin ME. Lymphomatoid papulosis and anaplastic large cell lymphomas of the skin. Semin Cutan Med Surg. 2000;19:109–17.
34. Willemze R, Beljaards RC. Spectrum of primary cutaneous CD30 (Ki-1)-positive lymphoproliferative disorders. A proposal for classification and guidelines for management and treatment. J Am Acad Dermatol. 1993;28:973–80.
35. Beljaards RC, Kaudewitz P, Berti E, et al. Primary cutaneous CD30-positive large cell lymphoma: definition of a new type of cutaneous lymphoma with a favorable prognosis. A European Multicenter Study of 47 patients. Cancer. 1993;71:2097–104.
36. Paulli M, Berti E, Rosso R, et al. CD30/Ki-1-positive lymphoproliferative disorders of the skin–clinicopathologic correlation and statistical analysis of 86 cases: a multicentric study from the European Organization for Research and Treatment of Cancer Cutaneous Lymphoma Project Group. J Clin Oncol. 1995;13:1343–54.
37. Brice P, Cazals D, Mounier N, et al. Primary cutaneous large-cell lymphoma: analysis of 49 patients included in the LNH87 prospective trial of polychemotherapy for high-grade lymphomas. Groupe d'Etude des Lymphomes de l'Adulte. Leukemia. 1998;12:213–9.
38. Rijlaarsdam JU, Huijgens PC, Beljaards RC, Bakels V, Willemze R. Oral etoposide in the treatment of cutaneous large-cell lymphomas. A preliminary report of four cases. Br J Dermatol. 1992;127:524–8.
39. The International T-Cell Lymphoma Project. International peripheral T-cell and natural killer/T-cell lymphoma study: pathology findings and clinical outcomes. J Clin Oncol. 2008;26:4124–30.
40. Falini B, Pileri S, Zinzani PL, et al. ALK+ lymphoma: clinico-pathological findings and outcome. Blood. 1999;93:2697–706.
41. de Jong D, Vasmel WL, de Boer JP, et al. Anaplastic large-cell lymphoma in women with breast implants. JAMA. 2008;300:2030–5.
42. Gascoyne RD, Aoun P, Wu D, et al. Prognostic significance of anaplastic lymphoma kinase (ALK) protein expression in adults with anaplastic large cell lymphoma. Blood. 1999;93:3913–21.
43. Suzuki R, Kagami Y, Takeuchi K, et al. Prognostic significance of CD56 expression for ALK-positive and ALK-negative anaplastic large-cell lymphoma of T/null cell phenotype. Blood. 2000;96:2993–3000.
44. Benharroch D, Meguerian-Bedoyan Z, Lamant L, et al. ALK-positive lymphoma: a single disease with a broad spectrum of morphology. Blood. 1998;91:2076–84.
45. Stein H, Foss HD, Durkop H, et al. CD30(+) anaplastic large cell lymphoma: a review of its histopathologic, genetic, and clinical features. Blood. 2000;96:3681–95.
46. Delsol G, Falini B, Muller-Hermelink HK, et al. Anaplastic large cell lymphoma (ALCL), ALK-positive in WHO Classification of Tumors of haematopoietic and Lymphoid Tissues. 4th ed. Lyon: WHO PRESS; 2008.
47. Morris SW, Kirstein MN, Valentine MB, et al. Fusion of a kinase gene, ALK, to a nucleolar protein gene, NPM, in non-Hodgkin's lymphoma. Science. 1995;267:316–7.
48. Tilly H, Gaulard P, Lepage E, et al. Primary anaplastic large-cell lymphoma in adults: clinical presentation, immunophenotype, and outcome. Blood. 1997; 90:3727–34.
49. Pfreundschuh M, Trumper L, Kloess M, et al. Two-weekly or 3-weekly CHOP chemotherapy with or without etoposide for the treatment of young patients with good-prognosis (normal LDH) aggressive lymphomas: results of the NHL-B1 trial of the DSHNHL. Blood. 2004;104:626–33.
50. Le Gouill S, Milpied N, Buzyn A, et al. Graft-versus-lymphoma effect for aggressive T-cell lymphomas in adults: a study by the Societe Francaise de Greffe de Moelle et de Therapie Cellulaire. J Clin Oncol. 2008;26:2264–71.
51. Schmitz N, Trumper L, Ziepert M, et al. Treatment and prognosis of mature T-cell and NK-cell lymphoma: an analysis of patients with T-cell lymphoma treated in studies of the German High-Grade Non-Hodgkin Lymphoma Study Group. Blood. 2010;116:3418–25.
52. Song KW, Mollee P, Keating A, Crump M. Autologous stem cell transplant for relapsed and refractory peripheral T-cell lymphoma: variable outcome according to pathological subtype. Br J Haematol. 2003; 120:978–85.
53. Fanin R, Ruiz de Elvira MC, Sperotto A, Baccarani M, Goldstone A. Autologous stem cell transplantation for T and null cell CD30-positive anaplastic large cell lymphoma: analysis of 64 adult and paediatric cases reported to the European Group for Blood and Marrow Transplantation (EBMT). Bone Marrow Transplant. 1999;23:437–42.
54. Whittaker SJ, Demierre MF, Kim EJ, et al. Final results from a multicenter, international, pivotal study of romidepsin in refractory cutaneous T-cell lymphoma. J Clin Oncol. 2010;28:4485–91.
55. Nickelsen M, Ziepert M, Zeynalova S, et al. High-dose CHOP plus etoposide (MegaCHOEP) in T-cell lymphoma: a comparative analysis of patients treated within trials of the German High-Grade Non-Hodgkin Lymphoma Study Group (DSHNHL). Ann Oncol. 2009;20:1977–84.
56. Corradini P, Cavo M, Lokhorst H, et al. Molecular remission after myeloablative allogeneic stem cell transplantation predicts a better relapse-free survival in patients with multiple myeloma. Blood. 2003;102:1927–9.
57. Dodero A, Spina F, Narni F, et al. Allogeneic transplantation following a reduced-intensity conditioning

regimen in relapsed/refractory peripheral T-cell lymphomas: long-term remissions and response to donor lymphocyte infusions support the role of a graft-versus-lymphoma effect. Leukemia. 2012;26:520–6.
58. O'Connor OA, Horwitz S, Hamlin P, et al. Phase II-I-II study of two different doses and schedules of pralatrexate, a high-affinity substrate for the reduced folate carrier, in patients with relapsed or refractory lymphoma reveals marked activity in T-cell malignancies. J Clin Oncol. 2009;27:4357–64.
59. Olsen EA, Kim YH, Kuzel TM, et al. Phase IIb multicenter trial of vorinostat in patients with persistent, progressive, or treatment refractory cutaneous T-cell lymphoma. J Clin Oncol. 2007;25:3109–15.
60. Dang NH, Pro B, Hagemeister FB, et al. Phase II trial of denileukin diftitox for relapsed/refractory T-cell non-Hodgkin lymphoma. Br J Haematol. 2007;136: 439–447.
61. Coiffier B, Pro B, Prince HM, et al. Final results from a pivotal, multicenter, international, open-label, phase 2 study of romidepsin in progressive or relapsed peripheral T-cell lymphoma (PTCL) following prior systemic therapy. Blood (ASH Annual Meeting Abstracts). 2010;116:114.
62. Piekarz R WJ, Frye R, et al. Results of a phase 2 NCI multicenter study of romidepsin in patients with relapsed peripheral T-cell lymphoma (PTCL). ASH Annual Meeting Abstracts. 2008;1567.
63. Damaj G, Bouabdallah R, Vey N, Bilger K, Mohty M, Gastaut JA. Single-agent thalidomide induces response in T-cell lymphoma. Eur J Haematol. 2005;74:169–71.
64. Dueck GS CN, Prasad A et al. Activity of lenalidomide in a phase II trial for T-cell lymphoma: report on the first 24 cases. ASCO Annual Meeting; 2009:8524.
65. Borchmann P, Treml JF, Hansen H, et al. The human anti-CD30 antibody 5F11 shows in vitro and in vivo activity against malignant lymphoma. Blood. 2003;102:3737–42.
66. Ansell SM, Horwitz SM, Engert A, et al. Phase I/II study of an anti-CD30 monoclonal antibody (MDX-060) in Hodgkin's lymphoma and anaplastic large-cell lymphoma. J Clin Oncol. 2007;25:2764–9.
67. Forero-Torres A, Leonard JP, Younes A, et al. A Phase II study of SGN-30 (anti-CD30 mAb) in Hodgkin lymphoma or systemic anaplastic large cell lymphoma. Br J Haematol. 2009;146:171–9.
68. Francisco JA, Cerveny CG, Meyer DL, et al. cAC10-vcMMAE, an anti-CD30-monomethyl auristatin E conjugate with potent and selective antitumor activity. Blood. 2003;102:1458–65.
69. Duvic M, Reddy SA, Pinter-Brown L, et al. A phase II study of SGN-30 in cutaneous anaplastic large cell lymphoma and related lymphoproliferative disorders. Clin Cancer Res. 2009;15:6217–24.
70. Younes A F-TA, Bartlett NL. Multiple complete responses in a phase I dose-escalation study of the antibody-drug conjugate SGN-35 in patients with relapsed or refractory CD-30 positive lymphomas. ASH Annual Meeting Abstracts; 2008.
71. Bartlett NL F-TA, Rosenblatt JD. Complete remissions with weekly dosing of SGN-35, a novel antibody-drug conjugate (ADC) targeting CD30, in a phase I dose-escalation study in patients with relapsed or refractory Hodgkin Lymphoma (HL) or systemic anaplastic large cell lymphoma. ASCO Annual Meeting Abstracts; 2009:8500.
72. Pro B, Advani R, Brice P, Bartlett N, Rosenblatt J, et al. Durable remissions with brentuximab vedotin (SGN-35): updated results of a phase II study in patients with relapsed or refractory systemic anaplastic large cell lymphoma (sALCL). J Clin Oncol. 2011;29:9032.

NK-Cell Neoplasms

6

Motoko Yamaguchi and Kensei Tobinai

Natural killer (NK) cell-derived neoplasms were first reported in the late 1980s, and the definition of this disease was established in the 1990s [1]. NK-cell neoplasms mainly arise in East Asia and Latin America and usually show an aggressive clinical course. In the 2000s, detailed clinicopathologic features and effective therapeutic approaches have been actively investigated. In this chapter, we provide an overview of the clinicopathologic and molecular features of NK-cell neoplasms and summarize the recent progress in the treatment of these diseases.

Definition, Subtypes, and Clinical Characteristics

Definition and Subtypes of NK-Cell Neoplasms in the 2008 WHO Classification

The 2008 World Health Organization (WHO) classification recognizes two NK-cell neoplasm categories: extranodal NK/T-cell lymphoma, nasal type (ENKL), and aggressive NK-cell leukemia (ANKL) [2]. The former edition of the WHO classification (2001) also recognized blastic NK cell lymphoma as an NK-cell neoplasm [3]. However, the cumulative evidence from detailed immunophenotyping, gene expression profiling studies [4], and characterization of blastic NK-cell lymphoma cell lines [5] strongly suggests that blastic NK cell lymphoma is derived from a plasmacytoid dendritic cell [2] and is classified as such in the 2008 WHO classification.

Definition and Subtypes of ENKL

ENKL is defined as "a predominantly extranodal lymphoma characterized by vascular damage and destruction, prominent necrosis, cytotoxic phenotype and association with the Epstein–Barr virus (EBV)" in the 2008 WHO classification [2]. It was formerly designated as lethal midline granuloma, angiocentric T-cell lymphoma, or polymorphic reticulosis. ENKL commonly occurs in the upper aerodigestive tract, with the nasal cavity being the most common site of involvement. ENKL also involves the extra-upper aerodigestive tract, such as the skin, soft tissue, gastrointestinal tract, lung, and testis [2]. In the 2001 WHO classification, two clinical subtypes of ENKL, nasal NK/T-cell lymphoma and nasal-type NK/T-cell lymphoma, were described [3]. The former was characterized by lymphomatous involvement of the nasal cavity and/or its adjacent sites. Conversely, nasal-type NK/T-cell lymphoma occurs outside the nasal cavity, such as in the skin or gastrointestinal tract [3]. There are also differences in the clinical characteristics and

M. Yamaguchi (✉)
Department of Hematology and Oncology, Mie University Graduate School of Medicine, 2-174 Edobashi, Tsu, Mie 514-8507, Japan
e-mail: waniwani@clin.medic.mie-u.ac.jp

K. Tobinai
Department of Hematology, National Cancer Center Hospital, Tokyo, Japan

F. Foss (ed.), *T-Cell Lymphomas*, Contemporary Hematology,
DOI 10.1007/978-1-62703-170-7_6, © Springer Science+Business Media New York 2013

therapeutic outcomes between these two subgroups. An international survey has revealed that extranasal NK/T-cell lymphoma is more frequent in Continental Asia than in Japan and is characterized by a shorter survival compared to nasal NK/T-cell lymphoma [6]. This latter finding was confirmed by a large retrospective survey from Korea [7]. The two subgroups have been managed with considerably different treatment strategies, as will be described later in this chapter. Moreover, it is known that extensive examinations, such as random biopsy of the nasal mucosa, occasionally reveal nasal involvement in patients with non-nasal NK/T-cell lymphoma [8]. It is noteworthy that the term "nasal NK-cell lymphoma" is not used in the 2008 WHO classification, although it is widely adopted in current research and in clinical practice.

ENKL rarely presents as a primary nodal lymphoma. Nodal NK/T-cell lymphoma is characterized by frequent CD8 expression and shows clinical features between ENKL and EBV-associated cytotoxic nodal T-cell lymphoma [9]. NK/T-cell lymphoma of the Waldeyer's ring is reported to be associated with frequent cervical node involvement and relatively longer survival [10]. Few cases of intravascular large cell lymphoma of the NK-cell phenotype have been reported [11]. However, additional validating studies are needed to determine the significant differences and thus discriminate between these particular ENKL subgroups.

Definition and Overview of ANKL

ANKL has been recognized as a subtype of large granular lymphocyte (LGL) leukemia since the 1980s and is now recognized as a distinct subtype in the WHO classification [2, 12]. It is characterized by the systemic proliferation of NK cells and has a highly aggressive clinical course, although it accounts for less than 1% of the lymphoid malignancies in East Asia. The leukemic cells in ANKL show an LGL morphology, a surface $CD3^-$ $CD2^+$ $CD16^+$ $CD56^+$ immunophenotype, and germline configurations of the T-cell receptor genes [13, 14]. The tumor cells express P-glycoprotein [15, 16] and are positive for EBV, as also seen in ENKL [13]. ANKL can be differentially diagnosed from chronic lymphoproliferative disorders of NK cells [2] (or chronic NK lymphocytosis [17]) by the presence of clonal cytogenetic abnormalities and/or analysis of the terminal repeat sequence of EBV by Southern blotting. Although there have been some reports of rare cases of ANKL transformed from chronic NK lymphocytosis [18], the etiology of this lymphoma subtype is still unknown.

ANKL displays the clinical features of leukemia, which include anemia and thrombocytopenia. Occasionally, patients with ANKL experience hepatosplenomegaly and/or lymph node swelling with no leukemic cells in either the bone marrow or peripheral blood. Some investigators have speculated that ANKL may be a leukemic subtype of ENKL (ANKL/lymphoma). However, there are some differences in the properties of the tumor cells between ANKL and ENKL. For example, neoplastic cells of ANKL express CD16 more frequently than those of ENKL, whereas CD3 epsilon expression is less frequent [13]. Genomic imbalances also differ between ENKL and ANKL [19].

Patients with ANKL have been treated with chemotherapeutic regimens for acute leukemia or aggressive lymphoma, but the response and prognosis are poor. The majority of patients die within 2 years, and many die within 6 months of their diagnosis [13]. Partly due to the rarity of the disease, the detailed clinicopathologic features and optimal treatment of ANKL have not been extensively investigated.

Clinical Characteristics of ENKL

The most frequent site of involvement in ENKL is the nasal cavity and its adjacent sites, such as the paranasal sinuses, nasopharynx, palate, Waldeyer's ring, and orbit. Nasal obstruction, nasal discharge, and epistaxis are common initial symptoms. An episode of unilateral epistaxis is often the stimulus for referral to a medical center. Eye symptoms may occur when ENKL involves the orbit or its adjacent sites. Also of note, ENKL is sometimes associated with complications such as hemophagocytic syndrome or fevers of unknown origin.

Table 6.1 Summary of the clinical characteristics at diagnosis from large retrospective studies of nasal NK/T-cell lymphoma and whole ENKL

	Nasal NK/T-cell lymphoma		Whole ENKL	
Parameter	Au (*n*=92) [6]	Suzuki (*n*=123) [20]	Lee (*n*=262) [21]	Kim (*n*=280) [7]
Male sex (%)	64	66	65	66
Median age	52	52	–	46
Age >60 years (%)	–	–	21	21
Performance status >1 (%)	9	20	13	23
Stage III/IV (%)	27	32	24	25
LDH >upper normal limit (%)	45	–	37	45
Number of sites of extranodal involvement >1 (%)	16	–	–	22
B symptoms (%)	39	46	35	42
High or high-intermediate risk of IPI (%)	–	26	19	21
NK-PI Group 3/4 (%)	–	46	42	42

IPI International Prognostic Index; *NK-PI* NK/T-cell lymphoma prognostic index

Table 6.1 summarizes the clinical characteristics of nasal NK/T-cell lymphoma and whole ENKL at diagnosis, based on studies of large patient cohorts [6, 7, 20, 21]. Because the incidence of extranasal (nasal-type or non-nasal) ENKL is 25% or less among cases with this lymphoma subtype, the principal clinical data that have been assembled for nasal NK/T-cell lymphoma and whole ENKL are very similar, as shown in Table 6.1. Approximately 65% of patients with ENKL are male, and the median age at diagnosis ranges from 46 to 52 years. Seventy-five percent of ENKL patients have stage I or II disease. The serum LDH levels are elevated in 45% of patients, whereas the relative frequency of a poor performance (PS) status (>1) is low. Based on these features, ~80% of patients with ENKL are classified as low or low-intermediate risk according to the International Prognostic Index (IPI) [22]. B symptoms of the Ann Arbor classification are present in ~45% of patients, which is more frequent than other localized aggressive lymphomas.

ENKL can disseminate preferentially to the skin, gastrointestinal tract, testis, and central nervous system (CNS). The initial symptoms of ENKL with gastrointestinal involvement often include perforation of the gastrointestinal tract, which can be a serious complication during chemotherapy.

Staging of ENKL

Because ENKL usually begins at extranodal sites, the staging of this lymphoma is often problematic. In the Ann Arbor classification system, stage IE is defined as the localized involvement of a single extralymphatic organ or site in the absence of any lymph node involvement. The diffuse or disseminated involvement of one or more extralymphatic organs is defined as stage IV. However, in most reports of ENKL, contiguous involvement extending to adjacent structures, such as the nasal cavity, paranasal sinuses, nasopharynx, oral cavity, or orbit, is considered to be stage IE (Table 6.2).

Regional lymph nodes in cases of localized nasal NK/T-cell lymphoma are considered to be equivalent to those in the cervical lymph node region using the Ann Arbor classification. In this regard, the tumor, node, metastasis (TNM) scheme for cancer of the nasal cavity and paranasal sinus defines regional lymph nodes as cervical lymph nodes. Mediastinal lymph node metastases are regarded as distant metastases. Stage IIIE disease usually accounts for <10% of nasal NK/T-cell lymphomas because it typically progresses rapidly to the bone marrow or other extranodal sites.

To evaluate the involvement of the nasal cavity and its adjacent sites in cases of ENKL, magnetic resonance imaging (MRI) of the nasal cavity is

Table 6.2 Staging of nasal NK/T-cell lymphoma[a]

IE	Contiguous involvement extending to adjacent structures (nasal cavity, paranasal sinuses, nasopharynx, oral cavity, and orbit)
IIE	Primary site with cervical lymph node involvement (contiguous stage IIE) with or without involvement of other supradiaphragmatic lymph node regions
	Primary site with isolated involvement of head and neck sites (Waldeyer's ring, oropharynx, hypopharynx, etc.)
IIIE (rare)	Primary site with cervical lymph node involvement with infradiaphragmatic lymph node involvement and/or involvement of the spleen
IV	Primary site (without cervical lymph node involvement) with isolated distant involvement
	Any involvement of the liver or bone marrow

[a]Summarized for this review using data from previous reports of ENKL and the current consensus in clinical practice

thought to be more useful that a CT scan alone. ENKL is a fluorodeoxyglucose (FDG)-avid lymphoma, and the usefulness of (18)F-FDG positron emission tomography (FDG-PET) in the staging of this lymphoma has also been reported in at least four independent studies [23–26]. To assess bone marrow involvement, in situ hybridization analysis of EBV-encoded RNA (EBER) has also been shown to be useful [27]. These new staging procedures are expected to allow for the discrimination of patients with advanced-stage disease who require different treatment strategies.

Epidemiology and Etiology of ENKL

Epidemiology

ENKL is much more common in Asia and Latin America than in the United States and Europe [28, 29]. In East Asia, its relative frequency among all lymphomas is approximately 3% in Japan [30], 6% in Hong Kong, 7% in Taiwan, and 9% in Korea [17]. In contrast, the relative frequency of ENKL is <1% in western countries.

Etiology

The etiology of ENKL has not yet been clarified. Because ENKL is almost always associated with EBV [31], it is regarded as one of the EBV-associated lymphoid malignancies [1]. A possible etiologic association between air pollution and ENKL was suggested by a previous Mexican study [32]. Further, a case–control study from East Asia has also revealed an etiologic association between ENKL and life-style or environmental factors, including farming, pesticide use, or residential proximity to garbage incineration facilities [33].

Pathology, Diagnosis, and Molecular Features of ENKL

Pathology and Diagnosis

Histopathologically, ENKL is characterized by an angiocentric or angiodestructive invasion of tumor cells, the formation of necroses, and infiltration by various types of inflammatory cells [2]. No definite mass formation is found in many cases. In such instances, a biopsy including normal-looking tissues or a random biopsy to obtain diagnostic tissue samples is recommended. It is known that the nuclei in the ENKL tumor cells are often elongated [2] and display a cucumber-like shape.

There are two lineages of tumor cells in ENKL, the NK- and cytotoxic T-cell immunophenotypes. In both types, CD56 is positive in most cases. However, NK-cell markers other than CD56, such as CD16 or CD57, are rarely positive in ENKL. CD5 expression strongly suggests a T-cell type of ENKL [34]. CD20 is usually negative in ENKL, but CD20-positive cases are known to exist [35]. In the NK-cell type of ENKL, the tumor cells express cytoplasmic CD3 epsilon only, whereas both surface CD3 and cytoplasmic CD3 epsilon are expressed in the T-cell type of ENKL [36–39]. NK-cell type ENKL shows germline configurations of the T-cell receptor genes. In addition, in situ hybridization analysis for EBER using paraffin-embedded material is a useful test, because the vast majority of these lymphomas show positive nuclear signals within the tumor cells. When CD56 is negative, both a positive EBV status and the expression of more than one cytotoxic molecule (e.g., perforin, granzyme B, or TIA-1) are required for a diagnosis of ENKL [2].

During the 1990s, the diagnosis of NK-cell neoplasms was facilitated by improvements in histopathologic diagnostic procedures. For example, anti-CD56 monoclonal antibodies that could be used for routinely processed formalin-embedded paraffin sections became available. The identification of disease-specific features, such as cytoplasmic CD3 epsilon expression and frequent detection of EBER by in situ hybridization, also contributed to a more accurate differential diagnosis from other lymphoma subtypes.

Molecular Features

ENKL lymphoma cells express the multidrug resistance (*MDR*) *1/ABCB1* gene and its product, P-glycoprotein [15, 16, 40]. This MDR phenomenon is thought to be the major reason why ENKL is resistant to CHOP (cyclophosphamide, doxorubicin, vincristine, and prednisone) or the CHOP-like chemotherapies that comprise mainly MDR-related agents. Immunohistochemical analyses have further revealed the prognostic significance of the expression of granzyme B-specific protease inhibitor 9 (PI9) [41], cyclooxygenase-2 (COX-2) [42], or high levels of Ki-67 in the tumor cells [6]. With respect to the EBV status, EBNA1 is expressed in the tumor cells of almost all nasal NK/T-cell lymphomas and most extranasal ENKL cases [1, 31]. Other EBNAs are not expressed, but latent membrane protein 1 is expressed in 50% of affected patients [43, 44]. Based on these data, ENKL is classified as a type II latency of an EBV infection. Sequence analysis has also identified a 30-bp deletion in LMP1 in ENKL [45].

Mutations of tumor suppressor genes have been reported in ENKL. *FAS* is mutated in 50% of patients [46], and *TP53* mutations are detectable in <50% of patients [44, 47]. Several cell lines from ENKL have also been established [12], and in vitro analyses suggest that endogenous IL-9, IL-10, and IP-10 may play important roles in ENKL cell proliferation and invasion via an autocrine mechanism [44, 48, 49]. A study that combined gene expression profiling and array-based comparative genomic hybridization analyses of ENKL revealed greater transcript levels for NK-cell and cytotoxic molecules compared with peripheral T-cell lymphoma, not otherwise specified [50]. ENKL tumor cells express more vascular biology-related genes, EBV-induced genes, and *PDGFRA* when compared to normal NK cells [50]. The Akt, JAK-STAT, NF-κB, and Wnt signaling pathways are also potentially relevant biological pathways in ENKL [50]. Del(6)(q21q25) or i(6)(p10) is the most common cytogenetic abnormality in ENKL [2]. Among the known genes at 6q21, *PRDM1* and *FOXO3* are considered to be the most likely target genes in NK-cell malignancies [50, 51].

Prognostic Factors and Prognostic Models

The IPI [22] is widely used to evaluate aggressive lymphomas. Because only 20% of patients with ENKL are classified as having an IPI score of 1 or less, most studies to date have concluded that the clinical significance of this score in ENKL is not high. However, a Hong Kong study reported that the IPI is still valid for patients with an NK-cell type ENKL [52]. A multicenter retrospective study of 262 patients with ENKL from Korea proposed a prognostic model for ENKL: the NK/T-cell lymphoma prognostic index (NK-PI) or "Korean index" [21]. Four independent prognostic factors were identified in this system that were associated with overall survival (OS) in terms of the presence of B symptoms, advanced stage, an elevated serum LDH level, and the regional lymph node involvement according to the TNM system. The clinical usefulness of NK-PI has been validated in an international cooperative study [6]. Conversely, NK-PI was found not to be a useful predictor of survival in two recent prospective studies of concurrent chemoradiotherapy (CCRT) [53, 54], which are discussed later in this chapter. Another Korean study reported the prognostic significance of local tumor invasiveness (LTI) in localized ENKL of the upper aerodigestive tract [55]. The authors defined LTI as bony invasion or perforation/invasion of the skin based on CT and physical findings and concluded that LTI is more predictive of survival than the IPI for patients with stage IE and IIE ENKL [55]. These two large retrospective studies [21, 55] indicate that high serum LDH levels, the presence of B symptoms, and LTI are important prognostic factors for ENKL, which partly differs from other aggressive lymphomas.

ENKL is an EBV-related disease, and the peripheral blood of affected patients contains fragmented EBV-DNA. Some retrospective studies suggest that measurement of the circulating viral DNA load is useful for the diagnosis, monitoring, and prognostication of this disease [56, 57]. The NK-Cell Tumor Study Group (NKTSG) conducted the first prospective study of EBV-DNA in ENKL using quantitative PCR [58]. A total of 33 patients were analyzed, and a significant correlation between the number of mononuclear cells and plasma EBV-DNA copy number was observed. The pretreatment plasma EBV-DNA levels were thus well correlated with several clinical parameters. Multivariate analysis showed that the clinical stage and pretreatment plasma EBV-DNA levels are significant prognostic factors. The plasma EBV-DNA copy number was found to be a valid indicator for both the response to treatment and OS [58]. Monitoring of EBV-DNA in the peripheral blood is already conducted routinely in some centers in East Asia [59].

Treatment of ENKL

Treatment of Localized Nasal NK/T-Cell Lymphoma

Background

Despite recent improvements in diagnostics, no standard therapy for ENKL has been established, and prior to 2009, no well-designed prospective trial for localized nasal NK/T-cell lymphoma had been reported. The 5-year OS rates for localized nasal NK/T-cell lymphoma in early reports ranged from 14 to 100% [60]. Although more than two-thirds of patients with nasal NK/T-cell lymphoma present with localized disease, their prognosis is poorer than that for individuals with a localized diffuse large B-cell lymphoma.

Most patients with localized nasal NK/T-cell lymphoma have been treated with radiotherapy with or without chemotherapy. However, the details of such treatments in many previous reports, particularly the timing of the radiotherapy and chemotherapy, have not been adequately described. Many early studies did not evaluate lymphomas arising in the nasal cavity and paranasal sinuses separately because it was believed that these were the same condition. In addition, "true" NK-cell, T-cell, and B-cell lymphomas were often intermingled in single studies due to the difficulties in immunophenotyping. Hence, the outcomes of therapeutic strategies specific for nasal NK-cell lymphoma have not been thoroughly examined to date. In this review, we focus on well-documented reports of each modality and the immunophenotyping of tumor cells.

Chemotherapy Followed by Radiotherapy

Anthracycline-containing chemotherapy followed by radiotherapy has been established as the standard treatment for localized aggressive lymphomas, mainly diffuse large B-cell lymphomas [61]. However, this therapeutic strategy is ineffective against localized nasal NK/T-cell lymphoma. The five-year OS rates of patients with localized diseases who were treated with chemotherapy followed by radiotherapy are <50% (Table 6.3) [41, 60, 62–68]. In these retrospective studies, various chemotherapeutic regimens were used. Kim et al. [69] conducted two clinical studies of the efficacy of CHOP chemotherapy for localized nasal NK/T-cell lymphoma [69]. Between 1995 and 1999, 17 patients were treated with 4 courses of CHOP chemotherapy followed by 45 Gy radiotherapy as a planned treatment. The planned sequential chemoradiotherapy could only be completed in six patients because of early disease progression during the chemotherapy phase. Subsequently, 17 patients

Table 6.3 Survival outcomes for patients with a localized nasal NK/T-cell lymphoma treated with conventional standard therapy for localized aggressive non-Hodgkin lymphomas

Modality	Stage	*n*	5 year-OS rate (%)	Reference
Cx→RT	I–II	7	14	Yu et al. [62]
Cx (→RT)	I	18	28	Kwong et al. [63]
Cx (→RT)	I/II	12	<50	Ribrag et al. [64]
Cx (→RT)	I/II	7	14	Yamaguchi et al. [60]
Cx (→RT)	I–II	61	40	Cheung et al. [65]
Cx	I–II	18	15	Li et al. [66]
Cx (→RT)	I–II	40	29	You et al. [67]
Cx (→RT)	I–IV	26	18	Pagano et al. [68]
Cx (→RT)	I–IV	48	49	Bossard et al. [41]

Cx CHOP(-like) chemotherapy; *RT* radiotherapy; *OS* overall survival

were treated more aggressively with intensified doses, dose dense CHOP and radiotherapy [70]. The complete response (CR) rate was improved, but five patients still experienced systemic failure. These results suggest that the efficacy of CHOP chemotherapy is not sufficient to treat ENKL, even at the maximal dose intensity. As previously discussed in this chapter, it has been speculated that CHOP(-like) chemotherapy comprises MDR-related agents (e.g., vincristine and doxorubicin, among others) is not effective against this disease, because ENKL tumor cells express P-glycoprotein.

EPOCH chemotherapy (etoposide, prednisone, vincristine, cyclophosphamide, and doxorubicin) was originally designed to overcome the MDR phenomenon by using continuous infusion of anticancer agents. In a retrospective study from China in which 76% of a 34-patient cohort had localized disease, EPOCH chemotherapy followed by radiotherapy produced CR and 3-year OS rates of 75% [71]. However, these favorable results must be further validated in a prospective trial setting before incorporating this treatment method into clinical practice.

Frontline Radiotherapy

Radiotherapy has frequently been used as the primary treatment for ENKL, because most patients present with localized disease. In patients treated with radiotherapy alone, the CR rate is >65% [72, 73], which is the best reported single modality outcome for this disease. The reported 5-year OS rates range from 42 to 83%, but this may be caused by several selection biases, that is, patients with a small tumor burden, no systemic symptoms, or no immunophenotypic or EBV data. Kim et al. previously examined the patterns of failure in 92 patients treated with radiotherapy alone at a median dose of 50 Gy (range, 40–60 Gy) [72]. After completion of this treatment, 61 patients (66%) achieved CR, and 16 (17%) showed a partial response (PR). However, ~50% of the patients ultimately displayed a local recurrence, and systemic failure was observed in 25% of cases. In addition, all patients with systemic failure (except one) died within 1 year [72]. The OS curve declined soon after diagnosis and reached a plateau at 2 years after diagnosis. The 5-year OS rate was 40%, and the 2-year OS rate was 45%. Hence, because both in-field and systemic relapses are frequent, radiotherapy alone is not sufficient to achieve a high cure rate for patients with localized nasal NK/T-cell lymphoma.

Radiotherapy for Localized Nasal NK/T-Cell Lymphoma

To determine the optimal radiotherapy and to achieve good local control of NK/T-cell lymphoma cases, radiation oncologists in East Asia have conducted several multicenter cooperative studies over the past decade. In terms of the radiation dose, these studies have suggested that >46 Gy is needed to obtain good local control [74, 75]. It is noteworthy that ENKL tumor cells are more resistant to radiotherapy than aggressive B-cell lymphomas. In terms of radiation volume, extension to include entire nasal cavities and sinuses is reported to be more effective than simply targeting the tumor volume with a small margin [76]. Moreover, CT- or MRI-based radiation planning is also recommended to achieve good local control [75]. However, it has been shown that late adverse events in the CNS escalate in patients who receive a total dose of >60 Gy. The optimal total dose is therefore likely to be 50 Gy. It must also be considered that there are several organs adjacent to the nasal cavity, such as the optic nerve, brain stem, and retina, that are at risk from radiotherapy. To minimize adverse events in these organs, treatments should be carefully planned using CT scanning and/or MRI by experienced radiation oncologists.

Intensity-modulated radiation therapy (IMRT) is expected to improve local control and reduce local toxicity in the treatment of ENKL. In western countries, IMRT has already been introduced as a routine treatment for localized nasal NK/T-cell lymphoma, at least in major centers. In East Asia, an attempt to substitute three-dimensional conformal radiotherapy with IMRT is ongoing [77], but conventional radiotherapy is still widely used in most institutes.

To prevent direct invasion of the brain, a sufficient margin to the side of the CNS should be established. There is also no firm evidence of any prophylactic benefit from the intrathecal administration of chemotherapeutic agents for localized nasal NK/T-cell lymphoma [78].

Frontline Radiotherapy Followed by Chemotherapy

Patients undergoing radiotherapy followed by chemotherapy have been reported to have a better prognosis [64, 79]. However, these results must be carefully evaluated because retrospective analyses may contain selection biases, and immunophenotypic analysis and the examination of the EBV status of the tumor cells were incomplete in many cases. It is also noteworthy that these earlier retrospective studies used anthracycline-containing chemotherapeutic regimens.

Concurrent Chemoradiotherapy

Overview

CCRT is expected to improve both local and systemic disease control and has been established as a standard therapy for several solid cancers. Conversely, this is not a standard treatment for lymphoma due to the generally good response of lymphomas to both chemotherapy and radiotherapy. In an earlier report from Mie University Hospital in Japan, two patients with localized nasal NK/T-cell lymphoma were successfully treated using CCRT [60]. DeVIC chemotherapy, which is a salvage chemotherapeutic regimen developed in Japan for relapsed or refractory aggressive lymphomas, was selected for concurrent use in these cases [80]. This therapy comprises dexamethasone, two MDR non-related chemotherapeutic agents (ifosfamide and carboplatin), and etoposide. Etoposide has been demonstrated to have both in vitro and in vivo efficacy against NK-cell neoplasms [81, 82] and is effective for both pediatric EBV-related hemophagocytic syndrome and pediatric EBV-associated lymphoproliferative disease [83]. The two patients [60] showed a high serum LDH level or B symptoms, which are known to be unfavorable prognostic factors in nasal NK/T-cell lymphoma [60]. However, they achieved CR and long-term survival, suggesting the potential efficacy of this treatment in high-risk patients. A Hong Kong study also reported a good therapeutic result from the use of frontline chemotherapy followed by CCRT with cisplatin and consolidative high-dose chemotherapy with autologous stem cell transplantation [84].

Because CCRT is a novel treatment modality for lymphomas, its toxicity and efficacy should be carefully evaluated in a prospective trial setting. Only one small phase II study of the use of CCRT in relapsed or refractory lymphomas with bulky disease was reported prior to 2006 [85]. In this study, radiotherapy at a median dose of 40 Gy and chemotherapy with cisplatin and etoposide were administrated concurrently. Because grade 3 or 4 hematologic toxicities were observed in 70% of the patients (14/21), the researchers concluded that hematologic toxicities and infection must be carefully managed when using this regimen.

A Prospective Trial for CCRT in a Japanese ENKL Cohort

To develop a more effective therapeutic strategy for newly diagnosed, localized nasal NK/T-cell lymphoma, the Lymphoma Study Group of the Japan Clinical Oncology Group (JCOG-LSG) conducted a phase I/II study to evaluate the

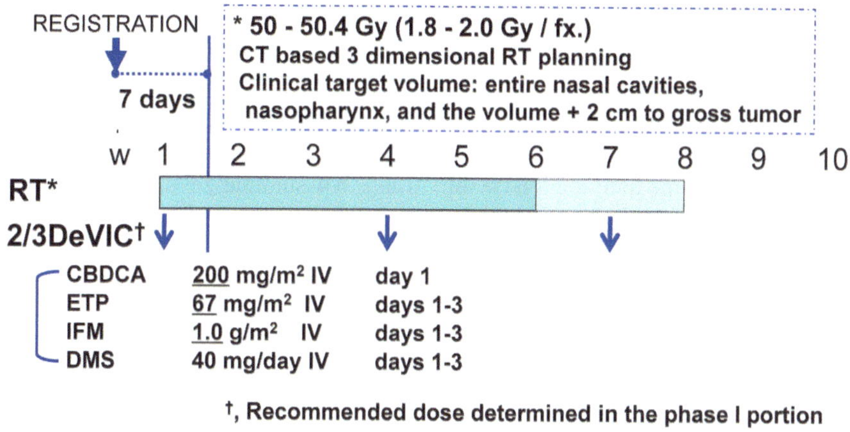

Fig. 6.1 Treatment protocol used in the JCOG0211 study. Radiotherapy at a 50 Gy dose and three courses of DeVIC chemotherapy were simultaneously initiated within 7 days of enrollment in the trial. Three dimensional conformal radiation planning using a CT scanner was performed for all patients. The clinical target volume included the entire nasal cavity, the nasopharynx, and the gross tumor volume with a margin of at least 2 cm. *RT* radiotherapy; *CBDCA* carboplatin; *ETP* etoposide; *IFM* ifosfamide; *DMS* dexamethasone

efficacy and toxicity of CCRT. This trial was designed to establish the optimal dose of DeVIC chemotherapy in combination with 50 Gy radiotherapy and then to historically compare the efficacy of this regimen with radiotherapy alone. This is the first prospective study for untreated, localized nasal NK/T-cell lymphomas that incorporated an adequate sample size and three central reviews (i.e., a central pathology review, a radiation quality assurance program, and a central CT review for efficacy assessments).

Patients with stage IE disease or contiguous stage IIE disease with cervical lymph node involvement were eligible for the trial. The protocol treatment comprised CCRT with relatively high-dose radiotherapy and chemotherapy with MDR-non-related agents and etoposide. Figure 6.1 depicts the treatment protocol for the trial (JCOG0211). In phase I, two dose levels of carboplatin, etoposide, and ifosfamide were evaluated. A two-thirds dose of DeVIC was then established as the recommended dose due to hematologic toxicity and infection.

In phase II of the trial, 27 patients who were treated with the recommended DeVIC dose (two-thirds) were evaluated. Compared to the historical control group [72], the median age was higher and B symptoms and cervical node involvement were more frequent in this study population. The median follow-up time was 32 months, with a range of 24–62 months. The primary endpoint, the 2-year OS, was 78% (90% CI, 61–88%; 95% CI, 57–89%), which was superior to the historical control of radiotherapy alone (45%) [72]. The 2-year progression-free survival (PFS) rate was 67%, the CR rate was 77%, and the overall response rate was 81%. The 2-year planning target volume control rate was 96%. Only one patient experienced loco-regional failure. Toxicity was mild and manageable in patients treated with the recommended dose, and no treatment-related deaths occurred. The most common grade 3 non-hematologic toxicity was mucositis related to radiation. From these data, it was concluded that CCRT using MDR non-related agents and etoposide is a safe and effective treatment for localized nasal NK/T-cell lymphoma, thus providing a basis for subsequent investigations.

A Prospective Trial of CCRT in a Korean ENKL Cohort

Subsequently to the aforementioned JCOG-LSG trial, a Korean group (Consortium for Improving Survival of Lymphoma; CISL) reported promising results from a phase II study of CCRT followed by ICE (ifosfamide, carboplatin, etoposide)-like chemotherapy for localized nasal NK/T-cell lymphoma [54]. Weekly cisplatin (30 mg/m^2, four treatments in total) was used for CCRT as a radiation sensitizer. The median total dose of radiotherapy was 40 Gy, ranging from 40 to 52.8 Gy. After 3–5 weeks, three courses of cisplatin-containing chemotherapy, a VIPD chemotherapeutic regimen (etoposide 100 mg/m^2, days 1–3; ifosfamide 1,200 mg/m^2, days 1–3; mesna 240 mg/m^2, days 1–3; cisplatin 33 mg/m^2, days 1–3; and dexamethasone 40 mg/day, days 1–4) was initiated. The protocol treatment was designated CCRT-VIPD.

Thirty patients were enrolled in this study. The CR rate at the best response was 80%, [54, 86] which was superior to the historical control group used [70]. At the median follow-up of 24 months, the estimated 3-year OS and PFS rates were 86 and 80%, respectively [54, 86]. Toxicities during CCRT were reported to be mild. However, grade 3 or 4 infections occurred in 60% of the patients during the VIPD therapy, and two patients died of infection. The researchers concluded that localized nasal NK/T-cell lymphoma is best treated with frontline CCRT [54].

Current Optimal Treatment Strategy for Localized Nasal NK/T-Cell Lymphoma

Table 6.4 summarizes the results from the two prospective studies of CCRT for localized nasal NK/T-cell lymphoma. The JCOG0211 study was characterized by relatively high-dose radiotherapy supported by a quality assurance program, short treatment duration, and acceptable local toxicities. The Korean study showed promising results in terms of the estimated PFS. However, because it was initiated 3 years later than the JCOG0211 study, the excellent estimated PFS may have been obtained by strict baseline evaluation using new diagnostic and staging procedures, such as FDG-PET or in situ hybridization for EBER in bone marrow material [27]. No patients experienced disease progression during the CCRT with cisplatin.

It is of interest that the profile of toxicity was quite different between the two studies. The most severe and frequent non-hematologic toxicity reported for the RT-2/3DeVIC therapy was mucositis due to radiation. In the Korean study, two treatment-related deaths due to infection

Table 6.4 Comparison of the results from two prospective clinical trials of concurrent chemoradiotherapy for localized nasal NK/T-cell lymphoma

	JCOG0211 study [53]	Korean study [54, 86]
Study design	Phase I/II	(Pilot study→) Phase II
Registration period	Sep 2003–Dec 2006	Apr 2006–Oct 2007
Median follow-up period (months, range)	32 (24–62)	24 (17–37)
Number of patients in Phase II	27	30
Total dose of radiotherapy	50 Gy (supported by quality assurance program)	40 Gy (median)
Concurrent chemotherapy regimen	2/3 DeVIC	Cisplatin alone
Time to completion of the treatment	9 weeks	16–18 weeks
CR rate (%)	77	80[a]
OS rate (%)	78 (2-year)	86 (3-year;estimated)
PFS rate (%)	67 (2-year)	80 (3-year;estimated)
Planning target volume (local) control rate (%)	96 (2-year)	93 (3-year;estimated)
Most common toxicity	Local toxicities due to radiation	Infection (two treatment-related deaths)

[a]At the best response

were observed during VIPD chemotherapy. It is likely that infection during CCRT-VIPD therapy is also more severe and frequent compared with the JCOG 0211 study.

Although there are several problems in analyzing the endpoints of the Korean study [86], these two trials showed promising results for CCRT in patients with localized nasal NK/T-cell lymphoma, particularly in terms of the excellent local control. From these data, CCRT using MDR non-related agents and etoposide is recommended for the current standard of care for this disease, partly because it is the first-line treatment that seems to be superior to radiotherapy alone in prospective studies of localized nasal NK/T-cell lymphoma. If it takes considerable time (e.g., more than 1 month) to prepare for frontline radiotherapy, chemotherapy with non-MDR-dependent drugs with sandwiched radiotherapy deserves consideration [59], although there is no prospective data regarding the efficacy of such a treatment strategy.

High-Dose Chemotherapy with Autologous Hematopoietic Stem Cell Transplantation

The benefits of consolidative high-dose chemotherapy with autologous hematopoietic stem cell transplantation (HSCT) as a first-line treatment have yet to be established. In a retrospective, multicenter study in a Korean cohort of 262 patients, 16 individuals underwent high-dose chemotherapy with autologous HSCT [87]. Subgroup analyses did not reveal any benefit of autologous HSCT in patients with localized disease, Group 1 or 2 NK-PI, or an involvement of the upper aerodigestive tract [87].

A multinational, matched, controlled study from East Asia suggested that high-dose chemotherapy is beneficial for patients in CR with a high NK-PI at diagnosis [88]. This study was based on long-term follow-up data, but no consideration was given to the heterogeneity of treatment, such as the chemotherapeutic regimen or the timing of the radiotherapy.

Treatment of Systemic, Relapsed or Refractory Cases of ENKL

Chemotherapy

The treatment outcomes for stage IV, relapsed or refractory patients with ENKL using conventional chemotherapy are extremely poor. For example, in the case of CHOP(-like) chemotherapy, the overall response rate is 36% for newly diagnosed stage IV diseases but <10% in relapsed or refractory cases. Two promising results for non-anthracycline-containing regimens in the treatment of nasal NK/T-cell lymphoma have been reported. The first is a prospective study of newly diagnosed advanced-stage ENKL with nasal involvement in a patient group from Mexico. In this trial, the patients were given six courses of CMED chemotherapy (cyclophosphamide, methotrexate, etoposide, and dexamethasone), with a sandwiched radiotherapy of 55 Gy after three courses, in patients with facial involvement [89]. The second study in a Chinese cohort involved treatment with a salvage chemotherapeutic regimen (L-asparaginase, vincristine, and dexamethasone) after a first-line anthracycline-containing chemotherapy followed by involved-field radiotherapy (median, 56 Gy) in patients with relapsed or refractory nasal NK/T-cell lymphoma [90]. Although the CR rates in these two studies exceeded 55%, this high level of efficacy has not been validated in other studies. The high-dose radiotherapy that was used in both studies makes it difficult to evaluate the efficacy of the chemotherapeutic regimens themselves. Moreover, high-dose radiotherapy is not a treatment option for patients who have already received involved-field radiotherapy during their first-line therapy for localized nasal NK/T-cell lymphoma. Because it is known that there are long-term survivors among patients with advanced-stage, relapsed or refractory ENKL who have undergone HSCT, development of an effective chemotherapeutic regimen for these patients may be an important initial step in improving the treatment outcome.

In 2004, Japanese core members of NKTSG and other colleagues in East Asia formulated a new chemotherapeutic regimen that comprises the steroid dexamethasone, methotrexate, ifosfamide, L-asparaginase, and etoposide (SMILE). The design of the SMILE regimen was based on several considerations. Etoposide was selected due to its in vitro and in vivo efficacy for NK-cell neoplasms and other EBV-associated diseases [81–83]. L-asparaginase is an anticancer drug that hydrolyzes serum asparagines and deprives lymphoid malignant cells of this required amino acid. This agent also induces the selective apoptosis of NK-cell lymphoma cells in vitro [91], and successful therapeutic results in NK-cell lymphoma have been reported using L-asparaginase, either alone or in combination with other drugs [90, 92, 93]. In a clinical trial for pediatric acute lymphoblastic leukemia, dexamethasone was reported to be more effective than prednisolone in ameliorating the adverse reactions to L-asparaginase [94]. Methotrexate and ifosfamide are unaffected by the MDR phenotype and are components of regimens that have been previously reported to be effective against ENKL. In the SMILE protocol, methotrexate was scheduled on day 1 to precede the other drugs because there is a possibility of antagonistic effects upon co-administration with etoposide and ifosfamide but synergic effects when preceding etoposide. The additional three drugs were scheduled for days 2–4 because the simultaneous use of etoposide and ifosfamide can lead to additive effects [95].

Given that advanced-stage ENKL and ANKL are extremely rare, a prospective therapeutic trial for these diseases is difficult to conduct. To overcome this problem, an international multicenter cooperative phase I study in East Asia was undertaken [95]. Patients with newly diagnosed stage IV, who had relapsed or refractory disease after first-line chemotherapy, and were between 15 and 69 years old with a PS of 0–2 were eligible. Six patients with ENKL were enrolled at Level 1 in the study. One treatment-related death due to infection occurred, but no other grade 4 non-hematologic toxicities were observed. After the first three patients were enrolled, a protocol revision stipulating the initiation of G-CSF from Day 6 was made. Major toxicities in six patients included grade 4 neutropenia and grade 3 hyponatremia. Three patients obtained a CR, with the remaining three cases showing PR, no response, and were not evaluable, respectively. The CR rate was 50% (3/6), and the overall response rate was 67% (4/6). The researchers concluded that a Level 1 dose with G-CSF support is recommended for further evaluation.

In the subsequent phase II study of SMILE, patients with ANKL were not eligible because none of these patients had been enrolled in phase I [95]. The primary endpoint was an overall response rate after two courses of SMILE chemotherapy thirty-nine patients were eventually enrolled and 38 patients were eligible. They had a median age of 47 years, and 20 of these patients had newly diagnosed stage IV disease. Because the first two patients died of a grade 5 infection, a protocol revision was made stipulating an awareness of infection and incorporating a lymphocyte count of 500/mm^3 or more into the eligibility criteria. There were no subsequent treatment-related deaths. The overall response rate, which was the primary endpoint of the trial, was 79% (95% CI, 65–89%), greatly superior to the historical control rate of 35%. The CR rate was 45%. The major toxicities were neutropenia, infection, and liver damage. These results indicate that SMILE chemotherapy is an effective induction therapy for newly diagnosed stage IV, relapsed or refractory ENKL [96]. Indeed, this regimen is now being used in clinical practice in East Asia [59]. However, careful monitoring for severe myelosuppression and infection is important when using this protocol.

Due to the high efficacy of this treatment against ENKL, a clinical trial incorporating a first-line use of SMILE chemotherapy for localized nasal NK/T-cell lymphoma may warrant investigation. However, because L-asparaginase can cause severe adverse drug reactions, such as thrombosis, hypofibrinogenemia, and pancreatitis, the efficacy and feasibility of first-line chemotherapeutic regimens containing this agent must be evaluated carefully.

Stem Cell Transplantation

To improve the therapeutic results in the treatment of ENKL, different HSCT settings have been attempted for patients with ENKL. The first case series were reported by Liang and colleagues in 1997 [97]. Three relapsed localized nasal NK/T-cell lymphoma patients underwent high-dose chemotherapy with cyclophosphamide, carmustine, and etoposide, supported by autologous bone marrow transplantation. Two of the patients were reported to be disease-free more than 12 months after transplantation. Subsequent reports provided data for small numbers of patients who had undergone various kinds of transplantation, such as autologous HSCT, tandem autologous HSCT, allogeneic HSCT, and cord blood transplantation. Two independent Japanese surveys of HSCT in the treatment of ENKL further revealed that some long-term survivors do emerge among patients with advanced-stage or relapsed/refractory disease following allogeneic HSCT [98, 99]. Survival curves for patients who underwent allogeneic HSCT often show a plateau, suggesting that this treatment may be curative for a fraction of patients.

Development of Novel Biological and Targeted Therapies

Because NK-cell neoplasms are rare, there have been very few clinical trials of novel agents specifically targeting ENKL. NK-cell neoplasms have been included in clinical trials of various kinds of novel agents for peripheral T-cell lymphomas or chemotherapy-resistant B-cell lymphomas in western countries. In East Asia, bortezomib and alemtuzumab have been investigated in terms of their efficacy against ENKL. Bortezomib induces apoptosis in the tumor cells of NK-cell leukemia and lymphoma [100]. Further, one of three patients with ENKL achieved CR in a previous phase I study of CHOP chemotherapy with bortezomib for advanced T or NK-cell lymphoma [101]. However, because CHOP is not effective against ENKL, other chemotherapy regimens in combination with bortezomib may warrant further study. Alemtuzumab, a humanized anti-CD52 antibody, is available in some countries in East Asia, and experience with this agent in the treatment of ENKL has been accumulating. However, its efficacy seems to be temporal in most patients with relapsed or refractory ENKL. The relatively low incidence (25%) of CD52 expression in the tumor cells of ENKL [102] may also diminish the clinical usefulness of this agent in ENKL.

Some of the new anticancer agents that have been developed in western countries are anticipated to show efficacy against ENKL. For example, pralatrexate is a folate antagonist that achieves a greater intracellular accumulation than other anti-folate drugs such as methotrexate. A relatively high response rate in patients with peripheral T-cell lymphomas in a phase II-I-II trial for relapsed or refractory peripheral T-cell lymphomas has been reported for this drug [103]. No patients with ENKL were enrolled in this trial, but because of its similarity with methotrexate (a key agent in the treatment of ENKL), pralatrexate is expected to be effective against this disease. Another example of a potentially effective new drug against ENKL is the histone deacetylase inhibitor vorinostat. This agent shows significant induction activity in the EBV lytic cycle in EBV-positive carcinoma cell lines [104]. In combination with azacitidine, vorinostat is being investigated in a clinical trial for the treatment of ENKL and nasopharyngeal carcinoma. Finally, siplizumab, a humanized monoclonal antibody against CD2, may be a viable candidate as a targeting therapy for ENKL, because CD2 is expressed in most ENKL tumors. A phase I trial of siplizumab in 29 patients with T-cell malignancies revealed that this agent could decrease the expression of CD2 and deplete both T-cells and NK-cells. However, this trial had to be terminated because of a high incidence of EBV-positive lymphoproliferative disease (14%) [105]. In an attempt to overcome this issue, a clinical trial of a rituximab-containing chemotherapy with siplizumab is now being conducted in the United States.

Conclusions

NK-cell neoplasms are rare and aggressive diseases, but an increased understanding and recognition of distinct disease entities, the emergence of better diagnostic procedures, recent multicenter prospective trials of new treatment strategies in East Asia, and the development of novel agents in western countries have all led to an improvement in the otherwise poor prognosis for these diseases. Further collaborative efforts on an international scale are needed to further improve the future treatments and outcomes for patients with NK-cell neoplasms.

References

1. Jaffe ES, Chan JK, Su IJ, et al. Report of the workshop on nasal and related extranodal angiocentric T/natural killer cell lymphomas. Definitions, differential diagnosis, and epidemiology. Am J Surg Pathol. 1996;20:103–11.
2. Swerdlow SH, Campo E, Harris NL, editors. WHO classification of tumours of haematopoietic and lymphoid tissues. Lyon: IARC; 2008.
3. Jaffe ES, Harris NL, Stein H, Vardiman JW. World Health Organization classification of tumours. Pathology and genetics of tumours of haematopoietic and lymphoid tissues. Lyon: IARC Press; 2001.
4. Dijkman R, van Doorn R, Szuhai K, Willemze R, Vermeer MH, Tensen CP. Gene-expression profiling and array-based CGH classify CD4+CD56+ hematodermic neoplasm and cutaneous myelomonocytic leukemia as distinct disease entities. Blood. 2007;109:1720–7.
5. Maeda T, Murata K, Fukushima T, et al. A novel plasmacytoid dendritic cell line, CAL-1, established from a patient with blastic natural killer cell lymphoma. Int J Hematol. 2005;81:148–54.
6. Au WY, Weisenburger DD, Intragumtornchai T, et al. Clinical differences between nasal and extranasal natural killer/T-cell lymphoma: a study of 136 cases from the International Peripheral T-Cell Lymphoma Project. Blood. 2009;113:3931–7.
7. Kim TM, Lee SY, Jeon YK, et al. Clinical heterogeneity of extranodal NK/T-cell lymphoma, nasal type: a national survey of the Korean Cancer Study Group. Ann Oncol. 2008;19:1477–84.
8. Tse E, Leung R, Khong PL, Lau WH, Kwong YL. Non-nasal natural killer cell lymphoma: not non-nasal after all. Ann Hematol. 2009;88:185–7.
9. Takahashi E, Asano N, Li C, et al. Nodal T/NK-cell lymphoma of nasal type: a clinicopathological study of six cases. Histopathology. 2008;52:585–96.
10. Li YX, Fang H, Liu QF, et al. Clinical features and treatment outcome of nasal-type NK/T-cell lymphoma of Waldeyer ring. Blood. 2008;112:3057–64.
11. Cerroni L, Massone C, Kutzner H, Mentzel T, Umbert P, Kerl H. Intravascular large T-cell or NK-cell lymphoma: a rare variant of intravascular large cell lymphoma with frequent cytotoxic phenotype and association with Epstein–Barr virus infection. Am J Surg Pathol. 2008;32:891–8.
12. Suzuki R. Leukemia and lymphoma of natural killer cells. J Clin Exp Hematop. 2005;45:51–70.
13. Suzuki R, Suzumiya J, Nakamura S, et al. Aggressive natural killer-cell leukemia revisited: large granular lymphocyte leukemia of cytotoxic NK cells. Leukemia. 2004;18:763–70.
14. Chan JK, Sin VC, Wong KF, et al. Nonnasal lymphoma expressing the natural killer cell marker CD56: a clinicopathologic study of 49 cases of an uncommon aggressive neoplasm. Blood. 1997;89: 4501–13.
15. Drenou B, Lamy T, Amiot L, et al. CD3- CD56+ non-Hodgkin's lymphomas with an aggressive behavior related to multidrug resistance. Blood. 1997;89:2966–74.
16. Egashira M, Kawamata N, Sugimoto K, Kaneko T, Oshimi K. P-glycoprotein expression on normal and abnormally expanded natural killer cells and inhibition of P-glycoprotein function by cyclosporin A and its analogue, PSC833. Blood. 1999;93:599–606.
17. Oshimi K. Progress in understanding and managing natural killer-cell malignancies. Br J Haematol. 2007;139:532–44.
18. Ohno Y, Amakawa R, Fukuhara S, et al. Acute transformation of chronic large granular lymphocyte leukemia associated with additional chromosome abnormality. Cancer. 1989;64:63–7.
19. Nakashima Y, Tagawa H, Suzuki R, et al. Genome-wide array-based comparative genomic hybridization of natural killer cell lymphoma/leukemia: different genomic alteration patterns of aggressive NK-cell leukemia and extranodal NK/T-cell lymphoma, nasal type. Genes Chromosomes Cancer. 2005;44:247–55.
20. Suzuki R, Suzumiya J, Yamaguchi M, et al. Prognostic factors for mature natural killer (NK) cell neoplasms: aggressive NK cell leukemia and extranodal NK cell lymphoma, nasal type. Ann Oncol. 2010;21:1032–40.
21. Lee J, Suh C, Park YH, et al. Extranodal natural killer T-cell lymphoma, nasal-type: a prognostic model from a retrospective multicenter study. J Clin Oncol. 2006;24:612–8.
22. A predictive model for aggressive non-Hodgkin's lymphoma. The International Non-Hodgkin's Lymphoma Prognostic Factors Project. N Engl J Med 1993;329:987–94.
23. Kako S, Izutsu K, Ota Y, et al. FDG-PET in T-cell and NK-cell neoplasms. Ann Oncol. 2007;18:1685–90.
24. Tsukamoto N, Kojima M, Hasegawa M, et al. The usefulness of (18)F-fluorodeoxyglucose positron emission tomography ((18)F-FDG-PET) and a comparison of (18)F-FDG-PET with (67)gallium scintigraphy in the evaluation of lymphoma: relation to histologic subtypes based on the World Health Organization classification. Cancer. 2007;110:652–9.

25. Khong PL, Pang CB, Liang R, Kwong YL, Au WY. Fluorine-18 fluorodeoxyglucose positron emission tomography in mature T-cell and natural killer cell malignancies. Ann Hematol. 2008;87:613–21.
26. Karantanis D, Subramaniam RM, Peller PJ, et al. The value of [(18)F]fluorodeoxyglucose positron emission tomography/computed tomography in extranodal natural killer/T-cell lymphoma. Clin Lymphoma Myeloma. 2008;8:94–9.
27. Lee J, Suh C, Huh J, et al. Effect of positive bone marrow EBV in situ hybridization in staging and survival of localized extranodal natural killer/T-cell lymphoma, nasal-type. Clin Cancer Res. 2007;13:3250–4.
28. Anderson JR, Armitage JO, Weisenburger DD. Epidemiology of the non-Hodgkin's lymphomas: distributions of the major subtypes differ by geographic locations. Non-Hodgkin's Lymphoma Classification Project. Ann Oncol. 1998;9:717–20.
29. Vose J, Armitage J, Weisenburger D. International peripheral T-cell and natural killer/T-cell lymphoma study: pathology findings and clinical outcomes. J Clin Oncol. 2008;26:4124–30.
30. The World Health Organization classification of malignant lymphomas in Japan: incidence of recently recognized entities. Lymphoma Study Group of Japanese Pathologists. Pathol Int. 2000;50:696–702.
31. Harabuchi Y, Yamanaka N, Kataura A, et al. Epstein–Barr virus in nasal T-cell lymphomas in patients with lethal midline granuloma. Lancet. 1990;335:128–30.
32. Calderon-Garciduenas L, Delgado R, Calderon-Garciduenas A, et al. Malignant neoplasms of the nasal cavity and paranasal sinuses: a series of 256 patients in Mexico City and Monterrey. Is air pollution the missing link? Otolaryngol Head Neck Surg. 2000;122:499–508.
33. Xu JX, Hoshida Y, Yang WI, et al. Life-style and environmental factors in the development of nasal NK/T-cell lymphoma: a case–control study in East Asia. Int J Cancer. 2007;120:406–10.
34. Emile JF, Boulland ML, Haioun C, et al. CD5-CD56+ T-cell receptor silent peripheral T-cell lymphomas are natural killer cell lymphomas. Blood. 1996;87:1466–73.
35. Hasserjian RP, Harris NL. NK cell lymphomas and leukemias: a spectrum of tumors with variable manifestations and immunophenotype. Am J Clin Pathol. 2007;127:860–8.
36. Yamaguchi M, Ohno T, Oka K, et al. Discordant reaction of Leu4 and rabbit anti-human CD3 epsilon in sinonasal "T"-cell lymphoma. Int J Hematol. 1993;59:25–30.
37. Suzumiya J, Takeshita M, Kimura N, et al. Sinonasal malignant lymphoma of natural killer cell phenotype associated with diffuse pancreatic involvement. Leuk Lymphoma. 1993;10:231–6.
38. Ohno T, Yamaguchi M, Oka K, Miwa H, Kita K, Shirakawa S. Frequent expression of CD3 epsilon in CD3 (Leu 4)-negative nasal T-cell lymphomas. Leukemia. 1995;9:44–52.
39. Chan JK, Tsang WY, Pau MY. Discordant CD3 expression in lymphomas when studied on frozen and paraffin sections. Hum Pathol. 1995;26:1139–43.
40. Yamaguchi M, Kita K, Miwa H, et al. Frequent expression of P-glycoprotein/MDR1 by nasal T-cell lymphoma cells. Cancer. 1995;76:2351–6.
41. Bossard C, Belhadj K, Reyes F, et al. Expression of the granzyme B inhibitor PI9 predicts outcome in nasal NK/T-cell lymphoma: results of a Western series of 48 patients treated with first-line polychemotherapy within the Groupe d'Etude des Lymphomes de l'Adulte (GELA) trials. Blood. 2007;109:2183–9.
42. Shim SJ, Yang WI, Shin E, et al. Clinical significance of cyclooxygenase-2 expression in extranodal natural killer (NK)/T-cell lymphoma, nasal type. Int J Radiat Oncol Biol Phys. 2007;67:31–8.
43. Chiang AK, Tao Q, Srivastava G, Ho FC. Nasal NK- and T-cell lymphomas share the same type of Epstein–Barr virus latency as nasopharyngeal carcinoma and Hodgkin's disease. Int J Cancer. 1996;68:285–90.
44. Harabuchi Y, Takahara M, Kishibe K, Moriai S, Nagato T, Ishii H. Nasal natural killer (NK)/T-cell lymphoma: clinical, histological, virological, and genetic features. Int J Clin Oncol. 2009;14:181–90.
45. Kim JE, Kim YA, Jeon YK, Park SS, Heo DS, Kim CW. Comparative analysis of NK/T-cell lymphoma and peripheral T-cell lymphoma in Korea: clinicopathological correlations and analysis of EBV strain type and 30-bp deletion variant LMP1. Pathol Int. 2003;53:735–43.
46. Takakuwa T, Dong Z, Nakatsuka S, et al. Frequent mutations of Fas gene in nasal NK/T cell lymphoma. Oncogene. 2002;21:4702–5.
47. Takahara M, Kishibe K, Bandoh N, Nonaka S, Harabuchi Y. P53, N- and K-Ras, and beta-catenin gene mutations and prognostic factors in nasal NK/T-cell lymphoma from Hokkaido, Japan. Hum Pathol. 2004;35:86–95.
48. Nagata H, Konno A, Kimura N, et al. Characterization of novel natural killer (NK)-cell and gammadelta T-cell lines established from primary lesions of nasal T/NK cell lymphomas associated with the Epstein–Barr virus. Blood. 2001;97:708–13.
49. Takahara M, Kis LL, Nagy N, et al. Concomitant increase of LMP1 and CD25 (IL-2-receptor alpha) expression induced by IL-10 in the EBV-positive NK lines SNK6 and KAI3. Int J Cancer. 2006;119:2775–83.
50. Huang Y, de Reynies A, de Leval L, et al. Gene expression profiling identifies emerging oncogenic pathways operating in extranodal NK/T-cell lymphoma, nasal type. Blood. 2010;115:1226–37.
51. Karube K, Nakagawa M, Tsuzuki S, et al. Identification of FOXO3 and PRDM1 as tumor-suppressor gene candidates in NK-cell neoplasms by genomic and functional analyses. Blood. 2011;118:3195–204.

52. Chim CS, Ma SY, Au WY, et al. Primary nasal natural killer cell lymphoma: long-term treatment outcome and relationship with the International Prognostic Index. Blood. 2004;103:216–21.
53. Yamaguchi M, Tobinai K, Oguchi M, et al. Phase I/II study of concurrent chemoradiotherapy for localized nasal natural killer/T-cell lymphoma: Japan Clinical Oncology Group Study JCOG0211. J Clin Oncol. 2009;27:5594–600.
54. Kim SJ, Kim K, Kim BS, et al. Phase II trial of concurrent radiation and weekly cisplatin followed by VIPD chemotherapy in newly diagnosed, stage IE to IIE, nasal, extranodal NK/T-Cell lymphoma: consortium for improving survival of lymphoma study. J Clin Oncol. 2009;27:6027–32.
55. Kim TM, Park YH, Lee SY, et al. Local tumor invasiveness is more predictive of survival than International Prognostic Index in stage I(E)/II(E) extranodal NK/T-cell lymphoma, nasal type. Blood. 2005;106:3785–90.
56. Lei KI, Chan LY, Chan WY, Johnson PJ, Lo YM. Quantitative analysis of circulating cell-free Epstein–Barr virus (EBV) DNA levels in patients with EBV-associated lymphoid malignancies. Br J Haematol. 2000;111:239–46.
57. Lei KI, Chan LY, Chan WY, Johnson PJ, Lo YM. Diagnostic and prognostic implications of circulating cell-free Epstein–Barr virus DNA in natural killer/T-cell lymphoma. Clin Cancer Res. 2002;8:29–34.
58. Suzuki R, Yamaguchi M, Izutsu K, et al. Prospective measurement of Epstein-Barr virus-DNA in plasma and peripheral blood mononuclear cells of extranodal NK/T-cell lymphoma, nasal type. Blood. 2011; 118:6018–22.
59. Kwong YL, Anderson BO, Advani R, Kim WS, Levine AM, Lim ST. Management of T-cell and natural-killer-cell neoplasms in Asia: consensus statement from the Asian Oncology Summit 2009. Lancet Oncol. 2009;10:1093–101.
60. Yamaguchi M, Ogawa S, Nomoto Y, et al. Treatment outcome of nasal NK-cell lymphoma: A report of 12 consecutively-diagnosed cases and a review of the literature. J Clin Exp Hematop. 2001;41:93–9.
61. Miller TP, Dahlberg S, Cassady JR, et al. Chemotherapy alone compared with chemotherapy plus radiotherapy for localized intermediate- and high-grade non-Hodgkin's lymphoma. N Engl J Med. 1998;339:21–6.
62. Yu KH, Yu SC, Teo PM, Chan AT, Yeo W, Chow J. Nasal lymphoma: results of local radiotherapy with or without chemotherapy. Head Neck. 1997;19: 251–9.
63. Kwong YL, Chan AC, Liang R, et al. CD56+ NK lymphomas: clinicopathological features and prognosis. Br J Haematol. 1997;97:821–9.
64. Ribrag V, Ell Hajj M, Janot F, et al. Early locoregional high-dose radiotherapy is associated with long-term disease control in localized primary angiocentric lymphoma of the nose and nasopharynx. Leukemia. 2001;15:1123–6.
65. Cheung MM, Chan JK, Lau WH, Ngan RK, Foo WW. Early stage nasal NK/T-cell lymphoma: clinical outcome, prognostic factors, and the effect of treatment modality. Int J Radiat Oncol Biol Phys. 2002;54:182–90.
66. Li CC, Tien HF, Tang JL, et al. Treatment outcome and pattern of failure in 77 patients with sinonasal natural killer/T-cell or T-cell lymphoma. Cancer. 2004;100:366–75.
67. You JY, Chi KH, Yang MH, et al. Radiation therapy versus chemotherapy as initial treatment for localized nasal natural killer (NK)/T-cell lymphoma: a single institute survey in Taiwan. Ann Oncol. 2004;15:618–25.
68. Pagano L, Gallamini A, Trape G, et al. NK/T-cell lymphomas 'nasal type': an Italian multicentric retrospective survey. Ann Oncol. 2006;17:794–800.
69. Kim WS, Song SY, Ahn YC, et al. CHOP followed by involved field radiation: is it optimal for localized nasal natural killer/T-cell lymphoma? Ann Oncol. 2001;12:349–52.
70. Lee SH, Ahn YC, Kim WS, Ko YH, Kim K, Park K. The effect of pre-irradiation dose intense CHOP on anthracyline resistance in localized nasal NK/T-cell lymphoma. Haematologica. 2006;91:427–8.
71. Huang H, Lin Z, Lin X, Cai Q, Xia Z, Jiang W. Long-term outcomes of patients with newly diagnosed extranodal natural killer/T-cell lymphoma treated by etoposide, prednisone, vincristine, cyclophosphamide, and doxorubicin regimen. Leuk Lymphoma. 2011;52:1041–8.
72. Kim GE, Cho JH, Yang WI, et al. Angiocentric lymphoma of the head and neck: patterns of systemic failure after radiation treatment. J Clin Oncol. 2000;18:54–63.
73. Li YX, Yao B, Jin J, et al. Radiotherapy as primary treatment for stage IE and IIE nasal natural killer/T-cell lymphoma. J Clin Oncol. 2006;24:181–9.
74. Shikama N, Ikeda H, Nakamura S, et al. Localized aggressive non-Hodgkin's lymphoma of the nasal cavity: a survey by the Japan Lymphoma Radiation Therapy Group. Int J Radiat Oncol Biol Phys. 2001;51:1228–33.
75. Koom WS, Chung EJ, Yang WI, et al. Angiocentric T-cell and NK/T-cell lymphomas: radiotherapeutic viewpoints. Int J Radiat Oncol Biol Phys. 2004; 59:1127–37.
76. Isobe K, Uno T, Tamaru J, et al. Extranodal natural killer/T-cell lymphoma, nasal type: the significance of radiotherapeutic parameters. Cancer. 2006;106: 609–15.
77. Tomita N, Kodaira T, Tachibana H, et al. A comparison of radiation treatment plans using IMRT with helical tomotherapy and 3D conformal radiotherapy for nasal natural killer/T-cell lymphoma. Br J Radiol. 2009;82:756–63.
78. Kim SJ, Oh SY, Hong JY, et al. When do we need central nervous system prophylaxis in patients with extranodal NK/T-cell lymphoma, nasal type? Ann Oncol. 2010;21:1058–63.

79. Aviles A, Diaz NR, Neri N, Cleto S, Talavera A. Angiocentric nasal T/natural killer cell lymphoma: a single centre study of prognostic factors in 108 patients. Clin Lab Haematol. 2000;22:215–20.
80. Okamoto M, Maruyama F, Tsuzuki M, et al. Salvage chemotherapy for relapsed/refractory aggressive non-Hodgkin's lymphoma with a combination of dexamethasone, etoposide, ifosfamide and carboplatin. Rinsho Ketsueki. 1994;35:635–41 (in Japanese).
81. Uno M, Tsuchiyama J, Moriwaki A, et al. In vitro induction of apoptosis for nasal angiocentric natural killer cell lymphoma-derived cell line, NK-YS, by etoposide and cyclosporine A. Br J Haematol. 2001;113:1009–14.
82. Lee KW, Yun T, Kim DW, et al. First-line ifosfamide, methotrexate, etoposide and prednisolone chemotherapy +/− radiotherapy is active in stage I/II extranodal NK/T-cell lymphoma. Leuk Lymphoma. 2006;47:1274–82.
83. Imashuku S, Kuriyama K, Teramura T, et al. Requirement for etoposide in the treatment of Epstein–Barr virus-associated hemophagocytic lymphohistiocytosis. J Clin Oncol. 2001;19:2665–73.
84. Au WY, Lie AK, Liang R, et al. Autologous stem cell transplantation for nasal NK/T-cell lymphoma: a progress report on its value. Ann Oncol. 2003;14:1673–6.
85. Girinsky T, Lapusan S, Ribrag V, Koscielny S, Ferme C, Carde P. Phase II study of concomitant chemoradiotherapy in bulky refractory or chemoresistant relapsed lymphomas. Int J Radiat Oncol Biol Phys. 2005;61:476–9.
86. Shimada K, Suzuki R. Concurrent chemoradiotherapy for limited-stage extranodal natural killer/T-cell lymphoma, nasal type. J Clin Oncol. 2010;28:e229. author reply e30.
87. Kim HJ, Bang SM, Lee J, et al. High-dose chemotherapy with autologous stem cell transplantation in extranodal NK/T-cell lymphoma: a retrospective comparison with non-transplantation cases. Bone Marrow Transplant. 2006;37:819–24.
88. Lee J, Au WY, Park MJ, et al. Autologous hematopoietic stem cell transplantation in extranodal natural killer/T cell lymphoma: a multinational, multicenter, matched controlled study. Biol Blood Marrow Transplant. 2008;14:1356–64.
89. Aviles A, Cleto S, Castaneda C, Nambo MJ. CMED in the treatment of nasal natural killer cell lymphoma with distant metastases. Hematology. 2007;12:241–4.
90. Yong W, Zheng W, Zhang Y, et al. L-asparaginase-based regimen in the treatment of refractory midline nasal/nasal-type T/NK-cell lymphoma. Int J Hematol. 2003;78:163–7.
91. Ando M, Sugimoto K, Kitoh T, et al. Selective apoptosis of natural killer-cell tumours by L-asparaginase. Br J Haematol. 2005;130:860–8.
92. Nagafuji K, Fujisaki T, Arima F, Ohshima K. L-asparaginase induced durable remission of relapsed nasal NK/T-cell lymphoma after autologous peripheral blood stem cell transplantation. Int J Hematol. 2001;74:447–50.
93. Jaccard A, Gachard N, Marin B, et al. Efficacy of L-asparaginase with methotrexate and dexamethasone (AspaMetDex regimen) in patients with refractory or relapsing extranodal NK/T-cell lymphoma, a phase 2 study. Blood. 2011;117:1834–9.
94. Nowak-Gottl U, Ahlke E, Fleischhack G, et al. Thromboembolic events in children with acute lymphoblastic leukemia (BFM protocols): prednisone versus dexamethasone administration. Blood. 2003;101:2529–33.
95. Yamaguchi M, Suzuki R, Kwong YL, et al. Phase I study of dexamethasone, methotrexate, ifosfamide, L-asparaginase, and etoposide (SMILE) chemotherapy for advanced-stage, relapsed or refractory extranodal natural killer (NK)/T-cell lymphoma and leukemia. Cancer Sci. 2008;99:1016–20.
96. Yamaguchi M, Kwong YL, Kim WS, et al. Phase II study of SMILE chemotherapy for newly diagnosed stage IV, relapsed, or refractory extranodal natural killer (NK)/T-cell lymphoma, nasal type: the NK-Cell Tumor Study Group study. J Clin Oncol. 2011;29:4410–6.
97. Liang R, Chen F, Lee CK, et al. Autologous bone marrow transplantation for primary nasal T/NK cell lymphoma. Bone Marrow Transplant. 1997;19:91–3.
98. Murashige N, Kami M, Kishi Y, et al. Allogeneic haematopoietic stem cell transplantation as a promising treatment for natural killer-cell neoplasms. Br J Haematol. 2005;130:561–7.
99. Suzuki R, Suzumiya J, Nakamura S, et al. Hematopoietic stem cell transplantation for natural killer-cell lineage neoplasms. Bone Marrow Transplant. 2006;37:425–31.
100. Shen L, Au WY, Guo T, et al. Proteasome inhibitor bortezomib-induced apoptosis in natural killer (NK)-cell leukemia and lymphoma: an in vitro and in vivo preclinical evaluation. Blood. 2007;110:469–70.
101. Lee J, Suh C, Kang HJ, et al. Phase I study of proteasome inhibitor bortezomib plus CHOP in patients with advanced, aggressive T-cell or NK/T-cell lymphoma. Ann Oncol. 2008;19:2079–83.
102. Jiang L, Yuan CM, Hubacheck J, et al. Variable CD52 expression in mature T cell and NK cell malignancies: implications for alemtuzumab therapy. Br J Haematol. 2009;145:173–9.
103. O'Connor OA, Horwitz S, Hamlin P, et al. Phase II-I-II study of two different doses and schedules of pralatrexate, a high-affinity substrate for the reduced folate carrier, in patients with relapsed or refractory lymphoma reveals marked activity in T-cell malignancies. J Clin Oncol. 2009;27:4357–64.
104. Hui KF, Chiang AK. Suberoylanilide hydroxamic acid induces viral lytic cycle in Epstein–Barr virus-positive epithelial malignancies and mediates enhanced cell death. Int J Cancer. 2010;126:2479–89.
105. O'Mahony D, Morris JC, Stetler-Stevenson M, et al. EBV-related lymphoproliferative disease complicating therapy with the anti-CD2 monoclonal antibody, siplizumab, in patients with T-cell malignancies. Clin Cancer Res. 2009;15:2514–22.

Rare Subtypes of Extranodal T-Cell Lymphoma

7

Frederick Lansigan, S. David Hudnall, and Francine Foss

Introduction

In 2008, two major publications clarified the importance of improving the diagnosis and outcomes of peripheral T-cell lymphoma. The first was the fourth edition of the World Health Organization (WHO) Classification of Tumours of the Haematopoietic and Lymphoid Tissues [1]. This project classified the mature T-cell and natural killer (NK)-cell neoplasms into over 20 subtypes, with six new subtypes added, in an effort to standardize the diagnostic criteria for these lymphomas which are often misdiagnosed due to unfamiliarity of the clinical picture from which they arise. The second was the International Peripheral T-Cell and Natural Killer/T-Cell Lymphoma Study: Pathology Findings and Clinical Outcomes by Vose et al. [2], which showed the distribution of the different subtypes (shown in Fig. 1.1) and reported outcomes. The extranodal group includes a number of less common entities described primarily by their tissue tropism. This includes the, including hepatosplenic T-cell lymphomas (HSTLs), intestinal T-cell lymphomas, and the panniculitis-like T-cell lymphomas. A new provisional entity included in this group is the primary cutaneous gamma delta T-cell lymphomas. The frequency of these subtypes is low, and treatment algorithms for most of the rare subtypes have not been well established. Outcomes for the rare subtypes of T-cell lymphomas are shown in Table 7.1.

Hepatosplenic T-Cell Lymphoma

Normal γ/δ T-cells are a small subset of cytotoxic T-cells that preferentially exhibit homing to epithelial rich tissue and sinusoidal areas of the splenic red pulp. These γ/δ T-cells originate from CD4 to CD8- (double negative) precursors, and have the potential to mature outside the thymus. When activated, γ/δ T-cells can express NK cell-associated surface and cytoplasmic molecules, suggesting a function similar to NK cells [3]. γ/δ T-cells also bear T-cell receptors (TCRs) with less discriminate antigen specificity and can recognize antigens of multiple pathogens. One hypothesis for the origin of the γ/δ T-cell lymphomas is that polyclonal expansion of the γ/δ T-cells due to external or internal stimuli occurs and may give rise to transforming events lead to the development of a monoclonal process, such as HSTL [3].

F. Lansigan
Department of Hematology and Oncology, Dartmouth-Hitchcock Medical Center, Norris Cotton Cancer Center, Lebanon, NH, USA

S.D. Hudnall
Department of Pathology, Yale University School of Medicine, New Haven, CT, USA

F. Foss (✉)
Department of Medical Oncology/Hematology, Yale University School of Medicine, 333 Cedar Street, FMP 130, PO Box 208032, New Haven, CT 06520, USA
e-mail: Francine.foss@yale.edu

F. Foss (ed.), *T-Cell Lymphomas*, Contemporary Hematology,
DOI 10.1007/978-1-62703-170-7_7, © Springer Science+Business Media New York 2013

Table 7.1 Outcomes for PTCL by histologic type (Based on data from Vose et al. [2])

Diagnosis	5-year OS	5-year FFS
PTCL-NOS	32	20
Angioimmunoblastic	32	18
ALCL ALK+	70	60
ALCL ALK−	49	36
Nasal NKT	42	29
Extranasal NKT	9	6
Enteropathy associated	20	4
Hepatosplenic	7	0
Subcutaneous panniculitis	64	24
Adult T-cell leukemia	14	12

OS overall survival; *FFS* failure-free survival; *PTCL* peripheral T-cell lymphoma; *NOS* not otherwise specified; *NKTCL* natural killer/T-cell lymphoma; *ATLL* adult T-cell leukemia/lymphoma; *ALCL* anaplastic large-cell lymphoma

HSTL was first described in 1990 by Farcet et al. [4]. Two patients with systemic symptoms, hepatosplenomegaly, thrombocytopenia, and absence of lymphadenopathy, were described. Both were found to have a sinusoidal pattern of infiltration of the liver with CD3 + TCRγ/δ T-cells. This was in contrast to the usual lymphomatous infiltration of the portal tracts of the liver and white pulp of the spleen in other types of T and B-cell lymphomas. These two patients had rapid progression of their disease despite treatment. HSTL comprises only 1.4% of peripheral and NK-cell lymphomas worldwide, but it is one of the most aggressive PTCL subtypes, with a dismal 7%, 5-year survival. Most patients succumb within one year [2]. HSTL most commonly occurs in males in the fourth decade of life and is more common in North America and Europe than in Asia.

Risk factors for HSTL include a history of immune suppression, and the disease occurs with increased frequency in the setting of organ transplant recipients and patient with autoimmune disorders, such as inflammatory bowel disease (especially those receiving thiopurines), lupus, Sjogren's syndrome, Hodgkin's lymphoma and malaria [5]. EBV does not appear to be associated with HSTL, though it has been associated with post-transplant lymphoproliferative disorder [5]. Recently, the incidence of HSTL has been reviewed in patients with inflammatory bowel disease. Schmidt et al. reported that eight cases were identified through the FDA's Adverse Event Reporting System [6]. Kotylar et al. reviewed 36 cases of HSTL in patients with inflammatory bowel disease, 20 of which received infliximab and a thiopurine and 16 received thiopurine therapy alone [7]. Most of the patients were under age 35 and only two were females. The median time from onset of thiopurine agents and diagnosis of HSTL was 5.5 years, and the median number of doses of infliximab was three. Of the 36 patients, only 8 are alive. They identified an increased risk of developing HSTL in patients receiving combination therapy with thiopurine an anti-TNF agents compared to those receiving monotherapy with thiopurines, but there was no increased risk identified in patients receiving only anti-TNF therapy.

The clinical features of HSTLs are described in Table 7.2. The morphology of HSTL demonstrates clusters of monomorphic medium-sized T-lymphoid cells with loosely condensed chromatin and a pale rim of cytoplasm. The infiltrate is seen in both the liver and the spleen. There is sinusoidal infiltration of the splenic red pulp with resultant atrophy of the white pulp, as shown in Fig. 7.1. The liver exhibits sinusoid expansion and sparing of the portal triads without hepatocyte destruction [1]. Bone marrow involvement is seen in two-thirds of patients with HSTL [8]. The immunohistochemical profile of this lymphoma is typically CD2+, CD3+, CD4−, CD5−, CD7+, CD8−, and either γ/δ or α/β, although the majority are γ/δ. Rare cases may be CD8 positive. The NK antigens, CD16 and CD56, are frequently expressed. Although the WHO 2008 does not distinguish γ/δ from α/β HSTL, the γ/δ phenotype predominates and contributes to the poor prognosis in HSTL similar to other non-hepatosplenic γ/δ T-cell lymphomas.

The HSTL cells exhibit clonality with gene rearrangements of the TCR. The TCR-Vδ expression is restricted to Vδ1, and Vδ1 associates with different Vγ regions. This is in contrast to the Vδ2 usage by non-HSTL such as primary cutaneous γ/δ T-cell lymphoma [7]. The majority of HSTL show recurrent cytogenetic abnormalities, namely

Table 7.2 Hepatosplenic T-cell lymphoma

Clinical features	Hepatosplenomegaly, no adenopathy
	Mostly occurs in young men
	Bone marrow involvement (cytopenias)
	Increased risk in IBD patients with thiopurine and anti-TNF agents
Immunophenotypic features	CD2+, CD3+, CD4−, CD5−, CD7+, CD8− Most are
	Some patients express CD8 or NK markers (CD16, CD56)
	Inactive cytotoxic phenotype (TIA-1+, perforin−)
Genetics	TCR $\gamma\delta$
	Isochromosome 7q in 40–70%
Outcome	Median survival 8–12 months

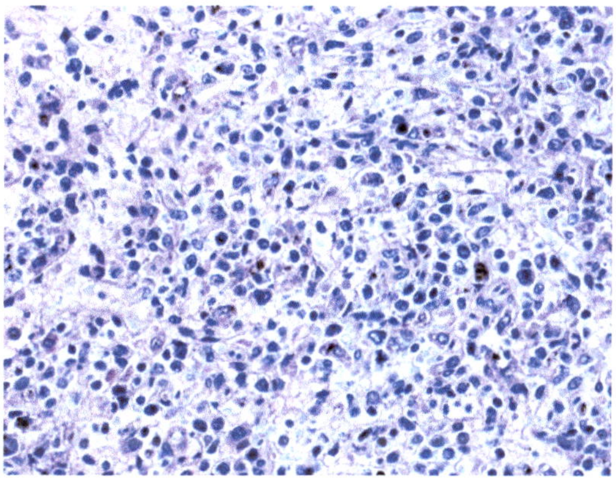

Fig. 7.1 Diffuse atypical T cell infiltrate of the splenic red pulp (hepatosplenic T cell lymphoma) (H&E stain)

isochromosome 7q which almost invariably is associated with trisomy 8 [6, 7]. These cytogenetic abnormalities while diagnostically useful do not have prognostic significance [8]. Recent data has shown that γ/δ HSTL shows a distinct gene expression profiling signature from PTCL including α/β PTCL and γ/δ PTCL. NK-associated molecules such as KIR and killer lectin-like receptors have been found to be overexpressed [9].

Published experience in treating HSTL include multiple induction regimens, most commonly CHOP-(cyclophosphamide, doxorubicin, vincristine, prednisone)-like and platinum-based lymphoma regimens [6, 7, 9]. Although responses have been seen in approximately two-thirds of HSTL, responses are brief. Platinum and cytarabine-based induction therapy has resulted in sustained responses [7]. There are also reports of patients responding to purine analog therapy, such as 2′deoxycoformycin [10]. One adolescent with HSTL treated with an aggressive pediatric T-cell leukemia regimen followed by allogeneic stem cell transplantation also has shown a sustained response [11]. Sequential combination chemotherapy such as IDSHAP/AMDBIDCOS/MINE, and monoclonal antibody combination therapy such as pentostatin/alemtuzumab have induced complete responses [12]. Falchook et al. reported 15 cases of HSTL [13]. Of these, seven had a complete response to chemotherapy and three underwent a stem cell transplant. The duration of CR was 8 months, and median OS was 13 months for the CR vs. 8 months for nonresponders. Adverse prognostic factors included male gender, failure to achieve a CR with chemotherapy, and absence of a detectable TCR rearrangement in the gamma chain. Due to demonstrable graft vs. lymphoma effect, allogeneic stem cell transplantation should be offered to all eligible patients, including those who are in first remission, as it seems to be the only chance for a durable remission [5]. With respect to newer agents, Piekerz et al. reported that one patient with relapsed HSTL had a partial response with a duration of 8 months with romidepsin.

Subcutaneous Panniculitis-Like T-Cell Lymphoma

Subcutaneous panniculitis-like T-cell lymphoma (SPTCL) is characterized by infiltration of malignant T-lymphocytes in subcutaneous tissue, often rimming the fat lobules. Although SPTCL has been recognized as a distinctive entity in the category of peripheral T-cell lymphoma in the WHO classification, its diagnostic criteria has been redefined by the recent WHO-European Organization for Research and Treatment of Cancer (EORTC) classification for primary cutaneous lymphomas. The term SPTCL is now restricted to primary tumors expressing the alpha/beta TCR

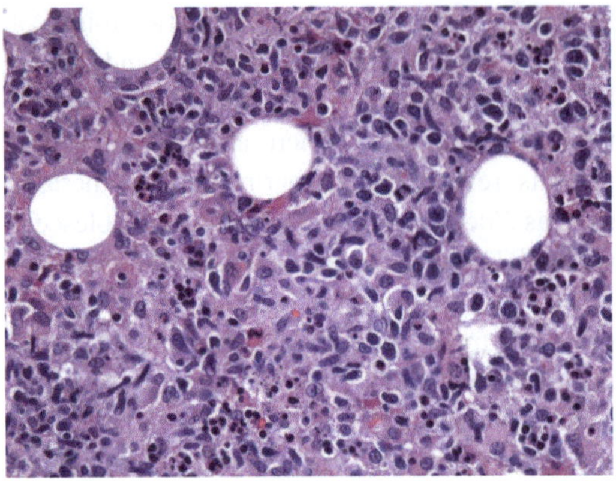

Fig. 7.2 Diffuse atypical T cell infiltrate of deep subcutaneous tissues of the thigh with growth around fat cells (subcutaneous panniculitis-like T cell lymphoma) (H&E stain)

phenotype. These lymphomas are usually CD3(+), CD4(−), CD8(+), and CD56(−), and usually have an indolent clinical course. The tumors expressing the gamma/delta phenotype have been reclassified as primary cutaneous gamma/delta T-cell lymphoma (PCGD-TCL) [14].

SPTCL usually presents with one or multiple subcutaneous nodules involving one or multiple areas of the body and often in the absence of extracutaneous disease. The nodules may resemble benign panniculitis and vary in size, but occasionally they may become necrotic and ulcerate. Systemic symptoms, including fevers, weight loss, and pancytopenia may also occur. The pancytopenia is often cytokine-mediated, as bone marrow involvement is rare [15, 16]. The histopathology is often distinctive, with atypical T-lymphocytes surrounding fat globules, as shown in Fig. 7.2.

Atypical lymphocyte lobular panniculitis is a benign entity which may be confused with SPTCL (Table 7.3). ALLP is manifest by the appearance of waxing and waning bruise-like plaques with no constitutional symptoms. The disease occurs in young women and is not ulcerative. The lesions demonstrate many of the same features as SPTCL but have less evidence of fat necrosis, and many cases are polyclonal. Another entity which overlaps SPTCL is lupus panniculitis. While clinical manifestations may be different, it is often difficult to distinguish between these entities based on histopathology. Microscopic findings that can help to distinguish LEP from SPTCL include vacuolar change at the dermal–epidermal interface, periadnexal lymphocytic infiltrates, and mucin deposition in the reticular dermis. Clusters of B-lymphocytes and plasma cells may also be seen in lupus panniculitis. Lupus panniculitis is often polyclonal and classically presents on the face or upper trunk. Studies have shown that there may be overlap between ALLP and lupus panniculitis and SPTCL, and the EORTC retrospective study reported that 19% of patients with SPTCL had autoimmune diseases, including four with lupus.

The clinical course for patients with SPTCL has been highly variable, due in part to the small number of cases reported and to the fact that until recently the distinction between the alpha/beta and gamma/delta subtypes had not been uniformly made at diagnosis. Other than alpha/beta vs. gamma/delta, Kong et al. have reviewed 22 cases of SPTCL in Asia and have identified angioinvasion as a poor prognostic marker [17]. In addition, the hemophagocytic syndrome may occur in up to one-third of patients and in some cases may be fulminant.

PCGD-TCL accounts for less than 1% of all cutaneous TCL and are believed to arise from the gamma/delta T-cell compartments within the skin and dermal appendages. PCGD-TCL most commonly presents as diffuse skin involvement with disseminated lesions that mainly affect the extremities and frequently are associated with ulceration and necrosis. The phenotype of PCGD patients is CD3+, CD8− with expression of cytotoxic markers in most cases (TIA-1, granzyme B, perforin). Unlike alpha/beta SPTCL, dissemination to other extranodal sites is frequently, and the majority of patients present with B-symptoms.

A retrospective review by Willemze et al. and the EORTC Cutaneous Lymphoma Group describes clinical features and outcomes of 63 patients with SPTCL and 20 with PCGD-TCL based on careful pathological review of the cases (Table 7.4) [14]. The median age was younger (39 years vs. 59 years) for the SPTCL patients, and there was no difference in the frequency of

Table 7.3 Differential diagnosis of panniculitis like disorders (Based on data from Magro et al. [22])

Atypical lymphocyte lobular panniculitis	SPTCLαβ	Cutaneous γδ T-cell lymphoma
Young women	All ages, 20% are children associated with SLE, RA	Median age 59
Deep plaques, legs frequently, no ulceration	Indurated, nonulcerated nodules	Ulcerative lesions
B symptoms rare	50% have constitutional symptoms, fevers, cytopenias Nodal and BM involvement rare	Most have constitutional symptoms Lymphadenopathy, hepatosplenomegaly, BM frequent
Infiltrate is less, hemorrhage, karyorrhexis, vasculitis absent	Infiltrate has fat necrosis and karyorrhexis without hemorrhage	Angiocentric, extensive hemorrhage and necrosis
No predominance of CD8 cells	CD8+ Nav3 mutation, perforin gene mutations noted	CD3+ CD56+ Few cases are CD8+
May be treated with steroids, methotrexate	Treatment with radiation, steroids, immunosuppressive agents, chemotherapy	Steroids, chemotherapy, denileukin diftitox, Allo BMT
Oligoclonal or clonal TCRR	Clonal TCRR	Clonal TCRR

Table 7.4 Characteristics of SPTCL and primary cutaneous gamma delta T-cell lymphoma (Based on data from Willemze et al. [14])

	SPTCL-AB	SPTCL-GD
PT characteristics	63	29
Age (median)	36	59
Skin ulceration (%)	6	45
Hemophagocytic syndrome (%)	17	45
Pathology		
CD8+ (%)	95	10
CD56+ (%)	0	60
Cytotoxic proteins (%)	100	100
Therapy		
CHOP (%)	49	70
Immunosuppressive (%)	38	10
Radiotherapy (%)	5	5
Response		
CR/PR (%)	67/13	30/35
5-year OS (%)	82	11
5-year EFS (%)	85	11

B-symptoms or bone marrow involvement between the groups. There was a higher frequency of hemophagocytic syndrome in the PCGD group compared to the SPTCL group (45% vs. 17%). When treatment and outcomes were reviewed, it was noted that 50–70% of patients received CHOP like regimens, 10–38% had immunosuppressive therapies, and a small number were treated with radiation or local excision of the nodules. With initial therapy, 80% of patients in the SPTCL group had a response, compared to 65% in the PCGD group. The 5-year OS for the SPTCL patients was 82% vs. 11% for the PCGD patients.

Treatment approaches for SPTCL and PCGD-TCL have not been clearly established. In the retrospective EORTC review, half of the patients were treated with aggressive chemotherapy and several had autologous stem cell transplantation as a consolidation. One-third of the patients were treated with single agent therapies such as methotrexate, prednisone, cyclosporine, chlorambucil, or cyclophosphamide. Sixteen of twenty-four had a complete response, but nine of these relapsed and five subsequently had a durable response on reinstitution of the same therapy. Eight of the patients received CHOP in relapse and three had a CR. Of five patients presenting with a solitary skin relapse, all were treated with local therapy (radiotherapy or surgery) and are in remission. In the PCGD group, 14 of 20 patients received multi-agent chemotherapy and only three had a CR; one patient went on to allogeneic transplant and had a CR after transplant. Seven patients developed visceral disease and at 12 months, 15 of 20 succumbed from hemophagocytic syndrome or progressive disease.

Other case reports and small series have described responses in SPTCL and PCGD patients. In one single institution review of ten consecutive patients, three (two SPTCL and one PCGD) were treated initially with denileukin diftitox; one each with SPTCL- and PCGD-disease had PR on therapy and have been maintained without PD [18]. Seven patients were treated with cytotoxic chemotherapy regimens. Four of seven achieved a remission after EPOCH (2), denileukin diftitox-CHOP (1) or pentostatin/cyclophosphamide followed by alemtuzumab (1). Four patients (one with refractory -SPTCL, two with refractory PCGD and one with PCGD in first CR after denileukin diftitox-CHOP) underwent allogeneic hematopoietic stem cell (HSCT) from matched-related donors. Two patients are alive 6–13 months after HSCT with no evidence of disease; one patient died in CR from infectious complications of HSCT, and one relapsed 6 month after HSCT and died from PD. At a median follow up of 3 year from diagnosis, eight patients (80%) are alive, including the two patients with SPTCL and six of eight patients with PCGD. In patients who were refractory to CHOP in one series, response to cyclosporine was reported in four [19]. Another report has demonstrated the efficacy of a fludarabine-based regimen in one patient with aggressive disease [20].

On the basis of these findings, the treatment approach to PCGD-TCL should be similar to that of other aggressive poor prognosis T-cell lymphomas and should include multi-agent chemotherapy followed by stem cell transplantation from an allogeneic donor if one is available. Patients with SPTCL with a benign clinical behavior may be managed with single agent therapies such as prednisone, cyclosporine, or methotrexate. For those with progressive or disseminated disease or with the hemophagocytic syndrome, multi-agents chemotherapy followed by autologous stem cell transplantation should be considered.

Enteropathy-Associated T-Cell Lymphomas

Enteropathy-type T-cell lymphoma (ETCL) is a rare primary extranodal T-cell lymphoma in characterized by infiltration of malignant T-cell within the gastrointestinal epithelium, as shown in Fig. 7.3. ETCL represents 4.7% of cases of PTCL around the world, but the incidence is higher in North America and Europe compared to Asia. While the WHO classification identifies ETCL as a distinct clinicopathologic entity, there are two distinct histolopathologic subtypes, EATL type 1, which is associated with a history of celiac sprue, and EATL type 2 (Table 7.5).

EATL type 1 is more frequent (80–90% of cases) and is a pleomorphic infiltrate of anaplastic T-lymphocytes with a phenotype that is CD3+, CD7+, CD5-CD8-CD4–, CD103+. The tumor cells may express cytotoxic markers such as TIA-1, and a subset may express CD30. EATL type 2 occurs sporadically and is composed of monomorphic populations of T-cells which are characteristically CD3+, CD8+ and CD56+. Chromosomal abnormalities found in EATL include gains at chromosome 9q33-q34 in up to 70% of cases. In the International T-cell Lymphoma Project, 69% of EATL patients had Stage III/IV disease at presentation. Bone marrow involvement was rare and occurred in only

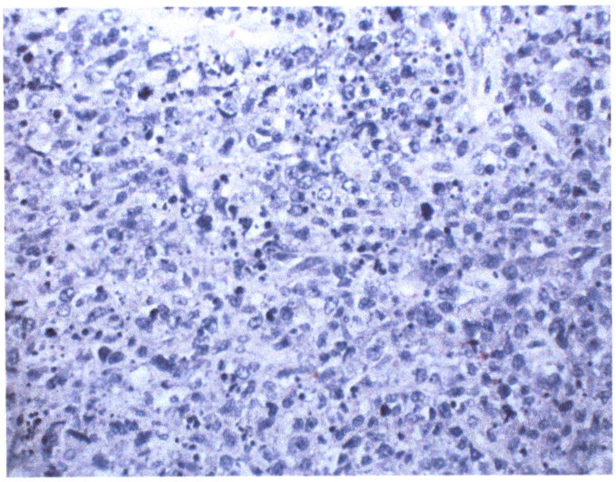

Fig. 7.3 Diffuse atypical T cell infiltrate infiltrating the wall of the small bowel (enteropathy-associated T cell lymphoma) (H&E stain)

Table 7.5 Enteropathy-associated T-cell lymphomas

EATL type1	EATL type 2
80–90% of cases	10–20%
Associated with celiac disease	Sporadic
Polymorphic lymphoid infiltrate	Monomorphic infiltrate
CD3+,CD7+, CD8− (20%+), TCRβ+/− Maybe CD30+	CD3+, CD4−, CD8+, CD56+, TCRβ+
Intraepithelial lymphocytes abnormal	Intraepithelial lymphocytes normal
9q+1q+5q+and 16q- abnormalities	9q+16q- 8q+(myc) abnormalities
Presents with weight loss	Presents with obstruction/ perforation

3% of cases, and only 25% of patients had a low IPI (0–1) [2].

The clinical approach for most patients is resection of the mass if the diagnosis is made at the time of laparotomy, followed by chemotherapy. The 5-year OS and PFS were 20% and 4% respectively. Even for the low IPI group, 5-year survival was only 29%. Recent strategies to improve outcomes have included more aggressive treatment regimens and introduction of non-anthracycline based regimens in the first line. The Nordic group reported results from 21 patients treated with CHOEP-14 followed by stem cell transplant. On that study, 33% of patients never made it to transplant due to progressive disease, and at 45 month follow up, 10 (45%) of patients were still alive [21]. Lennerd et al. have reported the use of CHOP×1 cycle followed by three cycles of ifosfamide/etoposide/epirubicin with intermediate dose methotrexate and then autologous stem cell transplantation. With this regimen, they have reported a response rate of 69% with a 5-year survival of 60%. Thus far there has been no data comparing outcomes with autologous vs. allogeneic stem cell transplantation in EATL, but patients with high IPI should be considered for clinical trials testing this approach. There is little data on efficacy of salvage therapy in EATL, so the treatment focus should be on effective first line therapy followed by a consolidation with stem cell transplantation.

Summary and Conclusions

The rare subtypes of aggressive T-cell lymphomas represent a diagnostic and a therapeutic challenge. The extranodal subtypes, including HSTL, enteropathy-associated T-cell lymphoma, and the panniculitis-like T-cell lymphomas have not been well-defined, and these patients are not well represented in multi-center trials due to their rarity. Therapeutic advances may be dependent on new insights into the biology of these diseases and identification of potential molecular targets.

References

1. Swerdlow SH, Campo E, Harris NL, et al. WHO classification of tumours of haematopoietic and lymphoid tissues. 4th ed. Lyon: IARC Press; 2008.
2. Vose J, Armitage J, Weisenburger D. International peripheral T-cell and natural killer/T-cell lymphoma study: pathology findings and clinical outcomes. J Clin Oncol. 2008;26:4124–30.
3. Tripodo C, Iannitto E, Florena AM, et al. Gamma-delta T-cell lymphomas. Nat Rev Clin Oncol. 2009;6:707–17.
4. Farcet JP, Gaulard P, Marolleau JP, et al. Hepatosplenic T-cell lymphoma: sinusal/sinusoidal localization of malignant cells expressing the T-cell receptor gamma delta. Blood. 1990;75:2213–9.
5. Roschewski M, Wilson WH. Biology and management of rare primary extranodal T-cell lymphomas. Oncology (Williston Park). 2010;24:94–100.
6. Schmidt LA, Lim MS. T cell lymphoproliferative disorders associated with anti-tumor necrosis factor alpha antibody therapy for ulcerative colitis: literature summary. J Hematop. 2009;2:121–6.
7. Kotlyar DS, Osterman MT, Diamond RH, et al. A systematic review of factors that contribute to hepatosplenic T-cell lymphoma in patients with inflammatory bowel disease. Clin Gastroenterol Hepatol. 2011; 9(1):36–41. e1.
8. Weidmann E. Hepatosplenic T cell lymphoma. A review on 45 cases since the first report describing the disease as a distinct lymphoma entity in 1990. Leukemia. 2000;14:991–7 (08876924).
9. Miyazaki K, Yamaguchi M, Imai H, et al. Gene expression profiling of peripheral T-cell lymphoma including gammadelta T-cell lymphoma. Blood. 2009;113:1071–4.
10. Bennett M, Matutes E, Gaulard P. Hepatosplenic T cell lymphoma responsive to 2'-deoxycoformycin therapy. Am J Hematol. 2010;85:727–9.
11. Schafer E, Chen A, Arceci RJ. Sustained first remission in an adolescent with hepatosplenic T-cell

lymphoma treated with T-cell leukemia induction, nucleoside analog-based consolidation, and early hematopoietic stem cell transplant. Pediatr Blood Cancer. 2009;53:1127–9.
12. Falchook GS, Champlin R, Hagemeister FB, et al. Hepatosplenic T-cell lymphoma: clinical characteristics and treatment outcome. ASH Annual Meeting Abstracts 2006;108:2460.
13. Falchook GS, Vega F, Dang NH, et al. Hepatosplenic gamma-delta T-cell lymphoma: clinicopathological features and treatment. Ann Oncol. 2009;20:1080–5.
14. Willemze R, Jansen PM, Cerroni L, et al. Subcutaneous panniculitis-like T-cell lymphoma: definition, classification, and prognostic factors: an EORTC Cutaneous Lymphoma Group Study of 83 cases. Blood. 2008;111:838–45.
15. Go RS, Wester SM. Immunophenotypic and molecular features, clinical outcomes, treatments, and prognostic factors associated with subcutaneous panniculitis-like T-cell lymphoma: a systematic analysis of 156 patients reported in the literature. Cancer. 2004;101:1404–13.
16. Salhany KE, Macon WR, Choi JK, et al. Subcutaneous panniculitis-like T-cell lymphoma: clinicopathologic, immunophenotypic, and genotypic analysis of alpha/beta and gamma/delta subtypes. Am J Surg Pathol. 1998;22:881–93.
17. Kong YY, Dai B, Kong JC, et al. Subcutaneous panniculitis-like T-cell lymphoma: a clinicopathologic, immunophenotypic, and molecular study of 22 Asian cases according to WHO-EORTC classification. Am J Surg Pathol. 2008;32:1495–502.
18. Alpdogan O, Ornstein D, Subtil T, et al. Outcomes in subcutaneous panniculitis-like T-cell lymphoma (STCL). Blood (ASH Annual Meeting Abstracts) 2008;112:3750.
19. Rojnuckarin P, Nakorn TN, Assanasen T, et al. Cyclosporin in subcutaneous panniculitis-like T-cell lymphoma. Leuk Lymphoma. 2007;48:560–3.
20. Chim CS, Loong F, Ng WK, et al. Use of fludarabine-containing chemotherapeutic, regimen results in durable complete remission of subcutaneous panniculitis-like T-cell lymphoma. Am J Clin Dermatol. 2008;9:396–8.
21. Jantunen E, Relander T, Lauritzsen GF, et al. Intensive induction chemotherapy followed by autologous stem cell transplantation (ASCT) In: Patients with enteropathy-associated T-cell lymphoma: a prospective study by the nordic lymphoma group (NLG-T-01). Blood (ASH Annual Meeting Abstracts) 116:3565.
22. Magro C, Segal J, Crowson A, Chadwick P. The phenotypic profile of dermatomyositis and lupus erythematosus: a comparative analysis. J Cutan Pathol. 2010;37(6):659–71.

8 HTLV-1-Associated T-cell Diseases

Kunihiro Tsukasaki and Kensei Tobinai

Introduction

Adult T-cell leukemia-lymphoma (ATL) was first described in 1977 by Uchiyama and Takatsuki as a distinct clinico-pathological entity with a suspected viral etiology because of the clustering of the disease in the southwest region of Japan [1]. Subsequently, a novel RNA retrovirus, human T-cell leukemia/lymphotropic virus type I (HTLV-1), was isolated from a cell line established from leukemic cells of an ATL patient, and the finding of a clear association with ATL led to its inclusion among human carcinogenic pathogens [2–5]. In the mid-1980s and 1990s, several inflammatory diseases were reported to be associated with HTLV-1 [6–10]. At the same time, endemic areas for the virus and diseases have been found [reviewed in 11–13]. Diversity in ATL has been recognized and the subtype classification of the disease was proposed [14]. This chapter will characterize HTLV-1 and review the current recognition of ATL focusing on treatment of the disease.

K. Tsukasaki, M.D., Ph.D. (✉)
Department of Hematology, National Cancer Centre Hospital East, Chiba, Japan
e-mail: ktsukash@east.ncc.gov.jp

K. Tobinai, M.D., Ph.D.
Department of Hematology, National Cancer Center Hospital, Tokyo, Japan

HTLV-1 Structure and Biology

HTLV-1 is a C-type oncovirus in the RNA retrovirus family [12, 13, 15]. Its genome of approximately 9 kb encodes three structural proteins, group angigen (gag), reverse transcriptase (pol), and envelop (env), the genes for which are flanked by 5′ and 3′ long terminal repeats (LTRs). In the 3′portion of the genome is a pX region that encodes the Tax, Rex, p21, p12, p13, and p30 proteins in its various reading frames [16, 17] (Fig. 8.1). Both Rex, a post-transcriptional regulator of viral expression, and Tax, a viral transcription factor co-operate with other viral products and cellular proteins to mediate viral replication [18, 19]. Antisense transcripts of the HTLV-1 provirus were reported. The transcripts can encode a novel basic leucine zipper protein, named HBZ, which interacts with several host genes and suppresses the activity of Tax [20–22]. Various isoforms of HBZ were reported to be steadily expressed in HTLV-1-infected cells and ATL cells in contrast to other viral genes, suggesting an important role in the development of ATL.

Methods of Detecting HTLV-1

Serological, virological, and molecular examinations can detect an HTLV-1 infection. As with other human retroviruses, HTLV-1 causes a persistent life-long infection after it synthesizes

F. Foss (ed.), *T-Cell Lymphomas*, Contemporary Hematology,
DOI 10.1007/978-1-62703-170-7_8, © Springer Science+Business Media New York 2013

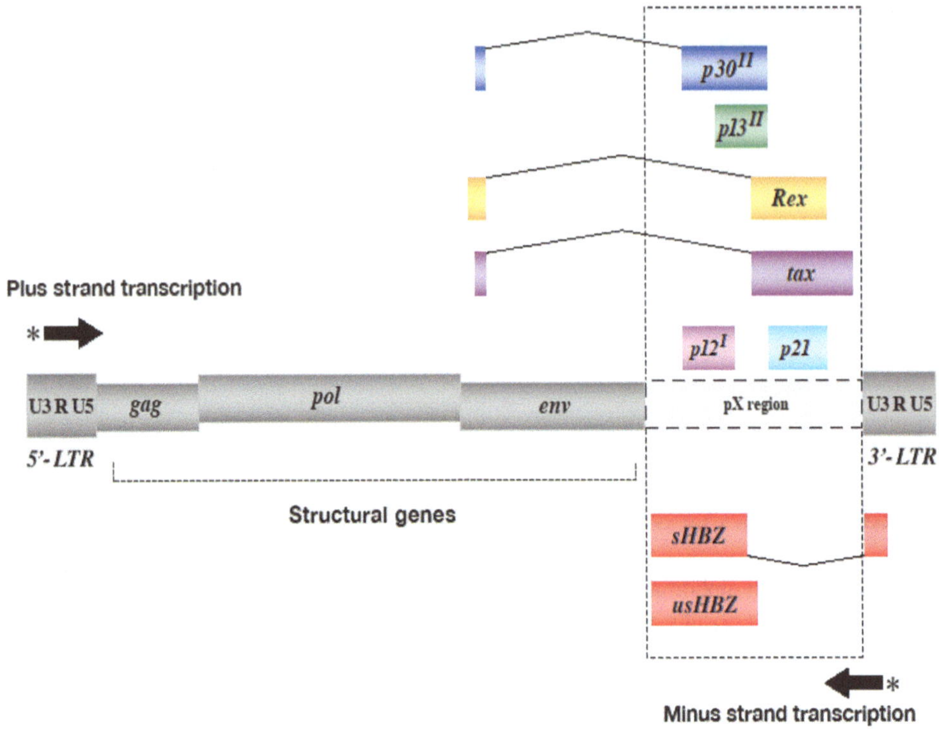

Fig. 8.1 Structure of HTLV-1. HTLV-1 encodes accessory and regulatory genes in the pXregion as well as viral structure genes. [Based on data from Satou Y, Matsuoka M. HTLV-1 and the host immune system: how the virus disrupts immune regulation, leading to HTLV-1-associated diseases. J Clin Exp Hematop. 2010; 50(1):1–8.]

copies of DNA by reverse transcriptase and integrates into the host's genome as a provirus.

Specific antibodies against HTLV-1 can be detected by enzyme-linked immunosorbent assay (ELISA), particle aggregation (PA), immunofluorescence microscopy, Western blotting (WB), or radioimmunoprecipitation. ELISA and PA are frequently used as screening assays [23–26]. To distinguish HTLV-1 from HTLV-2, which is less pathogenic, WB is usually necessary [27].

Fresh HTLV-1-infected cells from ATL patients or HTLV-1 carriers seldom express viral proteins except for HBZ [28, 29]. In contrast, in the presence of IL-2, short-term cultured HTLV-1-infected cells or established long-term T-cell lines usually produce viral particles and viral proteins, as demonstrated by electron microscopy and immunolabeling using antibodies to HTLV-1, respectively.

The clonal integration of HTLV-1 proviral DNA into infected T-cells can be demonstrated by Southern blot, inverse polymerase chain reaction (PCR), and/or ligation PCR assays [30–33]. Several investigators have analyzed the implications of the integration pattern of HTLV-I provirus in the progression of ATL [34, 35]. Neoplastic cells of ATL patients have only one complete copy of the HTLV-I provirus per cell in some cases (complete-type), but multiple complete copies in others (multiple-type). The HTLV-I proviruses in the remaining patients have a defective genome (defective-type). The median survival times for patients were 7 months, 24 months, and 33 months for defective-type, complete-type, and multiple-type ATL, respectively ($P=0.006$). Among the 52 patients examined, the HTLV-I integration patterns changed at disease progression in four patients (8%). In three of these four, the rearrangements of the TCR-β gene changed concomitantly, suggesting the appearance of a new ATL clone. The researchers concluded that the frequent clonal change of ATL reflects the emergence of multiple premalignant clones in viral leukemogenesis. Tamiya and coworkers reported the presence of two types of defective virus. Among them, the type 2 defective virus with a deletion that includes the 5′ LTR was found more frequently in the acute and lymphoma types (39%, 21 of 54) than in the chronic type (6%, 1 of 18). It is postulated that the high frequency of the type 2 virus is caused by the genetic instability of the HTLV-I provirus and that the defective virus is selected because it escapes from the immune surveillance system in the host. Southern blotting and inverse PCR assays have sensitivity to detect the clonal disease, being able to identify the virus in a population with at least 5% and 1% of cells infected, respectively [33]. Also, about 20% of patients with HTLV-1-associated myelopathy (HAM)/tropical spastic paraparesis (TSP) and a small proportion of healthy HTLV-1 carriers have monoclonal HTLV-1 integration which can be detected by Southern blotting and/or inverse PCR [36, 37].

Epidemiology of HTLV-1

The three major routes of HTLV-1 transmission are mother-to-child infections via breast milk, sexual intercourses, and blood transfusions. Otherwise, HTLV-1 is not easily transmittable, since cell-to-cell contact is presumably required. Vertical transmission from mother to child is caused by breast-feeding beyond 4 to 6 months of age, after which time the protective IgG maternal antibodies decline [38]. HTLV-1-infected mononuclear cells are present in breast milk [39]. The overall rate of infection among breast-fed children from carrier mothers has been estimated at 10–30% [40]. Sexual transmission of HTLV-1 more frequently occurs from men to women than women to men. Infection by transfusion of contaminated cellular blood products is presumably the most efficient mode of transmission [41]. In contrast, fresh frozen plasma, which is acellular, is not infectious [42]. The transmission of HTLV-1 between intravenous drug abusers has been reported [43].

The Southwestern district of Japan has the highest prevalence of HTLV-1 infection in the world, but this infection is also endemic in the Caribbean basin, parts of Africa, Latin America, the Middle East, and the Pacific region [41, 44–48]. Many of the HTLV-1 carriers and ATL patients in the USA and Europe are immigrants from the above described endemic areas [49].

The seroprevalence of HTLV-1 in endemic areas is low and stable among children, but increases gradually with age, especially in women over 50 year of age [50]. In a cohort study in an endemic region of Japan, the seroprevalence of HTLV-1 in individuals between 16 and 39 years of age was 10% in both sexes; in contrast, the prevalence sky-rocketed to 30% in men and 50% in women over the age of 70 [51]. For several decades, the prevalence of HTLV-1 has declined drastically in endemic areas in Japan, probably because of birth cohort effects [52]. The elimination of HTLV-1 in endemic areas is now considered possible due to the natural decrease in the prevalence as well as intervention of transmission through blood transfusion and breast feeding.

HTLV-1-Related Diseases

HTLV-1 is associated with the development of ATL [1–5, 11–13], as well as HAM/TSP, a progressive form of chronic spastic myelopathy with demyelination of the spinal cord motor neurons, and HTLV-1-associated uveitis (HAU), a subacute inflammatory condition in which vitreous opacities are associated with mild iritis and mild retinal vasculitis [6, 7, 9]. Staphylococcal and streptococcal skin infections are common in the infective dermatitis (ID) syndrome described in Jamaica in association with HTLV-I infections in childhood [8]. Those individuals with ID were reported to be susceptible to ATL and HAM/TSP. ID was reported first in Jamaica and subsequently in Brazil and other countries of South America but rarely in Japan. In contrast, HAU was first reported in Japan and rarely occur in other countries. Other conditions reportedly associated with HTLV-1 include Sjogren's syndrome, polymyositis, alveolitis, arthritis, thyroiditis, and immune suppression [53–56].

Adult T-Cell Leukemia-Lymphoma

ATL is a distinct peripheral T-lymphocytic malignancy associated with a retrovirus designated human T-cell leukemia virus type I or human T-cell lymphotropic virus type I (HTLV-1) [1, 11–13, 57, 58]. Major prognostic indicators for ATL, which have been elucidated in 854 patients with ATL in Japan by the Lymphoma Study Group (LSG) of the Japan Clinical Oncology Group (JCOG) using multivariate analysis, were advanced performance status (PS), high lactic dehydrogenase (LDH) level, age of 40 years or more, more than three involved lesions, and hypercalcemia [56]. Also, a subclassification was proposed based on prognostic factors and clinical features of the disease (Table 8.1) [14]. The leukemic subtypes include all of the acute and chronic types and most of the smoldering type. The acute type has a rapid course with leukemic manifestation (>=2% ATL cells) with or without lymphocytosis (>4×10^9/L) including ATL cells and most of the characteristic features of ATL-generalized lymphadenopathy, hepatosplenomegaly, skin involvement, other organ infiltration as shown in Figure 8.2, a high LDH value, and hypercalcemia. The symptoms and signs include abdominal pain, diarrhea, ascites, jaundice, unconsciousness, dyspnea, pleural effusion, cough, sputum, and chest X-ray abnormalities because of organ involvement, hypercalcemia, and/or opportunistic infections. The smoldering type shows an indolent course and 5% or more of leukemic cells in the peripheral blood without lymphocytosis, but may also include skin/lung involvement. The calcium level is less than the upper limit and LDH level is less than 1.5 times the upper limit in smoldering ATL. The chronic type, with absolute lymphocytosis (4×10^9/L) less frequently showing flower cell morphology than the acute type, is occasionally associated with skin involvement and lymphadenopathy and also

Table 8.1 Diagnostic Criteria for Clinical Subtypes of HTLV-1-associated ATL

	Smoldering	Chronic	Lymphoma	Acute
Anti-HTLV-I antibody	+	+	+	+
Lymphocyte (×103/μL)	<4	>=4‡	<4	*
Abnormal T lymphocytes	>=5%¶	+§	=<1%	+???
Flower cells with T-cell marker	†	†	No	+
LDH	=<1.5N	=<2N	*	*
Corrected Ca2+ (mEq/L)	<5.5	<5.5	*	*
Histology-proven lymphadenopathy	No	*	+	*
Tumor lesion A	*	*	*	*
Skin and/or lung	*	*	*	*
Lymph node	No	*		*
Liver	No	*	*	*
Spleen	No	*	*	*
Central nervous system	No	*	*	*
Bone	No	No	*	*
Ascites	No	No	*	*
Pleural effusion	No	No	*	*
Gastrointestinal tract	No	No	*	*

HTLV-I, human T-lymphotropic virus type I; LDH, lactate dehydrogenase; N normal upper limit
*No essential qualification except terms required for other subtype(s)
†Typical "flower cells" may be seen occasionally
‡Accompanied by T lymphocytosis (3.5×103/μL or more)
§If abnormal T lymphocytes are less than 5% in peripheral blood, histologically proven tumor lesion is required
Histologically proven skin and/or pulmonary lesion(s) is required if there are fewer than 5% abnormal T lymphocytes in peripheral blood
[Based on data from Shimoyama M, Members of the Lymphoma Study Group (1984–1987): Diagnostic criteria and classification of clinical subtypes of adult T-cell leukemia-lymphoma. Br J Haematol 1991;79:428.]

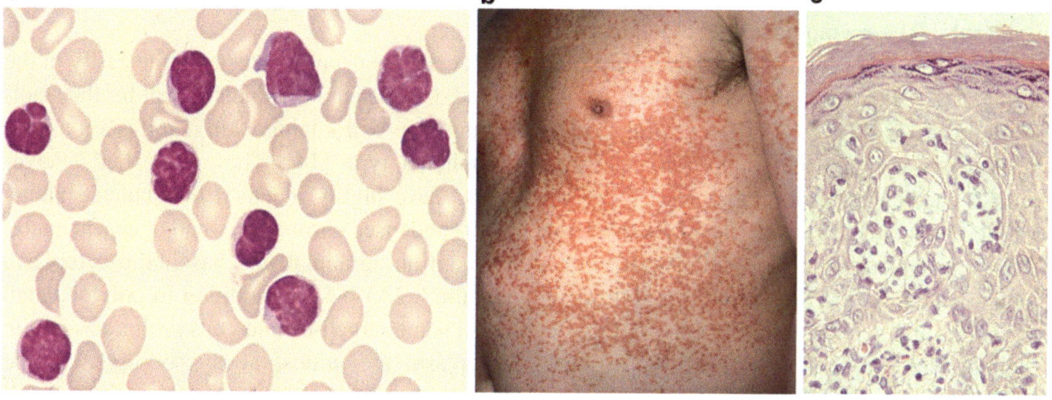

Fig. 8.2 (**a**) Leukemic cells (the so-called flower cells) showing characteristic polymorphic nuclei with condensed chromatin and agulanular and basophilic cytoplasm. (**b**) Photograph of skin lesion in a patient with acute-type ATL. (**c**) Histology of skin infiltration of ATL cells in the same patient; infiltrating ATL cells are present in the epidermis forming a Pautrer's micro-abscess.

usually shows a relatively indolent course. The calcium level is less than the upper limit and the LDH level is less than double the upper limit of the chronic type. The lymphoma type presents with the manifestations of a lymphoma without leukemic cells, frequently with high LDH/Ca levels, a rapid course, and symptoms and signs similar to the acute type. In case of ATL, clinical subtype is more important than Ann Arbor stage for predicting prognosis and deciding treatment.

Additional factors associated with a poor prognosis include thrombocytopenia, eosinophilia, bone marrow involvement, a high interleukin (IL)-5 serum-level, CC chemokine receptor 4 (CCR4) expression, lung resistance-related protein, p53 mutation, and p16 deletion by multivariate analysis [59–65]. Specific for the chronic type of ATL, high LDH, high blood urea nitrogen (BUN), and low albumin levels were identified as factors for a poor prognosis by multivariate analysis [11]. Primary cutaneous tumoral type, although generally included among smoldering ATL, had a poor prognosis in one uni-variate analysis [66].

Epidemiology of ATL

The average age at onset of ATL in Japan is 57 years, which is about 15 years older than in the Caribbean, South America, and Africa [67–69]. This may reflect unknown environmental or ethnic cofactors in the multi-step leukemogenesis of this disease. The estimated annual incidence in Japan is about 1 per 1,000 HTLV-1 carriers over 40 years of age, with males affected about twice as often [70]. The cumulative life time risk for ATL among HTLV-1 carriers has been estimated at 1–5% in both sexes in Japan and in Jamaica [71, 72]. HTLV-1 infection early in life, presumably from breast feeding, is crucial in the development of ATL; 100% of mothers of ATL patients examined were HTLV-1 carriers as compared to about 30% of mothers of HAM/TSP patients [73]. HTLV-1infection by blood transfusion is associated with a higher risk for the development of HAM/TSP than infection by other routes [74]. In contrast, very few cases of ATL after HTLV-1 infection by blood transfusion have been reported [75, 76]. Interestingly, those affected had blood transfusions for a preceding hematological malignancy, and developed ATL within 11 years after HTLV-1infection. Factors reportedly associated with the onset of ATL include: HTLV-1 infection early in life, increase in age, male sex, family history of ATL, past history of infective dermatitis, smoking of tobacco, serum titers of antibody against HTLV-1, and several HLA subtypes [77–82].

Recently, HTLV-1 proviral loads have been proposed as an important predictor of ATL, but only a few small prospective studies have been conducted. Recently, Iwanaga and colleagues evaluated 1,218 asymptomatic HTLV-1 carriers (426 males and 792 females) who were enrolled during 2002–2008 for a prospective study on the development of ATL [83]. The proviral load at enrollment was significantly higher in males than females (median, 2.10 vs. 1.39 copies/100 peripheral blood mononuclear cells (PBMC; $P < 0.0001$)), in those aged 40 or more years and in those with a family history of ATL. During the follow-up period, 14 participants developed acute ATL. Their baseline proviral loads were high (range, 4.17–28.58 copies/100 PBMC). Multivariate Cox regression analyses indicated that not only a higher proviral load but also advanced age, a family history of ATL, and the first opportunity for HTLV-1 testing during treatment for other diseases were independent risk factors for the progression of ATL from a carrier status.

Clinical Features

ATL patients show a variety of clinical manifestations because of various complications of organ involvement by ATL cells, opportunistic infections, and/or hypercalcemia [11–14]. These three often contribute to the extremely high mortality of the disease. Lymph node, liver, spleen, and skin lesions are frequently observed. Although less frequent, the digestive tract, the lungs, the central nervous system, bone, and/or other organs may be involved. Large nodules, plaques, ulcers, and erythroderma are common skin lesions [66, 84]. Immune suppression is common. Approximately 26% of 854 patients with ATL had active infections at diagnosis in a prior nationwide study in Japan [14]. The incidence was highest in the chronic and smoldering types (36%) and lower in the acute (27%) and lymphoma types (11%). The infections were bacterial in 43%, fungal in 31%, protozoal in 18%, and viral in 8% of patients. The immunodeficiency at presentation in ATL patients can be exacerbated by cytotoxic chemotherapy. Individuals with indolent ATL might have no manifestation of the disease and are identified only by health check-ups and laboratory examinations.

Laboratory Findings

ATL cells are usually detected quite easily in the blood of affected individuals except for the smoldering type with mainly skin manifestations and lymphoma type [14]. These so called "flower cells" have highly indented or lobulated nuclei with condensed chromatin, small or absent nucleoli, and an agranular and basophilic cytoplasm (Figure 8.2A) [85]. In addition to polylobulated cells, some large blastoid cells with a basophilic cytoplasm are almost always observed in the blood film. Furthermore, the diversity of cell morphology in ATL is associated with prognostic factors, an aberrant immmunophenotype, and a defective HTLV-1 genotype [86]. Five percent or more abnormal T-lymphocytes in peripheral blood confirmed by cytology and immunophenotyping are required to diagnose ATL in cases without histologically proven tumor lesions [14].

The histological analysis of aberrant cutaneous lesions or lymph nodes is essential for the diagnosis of the smoldering type with mainly skin manifestations and lymphoma type of ATL, respectively. Because ATL cells in the skin and lymph node can vary in size from small to large and in form from pleomorphic to anaplastic and Hodgkin-like cell with no specific histological pattern of involvement, differentiating between Sezary syndrome, other peripheral T-cell lymphomas (PTCLs), and Hodgkin lymphoma versus ATL can at times be difficult without examinations for HTLV-1 serotype/genotype [13, 87].

The white blood cell count ranges from normal to 500×10^9/L. Marked leukocytosis of >30 and lymphocytes of 15× have been observed in about 40% of acute ATLs and 25% of chronic ATLs, but not in the other two subtypes (lymphoma, smoldering) [14]. Granulocytosis of more than 8× is frequently observed (about 40% of acute type and 15% of the other three types) even in the absence of infection. Eosinophilia is frequent (21%) as compared to other T- or B-lymphomas. Neutrophilia and eosinophilia are presumably related to the release of cytokines {chiefly granulocyte-macrophage colony-stimulating factor (GM-CSF) and Interleukin (IL)-5} by malignant cells. Anemia and thrombocytopenia are less frequently observed, probably because much of the bone marrow is spared by the leukemia. Some of the hematological abnormalities were associated with the prognosis of ATL as described previously.

Hypercalcemia is the most distinctive laboratory abnormality in ATL as compared to other lymphoid malignancies and is observed in 31% of patients (50% in acute type, 17% in lymphoma type, and 0% in the other two types) at onset [14]. Individuals with hypercalcemia do not usually have osteolytic bone lesions. Parathyroid hormone-related protein or receptor activator of nuclear factor kappa B ligand produced by ATL cells is considered the main factor causing hypercalcemia [88, 89].

Similar to serum LDH, β2-microglobulin, and serum thymidine kinase levels reflecting disease bulk/activity, the level of the soluble form of interleukin (IL)-2 receptor alpha-chain is elevated in the order acute/lymphoma-type ATL, smoldering chronic-type ATL, and HTLV-1 carriers as compared with normal individuals, perhaps with better accuracy than the other markers [90–92]. These serum markers are useful for detecting the acute transformation of indolent ATL as well as the early relapse of ATL after achieving responses by therapy.

Prototypical ATL cells have a mature alpha–beta T-cell phenotype, that is, they are terminal deoxynucleotidyl transferase (TdT)-negative, CDla-negative, T-cell receptor alpha–beta-positive, CD2-positive and CD5, CD45RO and CD29-positive, and frequently do not express CD7 and CD26. A decline in the CD3 level with the appearance of CD25 indicates that the ATL cells are in an activated state. Most ATL cells are CD52-positive, but some are negative and this may correlate with the co-expression of CD30. About 90% of cases are CD4-positive and CD8-negative, and in rare cases either co-express CD4 and CD8, are negative for both markers, or are only CD8-positive [93]. CCR4 is expressed in more than 90% of cases and associated with a poor prognosis. Recent studies have suggested that the cells of some ATL may be the equivalent of regulatory T-cells because of the high frequency of expression of CD25/CCR4 and about half of FoxP3 [62, 94].

Chromosomal abnormalities detected by cytogenetics or comparative genomic hybridization are often more complex and more frequent in aggressive ATL than in indolent ATL, with aneuploidy and several hot spots such as 14q and 3p [95, 96]. A more sensitive array-CGH revealed that the lymphoma type had significantly more frequent gains at 1q, 2p, 4q, 7p, and 7q, and losses at 10p, 13q, 16q, and 18p, whereas the acute type showed a gain at 3/3p, but no specific pattern of abnormality has been identified which is in contrast to Burkitt leukemia/lymphoma with a *myc* gene rearrangement induced by Epstein–Barr virus [97, 98].

DNA microarray analyses of the transcriptomes of ATL cells at the chronic and acute stages to elucidate the mechanism of stage progression in this disease revealed that several hundred genes were modulated in expression including those for MET, a receptor tyrosine kinase for hepatocyte growth factor, and cell adhesion molecule, TSLC1 [99, 100].

Diagnosis of ATL

The diagnosis of typical ATL is not difficult and is based on clinical features, ATL cell morphology, mature helper-T-cell phenotype, and ant-HTLV-1 antibody in most cases [13, 55]. Those rare cases which might be difficult to diagnose can be shown to have the monoclonal integration of HTLV-1 proviral DNA in the malignant cells as determined by Southern blotting. However, the monoclonal integration of HTLV-1 is also detected in some HAM/TSP patients and HTLV-1 carriers [36, 37]. After the diagnosis of ATL, subclassification of the disease is necessary for the selection of appropriate treatment [14, 57].

Clinical Course and Treatment of ATL

Treatment decisions should be based on the ATL subclassification and the prognostic factors at onset including those related with ATL and co-morbidity [57]. As mentioned above, subclassification of this disease has been proposed based on the prognosis and clinical manifestations. Without treatment, most patients with acute-/lymphoma/type ATL die of the disease or infections within weeks or months. More than half of patients with smoldering ATL survive for more than 5 years without chemotherapy and transformation to aggressive ATL. Chronic ATL has the most diverse prognosis among the subtypes and could be divided into favorable and unfavorable by clinical parameters (serum albumin, BUN, and LDH levels) after a multivariate analysis [11].

Current treatment options for ATL include watchful waiting until disease progression, interferon alpha (IFN) and zidobudine (AZT) therapy, multi-agent chemotherapy, allogeneic hematopoietic stem cell transplantation (allo-HSCT), and a new agent [57].

Watchful Waiting

At present, no standard treatment for ATL exists. Therefore, patients with the smoldering or favorable chronic type, who may survive one or more years without chemotherapy, excluding topical therapy for cutaneous lesions, should be observed and therapy should be delayed until progression of the disease [57]. However, it was recently found that the long-term prognosis of such patients was poorer than expected. In a long-term follow-up study for 78 patients with indolent ATL (favorable chronic- or smoldering-type) with a policy of watchful waiting until disease progression at a single institution, the median survival time was 5.3 years with no plateau in the survival curve. Twelve patients remained alive for >10 years, 32 progressed to acute ATL, and 51 died [101]. These findings suggest that even "indolent" ATL patients should be carefully observed in clinical practice. Further study is required to establish appropriate management practices for indolent ATL.

Chemotherapy

Since 1978, chemotherapy trials have been consecutively conducted for patients newly diagnosed with ATL by JCOG's LSG (Table 8.2) [102–107]. Between 1981 and 1983, JCOG conducted a phase III trial (JCOG8101) to evaluate LSG1-VEPA (vincristine, cyclophosphamide, prednisone, and doxorubicin) vs. LSG2-VEPA-M (VEPA plus methotrexate (MTX)) for advanced non-Hodgkin lymphoma (NHL), including ATL [102, 103]. The complete response (CR) rate of LSG2-VEPA-M for ATL (37%) was higher than that of LSG1-VEPA (17%; $P=0.09$). However, the CR rate was significantly lower for ATL than for B-cell NHL and PTCL other than ATL ($P<0.001$). The median survival time of the 54 patients with ATL was 6 months, and the estimated 4-year survival rate was 8%.

In 1987, JCOG initiated a multicenter phase II study (JCOG8701) of a multi-agent combination chemotherapy (LSG4) for advanced aggressive NHL (including ATL). LSG4 consisted of three regimens: (1) VEPA-B (VEPA plus bleomycin),

Table 8.2 Results of sequential chemotherapeutic trials of untreated patients with ATL (JCOG-LSG)

	J7801	J8101	J8701	J9109		J9303	JCOG9801
	LSG1	LSG1/LSG2	LSG4	LSG11		LSG15	mLSG15/mLSG19
Pts. No.	18	54	43	62	96	57	61
CR (%)	16.7	27.8	41.9	28.3	35.5	40.4	24.6
CR+PR (%)	51.6	80.6	72.0	65.6			
MST (months)	7.5	7.5	8.0	7.4	13.0	12.7	10.9
2-year survival (%)	17.0	31.3					
3-year survival (%)	10.0	21.9	23.6	12.7			
4-year survival (%)	8.0	11.6					

CR complete remission, PR partial remission, MST median survival time

(2) M-FEPA (methotrexate, vindesine, cyclophosphamide, prednisone, and doxorubicin), and (3) VEPP-B, (vincristine, etoposide, procarbazine, prednisone, and bleomycin) [104]. The CR rate for ATL patients was improved from 28% (JCOG8101) to 43% (JCOG8701); however, the CR rate was significantly lower in ATL than in B-cell NHL and PTCL ($P<0.01$). Patients with ATL still showed a poor prognosis, with a median survival time of 8 months and a 4-year survival rate of 12%.

The disappointing results with conventional chemotherapies have led to a search for new active agents. Multicenter phase I and II studies of pentostatin (2′-deoxycoformycin, a inhibitor of adenosine deaminase) were conducted against ATL in Japan [108]. The phase II study revealed a response rate of 32% (10 of 31) in cases of relapsed or refractory ATL (two CRs and eight PRs).

These encouraging results prompted the investigators to conduct a phase II trial (JCOG9109) with a pentostatin-containing combination (LSG11) as the initial chemotherapy [105]. Patients with aggressive ATL—that is, of the acute, lymphoma, or unfavorable chronic type—were eligible for this study. Unfavorable chronic-type ATL, defined as having at least one of three unfavorable prognostic factors (low serum albumin level, high LDH level, or high BUN), has an unfavorable prognosis similar to that for acute- and lymphoma-type ATL. A total of 62 untreated patients with aggressive ATL (34 acute, 21 lymphoma, and 7 unfavorable chronic type) were enrolled. A regimen of 1 mg/m^2 vincristine on days 1 and 8, 40 mg/m^2 doxorubicin on day 1, 100 mg/m^2 etoposide on days 1 through 3, 40 mg/m^2 prednisolone (PSL) on days 1 and 2, and 5 mg/m^2 pentostatin on days 8, 15, and 22 was administered every 28 days for ten cycles. Among the 61 patients evaluable for toxicity, four patients (7%) died of infections, two from septicemia, and two from cytomegalovirus pneumonia. Among the 60 eligible patients, there were 17 CRs (28%) and 14 partial responses (PRs) (overall response rate [ORR] = 52%). The median survival time was 7.4 months, and the estimated 2-year survival rate was 17%. The prognosis in patients with ATL remained poor, even though they were treated with a pentostatin-containing combination chemotherapy.

In 1994, JCOG initiated a phase II trial (JCOG9303) of an eight-drug regimen (LSG15) consisting of vincristine, cyclophosphamide, doxorubicin, prednisone, ranimustine, vindesine, etoposide, and carboplatin for untreated ATL [106]. Dose intensification was attempted with the prophylactic use of granulocyte colony-stimulating factor (G-CSF). In addition, non-cross-resistant agents such as ranimustine and carboplatin, and intrathecal prophylaxis with MTX and PSL were incorporated. Ninety-six previously untreated patients with aggressive ATL were enrolled: 58 acute, 28 lymphoma, and 10 unfavorable chronic types. Approximately 81% of the 93 eligible patients responded (75/93), with 33 patients obtaining a CR (35%). The overall survival rate of the 93 patients at 2 years was estimated to be 31%, with a median survival time of 13 months. Grade 4 neutropenia and thrombocytopenia were observed in 65% and 53% of the patients, respectively, whereas grade 4 non-hematologic toxicity was observed in only one patient.

To confirm whether the LSG15 regimen is a new standard for the treatment of aggressive ATL, JCOG conducted a phase III trial comparing modified (m)-LSG15 with biweekly CHOP (cyclophosphamide, hydroxy-doxorubicin, vincristine [Oncovin], and prednisone), both supported with G-CSF and intrathecal prophylaxis [107].

mLSG15 in JCOG9801 was a modified version of LSG15 in JCOG9303, consisting of three regimens: VCAP [VCR 1 mg/m^2 (maximum 2 mg), CPA 350 mg/m^2, ADM 40 mg/m^2, PSL 40 mg/m^2] on day 1, AMP [ADM 30 mg/m^2, MCNU 60 mg/m^2, PSL 40 mg/m^2] on day 8, and VECP [VDS 2.4 mg/m^2 on day 15, ETP 100 mg/m^2 on days 15–17, CBDCA 250 mg/m^2 on day15, PSL 40 mg/m^2 on days 15–17] on days 15–17, and the next course was to be started on day 29 (Figure 8.3). The modifications in mLSG15 as compared to LSG15 were as follows; (1) the total number of cycles was reduced from seven to six because of progressive cytopenia, especially thrombocytopenia, after repeating the VCAP-AMP-VECP therapy, (2) cytarabine 40 mg was used with MTX 15 mg and PSL 10 mg for

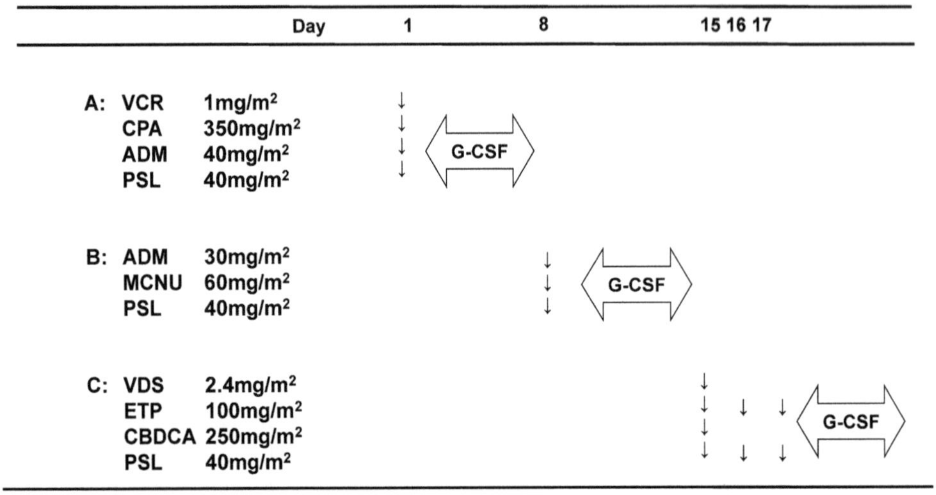

A→B→C is repeated every 28 days 6 times.
Intrathecal administration of cytarabine, methotrexate and is given just before the cycles 2, 4 and 6

Fig. 8.3 Regimen of VCAP-AMP-VECP. Ranimustinal (MCNU) and vindesine (VDS) are nitrosourea and vinca alkaloid, respectively, developed in Japan. A previous study on myeloma described that carmustine (BCNU), another nitrosourea, at 1 mg/kg is equivalent to MCNU at 0.8–1.0 mg/kg. VDS at 2.4 mg/m^2 can be substituted for VCR, another vinca alkaloid used in this regimen, at 1 mg/m^2 with possibly less myelosuppression and more peripheral neuropathy which can be managed by dose modification. VCAP=vincristine (VCR), cyclophosphamide (CPA), doxorubicin (ADM), prednisone (PSL); AMP=ADM, MCNU, PSL; VECP=VDS, etoposide (ETP), carboplatin (CBDCA) and PSL. [Based on data from Tsukasaki K, Utsunomiya A, Fukuda H, et al.: VCAP-AMP-VECP compared with biweekly CHOP for adult T-cell leukemia-lymphoma: Japan Clinical Oncology Group Study JCOG9801. J Clin Oncol 25:5,458–5,564, 2007.]

prophylactic intrathecal administration, at the recovery phases of courses 1, 3, and 5 because of the high frequency of central nervous system relapse in the JCOG9303 study. Untreated patients with aggressive ATL were assigned to receive either six courses of LSG15 every 4 weeks or eight courses of biweekly CHOP. The primary endpoint was overall survival. A total of 118 patients were enrolled. The CR rate was higher in the LSG15 arm than in the biweekly CHOP arm (40% vs. 25%, respectively; $P=0.020$). As illustrated in Figure 8.4, the median survival time and OS rate at 3 years were 12.7 months and 24% in the LSG15 arm and 10.9 months and 13% in the biweekly CHOP arm [two-sided $P=0.169$, and the hazard ratio was 0.75; 95% confidence interval (CI), 0.50 10 1.13]. A Cox regression analysis with performance status (PS 0 vs. 1 vs. 2–4) as the stratum for baseline hazard functions was performed to evaluate the effect on overall survival of age, B-symptoms, subtypes of ATL, LDH, BUN, bulky mass, and treatment arms. According to this analysis, the hazard ratio and two-sided P value for the treatment arms were 0.62 (95% CI, 0.38–1.01) and 0.056, respectively. The difference between the crude analysis and this result was because of unbalanced prognostic factors, such as PS 0 vs. 1, and the presence or absence of bulky lesions between the treatment arms. The progression-free survival rate at 1 year was 28% in the LSG15 arm compared with 16% in the biweekly CHOP arm (two-sided $P=0.200$).

In VCAP-AMP-VECP vs. biweekly CHOP, rate of grade 4 neutropenia, grade 4 thrombocytopenia, and grade 3/4 infection were 98% vs. 83%, 74% vs. 17%, and 32% vs. 15%, respectively. There were three toxic deaths in the former. Three treatment-related deaths (TRDs), two from sepsis and one from interstitial pneumonitis

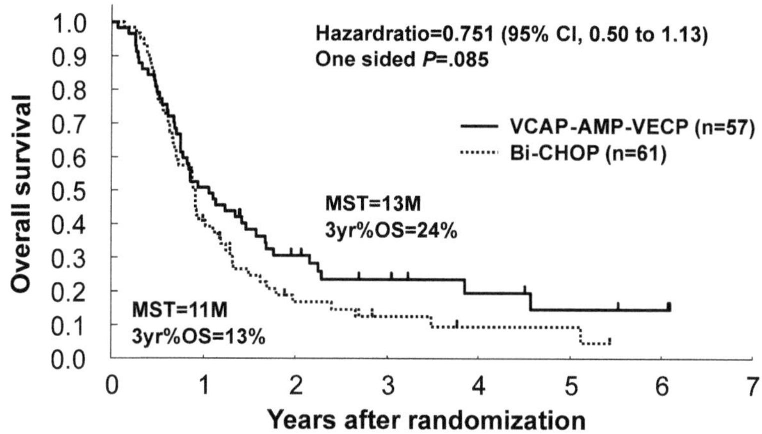

Fig. 8.4 Kaplan-Meier Estimate of Overall Survival for all Randomly Assigned Patients in JCOG9801. CI = confidential interval; VCAP = vincristine, cyclophosphamide, doxorubicin, prednisone; AMP = doxorubicin, ranimustine, prednisone; VECP = vindesine, etoposide, carboplatin, prednisone; MST = median survival time; OS = overall survival; [Based on data from Tsukasaki K, Utsunomiya A, Fukuda H, et al.: VCAP-AMP-VECP compared with biweekly CHOP for adult T-cell leukemia-lymphoma: Japan Clinical Oncology Group Study JCOG9801. J Clin Oncol 25:5,458–5,564, 2007.]

related to neutropenia, were reported in the VCAP-AMP-VECP arm. Two cases of myelodysplastic syndrome were reported, one each in both arms.

The longer survival at 3 years and higher CR rate with LSG15 compared with biweekly CHOP suggest that LSG15 is a more effective regimen at the expense of higher toxicity, providing the basis for future investigations in the treatment of ATL [107]. The superiority of VCAP-AMP-VECP to biweekly CHOP may be explained by the more prolonged, dose dense schedule of therapy in addition to four more drugs. In addition, agents such as carboplatin and ranimustine not affected by multidrug-resistance related genes, which were frequently expressed in ATL cells at onset, were incorporated [109]. Intrathecal prophylaxis, which was incorporated in both arms of the phase III study, should be considered for patients with aggressive ATL even in the absence of clinical symptoms because a previous analysis revealed that more than half of relapses at new sites after chemotherapy occurred in the CNS [110]. However, the median survival time of 13 months still compares unfavorably to other hematological malignancies, requiring further effort to improve the outcome.

Interferon-Alpha and Zidovudine

A small phase II trial in Japan of IFN alpha against relapsed/refractory ATL showed a response rate (all PR) of 33% (8/24), including five out of nine (56%) chronic type ATL [111]. In 1995, Gill and associates reported that 11 of 19 patients with acute- or lymphoma-type ATL showed major responses (five CR and six PR) to a combination of interferon-alpha (IFN) and zidovudine (AZT) [112]. The efficacy of this combination was also observed in a French study; major objective responses were obtained in all five patients with ATL (four with acute type and one with smoldering type) [113]. Although these results are encouraging, the OS of previously untreated patients with ATL was relatively short (4.8 months) compared with the survival of those in the chemotherapy trials conducted by the JCOG-LSG (7–8 months) [114]. After that, numerous small phase II studies using AZT and IFN have shown responses in ATL patients [115–117]. High doses of both agents are recommended: 6–9 million units of IFN in combination with daily divided AZT doses of 800–1,000 mg/day.

Recently, the results of a "meta-analysis" on the use of IFN and AZT for ATL were reported

[118]. A total of 100 patients received interferon-alpha and AZT as initial treatments. The ORR was 66%, with a 43% CR rate. In this worldwide retrospective analysis, the median survival time was 24 months and the 5-year survival rate was 50% for first-line IFN and AZT, vs. 7 months and 20% for 84 patients who received first-line chemotherapy. The median survival time of patients with acute-type ATL treated with first-line IFN/AZT and chemotherapy was 12 and 9 months, respectively. Patients with lymphoma-type ATL did not benefit from this combination. In addition, first-line IFN/AZT therapy in chronic- and smoldering-type ATL resulted in a 100% survival rate at a median follow-up of 5 years. While the results for IFN/AZT in indolent ATL appear to be promising compared to those with watchful-waiting policy until disease progression, recently reported from Japan [101], the possibility of selection bias cannot be ruled out. A prospective multicenter phase III study evaluating the efficacy of IFN/AZT as compared to watchful-waiting for indolent ATL is to be initiated in Japan.

Recently, a phase II study of the combination of arsenic trioxide, IFN, and AZT for chronic ATL revealed an impressive response rate and moderate toxicity [119]. Although the results appeared promising, the addition of arsenic trioxide to IFN/AZT, which might be sufficient for the treatment of chronic ATL as described above, caused more toxicity and should be evaluated with caution.

Allergenic Hematopoietic Stem-Cell Transplantation (allo-HSCT)

Allo-HSCT is now recommended for the treatment of young patients with aggressive ATL. Despite higher treatment-related mortality in a retrospective multicenter analysis of myeloablative allo-HSCT, the estimated 3-year OS of 33% is promising, possibly reflecting a graft versus ATL effect [120]. To evaluate the efficacy of allo-HSCT more accurately, especially in view of a comparison with intensive chemotherapy, a prospective multicenter phase II study of LSG15 chemotherapy followed by allo-HSCT will be initiated in Japan.

Feasibility studies of allo-HSCT with reduced intensity conditioning for ATL also revealed promising results, and a subsequent multicenter trial of RIST is being conducted in Japan [121, 122]. The minimal residual disease after allo-HSCT detected as HTLV-1 proviral load was much less extensive than that after chemotherapy or AZT/IFN therapy, suggesting the presence of a graft-versus-ATL effect as well as graft-versus-HTLV-1 activity [121]. It remains unclear which type of allo-HSCT (myeloablative or reduced intensity conditioning) is more suitable for the treatment of ATL. Furthermore, selection criteria with respect to responses to previous treatments, sources of stem cells, and HTLV-1 viral status of the donor remain to be determined. However, several other retrospective studies as well as those mentioned above on allo-HSCT showed a promising long-term survival rate of 20–40% with an apparent plateau phase despite significant treatment-related mortality.

Supportive Care

The prevention of opportunistic infections is essential in the management of ATL patients, nearly half of whom develop severe infections during chemotherapy. Some patients with indolent ATL develop infections during watchful waiting. Sulfamethoxazole/trimethoprim and antifungal agents have been recommended as prophylaxes for Pneumocystis jiroveci pneumonia and fungal infections, respectively, in the JCOG trials [105–107]. While cytomegalovirus infections are not infrequent among ATL patients, ganciclovir is not usually recommended as a prophylaxis [55]. In addition, in patients not receiving chemotherapy, antifungal prophylaxis may not be critical. An anti-strongyloides agent, such as ivermectin or albendazole, should be considered to avoid systemic infections in patients with a history of exposure to the parasite in the tropics. Treatment with steroids and proton pump inhibitors may precipitate a fulminant strongyloides infestation and warrants testing before these agents are used in endemic areas [55]. Hypercalcemia associated with aggressive ATL can be corrected using chemotherapy in combination with hydration and bisphosphonate even when the PS of the patient is poor.

Response Criteria in ATL

The complex nature of ATL, often with both leukemic and lymphomatous components, makes response assessment difficult. A modification of the JCOG response criteria was suggested reflecting those for CLL and NHL which had been published later [55, 123, 124]. Recently, revised response criteria were proposed for lymphoma, incorporating positron emission tomography (PET), especially for the assessment of CR. It is well known and described in the criteria that several kinds of lymphoma including PTCLs were variably [18F]fluorodeoxyglucose avid [125]. Meanwhile, PET or PET/CT is recommended for evaluations of response for ATL when the tumorous lesions are FDG-avid at diagnosis [57].

New Agents for ATL

Topoisomerase Inhibitors

MST-16, a new orally administered bis(2,6-dioxopiperazine) analogue and an inhibitor of topoisomerase II, showed some activity with little cross resistance toward lymphoid malignancies in vitro and in vivo. MST-16 at 1,200–2,800 mg/day was given orally daily for 7 days, with courses repeated at intervals of 2–3 weeks to 24 patients with ATL in a phase I–II study [126]. Two CRs and eight PRs were obtained in 23 (13 acute, 8 lymphoma, and 2 chronic ATL) evaluable patients. Remissions were obtained at 7–232 (median, 23) days and lasted 43–374 (median, 68) days. The major toxic effects were leukopenia (68%), anemia (52%), thrombocytopenia (35%), and gastrointestinal disorders (22%). Although this agent showed promising activity against ATL as a single agent, no further study in combination with other agents has been reported.

Irinotecan hydrochloride (CPT-11) is a semisynthetic camptothecin with inhibitory activity against topoisomerase I. Preclinical studies of CPT-11 have suggested a lack of cross-resistance between topoisomerase I inhibitors and other anticancer agents. Multicenter phase II studies of CPT-11 have been conducted against relapsed or refractory NHL [127]. In this study, 9 patients achieved a CR, and 17 patients achieved a PR (response rate 38%: 26 of 69), using a weekly intravenous administration of 40 mg/m^2/day for three consecutive days. Within this group, 5 of 13 patients with ATL (38%) responded to CPT-11 (one CR and four PR) [127]. The major toxic effects of CPT-11 were leukopenia, diarrhea, and nausea and/or vomiting. Subsequently, to develop a new chemo therapy regimen effective against NHL and ATL, two kinds of phase I/II studies of CPT-11 in combination with CBDCA or ETP were conducted for relapsed or refractory NHL. In both studies, however, dose escalation was halted because of hematologic toxicity (in combination with CBDCA) and hepatotoxicity (in combination with ETP).

Purine Analogs

Several purine analogs have been evaluated for ATL. Among them, pentostatin (deoxycoformycin) has been most extensively evaluated as a single agent and in combination as described above [105, 108]. Other purine analogs clinically studied for ATL are fludarabine and cladribine. Fludarabine is among standard treatments for B-chronic lymphocytic leukemia and other lymphoid malignancies. In a phase I study of fludarabine in Japan, five ATL patients and ten B-CLL patients with refractory or relapsed-disease were enrolled [128]. Six grade 3 non-hematological toxicities were only observed in the ATL patients. PR was achieved only in one of the five ATL patients and the duration was short. Cladribine is among standard treatments for hairy cell leukemia and other lymphoid malignancies. A phase II study of cladribine for relapsed/refractory aggressive-ATL in 15 patients revealed only one PR [129].

Forodesine, a purine nucleotide phosphorylase (PNP) inhibitor, is among purine nucleotide analogs. PNP is an enzyme in the purine salvage pathway that phosphorolysis 2′deoxyguanosine (dGuo). PNP deficiency in humans results in a severe combined immunodeficiency phenotype and the selective depletion of T cells associated with high plasma deoxyguanosine (dGuo) and high intracellular deoxyguanosine triphosphate levels in those cells with high deoxynucleoside kinase activity such as T cells, leading to cell death. Inhibitors of PNP, such as forodesine, mimic SCID in vitro and in vivo, suggesting a new targeting agent specific for T-cell malignancies [130]. A dose escalating phase I study of forodesine is being conducted for T-cell malignancies including ATL.

Histone Deacetylase Inhibitors

Gene expression governed by epigenetic changes is crucial to the pathogenesis of cancer. Histone deacetylases (HDACs) are enzymes involved in the remodeling of chromatin and play a key role in the epigenetic regulation of gene expression. Deacetylase inhibitors (DACi) induce the hyperacetylation of non-histone proteins as well as nucleosomal histones resulting in the expression of repressed genes involved in growth arrest, terminal differentiation, and/or apoptosis among cancer cells. Several classes of HDACi have been found to have potent anticancer effects in preclinical studies. HDACis such as vorinostat (suberoylanilide hydroxamic acid), romidepsin (depsipeptide), and panobinostat (LBH589) have also shown promise in preclinical and/or clinical studies against T-cell malignancies including ATL [131]. Vorinostat and romidepsin have been approved for cutaneous T-cell lymphoma (CTCL) by the Food and Drug Administration in the USA. LBH589 has a significant anti-ATL effect in vitro and in mice [132]. However, a phase II study for CTCL and indolent ATL was terminated because of severe infections associated with the shrinkage of skin tumors and formation of ulcers in patients with ATL. Further study is required to evaluate the efficacy of HDACIs for PTCL/CTCL including ATL.

Monoclonal Antibodies and Toxin Fusion Proteins

Monoclonal antibodies (MoAb) and toxin fusion proteins targeting several molecules expressed on the surface of ATL cells and other lymphoid malignant cells, such as CD25, CD2, CD52 and CCR4, have shown promise in recent clinical trials. Because most ATL cells express the alpha-chain of IL-2R (CD25), Waldmann et al. treated patients with ATL using monoclonal antibodies to CD25 [133]. Six (32%) of 19 patients treated with anti-Tac showed objective responses lasting from 9 weeks to longer than 3 years. One impediment to this approach is the quantity of soluble IL-2R shed by the tumor cells into the circulation. Another strategy for targeting IL-2R is conjugation with an immunotoxin (Pseudomonas exotoxin) or radioisotope (yttrium-90). Waldmann et al. developed a stable conjugate of anti-Tac with yttrium-90. Among the 16 patients with ATL who received 5- to 15-mCi doses, 9 (56%) showed objective responses. The response lasted longer than that obtained with unconjugated anti-Tac antibody [134, 135].

LMB-2, composed of the anti-CD25 murine MoAb fused to the truncated form of Pseudomonas toxin, was cytotoxic to CD25-expressing cells including ATL cells in vitro and in mice. Phase I/II trials of this agent showed some effect against hairy cell leukemia, CTCL, and ATL [136]. Six of thirty-five patients in the phase I study had significant levels of neutralizing antibodies after the first cycle. This drug deserves further clinical trials including in combination with cytotoxic agents.

Denileukin diftitox (DD; DAB(389)-interleukin-2 [IL-2]), an interleukin-2-diphtheria toxin fusion protein targeting IL-2 receptor-expressing malignant T lymphocytes, shows efficacy as a single agent against CTCL and PTCL [137]. Also, the combination of this agent with multi-agent chemotherapy, CHOP, was promising for PTCL [138]. ATL cells frequently and highly express CD25 as described above and several ATL cases successfully treated with this agent have been reported [139].

CD52 antigen is present on normal and pathologic B and T cells. In PTCL, however, CD52 expression varies among patients, with an overall expression rate lower than 50% in one study but not in another [140, 141]. ATL cells frequently express CD52 as compared to other PTCLs. The humanized anti-CD52 monoclonal antibody alemtuzumab is active against CLL and PTCL as a single agent. The combination of alemtuzumab with a standard-dose cyclophosphamide/doxorubicin/vincristine/prednisone (CHOP) regimen as a first-line treatment for 24 patients with PTCL showed promising results with CR in 17 (71%) patients, 1 had a partial remission, with an overall median duration of response of 11 months and was associated with mostly manageable infections but including CMV reactivation [142]. Major infections were Jacob–Creutzfeldt virus reactivation, pulmonary invasive aspergillosis, and Staphylococcus sepsis.

ATL cells express CD52, the target of alemtuzumab, which was active in a preclinical model of ATL and toxic to p53-deficient cells, and several ATL cases successfully treated with this agent have been reported [143–145].

Siplizumab is a humanized MoAb targeting CD2 and showed efficacy in a murine ATL model. P1 dose-escalating study of this agent in 22 patients with several kinds of T/NK-cell malignancy revealed six responses (two CR in LGL leukemia, three PR in ATL and one PR in CTCL). However, four patients developed EBV-associated LPD [146]. The broad specificity of this agent may eliminate both CD4- and CD8-positive T cells as well as NK cells without affecting B cells and predispose individuals to the development of EBV lymphoproliferative syndrome.

CCR4 is expressed on normal T helper type 27 and regulatory T (Treg) cells and on certain types of T-cell neoplasms [63, 94]. KW-0761, a next generation humanized anti-CCR4 mAb, with a defucosylated Fc region, exerts strong antibody-dependent cellular cytotoxicity due to increased binding to the Fcγ receptor on effecter cells [147]. A phase I study of dose escalation with four weekly intravenous infusions of KW-0761 in 16 patients with relapsed CCR4-positive T-cell malignancy (13 ATL and 3 PTCL) revealed that one patient, at the maximum dose (1.0 mg/kg), developed grade (G) three dose-limiting toxic effects, namely skin rashes and febrile neutropenia, and G4 neutropenia [148]. Other treatment-related G3-4 toxic effects were lymphopenia ($n=10$), neutropenia ($n=3$), leukopenia ($n=2$), herpes zoster ($n=1$), and acute infusion reaction/cytokine release syndrome ($n=1$). Neither the frequency nor severity of these effects increased with dose escalation or the plasma concentration of the agent. The maximum tolerated dose was not reached. No patients had detectable levels of anti-KW-0761 antibody. Five patients (31%; 95% CI, 11–59%) achieved objective responses: two complete (0.1; 1.0 mg/kg) and three partial (0.01; 2 at 1.0 mg/kg) responses. Three out of thirteen patients with ATL (31%) achieved a response (two CR and one PR). Responses in each lesion were diverse, that is, good in PB (six CR and one PR/seven evaluable cases), intermediate in skin (three CR and one PR/eight evaluable cases), and poor in LN (1 CR and 2 PR/11 evaluable cases). KW-0761 was well tolerated at all the doses tested, demonstrating potential efficacy against relapsed CCR4-positive ATL or PTCL. Recently, results of subsequent phase II studies at the 1.0 mg/kg in relapsed ATL, showing 50% of response rate with acceptable toxicity profiles, were reported [149]. Also, a phase II trial of single agent KW-0761 at the 1.0 mg/kg in relapsed PTCL/CTCL and a phase II trial of VCAP-AMP-VECP combined with KW-0761 for untreated aggressive ATL are ongoing.

Other Novel Agents

Pralatrexate (Folotyn) is a new agent with potent preclinical and clinical activity in T-cell malignancies including ATL [150–152]. The agent is a novel anti-folate with improved membrane transport and polyglutamylation in tumor cells and high affinity for the reduced folate carrier highly expressed in malignant cells. Other potential drugs for ATL under investigation include a proteasome inhibitor, bortezomib (Velcade), and an immunomodulatory agent, lenalidomide (Revlimid) [153–155].

Table 8.3 Strategy for the treatment of Adult T-Cell Leukemia-Lymphoma

Smoldering- or favorable chronic-type ATL
• Consider inclusion in
• Symptomatic patients (skin lesions, opportunistic infections, etc.): Consider AZT/IFN or Watch and Wait
• Asymptomatic patients: Consider Watch and Wait
Unfavorable chronic- or acute-type ATL
• If outside clinical trials, check prognostic factors (including clinical and molecular factors if possible):
– Good prognostic factors: consider chemotherapy (VCAP-AMP-VECP evaluated by a phase III trial against biweekly-CHOP) or AZT/IFN (evaluated by a meta-analysis on retrospective studies)
– Poor prognostic factors: consider chemotherapy followed by conventional or reduced intensity allo-HSCT (evaluated by retrospective and prospective Japanese analyses, respectively).
– Poor response to initial therapy: Consider conventional or reduced intensity allo-HSCT
Lymphoma-type ATL
• If outside clinical trials, consider chemotherapy (VCAP-AMP-VECP)
• Check prognostic factors (including clinical and molecular factors if possible) and response to chemotherapy:
– Good prognostic factors and good response to initial therapy: Consider chemotherapy followed by observation
– Poor prognostic factors or poor response to initial therapy: Consider chemotherapy followed by conventional or reduced intensity allo-HSCT

[Based on data from Tsukasaki K, Hermine O, Bazarbachi A, et al.: Definition, prognostic factors, treatment, and response criteria of adult T-cell leukemia-lymphoma: A proposal from an international consensus meeting. J Clin Oncol 27:453–459, 2009.]

Prevention of ATL

Two steps should be considered for the prevention of HTLV-1-associated ATL. The first is the prevention of HTLV-1 infections. This has been achieved in some endemic areas in Japan by screening for HTLV-1 among blood donors and asking mothers who are carriers to refrain from breast feeding. The second step is the prevention of ATL among HTLV-1 carriers. This has not been achieved partly because only about 5% of HTLV-1 carriers develop the disease in their life time, although several risk factors have been identified by a cohort study of HTLV-1 carriers (Joint Study of Predisposing Factors for ATL Development) [83]. Also, no agent has been found to be effective in preventing the development of ATL among HTLV-1 carriers.

Ongoing Clinical Trials

Clinical trials have been paramount to the recent advances in ATL treatment, including assessments of chemotherapy, AZT/IFN, and allo-HSCT. Recently, a strategy for ATL treatment, stratified by subclassification, prognostic factors, and the response to initial treatment as well as response criteria was proposed (Table 8.3) [57]. The recommended treatment algorithm for ATL is shown in Fig. 8.2. However, as described in this chapter, ATL still has a worse prognosis than the other T-cell malignancies [156]. There is no plateau with an initial steep slope and subsequent gentle slope without a plateau in the survival curve for aggressive or indolent ATL treated by watchful waiting and with chemotherapy, respectively, although the prognosis is much better in the latter [14, 61]. A prognostic model for each subgroup should be elucidated to properly identify the candidate for allo-HSCT which can achieve a cure of ATL despite considerable treatment-related mortality. Although several small phase II trials suggested IFN/AZT therapy to be promising, no confirmative phase III study has been conducted. Furthermore, as described in the other chapters in detail, more than ten promising new agents for PTCL/CTCL including ATL are now in clinical trials or preparation. Future clinical trials on ATL as described above should be incorporated to ensure that the strategy as shown in Table 8.3 is continually updated to establish evidence-based practical guidelines.

References

1. Uchiyama T, Yodoi J, Sagawa K, et al. Adult T-cell leukemia: clinical and hematologic features of 16 cases. Blood. 1977;50:481–92.
2. Poiesz BJ, Ruscetti FW, Gazdar AF, et al. Detection and isolation of type C retrovirus particles from fresh and cultured lymphocytes of a patient with cutaneous T-cell lymphoma. Proc Natl Acad Sci USA. 1980;77:7415–9.
3. Hinuma Y, Nagata K, Hanaoka M, Nakai M, Matsumoto T, Kinoshita KI, et al. Adult T-cell leukemia: antigen in an ATL cell line and detection of antibodies to the antigen in human sera. Proc Natl Acad Sci USA. 1981;78(10):6476–80.
4. Miyoshi I, Kubonishi I, Yoshimoto S, Akagi T, Ohtsuki Y, Shiraishi Y, et al. Type C virus particles in a cord T-cell line derived by co-cultivating normal human cord leukocytes and human leukaemic T cells. Nature. 1981;294(5843):770–1.
5. Yoshida M, Miyoshi I, Hinuma Y. Isolation and characterization of retrovirus from cell lines of human adult T-cell leukemia and its implication in the disease. Proc Natl Acad Sci USA. 1982;79:2031–5.
6. Gessain A, Barin F, Vernant JC, Gout O, Maurs L, Calender A, et al. Antibodies to human T-lymphotropic virus type-I in patients with tropical spastic paraparesis. Lancet. 1985;2(8452):407–10.
7. Osame M, Usuku K, Izumo S, Ijichi N, Amitani H, Igata A, et al. HTLV-I associated myelopathy, a new clinical entity. Lancet. 1986;1(8488):1031–2.
8. LaGrenade L, Hanchard B, Fletcher V, Cranston B, Blattner W. Infective dermatitis of Jamaican children: a marker for HTLV-I infection. Lancet. 1990;336(8727):1345–7.
9. Mochizuki M, Watanabe T, Yamaguchi K, Takatsuki K, Yoshimura K, Shirao M, et al. HTLV-I uveitis: a distinct clinical entity caused by HTLV-I. Jpn J Cancer Res. 1992;83(3):236–9.
10. Terada K, Katamine S, Eguchi K, Moriuchi R, Kita M, Shimada H, et al. Prevalence of serum and salivary antibodies to HTLV-1 in Sjögren's syndrome. Lancet. 1994;344(8930):1116–9.
11. Takatsuki K. Adult T-cell Leukemia. Oxford: Oxford University Press, New York; 1994.
12. IARC Working Group on the Evaluation of Carcinogenic Risks to Humans: Human immunodeficiency viruses and human T-cell lymphotropic viruses. IARC monographs on the evaluation of carcinogenic risks to humans, Geneva: IARCPress 1996
13. Ohshima K, Jaffe ES, Kikuchi M. Adult T-cell leukemia/lymphoma. In: Swerdlow SH, Campo E, Harris NL, et al., editors. WHO classification of tumour of haemaopoietic and lymphoid tissues. 4th ed. Lyon: IARC Press; 2008. p. 281–4.
14. Shimoyama M. Diagnostic criteria and classification of clinical subtypes of adult T- cell leukaemia-lymphoma: a report from the lymphoma study group (1984–87). Br J Haematol. 1991;79:428–37.
15. Matsuoka M, Jeang KT. Human T-cell leukaemia virus type 1 (HTLV-1) infectivity and cellular transformation. Nat Rev Cancer. 2007;7(4):270–80.
16. Satou Y, Matsuoka M. HTLV-1 and the host immune system: how the virus disrupts immune regulation, leading to HTLV-1 associated diseases. J Clin Exp Hematop. 2010;50(1):1–8.
17. Seiki M, Hattori S, Hirayama Y, Yoshida M. Human adult T-cell leukemia virus: complete nucleotide sequence of the provirus genome integrated in leukemia cell DNA. Proc Natl Acad Sci USA. 1983;80(12):3618–22.
18. Sodroski JG, Goh WC, Rosen CA, Salahuddin SZ, Aldovini A, Franchini G, et al. trans-Activation of the human T-cell leukemia virus long terminal repeat correlates with expression of the x-lor protein. J Virol. 1985;55(3):831–5.
19. Kiyokawa T, Seiki M, Iwashita S, Imagawa K, Shimizu F, Yoshida M. p27x-III and p21x-III, proteins encoded by the pX sequence of human T-cell leukemia virus type I. Proc Natl Acad Sci USA. 1985;82(24):8359–63.
20. Gaudray G, Gachon F, Basbous J, et al. The complementary strand of the human T-cell leukemia virus type 1 RNA genome encodes a bZIP transcription factor that down-regulates viral transcription. J Virol. 2002;76:12813.
21. Satou Y, Yasunaga J, Yoshida M, et al. HTLV-I basic leucine zipper factor gene mRNA supports proliferation of adult T cell leukemia cells. Proc Natl Acad Sci USA. 2006;103:720.
22. Murata K, Hayashibara T, Sugahara K, Uemura A, Yamaguchi T, Harasawa H, et al. A novel alternative splicing isoform of human T-cell leukemia virus type 1 bZIP factor (HBZ-SI) targets distinct subnuclear localization. J Virol. 2006;80(5):2495–505.
23. Kline RL, Brothers T, Halsey N, Boulos R, Lairmore MD, Quinn TC. Evaluation of enzyme immunoassays for antibody to human T-lymphotropic viruses type I/II. Lancet. 1991;337(8732):30–3.
24. Ikeda M, Fujino R, Matsui T, Yoshida T, Komoda H, Imai J. A new agglutination test for serum antibodies to adult T-cell leukemia virus. Gann. 1984;75(10):815–8.
25. Aoki T, Miyakoshi H, Koide H, Yoshida T, Ishikawa H, Sugisaki Y, et al. Seroepidemiology of human T-lymphotropic retrovirus type I (HTLV-I) in residents of Niigata Prefecture, Japan. Comparative studies by indirect immunofluorescence microscopy and enzyme-linked immunosorbent assay. Int J Cancer. 1985;35(3):301–6.
26. Aboulafia DM, Feigal E, Vranzian K, Bennett C, Blattner W, Moss A, et al. Human T cell leukemia virus (HTLV-I/II) serodiagnostic testing: disparate results among a cohort of intravenous drug users. AIDS Res Hum Retroviruses. 1993;9(10):1043–50.
27. Acquired immunodeficiency syndrome (AIDS). Proposed WHO criteria for interpreting results from western blot assays for HIV-1, HIV-2, and HTLV-I/HTLV-II. Wkly Epidemiol Rec. 1990 Sep 14;65(37):281–3.

28. Franchini G, Wong-Staal F, Gallo RC. Human T-cell leukemia virus (HTLV-I) transcripts in fresh and cultured cells of patients with adult T-cell leukemia. Proc Natl Acad Sci USA. 1984;81:6207.
29. Kinoshita T, Shimoyama M, Tobinai K, Ito M, Ito S, Ikeda S, et al. Detection of mRNA for the tax1/rex1 gene of human T-cell leukemia virus type I in fresh peripheral blood mononuclear cells of adult T-cell leukemia patients and viral carriers by using the polymerase chain reaction. Proc Natl Acad Sci USA. 1989;86(14):5620–4.
30. Yoshida M, Seiki M, Yamaguchi K, Takatsuki K. Monoclonal integration of human T-cell leukemia provirus in all primary tumors of adult T-cell leukemia suggests causative role of human T-cell leukemia virus in the disease. Proc Natl Acad Sci USA. 1984;81(8):2534–7.
31. Takemoto S, Matsuoka M, Yamaguchi K, Takatsuki K. A novel diagnostic method of adult T-cell leukemia: monoclonal integration of human T-cell lymphotropic virus type I provirus DNA detected by inverse polymerase chain reaction. Blood. 1994; 84(9):3080–5.
32. Wattel E, Vartanian JP, Pannetier C, Wain-Hobson S. Clonal expansion of human T-cell leukemia virus type I-infected cells in asymptomatic and symptomatic carriers without malignancy. J Virol. 1995;69(5):2863–8.
33. Yamaguchi K, Seiki M, Yoshida M, Nishimura H, Kawano F, Takatsuki K. The detection of human T cell leukemia virus proviral DNA and its application for classification and diagnosis of T cell malignancy. Blood. 1984;63(5):1235–40.
34. Tamiya S, Matsuoka M, Etoh K, Watanabe T, Kamihira S, Yamaguchi K, et al. Two types of defective human T-lymphotropic virus type I provirus in adult T-cell leukemia. Blood. 1996;88(8):3065–73.
35. Tsukasaki K, Tsushima H, Yamamura M, et al. Integration patterns of HTLV-I provirus in relation to the clinical course of ATL: frequent clonal change at crisis from indolent disease. Blood. 1997;89:948–56.
36. Furukawa Y, Fujisawa J, Osame M, Toita M, Sonoda S, Kubota R, et al. Frequent clonal proliferation of human T-cell leukemia virus type 1 (HTLV-1)-infected T cells in HTLV-1-associated myelopathy (HAM-TSP). Blood. 1992;80(4):1012–6.
37. Ikeda S, Momita S, Kinoshita K, Kamihira S, Moriuchi Y, Tsukasaki K, et al. Clinical course of human T-lymphotropic virus type I carriers with molecularly detectable monoclonal proliferation of T lymphocytes: defining a low- and high-risk population. Blood. 1993;82(7):2017–24.
38. Takahashi K, Takezaki T, Oki T, Kawakami K, Yashiki S, Fujiyoshi T, et al. Inhibitory effect of maternal antibody on mother-to-child transmission of human T-lymphotropic virus type I. The Mother-to-Child Transmission Study Group. Int J Cancer. 1991;49(5):673–7.
39. Kinoshita K, Hino S, Amagaski T, Ikeda S, Yamada Y, Suzuyama J, et al. Demonstration of adult T-cell leukemia virus antigen in milk from three sero-positive mothers. Gann. 1984;75(2):103–5.
40. Hino S, Katamine S, Miyata H, Tsuji Y, Yamabe T, Miyamoto T. Primary prevention of HTLV-1 in Japan. Leukemia. 1997;11 Suppl 3:57–9.
41. Tajima K, Tominaga S, Suchi T, Kawagoe T, Komoda H, Hinuma Y, et al. Epidemiological analysis of the distribution of antibody to adult T-cell leukemia-virus-associated antigen: possible horizontal transmission of adult T-cell leukemia virus. Gann. 1982;73(6):893–901.
42. Okochi K, Sato H, Hinuma Y. A retrospective study on transmission of adult T cell leukemia virus by blood transfusion: seroconversion in recipients. Vox Sang. 1984;46(5):245–53.
43. Schwebke J, Calsyn D, Shriver K, Saxon A, Kleyn J, Oluoch-Mitchell E, et al. Prevalence and epidemiologic correlates of human T cell lymphotropic virus infection among intravenous drug users. J Infect Dis. 1994;169(5):962–7.
44. Schaffar-Deshayes L, Chavance M, Monplaisir N, Courouce AM, Gessain A, Blesonski S, et al. Antibodies to HTLV-I p24 in sera of blood donors, elderly people and patients with hemopoietic diseases in France and in French West Indies. Int J Cancer. 1984;34(5):667–70.
45. Hunsmann G, Bayer H, Schneider J, Schmitz H, Kern P, Dietrich M, et al. Antibodies to ATLV/HTLV-1 in Africa. Med Microbiol Immunol. 1984;173(3):167–70.
46. Ohtsu T, Tsugane S, Tobinai K, Shimoyama M, Nanri S, Watanabe S. Prevalence of antibodies to human T-cell leukemia/lymphoma virus type I and human immunodeficiency virus in Japanese immigrant colonies in Bolivia and Bolivian natives. Jpn J Cancer Res. 1987;78(12):1347–53.
47. Achiron A, Pinhas-Hamiel O, Doll L, Djaldetti R, Chen A, Ziv I, et al. Spastic paraparesis associated with human T-lymphotropic virus type I: a clinical, serological, and genomic study in Iranian-born Mashhadi Jews. Ann Neurol. 1993;34(5):670–5.
48. Yanagihara R, Jenkins CL, Alexander SS, Mora CA, Garruto RM. Human T lymphotropic virus type I infection in Papua New Guinea: high prevalence among the Hagahai confirmed by western analysis. J Infect Dis. 1990;162(3):649–54.
49. Cruickshank JK, Rudge P, Dalgleish AG, Newton M, McLean BN, Barnard RO, et al. Tropical spastic paraparesis and human T cell lymphotropic virus type 1 in the United Kingdom. Brain. 1989;112(Pt 4):1057–90.
50. Tajima K, Kamura S, Ito S, Ito M, Nagatomo M, Kinoshita K, et al. Epidemiological features of HTLV-I carriers and incidence of ATL in an ATL-endemic island: a report of the community-based co-operative study in Tsushima, Japan. Int J Cancer. 1987;40(6):741–6.
51. Mueller N, Okayama A, Stuver S, Tachibana N. Findings from the Miyazaki Cohort Study. J Acquir Immune Defic Syndr Hum Retrovirol. 1996;13 Suppl 1:S2–7.

52. Iwanaga M, Chiyoda S, Kusaba E, Kamihira S. Trends in the seroprevalence of HTLV-1 in Japanese blood donors in Nagasaki Prefecture, 2000–2006. Int J Hematol. 2009;90(2):186–90.
53. Morgan OS, Rodgers-Johnson P, Mora C, Char G. HTLV-1 and polymyositis in Jamaica. Lancet. 1989;2(8673):1184–7.
54. Sugimoto M, Nakashima H, Watanabe S, Uyama E, Tanaka F, Ando M, et al. T-lymphocyte alveolitis in HTLV-I-associated myelopathy. Lancet. 1987; 2(8569):1220.
55. Nishioka K, Maruyama I, Sato K, Kitajima I, Nakajima Y, Osame M. Chronic inflammatory arthropathy associated with HTLV-I. Lancet. 1989; 1(8635):441.
56. Tachibana N, Okayama A, Ishizaki J, Yokota T, Shishime E, Murai K, et al. Suppression of tuberculin skin reaction in healthy HTLV-I carriers from Japan. Int J Cancer. 1988;42(6):829–31.
57. Tsukasaki K, Hermine O, Bazarbachi A, et al. Definition, prognostic factors, treatment, and response criteria of adult T-cell leukemia-lymphoma: a proposal from an international consensus meeting. J Clin Oncol. 2009;27:453–9.
58. Major prognostic factors of patients with adult T-cell leukemia- lymphoma: a cooperative study. Lymphoma Study Group (1984–1987): Leuk Res 1991;15:81–90.
59. Yamada Y, Hatta Y, Murata K, et al. Deletions of p15 and/or p16 genes as a poor-prognosis factor in adult T-cell leukemia. J Clin Oncol. 1997;15:1778–85.
60. Utsunomiya A, Ishida T, Inagaki A, et al. Clinical significance of a blood eosinophilia in adult T-cell leukemia/lymphoma: a blood eosinophilia is a significant unfavorable prognostic factor. Leuk Res. 2007;31:915–20.
61. Takasaki Y, Iwanaga M, Tsukasaki K, et al. Impact of visceral involvements and blood cell count abnormalities on survival in adult T-cell leukemia/lymphoma (ATLL). Leuk Res. 2007;31:751–7.
62. Inagaki A, Ishida T, Ishii T, et al. Clinical significance of serum Th1-, Th2- and regulatory T cells-associated cytokines in adult T-cell leukemia/lymphoma: high interleukin-5 and −10 levels are significant unfavorable prognostic factors. Int J Cancer. 2006;118:3054–61.
63. Ishida T, Utsunomiya A, Iida S, et al. Clinical significance of CCR4 expression in adult T-cell leukemia/lymphoma: its close association with skin involvement and unfavorable outcome. Clin Cancer Res. 2003;9:3625–34.
64. Ohno N, Tani A, Uozumi K, et al. Expression of functional lung resistance–related protein predicts poor outcome in adult T-cell leukemia. Blood. 2001;98:1160–5.
65. Tawara M, Hogerzeil SJ, Yamada Y, et al. Impact of p53 aberration on the progression of Adult T-cell Leukemia/Lymphoma. Cancer Lett. 2006;234: 249–55.
66. Bittencourt AL, da Graças Vieira M, et al. Adult T-cell leukemia/lymphoma in Bahia, Brazil: analysis of prognostic factors in a group of 70 patients. Am J Clin Pathol. 2007;128:875–82.
67. Statistical analyses of clinico-pathological, virological and epidemiological data on lymphoid malignancies with special reference to adult T-cell leukemia/lymphoma: a report of the second nationwide study of Japan. The T- and B-Cell Malignancy Study Group. Jpn J Clin Oncol. 1985 Sep;15(3):517–35.
68. Bartholomew C, Charles W, Saxinger C, Blattner W, Robert-Guroff M, Raju C, et al. Racial and other characteristics of human T cell leukemia/lymphoma (HTLV-I) and AIDS (HTLV-III) in Trinidad. Br Med J (Clin Res Ed). 1985;290(6477):1243–6.
69. Gérard Y, Lepere JF, Pradinaud R, Joly F, Lepelletier L, Joubert M, et al. Clustering and clinical diversity of adult T-cell leukemia/lymphoma associated with HTLV-I in a remote black population of French Guiana. Int J Cancer. 1995;60(6):773–6.
70. Tajima K, Kuroishi T. Estimation of rate of incidence of ATL among ATLV (HTLV-I) carriers in Kyushu, Japan. Jpn J Clin Oncol. 1985;15(2):423–30.
71. Kondo T, Kono H, Nonaka H, Miyamoto N, Yoshida R, Bando F, et al. Risk of adult T-cell leukaemia/lymphoma in HTLV-I carriers. Lancet. 1987;2(8551):159.
72. Murphy EL, Hanchard B, Figueroa JP, Gibbs WN, Lofters WS, Campbell M, et al. Modelling the risk of adult T-cell leukemia/lymphoma in persons infected with human T-lymphotropic virus type I. Int J Cancer. 1989;43(2):250–3.
73. Wilks R, Hanchard B, Morgan O, Williams E, Cranston B, Smith ML, et al. Patterns of HTLV-I infection among family members of patients with adult T-cell leukemia/lymphoma and HTLV-I associated myelopathy/tropical spastic paraparesis. Int J Cancer. 1996;65(2):272–3.
74. Osame M, Janssen R, Kubota H, Nishitani H, Igata A, Nagataki S, et al. Nationwide survey of HTLV-I-associated myelopathy in Japan: association with blood transfusion. Ann Neurol. 1990;28(1):50–6.
75. Chen YC, Wang CH, Su IJ, Hu CY, Chou MJ, Lee TH, et al. Infection of human T-cell leukemia virus type I and development of human T-cell leukemia lymphoma in patients with hematologic neoplasms: a possible linkage to blood transfusion. Blood. 1989;74(1):388–94.
76. Kanno M, Nakamura S, Matsuda T. Adult T-cell leukemia with HTLV-I-associated myelopathy after complete remission of acute myelogenous leukemia. N Engl J Med. 1998;338(5):333.
77. Kondo T, Kono H, Miyamoto N, Yoshida R, Toki H, Matsumoto I, et al. Age- and sex-specific cumulative rate and risk of ATLL for HTLV-I carriers. Int J Cancer. 1989;43(6):1061–4.
78. Kawano F, Tsuda H, Yamaguchi K, Nishimura H, Sanada I, Matsuzaki H, et al. Unusual clinical courses of adult T-cell leukemia in siblings. Cancer. 1984;54(1):131–4.

79. Tokudome S, Shimamoto Y, Sumida I. Smoking and adult T-cell leukemia/lymphoma. Eur J Cancer Prev. 1993;2(1):84–5.
80. Tsukasaki K, Yamada Y, Ikeda S, Tomonaga M. Infective dermatitis among patients with ATL in Japan. Int J Cancer. 1994;57(2):293.
81. Hisada M, Okayama A, Shioiri S, Spiegelman DL, Stuver SO, Mueller NE. Risk factors for adult T-cell leukemia among carriers of human T-lymphotropic virus type I. Blood. 1998;92(10):3557–61.
82. Usuku K, Sonoda S, Osame M, Yashiki S, Takahashi K, Matsumoto M, et al. Igata A HLA haplotype-linked high immune responsiveness against HTLV-I in HTLV-I-associated myelopathy: comparison with adult T-cell leukemia/lymphoma. Ann Neurol. 1988;23(Suppl):S143–50.
83. Iwanaga M, Watanabe T, Utsunomiya A, Okayama A, Uchimaru K, Koh KR, et al. Human T-cell leukemia virus type I (HTLV-1) proviral load and disease progression in asymptomatic HTLV-1 carriers: a nationwide prospective study in Japan. Blood. 2010 [Epub ahead of print].
84. Amano M, Kurokawa M, Ogata K, Itoh H, Kataoka H, Setoyama M. New entity, definition and diagnostic criteria of cutaneous adult T-cell leukemia/lymphoma: human T-lymphotropic virus type 1 proviral DNA load can distinguish between cutaneous and smoldering types. J Dermatol. 2008;35(5):270–5.
85. Bennett JM, Catovsky D, Daniel MT, et al. Proposals for the classification of chronic (mature) B and T lymphoid leukaemias. French-American-British (FAB) Cooperative Group. J Clin Pathol. 1989; 42:567–84.
86. Tsukasaki K, Imaizumi Y, Tawara M, et al. Diversity of leukaemic cell morphology in ATL correlates with prognostic factors, aberrant immunophenotype and defective HTLV-1 genotype. Br J Haematol. 1999;105:369–75.
87. Lennert K, Kikuchi M, Sato E, Suchi T, Stansfeld AG, Feller AC, et al. HTLV-positive and -negative T-cell lymphomas. Morphological and immunohistochemical differences between European and HTLV-positive Japanese T-cell lymphomas. Int J Cancer. 1985;35(1):65–72.
88. Watanabe T, Yamaguchi K, Takatsuki K, Osame M, Yoshida M. Constitutive expression of parathyroid hormone-related protein gene in human T cell leukemia virus type 1 (HTLV-1) carriers and adult T cell leukemia patients that can be trans-activated by HTLV-1 tax gene. J Exp Med. 1990;172(3):759–65.
89. Nosaka K, Miyamoto T, Sakai T, Mitsuya H, Suda T, Matsuoka M. Mechanism of hypercalcemia in adult T-cell leukemia: overexpression of receptor activator of nuclear factor kappaB ligand on adult T-cell leukemia cells. Blood. 2002;99(2):634–40.
90. Tsuda H, Sawada T, Sakata KM, Takatsuki K. Possible mechanisms for the elevation of serum beta 2-microglobulin levels in adult T-cell leukemia. Int J Hematol. 1992;55(2):179–87.
91. Sadamori N, Ikeda S, Yamaguchi K, et al. Serum deoxythymidine kinase in adult T-cell leukemia-lymphoma and its related disorders. Leuk Res. 1991;15:99–103.
92. Kamihira S, Atogami S, Sohda H, et al. Significance of soluble interleukin-2 receptor levels for evaluation of the progression of adult T-cell leukemia. Cancer. 1994;73:2753–8.
93. Kamihira S, Sohda H, Atogami S, Toriya K, Yamada Y, Tsukazaki K, et al. Phenotypic diversity and prognosis of adult T-cell leukemia. Leuk Res. 1992;16(5):435–41.
94. Kohno T, Yamada Y, Akamatsu N, Kamihira S, Imaizumi Y, Tomonaga M, et al. Possible origin of adult T-cell leukemia/lymphoma cells from human T lymphotropic virus type-1-infected regulatory T cells. Cancer Sci. 2005;96(8):527–33.
95. Kamada N, Sakurai M, Miyamoto K, Sanada I, Sadamori N, Fukuhara S, et al. Chromosome abnormalities in adult T-cell leukemia/lymphoma: a karyotype review committee report. Cancer Res. 1992;52(6):1481–93.
96. Itoyama T, Chaganti RS, Yamada Y, et al. Cytogenetic analysis and clinical significance in adult T-cell leukemia/lymphoma: a study of 50 cases from the human T-cell leukemia virus type-1 endemic area, Nagasaki. Blood. 2001;97:3612–20.
97. Tsukasaki K, Krebs J, Nagai K, Tomonaga M, Koeffler HP, Bartram CR, et al. Comparative genomic hybridization analysis in adult T-cell leukemia/lymphoma: correlation with clinical course. Blood. 2001;97(12):3875–81.
98. Oshiro A, Tagawa H, Ohshima K, Karube K, Uike N, Tashiro Y, et al. Identification of subtype-specific genomic alterations in aggressive adult T-cell leukemia/lymphoma. Blood. 2006;107(11):4500–7.
99. Choi YL, Tsukasaki K, O'Neill MC, Yamada Y, Onimaru Y, Matsumoto K, et al. A genomic analysis of adult T-cell leukemia. Oncogene. 2007;26(8): 1245–55.
100. Sasaki H, Nishikata I, Shiraga T, Akamatsu E, Fukami T, Hidaka T, et al. Overexpression of a cell adhesion molecule, TSLC1, as a possible molecular marker for acute-type adult T-cell leukemia. Blood. 2005;105(3):1204–13.
101. Takasaki Y, Iwanaga M, Imaizumi Y, Tawara M, Joh T, Kohno T, et al. Long-term study of indolent adult T-cell leukemia-lymphoma. Blood. 2010;115(22): 4337–43.
102. Shimoyama M, Ota K, Kikuchi M, et al. Chemotherapeutic results and prognostic factors of patients with advanced non-Hodgkins lymphoma treated with VEPA or VEPA-M. J Clin Oncol. 1988;6:128–41.
103. Shimoyama M, Ota K, Kikuchi M, et al. Major prognostic factors of adult patients with advanced T-cell lymphoma/leukemia. J Clin Oncol. 1988;6:1088–97.
104. Tobinai K, Shimoyama M, Minato K, et al. Japan Clinical Oncology Group phase II trial of

second-generation LSG4 protocol in aggressive T- and B-lymphoma: a new predictive model for T- and B-lymphoma (abstract). Proc Am Soc Clin Oncol. 1994;13:378a.
105. Tsukasaki K, Tobinai K, Shimoyama M, et al. Deoxycoformycin-containing combination chemotherapy for adult T-cell leukemia-lymphoma: Japan Clinical Oncology Group study (JCOG9109). Int J Hematol. 2003;77:164–70.
106. Yamada Y, Tomonaga M, Fukuda H, et al. A new G-CSF-supported combination chemotherapy, LSG15, for adult T-cell leukemia-lymphoma (ATL): Japan Clinical Oncology Group (JCOG) Study 9303. Br J Haematol. 2001;113:375–82.
107. Tsukasaki K, Utsunomiya A, Fukuda H, et al. VCAP-AMP-VECP compared with biweekly CHOP for adult T-cell leukemia-lymphoma: Japan Clinical Oncology Group Study JCOG9801. J Clin Oncol. 2007;25:5458–564.
108. Tobinai K, Shimoyama M, Inoue S, et al. Phase I study of YK-176 (2-deoxycoformycin) in patients with adult T-cell leukemia-lymphoma. Jpn J Clin Oncol. 1992;22:164–71.
109. Kuwazuru Y, Hanada S, Furukawa T, et al. Expression of p-glycoprotein in adult T-cell leukemia cells. Blood. 1990;76:2065–71.
110. Tsukasaki K, Ikeda S, Murata K, et al. Characteristics of chemotherapy-induced clinical remission in long survivors with aggressive adult T-cell leukemia/lymphoma. Leuk Res. 1993;17:157–66.
111. Ichimaru M, Kamihira S, Moriuchi Y, Kuraishi Y, Usui N, Toki H, et al. Clinical study on the effect of natural alpha-interferon (HLBI) in the treatment of adult T-cell leukemia. Gan To Kagaku Ryoho. 1988;15(10):2975–81. Japanese.
112. Gill PS, Harrington W, Kaplan MH, et al. Treatment of adult T-cell leukemia-lymphoma with a combination of interferon alfa and zidovudine. N Engl J Med. 1995;332:1744–8.
113. Hermine O, Blouscary D, Gessain A, et al. Treatment of adult T-cell leukemia-lymphoma with zidovudine and interferon alfa. N Engl J Med. 1995;332: 1749–51.
114. Tobinai K, Kobayashi Y, Shimoyama M, et al. Interferon alfa and zidovudine in adult T-cell leukemia-lymphoma (correspondence). N Engl J Med. 1995;333:1285–6.
115. White JD, Wharfe G, Stewart DM, et al. The combination of zidovudine and interferon alpha-2B in the treatment of adult T-cell leukemia/lymphoma. Leuk Lymphoma. 2001;40:287–94.
116. Matutes E, Taylor GP, Cavenagh J, et al. Interferon alpha and zidovudine therapy in adult T-cell leukaemia lymphoma: response and outcome in 15 patients. Br J Haematol. 2001;113:779–84.
117. Hermine O, Allard I, Levy V, et al. A prospective phase II clinical trial with the use of zidovudine and interferon-alpha in the acute and lymphoma forms of adult T-cell leukemia/lymphoma. Hematol J. 2002; 3:276–82.
118. Bazarbachi A, Plumelle Y, Ramos JC, Tortevoye P, Otrock Z, Taylor G, et al. Meta-analysis on the use of zidovudine and interferon-alfa in adult T-cell leukemia/lymphoma showing improved survival in the leukemic subtypes. J Clin Oncol. 2010;28(27): 4177–83.
119. Kchour G, Tarhini M, Kooshyar M-M, et al. Phase 2 study of the efficacy and safety of the combination of arsenic trioxide, interferon alpha, and zidovudine in newly diagnosed chronic adult T-cell leukemia/lymphoma (ATL). Blood. 2009;113:6528–32.
120. Hishizawa M, Kanda J, Utsunomiya A, Taniguchi S, Eto T, Moriuchi Y, et al. Transplantation of allogeneic hematopoietic stem cells for adult T-cell leukemia: a nationwide retrospective study. Blood. 2010 [Epub ahead of print].
121. Okamura J, Utsunomiya A, Tanosaki R, et al. Allogeneic stem-cell transplantation with reduced conditioning intensity as a novel immunotherapy and antiviral therapy for adult T-cell leukemia/lymphoma. Blood. 2005;105:4143–5.
122. Tanosaki R, Uike N, Utsunomiya A, Saburi Y, Masuda M, Tomonaga M, et al. Allogeneic hematopoietic stem cell transplantation using reduced-intensity conditioning for adult T cell leukemia/lymphoma: impact of antithymocyte globulin on clinical outcome. Biol Blood Marrow Transplant. 2008;14(6):702–8.
123. Cheson BD, Horning SJ, Coiffier B, et al. Report of an international workshop to standardize response criteria for non-Hodgkin's lymphomas. NCI Sponsored International Working Group. J Clin Oncol. 1999;17:1244.
124. Cheson BD, Bennett JM, Grever M, et al. National Cancer Institute-sponsored Working Group guidelines for chronic lymphocytic leukemia: revised guidelines for diagnosis and treatment. Blood. 1996;87:4990–7.
125. Cheson BD, Pfistner B, Juweid ME, et al. The International Harmonization Project on Lymphoma. Revised response criteria for malignant lymphoma. J Clin Oncol. 2007;25:579–86.
126. Ohno R, Masaoka T, Shirakawa S, Sakamoto S, Hirano M, Hanada S, et al. Treatment of adult T-cell leukemia/lymphoma with MST-16, a new oral antitumor drug and a derivative of bis(2,6-dioxopiperazine). The MST-16 Study Group. Cancer. 1993;71(7):2217–21.
127. Tsuda H, Takatsuki K, Ohno R, et al. A late phase II trial of a potent topoisomerase inhibitor, CPT-11, in malignant lymphoma [abstract]. Proc Am Soc Clin Oncol. 1992;11:316.
128. Arima N, Mizoguchi H, Shirakawa S, Tomonaga M, Takatsuki K, Ohno R. Phase I clinical study of SH L573 (fludarabine phosphate) in patients with chronic lymphocytic leukemia and adult T-cell leukemia/lymphoma. Gan To Kagaku Ryoho. 1999;26(5):619–29 [Article in Japanese].
129. Tobinai K, Uike N, Saburi Y, Chou T, Etoh T, Masuda M, et al. Cladribine/ATL Study Group, Japan. Phase

II study of cladribine (2-chlorodeoxyadenosine) in relapsed or refractory adult T-cell leukemia-lymphoma. Int J Hematol. 2003;77(5):512–7.
130. Duvic M, Forero-Torres A, Foss F, et al: Long-term treatment of CTCL with the oral PNP inhibitor, forodesine. ASCO annual meeting, Jun 2009; No. 8552.
131. O'Connor OA, Heaney ML, Schwartz L, et al. Clinical experience with intravenous and oral formulations of the novel histone deacetylase inhibitor suberoylanilide hydroxamic acid in patients with advanced hematologic malignancies. J Clin Oncol. 2006;24(1):166–73.
132. Hasegawa H, Yamada Y, Tsukasaki K, et al. LBH589, a deacetylase inhibitor, induces apoptosis in adult T-cell leukemia/lymphoma cells via activation of a novel RAIDD-caspase-2 pathway. Leukemia. 2011;25(4):575–87.
133. Waldmann TA. Multichain interleukin-2 receptor: a target for immunotherapy in lymphoma. J Natl Cancer Inst. 1989;81:914–23.
134. Waldmann TA, White JD, Carrasquillo JA, et al. Radioimmunotherapy of interleukin-2Ra-expressing adult T-cell leukemia with yttrium-90-labeled anti-Tac. Blood. 1985;86:4063–75.
135. Berkowitz JL, Janik JE, Stewart DM, Fioravanti S, Jaffe ES, Fleisher TA, et al. Phase II trial of daclizumab in human T-cell lymphotropic virus type-1 (HTLV-1)-associated adult T-cell leukemia/lymphoma (ATL). J Clin Oncol. 2010;28:7s (suppl; abstr 8043).
136. Kreitman RJ, Wilson WH, White JD, Stetler-Stevenson M, Jaffe ES, Giardina S, et al. Phase I trial of recombinant immunotoxin anti-Tac(Fv)-PE38 (LMB-2) in patients with hematologic malignancies. J Clin Oncol. 2000;18(8):1622–36.
137. Dang NH, Pro B, Hagemeister FB, et al. Phase II trial of denileukin diftitox for relapsed/refractory T-cell non-Hodgkin lymphoma. Br J Haematol. 2007;136(3):439–47.
138. Foss FM, Sjak-Shie NN, Goy A, Advani R, Jacobsen ED. Phase II study of denileukin diftitox with CHOP chemotherapy in newly-diagnosed PTCL: CONCEPT trial. J Clin Oncol. 2010;28:15s (suppl; abstr 8045).
139. Di Venuti G, Nawgiri R, Foss F. Denileukin diftitox and hyper-CVAD in the treatment of human T-cell lymphotropic virus 1-associated acute T-cell leukemia/lymphoma. Clin Lymphoma. 2003;4(3):176–8.
140. Rodig SJ, Abramson JS, Pinkus GS, Treon SP, Dorfman DM, Dong HY, et al. Heterogeneous CD52 expression among hematologic neoplasms: implications for the use of alemtuzumab (CAMPATH-1H). Clin Cancer Res. 2006;12(23):7174–9.
141. Jiang L, Yuan CM, Hubacheck J, Janik JE, Wilson W, Morris JC, et al. Variable CD52 expression in mature T cell and NK cell malignancies: implications for alemtuzumab therapy. Br J Haematol. 2009;145(2):173–9.
142. Gallamini A, Zaja F, Patti C, Billio A, Specchia MR, Tucci A, Levis A, Manna A, Secondo V, Rigacci L, Pinto A, Iannitto E, Zoli V, Torchio P, Pileri S, Tarella C. Alemtuzumab (Campath-1H) and CHOP chemotherapy as first-line treatment of peripheral T-cell lymphoma: results of a GITIL (Gruppo Italiano Terapie Innovative nei Linfomi) prospective multicenter trial. Blood. 2007 Oct 1;110(7):2316–23. Clin Cancer Res. 2006 Dec 1;12(23):7174–9.
143. Zhang Z, Zhang M, Goldman CK, Ravetch JV, Waldmann TA. Effective therapy for a murine model of adult T-cell leukemia with the humanized anti-CD52 monoclonal antibody, Campath-1H. Cancer Res. 2003;63(19):6453–7.
144. Mone A, Puhalla S, Whitman S, Baiocchi RA, Cruz J, Vukosavljevic T, et al. Durable hematologic complete response and suppression of HTLV-1 viral load following alemtuzumab in zidovudine/IFN-[alpha]-refractory adult T-cell leukemia. Blood. 2005; 106(10):3380–2.
145. Ravandi F, Faderl S. Complete response in a patient with adult T-cell leukemia (ATL) treated with combination of alemtuzumab and pentostatin. Leuk Res. 2006;30(1):103–5.
146. O'Mahony D, Morris JC, Stetler-Stevenson M, Matthews H, Brown MR, Fleisher T, et al. EBV-related lymphoproliferative disease complicating therapy with the anti-CD2 monoclonal antibody, siplizumab, in patients with T-cell malignancies. Clin Cancer Res. 2009;15(7):2514–22.
147. Niwa R, Shoji-Hosaka E, Sakurada M, Shinkawa T, Uchida K, Nakamura K, Matsushima K, Ueda R, Hanai N, Shitara K.: Defucosylated chimeric anti-CC chemokine receptor 4 IgG1 with enhanced antibody-dependent cellular cytotoxicity shows potent therapeutic activity to T-cell leukemia and lymphoma. Cancer Res. 2004 Mar 15;64(6):2127–33. Cancer Res. 2004 Mar 15;64(6):2127–33.
148. Yamamoto K, Utsunomiya A, Tobinai K, et al. Phase I study of KW-0761, a defucosylated humanized anti-CCR4 antibody, in relapsed patients with adult T-cell leukemia-lymphoma and peripheral T-cell lymphoma. J Clin Oncol. 2010;28(9):1591–8.
149. Ishida T, Joh T, Uike N, et al. Defucosylated anti-CCR4 monoclonal antibody (KW-0761) for relapsed adult T-cell leukemia-lymphoma: a multicenter phase II study. J Clin Oncol. 2012 [Epub ahead of print].
150. O'Connor OA, Horwitz S, Hamlin P, et al. Phase II-I-II study of two different doses and schedules of pralatrexate, a high-affinity substrate for the reduced folate carrier, in patients with relapsed or refractory lymphoma reveals marked activity in T-cell malignancies. J Clin Oncol. 2009;27(26):4357–64.
151. O'Connor OA, Pro B, Pinter-Brown L, et al. PROPEL: a multi-center phase 2 open-label study of pralatrexate (PDX) with vitamin B12 and folic acid supplementation in patients with replapsed or refractory peripheral T-cell lymphoma. Blood (ASH Annual Meeting Abstracts). 2008;112:261.
152. Marneros AG, Grossman ME, Silvers DN, Husain S, Nuovo GJ, MacGregor-Cortelli B, et al.

Pralatrexate-induced tumor cell apoptosis in the epidermis of a patient with HTLV-1 adult T-cell lymphoma/leukemia causing skin erosions. Blood. 2009;113(25):6338–41.
153. Lee J, Suh C, Kang HJ, Ryoo BY, et al. Phase I study of proteasome inhibitor bortezomib plus CHOP in patients with advanced, aggressive T-cell or NK/T-cell lymphoma. Ann Oncol. 2008;19(12):2079–83.
154. Satou Y, Nosaka K, Koya Y, et al. Proteasome inhibitor, bortezomib, potently inhibits the growth of adult T-cell leukemia cells both in vivo and in vitro. Leukemia. 2004;18:1357–63.
155. Dueck GS, Chua N, Prasad A, et al. Activity of lenalidomide in a phase II trial for T-cell lymphoma: report on the first 24 cases. J Clin Oncol. 2009;27:15s (suppl; abstr 8524).
156. Vose J, Armitage J, Weisenburger D. International peripheral T-cell and natural killer/T-cell lymphoma study: pathology findings and clinical outcomes. J Clin Oncol. 2008;26(25):4124–30.

The T-Cell Leukaemias

9

Elisabeth Grey-Davies and Claire Dearden

Introduction

The mature T-cell leukaemias are a rare and heterogeneous group of disorders derived from the mature or post-thymic T-cell. They comprise T-cell prolymphocytic leukaemia (T-PLL), T-cell large granular lymphocytic leukaemia (T-LGL) and Adult T-cell lymphoma/leukaemia (ATLL) [1]. There are also neoplastic T-cells in the peripheral blood in cases of Sézary syndrome (SS), the generalised, more aggressive variant of the mature T-cell cutaneous lymphoma mycosis fungoides. ATLL and SS are covered elsewhere in this text and this chapter will therefore focus on T-PLL and T-LGL leukaemia.

The diagnosis of the T-cell leukaemias is based on a multiparameter approach which encompasses clinical presentation, peripheral blood count and morphology, immunohistochemistry, flow cytometry, cytogenetics and molecular genetics. Thus, the recent advances in modern immunophenotypic and molecular tools have been crucial in characterising these disorders and in distinguishing them from their B-cell counterparts. Prognosis and response to conventional chemotherapy are generally poor, with the exception of T-LGL which is a more indolent disorder than the others in its class. The rarity of these conditions, their refractoriness to standard therapies, underlying immune suppression, multi-factorial aetiologies and lack of single identifiable therapeutic targets in the majority of cases all contribute to a great management challenge. An important aspect therefore in advancing treatment of these and other T-cell disorders is adopting an international approach to diagnosis, documentation and trial design and entry in order to recruit sufficient patient and clinico-pathological data to inform robust choices.

E. Grey-Davies (✉)
Department of Haemato-Oncology, The Royal Marsden Hospital and Institute of Cancer Research, Downs Road, Sutton, Surrey SM2 5PT, UK
e-mail: egrey-davies@nhs.net

C. Dearden
Department of Haemato-Oncology, The Royal Marsden Hospital and Institute of Cancer Research, London, UK

T-Cell Prolymphocytic Leukaemia

Introduction

Prolymphocytic leukaemias (PLL) of B- and T-cell subtype are rare diseases which together account for around 2% of all mature lymphoid leukaemias. When first described in 1974 [2], the different cells of origin were not appreciated and the disease was described as a variant of chronic lymphocytic leukaemia (CLL). T-PLL was first documented in a patient presenting with clinical features similar to B-PLL, but in whom the cells had a T-cell phenotype [3]. The recent availability of modern immunophenotypic and molecular tools has allowed a better distinction of this disorder from its B-cell counterpart and other mature

F. Foss (ed.), *T-Cell Lymphomas*, Contemporary Hematology,
DOI 10.1007/978-1-62703-170-7_9,

Table 9.1 Key characteristics of T-cell prolymphocytic leukaemia

	Characteristic Findings
Clinical features	Older adults
	M:F 1.2:1
	Splenomegaly, lymphadenopathy, skin rash, oedema and serous effusions
	Lymphocytosis often exceeding 100×10^9/l
Morphology	Prolymphocytes with prominent nucleoli, basophilic cytoplasm with blebs
	Small cell (20%) and Sézary variants (5%)
Immunophenotyping	CD2, CD3, CD5, CD7+, CD52+
	CD4/8 variable
	CD1a-ve, TdT-ve, CD25−/+
Cytogenetics	Inversion 14; t(14,14); t(X,14); iso8q; complex
Oncogenes	*TCL-1, MTCP-1, ATM*
Prognosis	Median survival <1 year with conventional chemotherapy
Treatment	Alemtuzumab alone or in combination with purine analogues
	Consolidation with HSCT

T-cell leukaemias. T-PLL is recognised in the WHO classification [1] as having three morphological variants—typical, small cell and cerebriform—all of which have a similar clinical course and identical molecular genetics. Recent studies have highlighted the role of specific oncogenes such as *TCL-1, MTCP-1* and *ATM*. However, despite better understanding of the underlying cell biology, prognosis for these patients remains poor with no curative therapy and short survival. The advent of monoclonal antibody therapy and the wider application of non-myeloablative allogeneic transplantation have improved the treatment options for this group of patients. Table 9.1 summarises the characteristic features of T-PLL.

Pathogenesis

T-PLL is a rare proliferation of mature or post-thymic lymphocytes. It has been described in the East and West without geographical or racial clustering and there are no reports of familial cases. There is no evidence that radiation or carcinogenic agents play a role in the pathogenesis of T-PLL and neither had it been thought that viruses such as HTLV1 are involved. However, a recent study found that the EBV genome was present in T-PLL cells by using polymerase chain reaction (PCR) analysis across multiple sites in the viral genome [4]. In addition, these T-PLL cells expressed a number of EBV latent antigens suggesting a potential link between T-PLL and EBV infection.

T-cell maturation is strictly controlled by the thymic cellular microenvironment and depends on complex interactions between various cytokines and growth factors [5]. T-cells rely on the T-cell receptor (TCR)-CD3 complex to present a specific antibody to bind to a foreign antigen, as opposed to B cells, which depend on immunoglobulin rearrangements. Mutations in the TCR subunits result in T-cell lymphoproliferative diseases derived from post-thymic immunocompetent lymphoid cells. In adults T-PLL arises sporadically. There is a close relationship between this sporadic form of T-PLL and the leukaemia that occurs in patients with the hereditary debilitating neurological disease ataxia telangiectasia (AT) [6]. Patients with AT have bi-allelic inactivation of the AT mutated gene (*ATM*) located at the 11q23 locus [7]. Approximately 10% of AT homozygotes develop cancer, mostly of the lymphoid system and in particular of the T-cell type [8]. Some of these patients develop abnormal clonal proliferation of T-cells with morphological, immunological, cytogenetic and molecular features (e.g. over-expression of the *TCL-1* oncogene) identical to T-PLL. Genetic abnormalities (mutations and deletions) of *ATM* are well documented in T-PLL [9–12]. *ATM* is therefore a candidate gene likely to be involved in the pathogenesis of both sporadic and AT-associated T-PLL, possibly through its role as a tumour suppressor.

Clinical Presentation

T-PLL is a disease affecting older adults with a male predominance. In the Royal Marsden Hospital series of 150 patients, the median age at presentation was 63 years (range 33–91 years) and the male: female ratio 3:1 [13]. Patients are characteristically symptomatic at presentation with a peripheral blood lymphocytosis often exceeding 100×10^9/l [14], generalised lymphadenopathy and splenomegaly. Dermal lymphoid infiltrates are present in a third of patients and peri-orbital oedema can be a feature. Serous effusions, particularly pleural effusions, are seen in 15% of patients at diagnosis but are common in relapsed or refractory disease. Anaemia and thrombocytopenia are less common at presentation than in B-PLL [15], occurring in 25% and 45% of patients, respectively. Central nervous system involvement is rare. Human T-lymphotrophic viruses I and II (HTLV-I/II) are invariably negative by both serology and PCR. A small proportion of patients have a more indolent or "smouldering" form of T-PLL which may mimic stage A CLL. Although these patients are generally asymptomatic at presentation and may exhibit a long latent phase, they will inevitably progress after a median period of 33 months [16] to follow the more aggressive course typical for T-PLL.

Morphology and Histopathology

T-PLL has a broad morphological spectrum [17]. In half of cases the cells have a round to oval nucleus, while in the remainder the nuclei are irregular, often with convolutions. The degree of nuclear irregularity, however, is less pronounced than that seen in Sézary Syndrome (SS) or ATLL cells. There are three subtypes: typical T-PLL, a small cell variant and a cerebriform variant accounting for 75%, 20% and 5%, respectively. All three share the same immunophenotypic and cytogenetic features and are thus classified as a single disorder [1]. Typical cases have a peripheral blood lymphocytosis with pro-lymphocytes of medium size with condensed nuclear chromatin, a single prominent nucleolus, intensely basophilic agranular cytoplasm and cytoplasmic protrusions or "blebs" in most cases (Fig. 9.1). In the small cell variant the pro-lymphocytes are considerably smaller and the nucleolus is less prominent and can often only be visualised under electron microscopy. In the rarest variant the pro-lymphocytes have a cerebriform nucleus resembling Sézary cells.

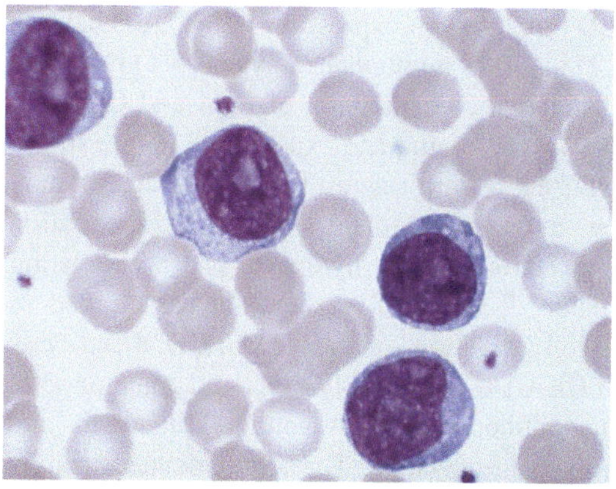

Fig. 9.1 Typical peripheral blood morphology in T-PLL showing small to medium sized lymphoid cells with a single nucleolus, basophilic cytoplasm and cytoplasmic protrusions

Although tissue histology is not essential for diagnosis, the bone marrow, lymph nodes and skin may be infiltrated. Diffuse and interstitial infiltration of the bone marrow is seen in the majority of cases and reticulin fibrosis is almost always present. Lymph nodes show paracortical expansion by T-prolymphocytes. The skin histology differs from that seen in mycosis fungoides (MF) and SS, showing dermal infiltration, preferentially around the appendages and without epidermotropism. Spleen histology shows a marked red pulp infiltration extending into the white pulp and capsule in contrast to T-cell large granular lymphocytic leukaemia which is confined to the red pulp.

Immunophenotype

T-PLL cells exhibit a mature, post-thymic phenotype and are, by definition, negative for terminal deoxynucleotidyl transferase (TdT) and the cortical thymic marker CD1a. They express the pan-T cell markers CD2, CD5 and CD7 [13]. CD7 is usually expressed with strong intensity in contrast to other mature T-cell malignancies where this marker may be weak or negative. CD3 and anti-TCR-α/β may be negative in the cell membrane but are always expressed in the cytoplasm, and the TCR-β and/or γ chain genes are rearranged in all cases. The majority (60%) have the CD4+/CD8– phenotype, but alternatively may have

CD4+/CD8+ co-expression (25%) or have a CD4–/CD8+ immunophenotype (15%) [14]. The distinctive co-expression of CD4 and CD8, the weak CD3 membrane expression and the strong CD7 expression suggest that the T-PLL cell may be at an intermediate stage of differentiation between a cortical thymocyte and a circulating mature T-cell. Cell surface antigens linked to T-cell activation such as CD25, CD38 and class II HLA-DR are variably expressed and monoclonal antibodies against natural killer cells and TIA-1 are negative. T-prolymphocytes strongly express the CD52 antigen at a high density [18], which can be targeted by the monoclonal antibody alemtuzumab. In most cases T-PLL patients express the TCR-αβ phenotype, although rare instances of TCR-γδ have been reported [19].

Molecular Features

In keeping with the aggressive clinical course of TPLL, patients usually have complex karyotypes and cytogenetic abnormalities which may occur progressively throughout the disease. The genetic hallmark of T-PLL is the inversion [inv(14)(q11;q32)] or its variant the tandem translocation [t(14;14)(q11;q32)] [20, 21]. These rearrangements of chromosome 14 are present in up to 80% of cases [22] and bring together the proto-oncogene *TCL-1* (T-cell leukaemia 1) located at 14q32.1 with the TCR α gene, located at 14q11. This results in deregulation of *TCL-1*, a gene physiologically expressed on CD4/CD8 double-negative thymocytes [23, 24]. In about 20% of patients the translocation [t(X;14)(q28;q11)] (Fig. 9.2) is reported, which results in the juxtaposition of the *MTCP-1* gene (a member of the *TCL-1* gene family) located at Xq28 with the TCR-α gene [25, 26]. Therefore, chromosomal rearrangements in T-PLL juxtapose *TCL-1* and *MTCP-1* to the TCR loci and lead to their activation. Genomic analyses of the 14q32.1 breakpoint region have revealed three additional genes; *TCL-1b, TNG1* (*TCL-1* neighbouring gene 1) and *TNG2*, which are also expressed on T-PLL cell lines and cells from patients with T-PLL but not on normal T-lymphocytes [27–29]. Activation of *TCL-1* through hypomethylation of its promoter has also been described [30]. The *TCL-1* oncoprotein is expressed in approximately 70% of T-PLL cases [31] and has been shown to associate with protein kinase B (Akt) resulting in the promotion of Akt-induced cell proliferation and survival [32].

In addition to the inversion rearrangement, which is regarded as the primary oncogenic event in T-PLL, the tumour cells usually harbour a high load of additional chromosomal aberrations. Abnormalities involving both arms of chromosome eight are frequent and over-expression of the c-myc protein is found in cases with iso8q. While the 14q abnormalities and trisomy 8q are common in western countries, they are rarely seen in Japan [33]. Although 11q23 abnormalities are seldom detected on cytogenetics, molecular analysis frequently detects mutations of the tumour suppressor gene *ATM*. Studies have demonstrated that T-PLL is associated with recurrent regions of chromosomal loss at 22q11, 13q, 6q, 9p, 12p, 11p11-p14 and 17p, as well as chromosomal gain at 8q, 14q32, 22q21 and 6p [22]. Recent single nucleotide polymorphism-based genomic mapping and global gene expression profiling has identified differential expression of a number of genes in T-PLL compared to normal CD3+T-cells [34]. These include functionally important genes involved in lymphomagenesis, cell cycle regulation, apoptosis and DNA repair, which are clustered in regions affected by known recurrent chromosomal aberrations in T-PLL. The upregulated genes were clustered on chromosome arms 6p and 8q, and the downregulated genes on 6q, 8p, 10p, 11q and 18p. This information suggests that a gene dosage effect may be involved in the pathogenesis of T-PLL and may also help to clarify the mechanisms involved in disease progression.

Differential Diagnosis

The morphology of prolymphocytes in the peripheral blood and cell markers are the vital requirements in order to make the diagnosis of T-PLL and distinguish it from other mature lymphoid leukaemias. T-PLL can be distinguished from B-PLL by immunological markers. Furthermore, skin infiltration and

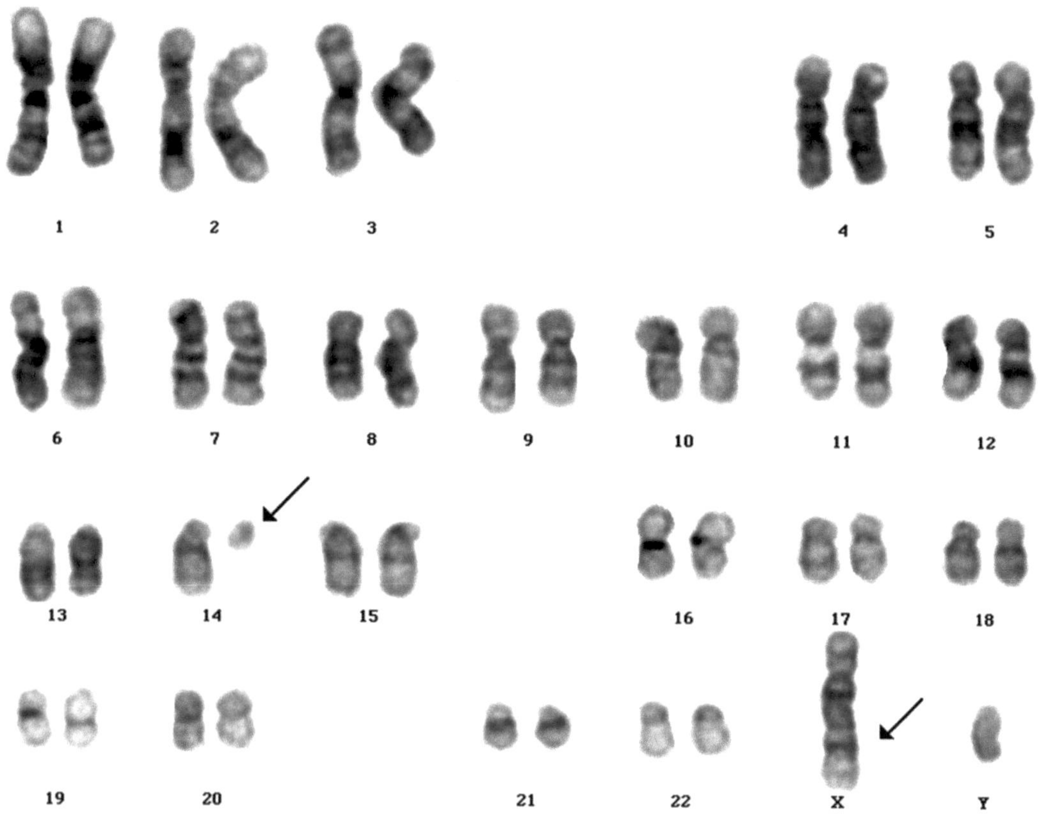

Fig. 9.2 Karyotype in T-PLL showing a t(X;14) translocation

lymphadenopathy are unusual in B-PLL, while they are present in a substantial proportion of T-PLL patients. Morphology, histology and immunological markers help to differentiate T-PLL from other mature T-cell malignancies such as T-LGL, ATLL and SS. The predominant population in T-cell LGL leukaemia is a granular lymphocyte, often with a CD8+ CD57+, CD16± phenotype, with or without expression of natural killer (NK) cell markers. The distinct geographical background, the clinical features (e.g. hypercalcemia) and positive HTLV-I serology distinguish ATLL from T-PLL. SS has distinct clinical features, skin histology and cell morphology.

Prognostic Factors

The prognosis for patients with T-PLL is poor. Data regarding specific disease variables which influence an individual's disease course and response to treatment are limited. A recent series of 84 cases reported a median overall survival of 24.7 months and a 5-year survival rate of 21% [35]. There was a highly significant correlation between poor outcome and high WBC count at presentation ($>40 \times 10^9$/l), shorter lymphocyte doubling time as well as with older age (>62 years) at presentation. Higher TCL-1 expression correlated with a higher WBC count at presentation, a rapid lymphocyte doubling time and a shorter overall survival [35]. The presence of hepatomegaly and serous effusions predict for a poor response to alemtuzumab [36]. Patients who do not respond to treatment have a median survival of only 4 months.

Treatment

T-PLL is an aggressive disease, which is often resistant to therapy. Overall prognosis is poor with a median overall survival historically of

Table 9.2 Summary of clinical trials in T-PLL

Study	Regimen	No	CR (%)	PR (%)	ORR (%)	MPFS months	MS months
Previously treated patients							
Mercieca [38]	Pentostatin[a]	55	9	36	45	6	9
Dearden [36]	Alemtuzumab	39	60	16	76	7	10
Keating [42]	Alemtuzumab[a,b]	76	38	12	50	4.5	7.5
Therapy-naive patients							
Dearden [43]	Alemtuzumab	11	100	0	100	10+	13+
Hopfinger [44]	FMC+Alemtuzumab	18	NA	NA	66 (FMC) 86 (after alemtuzumab)	10	19

[a]Retrospective analysis
[a]Compassionate-use trial
CR, Complete remission; *PR*, Partial remission; *ORR*, Overall response rate; *MPFS*, Median progression-free survival; *MS*, Median overall survival; *NA*, Not available

approximately 7 months in patients receiving conventional chemotherapy such as the alkylating agents [14]. However, survival has improved following the introduction of relatively new agents including the purine analogues and the anti-CD52 antibody (alemtuzumab; campath-1H). Pentostatin has been shown to be effective, particularly in patients who are CD25+, CD38+ and CD103+ [37]. A study of 55 patients performed in 1994 reported an overall response rate of 45% with 9% complete remissions and median response duration of 6 months [38]. This also resulted in an improvement in overall survival. Unlike standard approaches to the use of pentostatin in hairy cell leukaemia, initial doses of 4 mg/m^2 were given weekly for 4 weeks then every 2 weeks to maximum response. Interestingly, no significant difference in response rate was observed between previously treated and untreated patients rendering this agent a versatile option in treatment of T-PLL. Equally positive results have been reported with cladrabine, although study numbers are smaller [39, 40].

More recently, the anti-CD52 monoclonal antibody, alemtuzumab, has been utilised to target the CD52 antigen which is expressed at high density on the surface of T-prolymphocytes. An early study in 1997 of 14 patients reported an excellent response rate of 73% [41]. More recently, a European study of 39 patients with relapsed/refractory T-PLL, who received alemtuzumab intravenously three times a week after initial dose escalation, reported remarkable overall response rates of 76% with complete response rates of 60% [36]. Nine of the 39 patients were refractory to pentostatin. The median overall survival was 10 months and depth of response was positively associated with prolongation of survival; median overall survival was 16 months in those patients who achieved complete responses. Responses were poor in patients who had serous effusions, hepatic or CNS involvement. In the United States a retrospective analysis of 76 patients with T-PLL treated on a compassionate use with standard alemtuzumab therapy reported OR rates of 50% with 37.5% CR [42]. These patients, who had received one or more lines of treatment and had progressive and/or refractory disease, had a superior quality and duration of response to alemtuzumab compared to prior therapy. Alemtuzumab has subsequently been investigated in treatment naïve patients. In a preliminary study of 11 patients, all achieved a CR with 7 of 11 patients still alive at median follow up of 12 months (range 4–17 months) [43].

The successful use of chemo-immunotherapy in B cell malignancies has prompted similar studies in T-PLL. The German CLL study group has reported results of a prospective phase II trial of fludarabine, mitoxantrone and cyclophosphamide (FMC) followed by alemtuzumab consolidation in 18 patients [44]. The ORR was 66% following FMC, increasing to 86% after alemtuzumab, with a median progression-free survival of 10.6 months and OS of 19.2 months. Table 9.2 summarises the results of clinical trials in T-PLL.

Weidmann et al. have used a regimen consisting of fludarabine (days 1–4), cyclophosphamide (day 3), doxorubicin (day 4) together with alemtuzumab in escalating doses (days 1–4) to treat 23 patients with a range of peripheral T-cell malignancies [45]. Overall response rate in this series was 61% with a CR rate of 78% in the newly diagnosed patients. However, this cohort only included a single case of T-PLL. Anecdotal experience with the combination of alemtuzumab and pentostatin suggest that this combination may be more active than these agents used singly.

The introduction of alemtuzumab has significantly improved the outcome in T-PLL and it should be considered the treatment of choice. However, its use is not without risk. It causes prolonged T-cell depletion with significant immunosuppression and infective complications reported in approximately 13% of patients [42]. Prophylaxis for pneumocytsis and herpetic infections is required both during treatment and for a protracted period beyond completion and screening for cytomegalovirus (CMV) reactivation is advocated. Use of alemtuzumab in heavily pre-treated, often elderly patients is associated with increased risk of infectious and other treatment-related complications, although it can be well tolerated in elderly patients because of lack of organ toxicity. Tolerability is improved when alemtuzumab is used as first line therapy. Responses to alemtuzumab are still transient and further disease progression is inevitable. Furthermore, patients may down-regulate expression of CD52 at relapse making treatment with alemtuzumab ineffective. Hence, all patients who achieve a response to therapy should be considered for consolidation with a haematopoietic stem cell transplant (HSCT) to prolong disease-free and overall survival.

In a recent study 22 patients with T-PLL received a HSCT in first complete response, in second complete response or with a good partial response (PR) following alemtuzumab therapy. Thirteen were consolidated with an autologous HSCT and nine with an allogeneic HSCT (five sibling and four unrelated donor) [46]. In the patients who were autografted, 38% remain alive with median disease-free survival of 20 months (range 8–78 months). Of the nine patients who had an allograft, four had full intensity conditioning and five reduced intensity conditioning. Fifty-six percent remain alive, one patient in continued CR 7 years post-SCT. Two patients died from transplant-related mortality (TRM) and both had received full intensity conditioning. Two patients relapsed. These results demonstrate that autologous HSCT can increase disease-free survival, but two thirds of patients still relapse. While allogeneic HSCT is an attractive option, TRM with full intensity conditioning is high. There are other case reports of successful outcome with reduced intensity conditioning [47, 48], and this is a strategy which merits further study.

Treatment regimens in the future are likely to be based on intravenous alemtuzumab with the addition of purine analogues such as pentostatin, gemcitabine or nelarabine. The role of new agents like bortezomib and pralatrexate will also need to be explored. Better understanding of the molecular pathogenesis may also lead to the introduction of new therapeutic approaches targeting specific pathways such as Akt activation, ATM mutations (PARP inhibitors) and telomerase, all of which may be active in T-PLL.

T-Cell Large Granular Lymphocyte Leukaemia

Introduction

The term T-LGL was coined by Loughran in 1993 [49] to describe this clonal proliferation of mature, post-thymic T-cells. LGLs make up 10–15% of the total peripheral blood mononuclear cell count in normal adults [50]. The majority of these cells are of the CD3-natural killer (NK) lineage, with the minority of the CD3+ T-cell lineage (15%). T-cell LGLs are post-thymic, antigen-primed cytotoxic CD8+ T lymphocytes and NK-cell LGLs belong to the innate immune system with the capability of non-major histocompatibility complex (MHC)–restricted cytotoxicity [51]. LGL proliferations are clonally derived from either CD3–/CD56+ or CD3/CD8+ LGLs and are designated natural killer LGL leukaemia or T-cell LGL leukaemia, respectively. The WHO classifies NK-LGL leukaemia within the spectrum of NK cell disorders, which are covered elsewhere in the text. This chapter will therefore focus on T-LGL leukaemia, which makes up approximately 85% of cases of LGL leukaemias.

In contrast to the other T-cell disorders, T-LGL leukaemia is generally an indolent condition with a median survival in excess of 10 years. The aetiology is not fully understood, but there is a strong association with autoimmune disorders, suggesting a common immunogenetic pathogenesis. The most common presenting features are cytopenias, characteristically neutropenia which may manifest as increased susceptibility to and severity of infection. There is no genetic hallmark of T-cell LGL and diagnosis relies on morphology, characteristic cell surface markers and demonstration of clonality. Treatment modalities are predominantly immunosuppressive in nature and are only indicated for symptomatic patients. Table 9.3 summarises the key features of T-LGL leukaemia.

Table 9.3 Key characteristics of T-cell large granular lymphocyte leukaemia

	Characteristic findings
Clinical features	Median age 55–60 years M=F 60% symptomatic LGLs in peripheral blood 2–20 × 10^9 Cytopenias, characteristically neutropenia. Recurrent infection. Strong association with autoimmune disorders (e.g. rheumatoid arthritis)
Morphology	LGLs with abundant cytoplasm Fine or coarse azurophilic granules
Immunophenotyping	CD3+, TCR-αβ, CD8+, CD57+,CD16+
Cytogenetics	Clonal rearrangement of TCR-β chain gene No characteristic cytogenetic abnormality
Oncogenes	Abnormalities of Fas/Fas-ligand pathway, dysregulated apoptosis
Prognosis	Generally an indolent disorder Median survival >10 years
Treatment	Only if symptomatic Immunosuppression—methotrexate, cyclophosphamide, cyclosporine A

Pathogenesis

The aetiology of T-LGL leukaemia is not clear. There is a strong association with autoimmune disorders suggesting a common immunogenetic pathogenesis. A polyclonal immune response with chronic activation of T-cells by an autoreactive or viral antigen is believed to be the initial stimulus to expansion of LGLs [52–54]. It is not clear whether a second molecular event is necessary to establish the neoplastic phenotype. There has been much debate in the literature as to whether T-LGL leukaemia represents a neoplastic or reactive condition; however, the demonstration of clonality supports a neoplastic proliferation. It has been suggested, however, that T-cell LGL leukaemia could represent an autoimmune disorder caused by chronic antigenic stimulation leading to extreme expansion of only one clone of CD8+ cytotoxic T-cells [54, 55]. There have been several reports of detection of HTLV-1 antibodies in cases of T-LGL leukaemia [56, 57], but in contrast to ATLL, these represent just a few cases and there is no universal association. Recent studies have demonstrated involvement of hCMV in the ontogeny of CD4+ T-LGL leukaemia, and it has been suggested that it could be the antigenic stimulus responsible for the initiation and maintenance of the disease [58]. There is no evidence that any other virus is involved in the pathogenesis of T-LGL leukaemia. Rare cases of T-LGL have been reported as a form of lymphoproliferative disorder after autologous or allogeneic transplant [59, 60], which must be distinguished from the oligoclonal T-cell populations frequently present in transplant patients at the point of lymphocyte reconstitution [61]. Clonal T-LGL populations have also been reported in association with low grade B-cell dyscrasias such as hairy cell leukaemia, CLL and monoclonal gammopathy of unknown significance [62–64]. These do not usually progress to clinically significant disease and appear to represent a type of host response. The co-association of B-cell pathology with T-LGL leukaemia suggests that either a common antigen drives clonal B- and T-cells, or that humoral malignancy could serve as the stimulus for lymphocyte expansion representing an overactive anti-tumour surveillance [64].

Dysregulation of several intracellular signalling pathways may account for the inherent resistance to apoptosis of LGL cells in vitro [65] including Fas/Fas ligand [66, 67], phosphatidylicnositol-3-kinase [68] and mitogen-activated protein kinase/extracellular signal-regulated kinase/Ras [69]. The degree of cytopenias (most commonly neutropenia) is usually out of proportion to the level of bone marrow infiltration, supporting an immune component to the pathogenesis. Possible mechanisms for neutropenia include deregulated Fas/Fas ligand induced apoptosis of myeloid cells, immune complex or antibody mediated neutrophil destruction, hypersplenism or direct inhibition of myeloid maturation [51, 70, 71].

Clinical Features

In contrast to the other T-cell leukaemias, T-cell large granulocyte leukaemia is a relatively indolent condition, with a median survival in excess of 10 years [51]. It is a rare disorder, accounting for 2–3% of cases of small lymphocytic leukaemia [1]. The median age at diagnosis is 55–60 years, but cases are reported in all age groups [72, 73] and there is no reported gender predilection or geographical distribution. The total lymphocyte count is normal or slightly raised, usually under 15×10^9/l, and the majority are LGLs. Traditionally, an increase in peripheral blood LGLs to greater than 2×10^9/l for more than 6 months was required to make the diagnosis of LGL leukaemia. However, these criteria are not strictly necessary if T-cell clonality can be demonstrated. Sixty percent of patients are symptomatic at presentation [74] and the most common presenting feature is neutropenia, which is manifest in the form of increased frequency and severity of infection and oral ulceration. Opportunistic infections are uncommon. At diagnosis 85% of patients are neutropenic of whom 50% are within the severe range ($<0.5 \times 10^9$/l) [73]. Anaemia and thrombocytopenia are present in 50% and 20%, respectively [73]. Severe anaemia due to red cell hypoplasia has been reported in the context of T-LGL [75]. B symptoms are present in 20–40% of patients [51]. Lymphadenopathy is very rare but mild-to-moderate splenomegaly and hepatomegaly are found in 20–50% and 10–20% of patients, respectively [51].

There is a strong association with autoimmune disorders, most commonly rheumatoid arthritis, which co-exists in up to 30% of patients with T-LGL leukaemia [70]. Systemic lupus erythematosus, Hashimoto's thyroiditis, immune-mediated cytopenias and pulmonary artery hypertension have also been described in patients with T-LGL leukaemia [49, 76, 77]. A polyclonal autoimmune response may represent the initiating element and explain this association and hypergammaglobulinaemia is common. Based on the tissue infiltration in the bone marrow and spleen as well as demonstration of clonality and the occasional finding of non-recurring cytogenetic abnormalities, T-LGL leukaemia has been classified as a leukaemia rather than a reactive condition [78].

Morphology and Histopathology

There is a peripheral blood lymphocytosis due to an increased number of LGLs beyond the 10–15% of total peripheral blood mononuclear cells that LGLs account for in normal adults. Neoplastic cells are similar to normal LGLs; medium to large cells with eccentrically placed nuclei, moderately condensed chromatin and abundant, weakly basophilic cytoplasm with coarse azurophilic granules [1] (Fig. 9.3). The granules often exhibit a characteristic ultrastructural appearance described as parallel tubular arrays and contain a number of proteins such as perforin and granzyme B that play a role in the cytotoxic function of these lymphocytes [79]. Macrocytosis can sometimes be a feature but smear cells are rare.

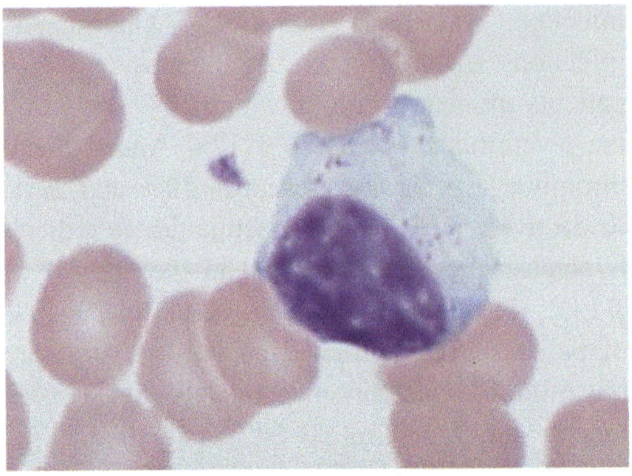

Fig. 9.3 Typical peripheral blood morphology in T-LGL Leukaemia showing large lymphoid cells with eccentric nucleus and abundant pale cytoplasm containing coarse azurophilic granules

Tissue histology is rarely essential for diagnosis. The bone marrow shows a variable, often low level, infiltrate by cells of similar morphology to those in the peripheral blood. The degree of cytopenias (most commonly neutropenia) is usually out of proportion to the level of bone marrow infiltration, supporting an immune component to the pathogenesis. In patients with severe neutropenia, there is often a picture of maturation block at the myelocyte stage, with mature granulocytic cells poorly represented. It is usual for there to be a normal number of megakaryocytes even in cases with significant thrombocytopenia. Cases with marked anaemia often show either a lack of maturing erythroblasts or megaloblastic erythropoiesis. Histologically, the pattern of infiltration may be interstitial, random focal, diffuse or nodular [80]. Nodules with non-clonal B-cell centres surrounded by CD4+ cells, with interstitial CD8+ cells, are a characteristic finding in T-LGL [81]. Care must be taken to examine the cell morphology to distinguish T-LGL from the low-grade B-cell lymphoproliferative disorders. The infiltrates are composed of small to medium lymphocytes, the nuclei of which have irregular contours, condensed nuclear chromatin and inconspicuous nucleoli [80]. The granules are not visible on the thin rim of cytoplasm. An association with trilineage dysplasia has been noted in a significant minority of patients [82]. Diffuse infiltration of red splenic pulp with preservation of sinuses and white pulp cords is characteristic of T-cell LGL leukaemia.

Immunophenotype

Neoplastic proliferations of LGLs are classified as T-cell or NK-cell according to their expression of T-cell markers such as CD3. T-LGL leukaemias have a mature T-cell phenotype and usually express surface CD3, CD8, CD16 and CD57, whereas NK-LGL leukaemias express CD2 and cytoplasmic but not surface CD3 and are variably positive for CD16, CD56 and CD57 [83]. CD57 is a 110-kDa glycoprotein found on NK cells and activated, effector CD8+ T-cells and is a characteristic marker for LGL leukaemia [51]. TIA-1 is also usually expressed. T-cell activation markers such as HLA-DR determinants and CD38 are expressed in a variable number of cases. Most cases of T-LGL leukaemia involve CD8+ cytotoxic T-cells; however, rarer incidences of CD4+ CD8–, CD4+ CD8+ and even CD4– CD8– disease are reported [50, 84]. Abnormally diminished or lost expression of CD5 and/or CD7 is common [85, 86]. The most common immunophenotype is therefore CD3+, TCR-$\alpha\beta$, CD8+, CD57+ and CD16+. Expression of the CD94/NKG2 and KIR families of NK-associated MHC-class I receptors can be detected in 50% or more of cases of T-LGL leukaemias [1]. All KIR positive cases expressed a single KIR isoform [86] and this finding can serve as a surrogate marker of clonality.

Molecular Features

The diagnosis of T-LGL leukaemia requires demonstration of clonality of the expanded LGL population by TCR gene rearrangement studies to distinguish the neoplastic proliferation from a reactive lymphocytosis [87]. This can be achieved using southern blot and/or PCR studies using primers specific to the variable regions of the TCR-β or -γ chain genes or by flow cytometry using monoclonal antibodies against the variable regions of the TCR-β or -γ chain. The majority of cases have TCR-β chain gene rearrangement. Only in a minority the TCR-β is in germline configuration and there is rearrangement of the TCR-γ chain gene [88]. There is no characteristic chromosomal abnormality detected in patients with T-LGL leukaemia and the majority will have normal cytogenetics. In those patients (<10%) with chromosomal abnormalities, inversion of 12p and 14q, deletion of 5q and trisomy 3, 8 and 14 have been reported [89–91]. T-LGL leukaemia cells constitutively express Fas (CD95) and Fas-ligand, which is found at high levels in the patient's sera [92]. Activated cytotoxic T-cells are usually eliminated by Fas-mediated apoptosis. However, a defective CD95 apoptotic pathway confers resistance to the leukaemia cells [74]. The serum level of Fas-ligand has been shown to be a marker of disease activity and to fall on successful treatment [93].

Differential Diagnosis

The diagnosis is made by a combination of morphological examination and the demonstration of T-cell clonality in the context of a characteristic immunophenotype: CD3, CD8, CD16 and CD57 positivity. Morphology and membrane markers distinguish T-LGL leukaemia from other B- and T-cell disorders. Cases morphologically resembling T-LGL leukaemia but with an NK immunophenotype are classified with the NK disorders. There is no agreement on the level of lymphocytosis required for the diagnosis of T-LGL [84], but a reactive lymphocytosis often has a value of $<5\times10^9$ and T-LGL leukaemia $>5\times10^9$. However, values of LGLs greater than 2×10^9 are consistent with this diagnosis [1]. Traditionally, the LGL lymphocytosis should be present for at least 6 months in order to make the diagnosis, but this criterion takes on a lesser importance with the advent of TCR rearrangement studies and the ability to demonstrate clonality. Reactive causes of LGL lymphocytosis such as following splenectomy or viral infection can be distinguished by the germline configuration of the TCR chain genes.

Prognostic Factors

The uniformity of clinical, morphological and laboratory features contrasts with phenotypic, functional and genotypic heterogeneity and hence clinical course for an individual is difficult to predict. The overall prognosis is good with a median survival in excess of 10 years [51]. The clinical course of T-LGL leukaemia is often stable or slowly progressive and the cause of death is most frequently infection and rarely progressive disease. Spontaneous remissions have been reported [94]. Transformation of T-LGL to high-grade large T-cell lymphomas has been reported in a minority of cases [95]. Rare cases of an aggressive CD56+ variant of T-LGL leukaemia have been described [96], but are not classified separately by the WHO. The expression of CD26, a surface glycoprotein with an essential role in T-cell function, including being a marker of T-cell activation and a mediator of T-cell activating signals, has also been associated with a more aggressive disease course [97]. There is no data regarding disease features which are predictive of a response to any particular treatment modality other than HLA DR4 positivity, which is highly predictive of response to Ciclosporin A [98].

Treatment

T-LGL leukaemia is an indolent disorder and is usually managed with immunosuppressive medications at doses similar to those used in the treatment of autoimmune disorders [78]. Approximately 60–70% of patients will require treatment at some point during the course of their illness [99]. The main indication for treatment is neutropenia leading to recurrent infection, with other indications including symptomatic anaemia or thrombocytopenia, massive splenomegaly and systemic features. Symptomatic improvement may occur despite failure to normalise neutrophil counts and cytopenias may improve without eradication of the malignant clone [51, 98, 100]. Therefore the aim of treatment, in contrast to the other T-cell leukaemias, is primarily to alleviate cytopenias without necessarily eliminating the clone. A substantial proportion of patients are asymptomatic and should be monitored closely but do not require treatment.

Because of the rarity of T-cell LGL leukaemia, there have been no prospective clinical trials reported and treatment data is derived from retrospective case series and single institution studies, with no established "gold standard" therapy. First line therapy is usually with single line immunosuppressive agents such as low dose methotrexate (10 mg/m^2 weekly), cyclophosphamide (50–100 mg daily) or cyclosporine A (5–10 mg/kg daily) with response rates in the order of 50–60% [101–103]. There are no randomised controlled trials to compare these agents. The onset of response to treatment is generally slow, with a median response time reported as 4 months in a recent study, although one patient had a delayed response at 14 months [104]. Cross resistance is absent among these agents which have all demonstrated good overall safety, efficacy and tolerability in the majority of patients. Responses can be sustained with continued treatment. However, reports of second malignancies (*Error! Bookmark not defined.*), taken in conjunction with the intrinsic potential for high grade transformation in T-cell LGL leukaemia [95], raise a note of caution. HLA-DR4 positivity has been shown to be highly predictive of responsiveness to cyclosporine A [98], but there are no other data to predict an individual's response to a particular agent. In the majority of cases there is no correlation between clinical response and reduction in the degree of bone marrow infiltration and number of circulating LGLs, in keeping with immunosuppressive or immunomodulatory rather than cytotoxic mechanism of action of these agents. Accordingly, there is no evidence that high dose therapy will benefit these patients by eradicating the clone.

The purine analogues including fludarabine, cladribine and pentostatin have also demonstrated efficacy in T-cell LGL leukaemia [38, 105, 106] and have the advantage of being administered as single discrete courses without the need for long-term maintenance therapy. As such they offer potentially attractive alternatives for younger symptomatic patients with T-cell LGL leukaemia. There are reports of the successful use of alemtuzumab in T-LGL [107, 108], which has been shown to strongly express the CD52 antigen [109]. The use of alemtuzumab would have associated increased expense and infective complications compared to other agents. Other monoclonal antibodies including anti-CD2 (Siplizumab, MedImmune, Gaitherburg, MD) and the humanised MiK-beta-1 monoclonal antibody (anti-CD122—the beta subunit of both interleukin-2 and interleukin-15 receptors) are being evaluated in phase I studies for T-LGL leukaemia and other T-cell disorders. Both interleukin-2 and interleukin-15 are thought to impact on the proliferation, survival and activity of LGLs [50, 110]. Though well tolerated, Mikβ1 monoclonal antibody treatment for T-cell LGL leukaemia did not result in amelioration of cytopenias in any of 12 patients treated with this agent, despite down-regulation of surface receptors seen in seven patients [111].

Haematopoietic growth factors are useful primarily in the early weeks to months required to see remissions with immunosuppressive therapies and as adjuvants to other treatments. Long-term steroid therapy should be avoided due to adverse effects. It is largely accepted that splenectomy, in the absence of splenic bulk and/or immune thrombocytopenia, has little to add to the management of T-cell LGL leukaemia and often induces a transient response in neutrophil count at the expense of increasing lymphocytosis [112, 113]. Haematopoietic stem cell transplantation would rarely be indicated in this indolent disorder, but both autologous and allogeneic transplants have been undertaken in younger patients who are refractory to other therapies [114]. The heavily immunosuppressive conditioning regimens and GVHD prophylaxis regimens may have contributed to the responses observed.

Conclusion

The mature T-cell leukaemias are a rare and heterogenous group of post-thymic T-cell lymphoproliferative disorders which encompass T-PLL, T-LGL and ATLL. Unfortunately, with the exception of the more indolent T-LGL, they have in common their unresponsiveness to conventional chemotherapy, lack of randomised controlled trials to guide management and poor prognosis. New understanding of these diseases on a cellular and molecular level has paved the way for targeted therapies which may circumvent the treatment challenges for which the diseases in this category are renowned. It is crucial that a collaborative international approach to trial design and the introduction of new therapies is undertaken in order to achieve the goal of improving the outlook for patients diagnosed with these rare and aggressive disorders.

References

1. Swerdlow SH, Campo E, Harris N, Jaffe ES, Puleri SA. WHO classification of tumours of haemopoietic and lymphoid tissues. world health organisation classification of tumours. Lyon: IARC Press; 2008.
2. Galton DA, Goldman JM, Wiltshaw E, Catovsky D, Henry K, Goldenberg GJ. Prolymphocytic leukaemia. Br J Haematol. 1974;27:7–23.
3. Catovsky D, Galetto J, Okas A, Galton DA, Wiltshaw E, Stathopoulos G. Prolymphocytic leukaemia of B and T cell type. Lancet. 1973;2(7823):232–4.
4. Lan K, Murakami M, Choudhuri T, Tsai DE, Schuster SJ, Wasik MA, et al. Detection of Epstein-Barr virus in T-cell prolymphocytic leukemia cells in vitro. J Clin Virol. 2008;43(3):260–5.
5. Bommhardt U, Beyer M, Hunig T, Reichardt HM. Molecular and cellular mechanisms of T cell development. Cell Mol Life Sci. 2004;61:263–80.
6. Brito-Babapulle V, Catovsky D. Inversions and tandem translocations involving chromosome 14q11 and 14q32 in T-prolymphocytic leukemia and T-cell leukemias in patients with ataxia telangiectasia. Cancer Genet Cytogenet. 1991;55:1–9.
7. Xu Y, Ashley T, Brainerd EE, Bronson RT, Meyn MS, Baltimore D. Targeted disruption of ATM leads to growth retardation, chromosomal fragmentation during meiosis, immune defects and thymic lymphoma. Genes Dev. 1996;10:2411–22.
8. Taylor AM, Metcalfe JA, Thick M, Mak YF. Leukaemia and lymphoma in ataxia telangiectasia. Blood. 1986;87:423–38.
9. Stilgenbauer S, Schaffner C, Litterst A, Liebisch P, Gilad S, Bar-Shira A, et al. Biallelic mutations in the ATM gene in T-prolymphocytic leukemia. Nat Med. 1997;3:1155–9.
10. Stoppa-Lyonnet D, Soulier J, Lauge A, Dastot H, Garand R, Sigaux F, et al. Inactivation of the ATM gene in T-cell prolymphocytic leukemias. Blood. 1998;91:3920–6.
11. Yuille MA, Coignet LJ. The ataxia telangiectasia gene in familial and sporadic cancer. Recent Results Cancer Res. 1998;154:156–73.
12. Yamaguchi M, Yamamoto K, Miki T, Mizutani S, Miura O. T-cell prolymphocytic leukemia with del(11)t(1;11)(q21;q23) and ATM deficiency. Cancer Genet Cytogenet. 2003;146:22–6.
13. Matutes E, Brito-Babapulle V, Yullie MR, Catovsky D. Prolymphocytic leukemia of B- and T-cell types. In: Cheson BD, editor. Chronic lymphoid leukemias. New York: Marcel Dekker; 2001. p. 525–41.
14. Matutes E, Brito-Babapulle V, Swansbury J, Ellis J, Morilla R, Dearden C. Clinical and laboratory features of 78 cases of T-prolymphocytic leukemia. Blood. 1991;78:3269–74.
15. Catovsky D, Galetto J, Okos A, Galton DA, Wiltshaw E, Stathopoulos G. Prolymphocytic leukaemia of B and T cell type. Lancet. 1973;2:232–4.
16. Garand R, Goasguen J, Brizard A, Buisine J, Charpentier A, Claisse JF. Indolent course as a relatively frequent presentation in T-prolymphocytic leukaemia. Groupe Francais d'Hematologie Cellulaire. Br J Haematol. 1998;103:488–94.
17. Matutes E, Talavera GJ, O'Brien M, Catovsky D. The morphological spectrum of T-prolymphcytic leukaemia. Br J Haematol. 1986;64:111–24.
18. Ginaldi L, De Martinis M, Matutes E, Farahat N, Morilla R, Dyer MJ, et al. Levels of expression of CD52 in normal and leukemic B and T cells: correlation with in vivo therapeutic responses to Campath-1H. Leuk Res. 1998;22:185–91.
19. Sugimoto T, Imoto S, Matsuo Y, et al. T-cell receptor gammadelta T-cell leukemia with the morphology of T-cell prolymphocytic leukemia and a postthymic immunophenotype. Ann Hematol. 2001;80:749–51.
20. Croce CM. Role of chromosome translocations in human neoplasia. Cell. 1987;49:155–6.
21. Croce CM, Isobe M, Palumbo A, Puck J, Ming J, Tweardy D, et al. Gene for alpha-chain of human T-cell receptor: location on chromosome 14 region involved in T-cell neoplasms. Science. 1985;227:1044–7.
22. Soulier J, Pierron G, Vecchione D, Garand R, Brizard F, Sigaux F, et al. A complex pattern of recurrent chromosomal losses and gains in T-cell prolymphocytic leukemia. Genes Chromosomes Cancer. 2001;31:248–54.
23. Virgilio L, Narducci MG, Isobe M, Billips LG, Cooper MD, Croce CM. Identification of the TCL1 gene involved in T-cell malignancies. Proc Natl Acad Sci USA. 1994;91:12530–4.
24. Narducci MG, Stoppacciaro A, Imada K, Uchiyama T, Virgilio L, Lazzeri C, et al. TCL1 is overexpressed in patients affected by adult T-cell leukemias. Cancer Res. 1997;57:5452–6.
25. Stern MH, Soulier J, Rosenzwajg M, Nakahara K, Canki-Klain N, Aurias A, et al. MTCP-1: a novel gene on the human chromosome Xq28 translocated to the T cell receptor alpha/delta locus in mature T cell proliferations. Oncogene. 1993;8:2475–83.
26. Madani A, Choukroun V, Soulier J, Cacheux V, Claisse JF, Valensi F, et al. Expression of p13MTCP1 is restricted to mature T-cell proliferations with t(X;14) translocations. Blood. 1996;87:1923–7.

27. Hallas C, Pekarsky Y, Itoyama T, Varnum J, Bichi R, Rothstein JL, et al. Genomic analysis of human and mouse TCL1 loci reveals a complex of tightly clustered genes. Proc Natl Acad Sci USA. 1999;96: 14418–23.
28. Pekarsky Y, Hallas C, Isobe M, Russo G, Cruce CM. Abnormalities at 14q32.1 in T cell malignancies involve two oncogenes. Proc Natl Acad Sci USA. 1999;96:2949–51.
29. Sugimoto J, Hatakeyama T, Narducci MG, Russo G, Isobe M. Identification of the TCL1/MTCP1-like 1 (TML1) gene from the region next to the TCL1 locus. Cancer Res. 1999;59:2313–7.
30. Yuille MR, Condie A, Stone EM, Wilsher J, Bradshaw PS, Brooks L, et al. TCL1 is activated by chromosomal rearrangement or by hypomethylation. Genes Chromosomes Cancer. 2001;30:336–41.
31. Herling M, Khoury JD, Washington LT, Duvic M, Keating MJ, Jones D, et al. A systematic approach to diagnosis of mature T-cell leukemias reveals heterogeneity among WHO categories. Blood. 2004;104: 328–35.
32. Laine J, Kunstle G, Obata T, Sha M, Noguchi M. The protooncogene TCL1 is an Akt kinase coactivator. Mol Cell. 2000;6:395–407.
33. Kojima K, Kobayashi H, Imoto S, Matsuo Y, Kobayashi H, Yano T, et al. 14q11 abnormality and trisomy 8q are not common in Japanese T-cell prolymphocytic leukemia. Int J Hematol. 1998;68: 291–6.
34. Durig J, Bug S, Klein-Hitpass L, Boes T, Jons T, Martin-Subero JI, et al. Combined single nucleotide polymorphism-based genomic mapping and global gene expression profiling identifies novel chromosomal imbalances, mechanisms and candidate genes important in the pathogenesis of T-cell prolymphocytic leukaemia with inv (14)(q11q32). Leukaemia. 2007;21(10):2153–63.
35. Herling M, Patek KA, Teitell MA, Konopleva M, Ravandi F, Kobayashi R, et al. High TCL1 expression and intact T-cell receptor signalling define a hyperproliferative subset of T-cell prolymphocytic leukaemia. Blood. 2008;111:328–37.
36. Dearden CE, Matutes E, Cazin B, Tjønnfjord GE, Parreira A, Nomdedeu B, et al. High remission rate in T-cell prolymphocytic leukemia with Campath-1H. Blood. 2001;98:1721–6.
37. Delgado J, Bustos JG, Jimenez MC, Quevedo E, Hernandez-Navarro F. Are activation markers (CD25, CD38 and CD103) predictive of sensitivity to purine analogues in patients with T-cell prolymphocytic leukemia and other lymphoproliferative disorders? Leuk Lymphoma. 2002;43:2331–4.
38. Mercieca J, Matutes E, Dearden C, MacLennan K, Catovsky D. The role of pentostatin in the treatment of T-cell malignancies: analysis of response rate in 145 patients according to disease subtype. J Clin Oncol. 1994;12:2588–93.
39. Palomera L, Domingo JM, Agullo JA, Soledad Romero M. Complete remission in T-cell prolymphocytic leukemia with 2-chlorodeoxyadenosine. J Clin Oncol. 1995;13:1284–5.
40. Delannoy A. 2-chloro-2'-deoxyadenosine: clinical applications in hematology. Blood Rev. 1996;10: 148–66.
41. Pawson R, Dyer MJ, Barge R, Matutes E, Thornton PD, Emmett E, et al. Treatment of T-cell prolymphocytic leukemia with human CD52 antibody. J Clin Oncol. 1997;15:2667–72.
42. Keating MJ, Cazin B, Coutre S, Birhiray R, Kovacsovics T, Langer W, et al. Campath-1H treatment of T-cell prolymphocytic leukaemia in patients for whom at least one prior chemotherapy regimen has failed. J Clin Oncol. 2002;20:205–13.
43. Dearden C, Matutes E, Cazin B, Tjønnfjord GE, Parreira A, Nomdedeu B, et al. Very high response rates in previously untreated T-cell Prolymphocytic leukaemia patients receiving alemtuzumab (Campath-1H) therapy. Blood. 2003;102, Abstract 2378.
44. Hopfinger G, Kandler G., Koller E, et al. (2007) T-PLL 1 protocol of the German CLL Study Group (GCLLSG)-A Prospective phase 2 trial of fludarabine phosphate, Mitoxantrone and cyclophosphamide (FCM) followed by alemtuzumab consolidation as first line treatment in T-PLL. Blood. 2007;110, abstract 2130.
45. Weidmann E, Hess G, Krause SW et al. Combination chemoimmunotherapy using alemtuzumab, fludarabine, cyclophosphomide and doxorubicin (FCD) is an effective first line regimen in peripheral T-cell lymphoma (PTCL). Blood. 2004;104, abstract 2460.
46. Krishnan B, Cazin B, Ireland R, et al. Improved survival for patients with T-cell prolymphocytic leuk receiving alemtuzumab therapy followed by stem cell transplantation. IWCLL. Leuk Lymphoma. 2007;48 Suppl 1:S180.
47. Garderet L, Bittencourt H, Kaliski A, Daniel M, Ribaud P, Socié G, et al. Treatment of T-prolymphocytic leukaemia with nommyeloablative allogeneic stem cell transplantation. Eur J Haematol. 2001;66:137–9.
48. De Lavallade H, Faucher C, Furst S, El-Cheikh J, Vey N, Coso D, et al. Allogeneic stem cell transplantation after reduced-intensity conditioning in a patient with T-cell prolymphocytic leukaemia: graft-versus-tumor effect and long-term remission. Bone Marrow Transplant. 2006;37:709–10.
49. Loughran Jr TP. Clonal diseases of large granular lymphocytes. Blood. 1993;82:1–14.
50. Lamy T, Loughran TP. Large granular lymphocyte leukemia. Cancer Control. 1998;5:25–33.
51. Sokol L, Loughran Jr TP. Large granular lymphocyte leukemia. Oncologist. 2006;11(3):263–73.
52. Zambello R, Trentin L, Facco M, Cerutti A, Sancetta R, Milani A, et al. Analysis of the T cell receptor in the lymphoproliferative disease of granular lymphocytes: superantigen activation of clonal CD3+ granular lymphocytes. Cancer Res. 1995;55:6140–5.

53. Kanchan K, Loughran Jr TP. Antigen-driven clonal T cell expansion in disorders of hematopoiesis. Leuk Res. 2003;27:291–2.
54. O'Keefe CL, Plasilova M, Wlodarski M, Risitano AM, Rodriguez AR, Howe E, et al. Molecular analysis of TCR clonotypes in LGL: a clonal model for polyclonal responses. J Immunol. 2004;172:1960–9.
55. Wlodarski MW, O'Keefe C, Howe EC, Risitano AM, Rodriguez A, Warshawsky 1, et al. Pathologic clonal cytotoxic T-cell responses: nonrandom nature of the T-cell-receptor restriction in large granular lymphocyte leukemia. Blood. 2005;106:2769–80.
56. Loughran Jr TP, Coyle T, Sherman MP, Starkebaum G, Ehrlich GD, Ruscetti FW, et al. Detection of human T-cell leukemia/lymphoma virus, type II, in a patient with large granular lymphocyte leukemia. Blood. 1992;80:1116–9.
57. Loughran Jr TP, Hadlock KG, Perzova R, Gentile TC, Yang Q, Foung SK, et al. Epitope mapping of HTLV envelope seroreactivity in LGL leukaemia. Br J Haematol. 1998;101:318–24.
58. Rodriguez-Caballero A, Garcia-Montero A, Barcena P, Almeida J, Ruiz-Cabello F, Tabernero MD, et al. Expanded cells in monoclonal TCRβ+/CD4+/NKa+/CD8−/+dim T-LGL lymphocytosis recognize hCMV antigens. Blood. 2009;112(12):4609–17.
59. Narumi H, Kojima K, Matsuo Y, Shikata H, et al. T-cell large granular lymphocytic leukemia occurring after autologous peripheral blood stem cell transplantation. Bone Marrow Transplant. 2004; 33(1):99–101.
60. Au WY, Lam CC, Lie AK, Pang A, Kwong YL, et al. T-cell large granular lymphocyte leukemia of donor origin after allogeneic bone marrow transplantation. Am J Clin Pathol. 2003;120(4):626–30.
61. French LE, Alcindor T, Shapiro M, McGinnis KS, Margolis DJ, Porter D, et al. Identification of amplified clonal T cell populations in the blood of patients with chronic graft-versus-host disease: positive correlation with response to photopheresis. Bone Marrow Transplant. 2002;30(8):509–15.
62. Arons E, Sorbara L, Raffeld M, Stetler-Stevenson M, Steinberg SM, Liewehr DJ, et al. Characterization of T-cell repertoire in hairy cell leukemia patients before and after recombinant immunotoxin BL22 therapy. Cancer Immunol Immunother. 2006;55(9):1100–10.
63. Martinez A, Pittaluga S, Villamor N, Colomer D, Rozman M, Raffeld M, et al. Clonal T-cell populations and increased risk for cytotoxic T-cell lymphomas in B-CLL patients: clinicopathologic observations and molecular analysis. Am J Surg Pathol. 2004;28(7):849–58.
64. Viny AD, Lichtin A, Pohlman B, Loughran T, Maciejewski J. Chronic B-cell dyscrasias are an important clinical feature of T-LGL leukemia. Leuk Lymphoma. 2008;49(5):932–8.
65. Yang J, Epling-Burnette P, Painter J, Zou J, Bai F, Wei S, et al. Antigen activation and impaired Fas-induced death-inducing signaling complex formation in T-large-granular lymphocyte leukemia. Blood. 2008;111(3):1610–6.
66. Lamy T, Liu JH, Landowski TH, Dalton WS, Loughran Jr TP. Dysregulation of CD95/CD95 ligand-apoptotic pathway in CD3(+) large granular lymphocyte leukemia. Blood. 1998;92:4771–7.
67. Schade AE, Wlodarski MW, Maciejewski JP. Pathophysiology defined by altered signal transduction pathways; the role of JAK-STAT and P13K signalling in large granular lymphocytes. Cell Cycle. 2006;5:2571–4.
68. Schade AE, Powers JJ, Wlodarski MW, Maciejewski JP. Phosphatidylinositol-3-phosphate kinase pathway activation protects leukemic large granular lymphocytes from undergoing homeostatic apoptosis. Blood. 2006;107:4834–40.
69. Epling-Burnette PK, Bai F, Wei S, Chaurasia P, Painter JS, Olashaw N, et al. ERK couples chronic survival of NK cells to constitutively activated Ras in lymphoproliferative disease of granular lymphocytes (LDGL). Oncogene. 2004;23:9220–9.
70. Lamy T, Loughran Jr TP. Clinical features of large granular lymphocyte leukemia. Semin Hematol. 2003;40:185–95.
71. Liu JH, Wei S, Lamy T, Epling-Burnette PK, Starkebaum G, Djeu JY, et al. Chronic neutropenia mediated by fas ligand. Blood. 2000;95:3219–22.
72. Rose MG, Berliner N. T-cell large granular lymphocyte leukemia and related disorders. Oncologist. 2004;9:247–58.
73. Miranda EG, Loughran Jr TP. Chronic T-cell and NK-cell leukemias. In: Cheson BD, editor. Chronic lymphoid leukemias. New York: Marcel Dekker; 2001. p. 543–65.
74. Lamy T, Loughran Jr TP. Current concepts: large granular lymphocyte leukaemia. Blood Rev. 1999; 13:230–40.
75. Kwong Y, Wong K. Association of pure red cell aplasia with T large granular lymphocyte leukaemia. J Clin Pathol. 1998;51:672–5.
76. Sampalo Lainz A, Lopez-Gomez M, Jimenez-Alonso J. Proliferation of large granular lymphocytes in patients with systemic lupus erythematosus. Rev Clin Esp. 1995;195:373–9.
77. Starkebaum G. Chronic neutropenia associated with autoimmune disease. Semin Hematol. 2002;39:121–7.
78. Burks EJ, Loughran Jr TP. Pathogenesis of neutropenia in large granular lymphocyte leukemia and Felty syndrome. Blood Rev. 2006;20(5):245–66.
79. McKenna R, Parkin J, Kersey J, Gajl-Peczalsca K, Peterson L, Brunnign R. Chronic lymphoproliferative disorder with unusual clinical, morphologic, ultrastructural and surface marker characteristics. Am J Med. 1977;62:588–96.
80. Argnasson B, Loughran T, Starkebaum G, Kadin M. The pathology of large granular lymphocyte lymphoma. Hum Pathol. 1989;20:643–51.
81. Osuji N, Beiske K, Randen U, Matutes E, Tjonnfjord G, Catovsky D, et al. Characteristic appearances of

the bone marrow in T-cell large granular lymphocyte leukaemia. Histopathology. 2007;50:547–54.
82. Dhodapkar M, Li CY, Lust J, Tefferi A, Phyliky RL. Clinical spectrum of clonal proliferations of T-large granular lymphocytes: a T-cell clonopathy of undetermined significance? Blood. 1994;84(5):1620–7.
83. Chan WC, Catovsky D, Foucar K, Montserrat E. T-cell large granular lymphocyte leukemia. In: Jaffe ES, Harris NL, Stein H, Vardiman JW, editors. World Health Organization classification of tumours: tumours of haematopoietic and lymphoid tissues. Lyon: IARC Press; 2001. p. 197–8.
84. Semenzato G, Zambello R, Starkebaum G, Oshimi K, Loughran Jr TP. The lymphoproliferative disease of granular lymphocytes: updated criteria for diagnosis. Blood. 1997;89:256–60.
85. Lundell R, Hartung L, Hill S, Perkins SL, Bahler DW. T-cell large granular lymphocyte leukaemias have multiple phenotypic abnormalities involving pan-T-cell antigens and receptors for MHC molecules. Am J Clin Pathol. 2005;124(6):937–46.
86. Morice WG, Kurtin PJ, Leibson PJ, Tefferi A, Hanson CA. Demonstration of aberrant T-cell and natural killer-cell antigen expression in all cases of granular lymphocytic leukaemia. Br J Haematol. 2003;120(6):1026–36.
87. Rambaldi A, Pelicci P, Allavena P, Knowles 2nd DM, Rossini S, Bassan R. T cell receptor beta gene rearrangements in lymphoproliferative disorders of large granular lymphocytes / natural killer cells. J Exp Med. 1985;162:2156–62.
88. Vie H, Chevalier S, Garand R, Moisan JP, Praloran V, Devilder MC. Clonal expansion of lymphocytes bearing the gamma delta T-cell receptor in a patient with large granular lymphocyte disorder. Blood. 1989;74:285–90.
89. Loughran Jr TP, Kadin ME, Starkebaum G, Abkowitz JL, Clark EA, Disteche C. Leukemia of large granular lymphocytes: association with clonal chromosomal abnormalities and autoimmune neutropenia, thrombocytopenia, and hemolytic anemia. Ann Intern Med. 1985;102:169–75.
90. Oshimi K, Yamada O, Kaneko T, Nishinarita S, Iizuka Y, Urabe A. Laboratory findings and clinical courses of 33 patients with granular lymphocyte-proliferative disorders. Leukemia. 1993;7:782–8.
91. Wong KF, Chan JC, Liu HS, Man C, Kwong YL. Chromosomal abnormalities in T-cell large granular lymphocyte leukaemia: report of two cases and review of the literature. Br J Haematol. 2002;116:598–600.
92. Liu JH, Wei S, Lamy T, Li Y, Epling-Burnette PK, Djeu JY, et al. Blockade of Fas-dependent apoptosis by soluble Fas in LGL leukemia. Blood. 2002; 100(4):1449–53.
93. Saitoh T, Karasawa M, Sakuraya M, Norio N, Junko T, Shirakawa K. Improvement of extrathymic T cell type of large granular lymphocyte (LGL) leukemia by cyclosporin A: the serum level of Fas ligand is a marker of LGL leukemia activity. Eur J Haematol. 2000;65:272–5.
94. Takeuchi M, Tamaoki A, Soda R, Takahashi K. Spontaneous remission of large granular lymphocyte T cell leukemia. Leukemia. 1999;13:313–4.
95. Matutes E, Wotherspoon A, Parker N, Osuji N. Transformation of T-cell large granular lymphocyte leukaemia into a high-grade large T-cell lymphoma. Br J Haematol. 2001;115(4):801–6.
96. Gentile TC, Uner AH, Hutchison RE, Wright J, Ben-Ezra J, Russell EC. CD3+, CD56+ aggressive variant of large granular lymphocyte leukemia. Blood. 1994;84:2315–21.
97. Dang NH, Aytac U, Sato K, O'Brien S, Melenhorst J, Morimoto C. T-large granular lymphocyte lymphoproliferative disorder: expression of CD26 as a marker of clinically aggressive disease and characterization of marrow inhibition. Br J Haematol. 2003;121:857–65.
98. Osuji N, Matutes E, Tjonnfjord G, Grech H, Del Giudice I, Wotherspoon A. T-cell large granular lymphocyte leukemia: a report on the treatment of 29 patients and a review of the literature. Cancer. 2006;107:570–8.
99. Pandolfi F, Loughran Jr TP, Starkebaum G, Chisesi T, Barbui T, Chan WC, et al. Clinical course and prognosis of the lymphoproliferative disease of granular lymphocytes. A multicenter study. Cancer. 1990; 65:341–8.
100. Sood R, Stewart CC, Aplan PD, Murai H, Ward P, Barcos M. Neutropenia associated with T-cell large granular lymphocyte leukemia: long-term response to cyclosporine therapy despite persistence of abnormal cells. Blood. 1998;91:3372–8.
101. Battiwalla M, Melenhorst J, Saunthararajah Y, Nakamura R, Molldrem J, Young NS. HLA-DR4 predicts haematological response to cyclosporine in T-large granular lymphocyte lymphoproliferative disorders. Br J Haematol. 2003;123:449–53.
102. Loughran Jr TP, Kidd PG, Starkebaum G. Treatment of large granular lymphocyte leukemia with oral low-dose methotrexate. Blood. 1994;84:2164–70.
103. Matrai Z, Lelkes G, Milosevits J, Páldiné HP, Pecze K. T-cell large granular lymphocytic leukemia associated with pure red cell aplasia, successfully treated with cyclophosphamide. Orv Hetil. 1997;138: 2075–80.
104. Aribi A, Huh Y, Keating M, O'brien S, Ferrajoli A, Faderl S. T-cell large granular lymphocytic (T-LGL) leukemia: experience in a single institution over 8 years. Leuk Res. 2007;31(7):939–45.
105. Witzig TE, Weitz JJ, Lundberg JH, Tefferi A. Treatment of refractory T-cell chronic lymphocytic leukemia with purine nucleoside analogues. Leuk Lymphoma. 1994;14:137–9.
106. Dincol G, Diz-Kuçukkaya R, Bicakci E. T-cell large granular lymphocytic leukaemia: successful response to 2-deoxycoformycin. Neth J Med. 2008;66(2):85–7.
107. Rosenblum MD, LaBelle JL, Chang CC, Margolis DA, Schauer DW, Vesole DH. Efficacy of alemtuzumab treatment for refractory T-cell large granular lymphocytic leukemia. Blood. 2004;103:1969–71.

108. Ru X, Liebman HA. Successful treatment of refractory pure red cell aplasia associated with lymphoproliferative disorders with the anti-CD52 monoclonal antibody alemtuzumab (Campath-1H). Br J Haematol. 2003;123:278–81.
109. Osuji N, Del Giudice I, Matutes E, Morilla A, Owusu-Ankomah K, Morilla R. CD52 expression in T-cell large granular lymphocyte leukemia-Implications for treatment with alemtuzumab. Leuk Lymphoma. 2005;46:723–7.
110. Aprile JA, Russo M, Pepe MS, Loughran Jr TP. Activation signals leading to proliferation of normal and leukemic CD3+ large granular lymphocytes. Blood. 1991;78:1282–5.
111. Morris JC, Janik JE, White JD, Fleisher TA, Brown M, Tsudo M. Preclinical and phase I clinical trial of blockade of IL-15 using Mikbeta1 monoclonal antibody in T cell large granular lymphocyte leukemia. Proc Natl Acad Sci USA. 2006;103:401–6.
112. Loughran Jr TP, Starkebaum G, Clark E, Wallace P, Kadin ME. Evaluation of splenectomy in large granular lymphocyte leukaemia. Br J Haematol. 1987;67:135–40.
113. Gentile TC, Loughran Jr TP. Resolution of autoimmune hemolytic anemia following splenectomy in CD3+ large granular lymphocyte leukemia. Leuk Lymphoma. 1996;23:405–8.
114. Toze CL, Shepherd JD, Connors JM, Voss NJ, Gascoyne RD, Hogge DE. Allogeneic bone marrow transplantation for low-grade lymphoma and chronic lymphocytic leukemia. Bone Marrow Transplant. 2000;25:605–12.

Cutaneous T-Cell Lymphomas

10

Farah Rukhsana Abdulla, Madeleine Duvic, and Youn H. Kim

Introduction

Cutaneous T cell lymphomas (CTCL) are T cell non-Hodgkin lymphomas (NHL) with primary cutaneous involvement. Mycosis fungoides (MF) and Sézary syndrome (SS) are subsets of CTCL [1]. Although MF and SS are uncommon forms of NHL, they are the most common lymphomas with primary involvement of the skin. The annual incidence in the United States is estimated at 0.96 cases per 100,000 with approximately 3,000 new cases per year in the United States [2]. While MF and SS occur in children and young adults, the median age at diagnosis is between 55 and 60 years [3]. There is 2:1 male predominance, and black patients have a twofold greater risk for developing MF/SS than white. The diagnosis and work-up for MF and SS are outlined in the National Comprehensive Cancer Network (NCCN) practice guidelines.

F.R. Abdulla
Department of Dermatology, Southern California Permanente Medical Group, Fontana, CA, USA

M. Duvic
Department of Dermatology, UT-MD Anderson Cancer Center, Houston, TX, USA

Y.H. Kim (✉)
Department of Dermatology, Stanford Cancer Center/Stanford University School of Medicine, 900 Blake Wilbur Drive, Room 1010, Stanford, CA 95014, USA
e-mail: younkim@stanford.edu

Clinical Presentation

MF is the most common type of CTCL with a unique clinical–pathologic presentation. The initial cutaneous presentation of MF can be as patches or plaques that may subsequently evolve into tumors or generalized erythroderma; however, some patients may present with tumors or generalized erythroderma (Fig. 10.1). The most common initial cutaneous presentation is patch and plaque disease with approximately 30% of patients presenting with limited patch and plaque disease (less than 10% of the skin surface involved) and 35–40% with generalized patch and plaque (greater than or equal to 10% of the skin surface involved) [4]. Patches or plaques in MF are often localized, typically affecting flexural areas and the buttocks ("bathing trunk" distribution), although any cutaneous area of the body can be involved. The typical patches of mycosis fungoides are slightly scaling and mildly erythematous. More infiltrated lesions evolve into palpable plaques. These plaques are erythematous and slightly scaling, with well-defined borders. The shape and distribution of lesions are variable. Pruritus is the most common symptom even in the early phases of the disease and is often the problem that prompts a visit to the dermatologist.

However, the skin involvement can be much more extensive with infiltrated plaques evolving into ulcerating or fungating tumors or generalized erythroderma involving the entire skin surface. Fifteen to 20% of patients with MF present

F. Foss (ed.), *T-Cell Lymphomas*, Contemporary Hematology,
DOI 10.1007/978-1-62703-170-7_10,

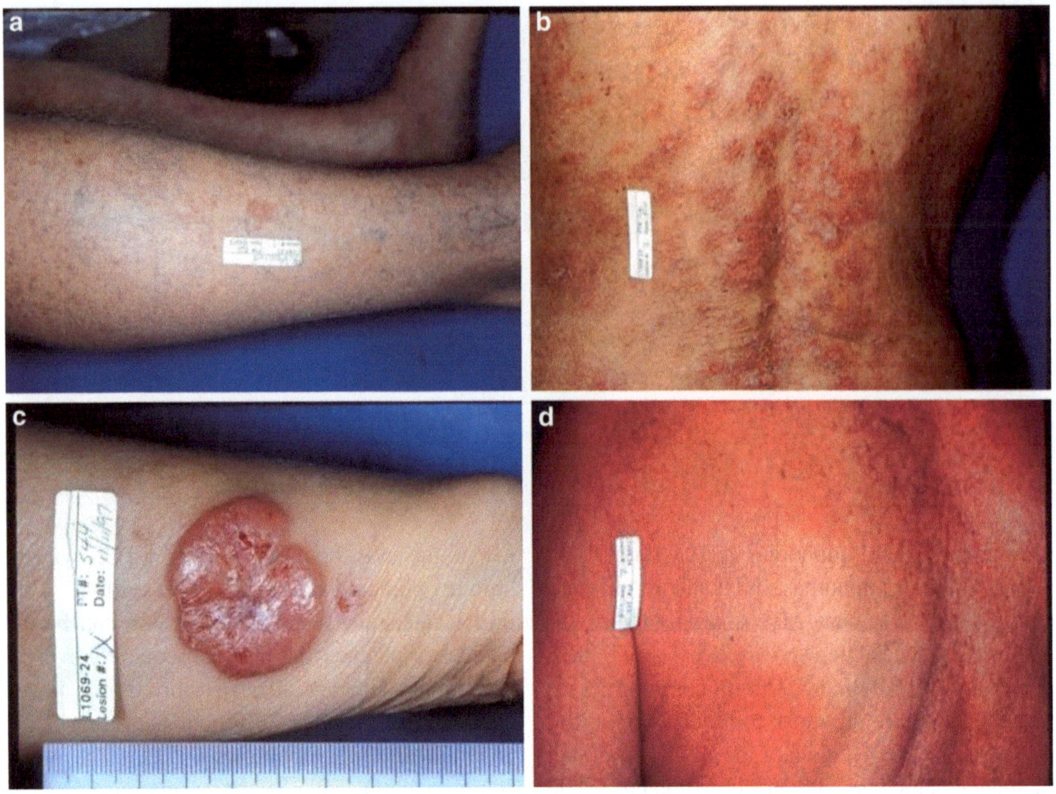

Fig. 10.1 Clinical manifestations of mycosis fungoides. (**a**) Patch stage disease. (**b**) Cutaneous plaques and patches. (**c**) Tumor stage disease. (**d**) Erythroderma

with tumorous lesions [4]. Tumors often become infected, and sepsis secondary to infection is often the cause of death in individuals so affected. Generalized dermal thickening from infiltrative disease may cause the classic but very unusual leonine facies of mycosis fungoides.

Another manifestation of skin involvement in mycosis fungoides is generalized erythroderma, with 15% of patients presenting as such [4]. The erythema may be accompanied by either atrophic or lichenified plaques or tumors. In the more generalized presentations, keratoderma may develop, nails may become dystrophic, and scalp involvement can result in alopecia [1]. These patients are almost always intensely symptomatic from pruritus and scaling and often have lymphadenopathy due to diffuse and severe skin involvement. SS is a distinct subtype of CTCL which is characterized by the triad of erythroderma, lymphadenopathy, and neoplastic T cells (or Sézary cells). The presence of all three is not required for the diagnosis. However, the presence of blood involvement is required for the definitive diagnosis of this syndrome. Sézary cells have the same microscopic appearance and immunophenotypic and genotypic characteristics as the cells that infiltrate the epidermis. Sézary cells in the peripheral blood meet the criteria of significance either by morphology, flow cytometry, or molecular analysis [5, 6]. For a definitive diagnosis, Sézary cells should number at least 1,000 per mm^3 [3, 5]. Additional ancillary tests, which help to define the diagnosis, include an expanded peripheral blood $CD4^+$ population with increased ratio of CD4 to CD8 T lymphocytes (greater than 10:1), expanded populations of abnormal T-cells with $CD4^+/CD7^-$ or $CD4^+/CD26^-$ phenotype, and molecular evidence of a relevant T-cell receptor gene rearrangement in the peripheral blood [5]. Patients may present initially with all components of SS or with only one component, e.g., generalized erythroderma, and subsequently progress to develop other clinical features of SS [7]. Patients with SS have a worse prognosis than erythrodermic patients with mycosis fungoides who do not have the other findings of the SS [7].

The median duration from the onset of skin symptoms to a diagnosis of mycosis fungoides may be 5 years or longer [8]. In many patients, the disease presents initially in a premycotic phase with nonspecific, slightly scaling skin lesions that wax and wane over a period of years. Biopsies are generally nondiagnostic during this phase of disease, and patients may respond to treatment with topical corticosteroids. Clinically and histologically, the patients may be confused with a nonspecific dermatitis. Some of these patients will experience an evolution of their disease and develop more typical patches or infiltrated plaques, from which a definitive diagnostic biopsy may be obtained. Repeated biopsies must be obtained from patients suspected of having mycosis fungoides, even when an initial biopsy is negative. In addition, ancillary tests such as immunohistochemistry and T-cell receptor gene rearrangements may be helpful (Fig. 10.1).

Pathogenesis, Histology, Immunophenotype, and Molecular Diagnosis

The etiology of MF and SS remains undetermined. Various studies and case reports have suggested an association with genetic factors, environmental exposure, or an infectious etiology, but none has confirmed a causal association. The immunopathogenesis has been a focus of much research in the last decade. The malignant lymphocytes in mycosis fungoides are $CD4^{+}$ T cells that express the skin-homing receptors CLA and CCR4. The malignant cells are associated with increased T helper type 2 and reduced T helper type 1 cytokine production [9]. However, whether cytokine abnormalities are primarily involved or are secondary processes in the pathogenesis is unclear. The trigger of T cell activation and subsequent clonal expansion of the malignant T cells in the skin remains unclear.

Genetic aberrations that contribute to the development and progression of mycosis fungoides or SS are becoming better elucidated. Cytogenetic studies have yet to disclose a consistent chromosomal change in all patients with mycosis fungoides, but alterations to 10q, including loss of heterozygosity and microsatellite instability, are reported [10]. These may result in the loss of function of a tumor suppressor gene (or genes) found in this region, such as PTEN. Other studies have found evidence that p16(INK4a), a tumor suppressor gene located on 9p, may be selectively inactivated with progression of mycosis fungoides from patch to tumor stage [11]. Recurrent chromosomal or genetic abnormalities have been reported in SS. In particular, utilizing high-resolution array-based comparative genomic hybridization, the SS genome was characterized by gross chromosomal instability with highly recurrent gains and losses. Prominent among deregulated genes are those encoding c-myc, c-myc regulating proteins, mediators of myc-induced apoptosis, and IL-2 signaling pathways components [12]. Preliminary data from transcriptional analysis with oligonucleotide microarrays in mycosis fungoides revealed promising clinically relevant gene signatures predictive of survival, disease progression, and response to therapy [13]. However, further prospective long-term studies are needed to validate these early findings.

In patch lesions of mycosis fungoides, there is a perivascular or band-like infiltrate of small- to medium-sized atypical lymphocytes with hyperchromatic and convoluted (cerebriform) nuclei. The atypical cells exhibit epidermotropism, with individual lymphocytes arranged along the dermal–epidermal junction in a single-file pattern or scattered throughout all layers of the epidermis in the absence of spongiosis. There may also be small intraepidermal collections of neoplastic lymphocytes known as Pautrier's microabscesses (Fig. 10.2a). Although such collections are virtually pathognomonic of mycosis fungoides, in early patch-stage lesions, Pautrier's microabscesses may not be present (Fig. 10.2b). As lesions evolve from patches to plaques, the density of neoplastic cells within the dermis

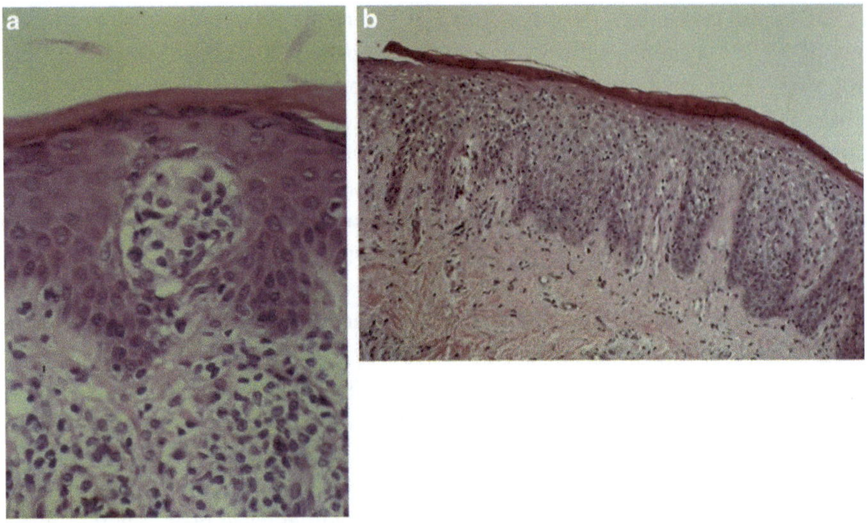

Fig. 10.2 Histopathologic features of mycosis fungoides. (**a**) Epidermotropism, Pautrier microabscesses, atypical cells with hyperconvoluted nuclei. (**b**) Epidermotropism, spongiosis, no Pautrier's microabscesses, minimal dermal infiltrate

increases, and the degree of epidermotropism becomes more exaggerated. In tumorous lesions, the dermal infiltrate is very dense, involving the full breadth of the dermis, often extending into the subcutaneous fat, and epidermotropism tends to diminish. Biopsies of patients with erythroderma show very similar histology to that of patch mycosis fungoides, but the infiltrate is typically more sparse, and the diagnosis is more difficult to establish [14]. Most cases of conventional mycosis fungoides exhibit the following immunophenotype: $CD2^+$, $CD3^+$, $CD4^+$, $CD8^-$, $CD5^+$, $CD7^-$, $CD25^{-/+}$, $CD30^{-/+}$, and T-cell receptor alpha/beta$^+$. Some cases exhibit a $CD8^+$/$CD4^-$ immunophenotype.

Both Southern blot and polymerase chain reaction analyses are capable of detecting clonally rearranged T-cell receptor gene sequences in clinical material from patients with mycosis fungoides. In normal and neoplastic T-cell ontogeny, the γ region of the T-cell receptor gene is rearranged early on, such that most T-cell malignancies have detectable T-cell–receptor γ chain rearrangements, despite the fact that the alpha/beta heterodimer is more often expressed at the cell surface. For various practical reasons, polymerase chain reaction analysis of the gamma-chain region of the T-cell receptor (T-cell receptor gamma) has proved more useful than Southern blot analysis in the evaluation of T-cell lymphoproliferative disorders. Polymerase chain reaction of T-cell receptor gamma represents a very useful adjunct to the histopathologic diagnosis of various cutaneous T-cell malignancies, especially early patch-stage mycosis fungoides, and, at present, the sensitivity of the assay is approximately 70%. Beta-chain region of the T-cell receptor is also rearranged early on in T-cell development. However, the beta-chain region is much larger with more possible rearrangements. The T-cell receptors rearrangements in both the beta region and the gamma region have identical sensitivity (64%) and specificity (84%) when analyzed as individual assays [15]. It is well established that nonneoplastic inflammatory dermatoses can exhibit detectable T-cell receptor gene rearrangements. The false-positive rate reported in the literature is quite variable, but the overall specificity is probably approximately 80–90% [16]. Recently reported data suggest that the false-positive rate becomes lower when tissue samples from two anatomically different sites or different time points demonstrate presence of identical clones [17].

Involved lymph nodes in mycosis fungoides or SS show a range of histologic features. The disease may cause regional nodes to develop the changes of dermatopathic lymphadenitis, with or without scattered individual atypical cerebriform lymphocytes (category N_1). Category N_2 lymph nodes demonstrate dermatopathic lymphadenitis with clusters of more than ten cytologically atypical lymphocytes confined to the paracortex. Category N_3 is reserved for lymph nodes that demonstrate partial or total effacement of lymph node architecture by atypical lymphocytes [5]. Because reactive lymph nodes can sometimes exhibit non-neoplastic lymphocytes with cerebriform nuclei, and because the diagnosis of early lymph node involvement by mycosis fungoides (i.e., category I) can be very difficult on histologic grounds alone, molecular methods for demonstrating T-cell clonality are gaining wide acceptance. Recent studies even suggest that patients with lymph nodes exhibiting rearranged T-cell receptor genes by molecular methods have a worse prognosis, regardless of the histologic grade [5].

Staging of Mycosis Fungoides/Sézary Syndrome

Along with a revised clinical staging system for patients with mycosis fungoides and SS, a consensus recommendation for staging evaluation has been established [5]. Accurate staging is important because therapeutic approaches in MF are largely based on the clinical stage of the disease. The standard clinical staging system for MF and SS is based on the extent and type of skin involvement (T classification), the presence of lymph node (N classification) or visceral disease (M classification), and the detection of abnormal (Sézary) cells in the peripheral blood (B classification) [5]. Tables 10.1 and 10.2 summarize the revised TNMB categories and staging classification.

Many patients with mycosis fungoides have only cutaneous disease. Only 15–20% of patients with mycosis fungoides develop clinical problems related to extracutaneous disease. The most commonly identified site of extracutaneous disease is the regional lymphatics, usually in areas that drain significant sites of skin involvements and the blood compartment. Visceral disease may be identified subsequently. Any visceral site can be involved with MF and SS, the most common of which are the lungs, bone marrow, gastrointestinal tract, liver, and central nervous system [18].

The risk of extracutaneous disease tends to correlate with the extent and type of skin involvement [19, 20]. The extent and type of skin involvement are defined in the T-classification in the revised staging system [5]. T1 disease is defined as less than 10% of the skin surface involved with patches or plaques while T2 disease is defined as greater than 10% but less than 80% of the skin surface involved with patches or plaques. T3 disease is defined as tumor (nodular) disease, and T4 disease is erythroderma with at least 80% of the skin surface diffusely involved. Extracutaneous involvement at presentation is exceedingly rare in patients with T1 disease, infrequent in patients with T2 disease (2%), and (more) likely in patients with T3 (13%) or T4 (24%) disease [4, 20]. Patients who present with limited cutaneous involvement (T1) may never progress to more advanced T classification, especially when appropriate treatment is administered [19, 21, 22]. Although MF may be a systemic disease from the outset, the clinical behavior is such that progression of skin disease precedes onset of clinical symptoms at extracutaneous sites.

Conventional staging for patients with mycosis fungoides includes a comprehensive physical examination with careful examination of the skin (including the scalp, palms, soles, and perineum) and lymph nodes, a complete blood count with Sézary cell studies, screening chemistries (including lactate dehydrogenase), and chest X-ray. Additional imaging studies for patients with T1 or T2 skin involvement are not recommended unless the patient has very extensive skin disease, lymphadenopathy or parameters associated with worse clinical outcome, such as folliculotropic disease, large cell transformation, or blood involvement. However, patients with T3 or T4 disease are at increased risk for extracutaneous involvement, and further imaging, such as a contrast-enhanced chest/abdomen/pelvis computed tomography (CT) scan or whole body FDG-PET/CT, is appropriate. The usefulness of added functional information with FDG-PET (positron emission tomography) has been demonstrated in

Table 10.1 TNMB classification and Staging of mycosis fungoides/Sézary syndrome according to ISCL/EORTC

TNMB stages	Description
Skin (T)	
T1	Limited patches, papules, plaques covering <10% of the skin surface
T2	Patches, papules, plaques covering ≥10% of the skin surface
T3	One or more tumors
T4	Confluent erythema covering >80% BSA
Node (N)	
N0	No abnormal nodes; biopsy not required
N1	Abnormal lymph nodes; histopathology Dutch grade I or NCI LN0-2
N1a	Clone negative
N1b	Clone positive
N2	Abnormal lymph nodes; histopathology Dutch grade 2 or NCI LN3
N2a	Clone negative
N2b	Clone positive
N3	Abnormal lymph nodes; histopathology Dutch grades 3–4 or NCI LN4; clone positive or negative
Nx	Abnormal lymph nodes; no histologic confirmation
Visceral (M)	
M0	No visceral organ involvement
M1	Visceral involvement (must have pathology confirmation and organ involved should be specified)
Blood (B)	
B0	Absence of significant blood involvement: <5% of peripheral blood lymphocytes are atypical (Sézary cells)
B0a	Clone negative
B0b	Clone positive
B1	Low blood tumor burden: >5% of peripheral blood lymphocytes are atypical (Sézary cells) but do not meet the criteria of B2
B1a	Clone negative
B1b	Clone positive
B2	High blood tumor burden: >1,000/μL Sézary cells on ≥ 407.$CD4^+/CD7^-$ or ≥ 307.$CD4^+$ /$CD26^-$ cells with positive clone

Table 10.2 Clinical Staging of mycosis fungoides/Sézary syndrome according to ISCL/EORTC

Stage	T	N	M	B
IA	1	0	0	0, 1
IB	2	0	0	0, 1
IIA	1, 2	1, 2	0	0, 1
IIB	3	0–2	0	0, 1
IIIA	4	0–2	0	0
IIIB	4	0–2	0	1
IVA_1	1–4	0–2	0	2
IVA_2	1–4	3	0	0–2
IVB	1–4	0–3	1	0–2

mycosis fungoides and SS [23]. Lymph node biopsies should be obtained if lymphadenopathy is present. Suspected sites of visceral involvement should be confirmed by appropriate biopsy. Bone marrow involvement may often be detected in patients who meet the clinical criteria for SS but is extremely uncommon in classic mycosis fungoides [24]. Therefore, a bone marrow biopsy is not routinely used as part of the initial staging.

The updated classification also eliminated the need for biopsy of lymph nodes that are not enlarged on physical examination or imaging for staging purposes. A clinically abnormal peripheral node is now defined as measuring 1.5 cm in the longest transverse diameter, or any size of palpable peripheral node that is firm, irregular, clustered, or fixed on physical examination [5]. The revision also further specified histopathologic grading systems for lymph nodes.

The ISCL/EORTC revision also considers visceral involvement to include splenomegaly on physical examination and by imaging that shows either enlargement or focal defects that are not cystic or vascular, even without biopsy confirmation. On the other hand, liver disease should be confirmed with biopsy. However, hepatic enlargement or focal defects that are not cystic or vascular on at least two imaging techniques may be considered to show tumor involvement. Any abnormalities found on imaging of the lungs or visceral organs other than the above would still warrant pathological evaluation, since they could be secondary to another malignancy or infectious disease [5].

Prognostic Factors

The T classification and presence of extracutaneous disease are the most important predictors of survival in patients with mycosis fungoides [4, 25]. Among patients with T4 disease (erythroderma), age older than 60 years, peripheral blood involvement, and extracutaneous disease are independent adverse predictive factors for survival [26]. Other worse prognostic factors include folliculotropic or large cell transformed disease [22, 27]. Mycosis fungoides may be associated with follicular involvement with or without mucin deposit. In these cases, involvement of the hair follicles is clinically prominent, and biopsy shows a heavy infiltration of the hair follicle epithelium by atypical cerebriform lymphocytes with sparing of the interfollicular epidermis [7].

Histologically, transformation to large-cell lymphoma is defined on the basis of either an infiltrate of large atypical lymphocytes that comprise greater than 25% of the dermal infiltrate, or nodular expansile aggregates of atypical large lymphocytes [28, 29]. This large cell transformation is associated with worse clinical outcome [27]. In the majority of cases, increased mitotic activity is readily observed, and the Ki-67 proliferation rate by immunohistochemistry is greater than 25% [28]. Immunophenotypically, the transformed large lymphocytes can exhibit variable loss of one or more T-cell–associated antigens such as CD3, CD5, CD4, CD8, CD45RO, or CD43. Also, the large cells may express lymphocyte activation markers such as CD30 and CD25 [28]. In some cases, there are intermixed aggregates of small, medium, or large-sized B lymphocytes, which are presumably reactive and should not be erroneously interpreted as a secondary B-cell lymphoproliferative disorder [28]. When CD30 expression is prominent among the transformed large lymphocytes, $CD30^+$ lymphoproliferative disorders (especially $CD30^+$ anaplastic large-cell lymphoma) must be considered in the differential diagnosis. Histologic findings that favor a diagnosis of transformed mycosis fungoides include an accompanying infiltrate of smaller-sized lymphocytes that exhibit epidermotropism (as seen in earlier-stage mycosis fungoides lesions), epidermotropism by $CD30^+$ lymphocytes (which is usually not a feature of anaplastic large-cell lymphoma), and a relatively low percentage of $CD30^+$ lymphocytes (as compared to cases of anaplastic large-cell lymphoma in which $CD30^+$ large lymphocytes are greater than 75%). In many cases, correlation with the clinical findings is essential for a definitive diagnosis.

General Principles of Therapy

While there are multiple therapeutic options for MF and SS, there is a lack of well-designed, prospective, controlled clinical trials comparing the efficacy and safety of various therapies. Many studies use skin response as the primary endpoint only while others used composite or global responses as the primary endpoint. As a result, caution is needed when interpreting efficacy data such as duration of response and time to response. The most important factor in designing a treatment plan is the clinical stage (Figs. 10.3, 10.4, 10.5, 10.6, 10.7, and 10.8). Selection of a specific treatment plan is based on the clinical stage, additional prognostic factors (e.g., folliculotropism or large cell transformation), toxicities associated with the treatment options, the patient's age, and other social and medical problems. The NCCN as well as the European Organisation for the Research and Treatment of Cancer (EORTC)

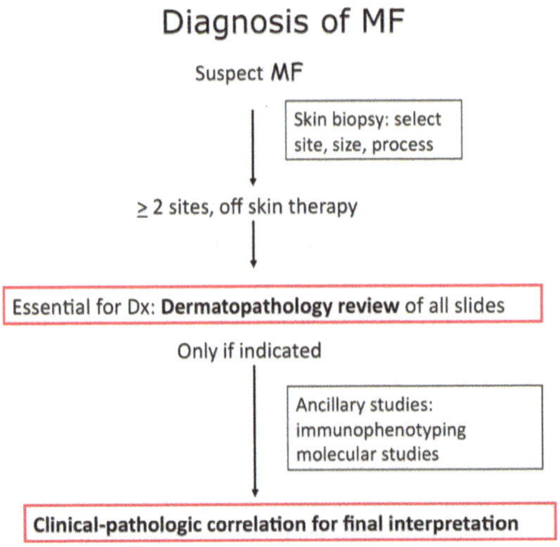

Fig. 10.3 Diagnosis of MF

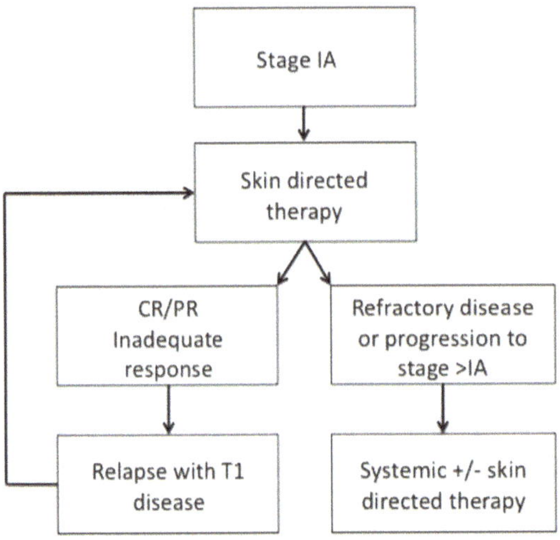

Fig. 10.4 Therapy schematic for mycosis fungoides, IA

outline the treatment guidelines for MF and SS according to stage of disease [30]. In considering all possible therapeutic options for a given stage of disease, retrospective cohort as well prospective studies were reviewed. Subsequently, the studies were evaluated using the U.S. Preventive Services Task Force: Hierarchy of Evidence [31].

In general, the treatment options in MF/SS are categorized into skin-directed treatments, systemic biologic/non-cytotoxic therapies, and systemic cytotoxic chemotherapies. For patients with T1 and T2 disease without extracutaneous involvement, stages IA–IIA, the primary treatment plan will usually be limited to skin-directed therapies. However, if these fail or there is histologic evidence of either large cell transformation or folliculotropism, a more intensive regimen is usually indicated. With respect to tumor disease, stage IIB, the treatment plan depends on the extent of the tumor lesions. If the tumor lesions are few in number, the skin-directed treatment options for stage IA-IIA are indicated, and the tumor lesions should be treated with local radiation. In cases with extensive tumor involvement, total skin electron beam therapy (TSEBT) or systemic therapies are considered. The affected skin in patients with erythroderma (T4) is very sensitive and may not tolerate skin-directed treatment. Hence, primary therapy for patients with erythroderma consists of the use of systemic biologic response modifiers (e.g., photopheresis, and oral retinoids/rexinoids, interferons [IFNs]), histone deacetylase inhibitors (HDAC-i), denileukin diftitox (fusion toxin), or low-dose methotrexate monotherapy or in combination. When biologic therapies fail in patients with refractory stage IIB to IV disease, single-agent chemotherapy such as gemcitabine, liposomal doxorubicin or Pralatrexate is considered.

Effective supportive care is critical in the management of patients with T4 disease. Increased susceptibility to bacterial and viral infection is a considerable source of morbidity and mortality. Patients with this type of compromise to the skin barrier should have diligent surveillance for skin infections, especially *Staphylococcus aureus* and herpes simplex virus. There is a low threshold for beginning systemic and skin-directed antibacterial agents with the appropriate susceptibilities.

Mycosis Fungoides and SS are associated with severe pruritus, which can be a serious detriment to patient quality of life. The measurement of this very subjective symptom is important to assess improvements in itching. It is important to attempt to quantify the severity of pruritus using a tool such as a visual analog scale. The Visual Analog Scale is a line with the numbers one (representing minimal itch) through ten (representing the worst itch), and it is the most common assessment tool utilized in the assessment of pruritus in clinical trials. However,

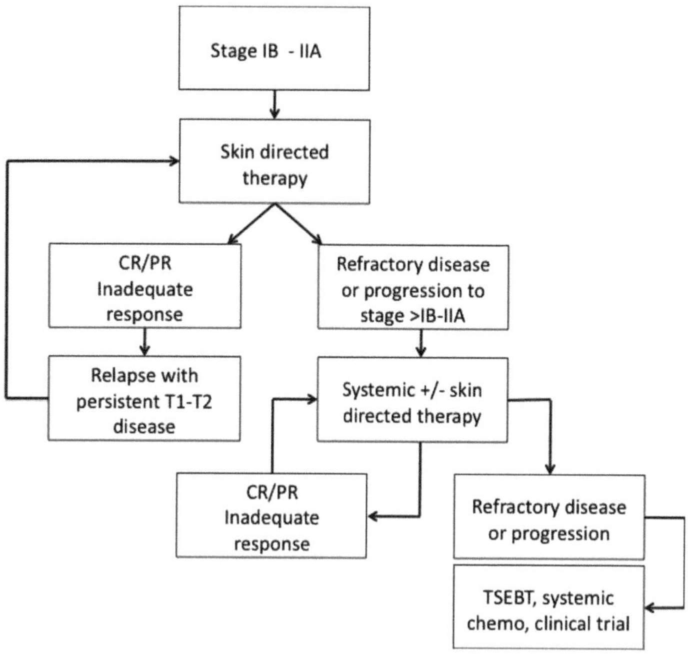

Fig. 10.5 Therapy schematic for mycosis fungoides, IB-IIA

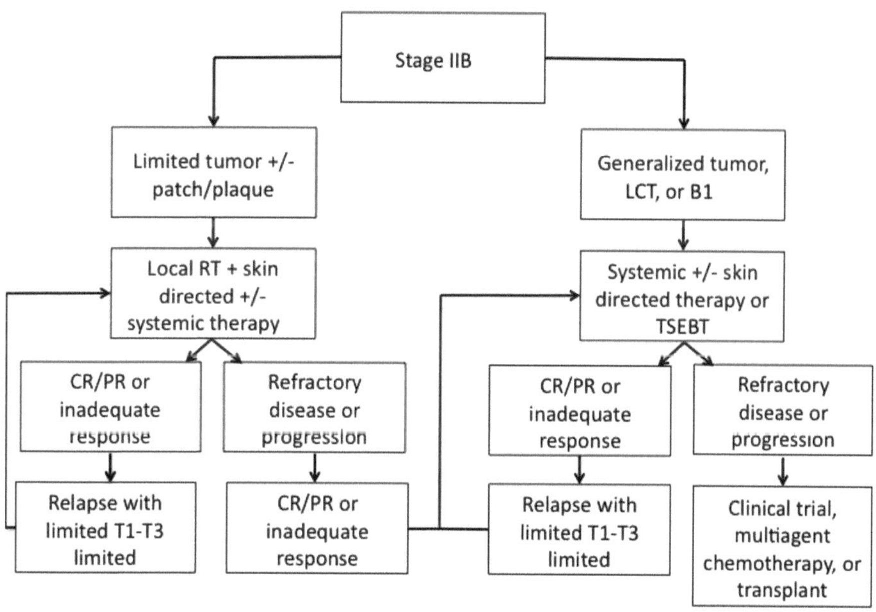

Fig. 10.6 Therapy schematic for mycosis fungoides, IIB

a more rigorous validated tool is needed for clinical trials. The effective symptomatic treatment of pruritus is of utmost importance, especially in SS. Most often, occlusive medium potency topical steroids and oral anti-itch measures such as gabapentin and mirtazapine are used [32].

Combination chemotherapy is generally reserved for patients with refractory lymph node

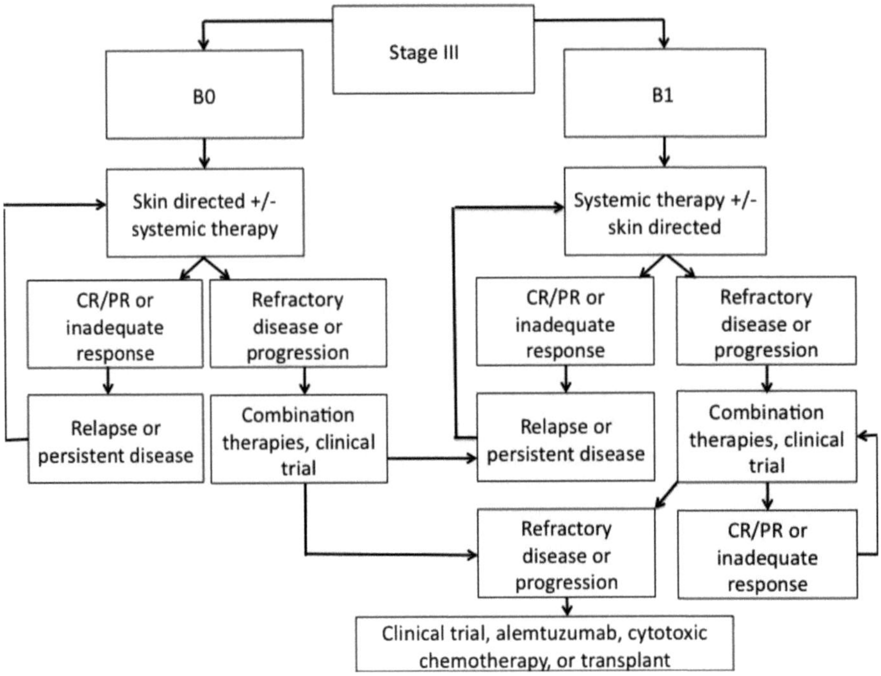

Fig. 10.7 Therapy schematic for mycosis fungoides, III

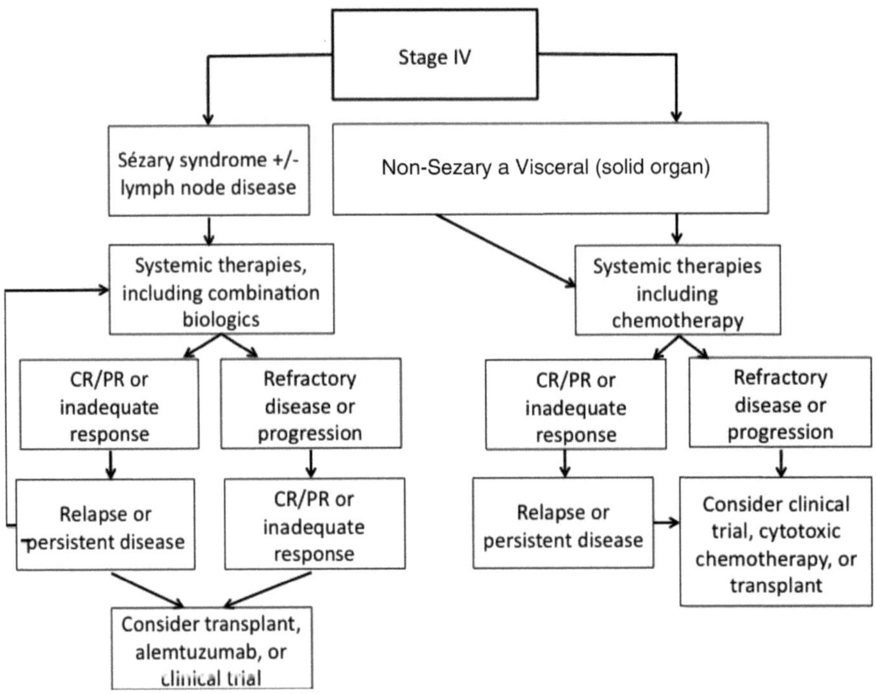

Fig. 10.8 Therapy schematic for mycosis fungoides, IV

or visceral (solid organ) disease. Patients with advanced disease in whom primary treatment fails are candidates for potential allogeneic stem cell transplantation. There is no evidence that early aggressive systemic therapy is better than conservative therapy in the management of limited disease. There is a definite need for more reliably effective therapies, especially in advanced cases of the disease. As a result, participation in clinical trials is critical for patients with advanced disease who have failed primary systemic therapies. It is important to consider allogenic stem cell transplant in patients with advanced disease as this may offer a long-lasting remission or possible cure.

Skin-Directed Therapies

Despite advances in treatment for MF and SS, traditional skin-directed therapies are still used as the primary therapeutic modality in the majority of patients with stage I–IIA disease. In patients where initial skin-directed therapy has failed or in those with severely symptomatic disease, skin-directed therapies can be combined with systemic treatments, or the patients may be referred for experimental therapy.

Topical Corticosteroid Therapy

Topical steroids can be used either as primary treatment in patients with limited patch or thin plaque disease, or they can be combined with other skin-directed treatments for added symptomatic control. The rationale for use of corticosteroids in MF is that they inhibit lymphocyte binding to endothelium and intercellular adhesion [33]. In addition, they also induce apoptosis of neoplastic lymphoid cells [34].

For patients with very limited skin involvement, topical corticosteroids can be a very cost-effective option for disease control. Application of topical steroids as treatment is generally performed once to twice a day to affected areas [35]. The percentage of complete clearance in patients with T1 disease is 63% and in T2 disease is 25% [35]. However, all patients with complete clearance had patch disease only [35]. The efficacy of topical steroids it not diminished over time and can be used again in the event of disease relapse. The benefit is that topical steroids can be used again for relapse of disease. However, long-term use of topical corticosteroids in any disease may lead to epidermal atrophy, striae, dyspigmentation, and steroid addiction. In particular clinical morphologic subsets of MF, such as the poikilodermatous MF, it may be difficult to interpret resolution of disease when topical steroids are used. In this variant, the clinical findings of telangiectasias and atrophy are the same as the side effects induced by prolonged use of topical corticosteroids. Hence, caution should be used in interpretation of disease vs. side effect of therapy.

Topical Chemotherapy

Topical nitrogen mustard (mechlorethamine hydrochloride) is the major form of topical chemotherapy used for MF and SS [36]. Topical carmustine (BCNU) has also been used [37].

Nitrogen mustard is the most widely utilized topical chemotherapeutic agent for MF because of its well-demonstrated efficacy, safety, and ease of application. The mechanism of action of nitrogen mustard in MF is unclear but may be mediated by immune mechanisms (e.g., immune stimulation) or by interaction with the epidermal Langerhans cell [36].

Topical nitrogen mustard preparation is applied to the skin once daily as initial therapy. If the disease is localized, the application field may be limited to the regional area of involvement or to the entire skin surface for those patients with generalized skin involvement. The initial concentration used is usually 20 mg%. Other areas of disease activity may become evident secondary to the inflammatory reaction provoked by the nitrogen mustard. After a period of several weeks, treatment may be limited to the affected region. Alternatively, if the disease is initially limited in distribution, the nitrogen mustard may be applied only to the affected anatomic region or regions, with careful follow-up to detect any new areas of involvement. Treatment is continued on a daily basis until skin clearance is complete. This may require 6 months or longer and is then followed by a variable duration of maintenance therapy

(3–6 months). If response is particularly slow, the concentration of the topical nitrogen mustard may be increased to 30 or 40 mg%. In addition, the frequency of application may be increased. The complete response rate for topical nitrogen mustard for limited patch or plaque (T1) disease is 70–80%. The median time to skin clearance is 6–8 months. When treatment is discontinued, more than one-half of patients will relapse in the skin, but most will respond to a resumption of therapy. The proportion of patients treated with topical nitrogen mustard who have a durable complete response (longer than 10 years) is 20–25%. In patients with a discrete number of refractory lesions, treatment may be supplemented with local irradiation. Once complete skin clearance is achieved with topical nitrogen mustard, a maintenance regimen of some kind is usually instituted, but there is no evidence that more prolonged maintenance is beneficial [36, 38, 39].

Both acute and chronic complications have been associated with topical nitrogen mustard therapy. The most frequent acute complication is an immediate or delayed cutaneous hypersensitivity reaction. It occurs in less than 10% of patients treated with the ointment-based preparation of nitrogen mustard. However, patients can be desensitized with a variety of topical or systemic desensitizing regimens [36, 39].

Chronic use of topical nitrogen mustard is not associated with increased risk of secondary cutaneous malignancies [36]. However, in patients who have used topical nitrogen mustard in combination or sequentially with other skin-damaging therapies (e.g., ultraviolet [UV] phototherapy, radiation therapy), there is an increased risk for non-melanoma skin cancers [40, 41]. Application of nitrogen mustard in the genital areas should be strictly avoided since genital application has been linked with development of secondary skin cancers. Topical Nitrogen Mustard can be used safely in pediatric patients, and studies have not shown worse adverse effects in children [36]. There is no evidence of significant systemic absorption of the medication.

Another topical chemotherapeutic agent that has been used for patients with limited disease is carmustine (BCNU). The efficacy of topical BCNU is similar to topical nitrogen mustard. BCNU can be used in solution or ointment form [37, 38]. Similar to nitrogen mustard, it can be applied to regional areas for localized disease or to the entire skin surface for generalized disease. 86% of patients with T1 were completely clear after a median of 9 weeks of use, while 47% with T2 disease were clear after a median of 11.5 weeks [42]. Contact should be avoided with the eyes or orifices [42]. There are both cutaneous and hematologic side effects. The majority of patients experience a degree of erythema accompanied by a burning sensation. This tends to localize to the intertriginous areas. It usually subsides with the use of topical corticosteroids and cool compresses. More severe erythematous reactions can lead to the development of telangiectasias that can persist for several years. Because of the systemic absorption of BCNU, the potential hematologic complications are greater, and the maximum duration of treatment is limited. Five percent of patients treating the general body surface had mild leukopenia. Other adverse hematological side effects have not been observed [42].

Topical corticosteroids, nitrogen mustard, and BCNU are indicated as initial primary therapy for patients with stage IA or IB disease. Topical chemotherapy should be considered as an alternative for those patients who are candidates for phototherapy but prefer the convenience of home application or already have a significant amount of photodamage.

Phototherapy

Phototherapy involves using UV radiation in the form of UVA or UVB wavelengths. It can be used alone or in combination with psoralen, a photosensitizing agent. Psoralen used with UVA (PUVA) is also referred to as photochemotherapy. PUVA therapy is widely used in dermatology for various dermatoses such as psoriasis. Psoralens intercalate between pyrimidines within DNA and, upon exposure to UVA, form photoadducts and DNA crosslinks [43]. This process results in cytotoxic, antiproliferative, and immunomodulatory effects. The long-wave UVA has an advantage over UVB because of its greater depth of penetration. This is useful in that while MF is defined as an epidermotropic process, a considerable amount of neoplastic infiltrate is still in the dermis.

PUVA is indicated as primary therapy in generalized plaque and erythrodermic MF without evidence of extracutaneous disease. It is also used as palliative therapy in combination with another treatment in patients with advanced disease. Initially, PUVA treatments are given 2–3 times per week, with a minimum of 48 h between treatments to monitor the delayed erythema reaction [44]. The initial dose of UVA and the rate at which the dose is increased are generally dependent upon the skin type. Erythrodermic patients tend to require very low starting doses with very small dose increments. After maximal response, the frequency of PUVA treatments is decreased.

Both acute and chronic adverse effects have been observed with PUVA therapy [44]. Nausea from psoralen ingestion is observed in 10–20% of patients and can be managed by ingesting the drug with food or milk, or with appropriate antiemetics [43]. Phototoxic reactions can range from erythema to the development of bullae. Ultraviolet-opaque goggles must be worn during the UVA irradiation. Long-term PUVA therapy with high cumulative doses has been linked to an increased risk for the development of squamous cell carcinomas [45, 46], pigmented macules [47], and cataract formation [45]. Up to one-third of patients treated with PUVA develop signs of chronic photodamage and secondary cutaneous malignancies. After each PUVA treatment, appropriate photoprotection, including application of sunscreens, protective clothing, and UV-shielding glasses, should be used for a minimum of 24 h.

UVB therapy is a widely used alternative to PUVA. While broadband has been used, it has been supplanted with light limited to the 311 nm wavelength known as narrowband UVB (NBUVB). The use of NBUVB does not require the ingestion of psoralen prior to therapy, which is advantageous in patients that have problems tolerating the medication. Similar to PUVA, it is performed 2–3 times per week with 24 h between treatments. NBUVB is considered to have less toxicity than broadband UVB or PUVA since the penetration of UVB is reduced. The clearance rate of NBUVB is T1 and T2 disease is 70–80% and is the same with PUVA [48].

Topical Retinoid and Rexinoid Therapy

Retinoids modulate gene expression by activating nuclear retinoic acid receptors (RARs) and retinoid X receptors (RXRs). This leads to alterations in cell differentiation, proliferation, and apoptosis [49]. These properties have prompted investigation into their use as antineoplastic agents. Broad-spectrum retinoids have an affinity for RARs but exhibit poor tissue specificity and low activity. There is a derivative category of agents, known as rexinoids, which specifically activate the RXR receptors and have a lower affinity for RAR receptors. A rexinoid agent commonly used in MF is bexarotene. Although the molecular basis of bexarotene has not been clearly elucidated, it has been shown to induce apoptosis in CTCL lines [50].

Bexarotene 1% gel, a rexinoid, is the most commonly used topical retinoid for treating MF. The medication is typically applied as a thin film to the patches or plaques. It is most effective and best tolerated when used twice daily [51]. The reported overall response rate is 63%, with a complete response rate of 21% [52]. Due to the irritant effect of the rexinoids, it is only feasible to use this agent when there is limited number of patches or plaques. It is not intended for generalized application. The most common toxicity of bexarotene gel is irritation at the sites of application and occurs in the majority of patients [51]. The irritation commonly occurs in flexural areas affected by MF. Because of the erythema from the irritant reaction, it may be necessary to withhold therapy for a few weeks to assess disease activity.

Tazarotene 0.1% gel, a RAR agonist, has also been evaluated in a pilot study [53]. The gel was applied daily to discrete lesions only. Use of the gel to lesions resulted in a 35% clearance rate [53]. Mild to moderate local irritation was the most common adverse event in the majority of patients (84%). Any associated irritation was relieved by decreasing the frequency to every other day application or the use of a mid-potency steroid [53].

Imiquimod

Imiquimod is a topical immunomodulator that has been approved by the Food and Drug Administration (FDA) for the treatment of genital warts. The drug is believed to function in part through the induction of local IFN production [54]. Because systemic IFN is effective in the treatment of MF, it has been hypothesized that topical imiquimod might also be effective while sparing patients the systemic side effects of IFN treatment. An open-label, pilot study used 5% imiquimod cream to localized patches and plaques of MF. Of the six patients, three had complete histologic clearance [55]. Imiquimod was generally well-tolerated, and skin irritation was limited to lesions, which ultimately cleared with treatment.

Radiation Therapy

Mycosis fungoides is an extremely radiosensitive neoplasm. Individual plaques or tumors can be treated with local electron beam therapy (EBT) to total doses of 12–36 Gy, with a high complete response rates. The widespread use of total-skin EBT (TSEBT) was facilitated by the development of the modern medical linear accelerator. TSEBT has been developed to treat patients with extensive cutaneous disease [56]. Radiation is administered four times a week to a total dose of 30–36 Gy. A full "cycle" of treatment is administered over a 2-day period. The dose administered with each cycle is 1.5–2.0 Gy. Most patients will tolerate 2.0 Gy per cycle, but lower doses are used for patients with erythroderma, atrophic skin, or a previous course of EBT.

The treatment course is 8–10 weeks in duration. During each treatment session, patients assume multiple positions to ensure that the entire skin surface is irradiated. Supplementary treatment is required for the soles of the feet, perineum, and inframammary areas. Also, some patients with a discrete number of tumorous lesions will receive boost treatment to these tumors at the outset of EBT to reduce their thickness and permit better penetration by the electrons. The eyes are shielded routinely, but other areas may be protected over the course of the treatment to help control localized skin reactions.

TSEBT should be considered as initial therapy for patients with generalized very thickened plaque or tumorous disease, because the effective depth of treatment of EBT is more substantial than either topical nitrogen mustard or phototherapy. It is also appropriate palliative therapy for patients with a recent history of rapid progression of disease and for those patients for whom topical nitrogen mustard, bexarotene gel, or phototherapy was not effective. Although the curative potential of this treatment remains disputed, there is no doubt that it provides an important palliative benefit, especially for patients with extensive disease. Often, when disease recurs, it is in a more limited distribution and may be controlled more readily with localized topical therapies. Generally, after completion of TSEBT, adjuvant treatment with topical nitrogen mustard with or without systemic adjuvant (e.g., oral bexarotene, photopheresis) is indicated and may be continued for up to 6–12 months. Several centers have developed expertise in the use of TSEBT [56]. Overall response rates are nearly 100%, with complete response rates ranging from 40 to 98% depending on the extent of skin involvement. As many as 50% of patients with limited plaque disease and 25% of patients with generalized plaque disease may remain free of disease for longer than 5 years after completion of a single course of EBT [1, 56, 57]. Up to two courses of TSEBT may be administered over the course of a lifetime, which can limit its use in long-term management of the disease [58].

In patients who have lymph node involvement or in some situations of localized visceral disease, megavoltage (4–15 MeV) photon irradiation may be helpful in providing important additional palliation. Doses of 24–36 Gy in 3–4 weeks are often sufficient to achieve local control of lymph nodes or other extracutaneous sites of disease. This is often combined with systemic chemotherapy or biologic therapy (IFN-α or bexarotene), depending on the extent of the extracutaneous involvement.

Short-term side effects associated with TSEBT include acute erythema, desquamation, temporary nail and hair loss, and an impaired ability to perspire properly for up to 12 months. Long term, there is an increased risk of secondary squamous cell and basal cell carcinomas of the skin. The risk of secondary malignancies is greatest in those who have received long courses of therapy with other skin-damaging therapies such as phototherapy [43].

Systemic Therapies

Systemic therapies are indicated when skin-directed primary therapies fail or in aggressive or advanced MF cases. Patients with significant numbers of circulating Sézary cells should also be placed on a systemic therapy as part of their treatment regimen. Therapeutic efforts are focused on targeted biologic agents that promote apoptosis and manipulate the host immune response. The combination of either a biologic agent with a skin-directed therapy or the combination of multiple biologic agents results in improved disease control by acting in a synergistic manner. Toxicity can also be reduced in combination regimens as lower doses are required for each therapeutic modality.

Biologic Therapies

Extracorporeal Photopheresis

Extracorporeal photopheresis (ECP) is considered first line therapy for patients with Sézary cell blood involvement. ECP delivers psoralen and UVA radiation systemically by utilizing an extracorporeal technique [59]. White blood cells are collected in a clear container (leukapheresis) and exposed to psoralen. The cells are then irradiated with UVA (PUVA). The irradiated cells are returned to the patient in a closed system. The ECP instrument performs the leukapheresis and delivers the UVA. The mechanism of action of ECP involves induction of malignant T cell apoptosis with PUVA, which is accompanied by the enhancement of a tumor-specific immune response. ECP also induces monocytes to differentiate into dendritic cells capable of phagocytosing and processing the apoptotic tumor cell antigens [9, 60].

A standard complete ECP regimen for CTCL consists of 2 consecutive days of therapy repeated at 2–4-week intervals. The frequency of administration is adjusted according to disease severity and/or clinical response. After a maximal, stable response has been achieved, the frequency of treatments is gradually decreased, and then stopped completely, unless the disease relapses or flares during the weaning process, or when maintenance therapy is given. Maintenance therapy is given every 4–6 weeks; a repeat attempt at weaning can be made at a later time. If an adequate response is not attained with ECP monotherapy, or if patients have a significant level of circulating Sézary cells, additional biologic agents should be added. These can include IFN or systemic retinoid. A minimum of 4–6 months of treatment should be given before ECP is considered a failure. The overall response rate is 70–80% [61, 62].

An advantage of ECP is its limited side effect profile. One of the greatest advantages of ECP is that the adverse effects are minimal [59]. Common side effects include mild fatigue associated with leukapheresis and fluid shifts. Peripheral intravenous access for treatment is preferable to central access to minimize complications. There are no significant side effects in terms of laboratory parameters. Patients receive psoralen, and need to protect their eyes and skin from UV exposure for 24 h after treatment. ECP has been shown to be most effective in patients with blood involvement, particularly those with SS [61, 63].

Interferon-Alpha

IFN therapy is indicated for refractory or advanced disease and is often combined with other skin directed or systemic therapies. IFN was originally discovered by Isaacs and Lindenmann [64]. It is a protein expressing virus non-specific antiviral activity [65]. Based on antigenic proteins, IFNs are divided into three main groups: IFN-alpha, IFN-beta, and IFN-gamma. IFN-alpha and beta bind to IFN type I receptor while IFN-gamma binds to the IFN type II receptor. IFN-alpha preparations are primarily used in the treatment of CTCL [66]. IFN-gamma has been used rarely as an alternative in patients who have developed resistance to IFN-alpha [66].

IFN-alpha induces a variety of immunologic effects that may lead to clinical response [9]. It directly enhances cell-mediated cytotoxicity by $CD8^+$ T cells and NK cells which augments the antitumor response. It also suppresses TH2 cytokine production by malignant T cells, which can lead to enhanced immunomodulation.

IFNs are administered intramuscularly or subcutaneously with a maximum plasma concentration 6–8 h after administration [66]. There are multiple regimens used. Traditionally, IFN-alpha is started at lower doses, such as 1–3 MU three times per week subcutaneously and titrated up as tolerated. However, because of the numerous associated side effects, it is typically not used as monotherapy. Rather, it is used in combination with ECP, systemic retinoids, methotrexate, and phototherapy in an effort to limit side effects. When used in combination, it is a first line therapy for advanced MF and SS.

The dosage of IFN-a for mycosis fungoides is usually initiated at 3–5 million units daily or three times per week and is gradually increased, depending on the clinical response and the severity of adverse effects. Reported overall response rates when used as monotherapy are 53–74%, with complete response rates of 21–35% [67, 68].

The adverse effects of IFN can prohibit its use in some patient populations such as the elderly. The most common side effects include fevers, chills, tachycardia, malaise, myalgias, and headaches that are part of the general flu-like syndrome [69]. The flu-like syndrome seems to decrease in intensity with time [68]. However, in patients on low-dose intermittent therapy, acetaminophen is able to control the symptoms. Hematological side effects primarily involve leukocytes, platelets and erythrocytes. Leukopenia occurs within hours of exposure, and often stabilizes around 40–60% of the normal leukocyte count. The recovery of granulocyte and lymphocyte counts is rather rapid after discontinuation of IFN therapy [69]. Prolonged IFN therapy often results in normocytic normochromic anemia, which in contrast to the IFN-induced leukopenia, has a slow recovery. Thrombocytopenia is also an observed side effect especially in patients with hematological malignancies [69].

Retinoids

Systemic retinoids are indicated primarily in patients with advanced disease and can be used as monotherapy or as part of combination regimens with skin-directed or other biologic therapies. They are also used in early stage, refractory disease.

The most commonly used systemic retinoid is a RXR agonist, bexarotene; however, RAR agonists, such as isotretinoin, acitretin, or all-*trans* retinoic acid, are available as alternative agents [70]. Much of the molecular basis of the mechanism of action of bexarotene is unknown. However, it has been shown to induce apoptosis in CTCL lines and T lymphocytes from Sézary patients [50, 71]. In addition, patients who have responded to bexarotene had higher $CD8^+$ cell counts after therapy [72]. The initial dose of oral bexarotene is 300 mg/m^2/day, which can be adjusted according to the clinical response, patients; comorbidity risk, and the severity of adverse effects.

The reported response rate is approximately 45–55%, with a 10–20% complete response rate depending on the dose of bexarotene and the severity of disease [52, 73].

There is a common toxicity profile for the different forms of retinoids, and many of these adverse effects are dose dependent. Most commonly, patients experience photosensitivity and dryness of the skin and mucous membranes. Other adverse effects include myalgia, arthralgia, hyperlipidemic, and fatigue, and less commonly, headaches. On rare occasions, headaches can be caused by pseudotumor cerebri. The well-known teratogenic effects of retinoids must be carefully addressed in female patients of childbearing age. Potential long-term, cumulative toxicity of retinoids includes the development of bony changes such as hyperostosis. Bexarotene also has unique effects on the pituitary-thyroid axis, which results in hypothyroidism with low free thyroxine (FT4) and low thyroid-stimulating hormone (TSH) levels.

Bexarotene is a selective agonist for RXR receptors. The receptors can form homodimers and heterodimers with RARs as well as with other nuclear receptors such as vitamin D receptors and thyroid receptors. Due to the formation of heterodimers, the use of bexarotene affects the thyroid receptors leading to central hypothyroidism.

Because of their potential hepatotoxic and hyperlipidemic effects, liver function and serum lipid levels (triglycerides/cholesterol) should be monitored during treatment. Bexarotene also has more profound effects on serum lipid levels, especially triglycerides, than any other retinoid. Thus, it is conventional to have patients on lipid-lowering agents and thyroid supplements during bexarotene therapy. These are ideally started in the week prior to beginning bexarotene therapy. Gemfibrizol is contraindicated with bexarotene due to increased plasma levels of bexarotene and higher triglyceride levels. In addition, several patients were known to develop pancreatitis in early clinical trials [73]. The preferred lipid-lowering drugs are of the statin or fenofibrate class of agents [74]. Toxicities associated with systemic retinoids are usually reversible upon cessation of therapy.

Retinoids can be combined with skin-directed such as PUVA or with other systemic agents including IFN-alpha, ECP, or denileukin diftitox therapy. Combination therapies often have better efficacy and safety profiles when compared to the use of individual biologic agents alone [9].

Recombinant Fusion Proteins

Denileukin difitox is a recombinant cytotoxic fusion protein that targets the IL-2 receptor on T-cells. It is indicated for use in patients with advanced, persistent and recurrent MF and SS [75–77]. This recombinant fusion protein combines the receptor-binding domain of IL-2 with diphtheria toxin. Once the molecule is bound to the IL-2 receptor, it is taken up by endocytosis, and the diphtheria toxin is cleaved. This leads to inhibition of protein synthesis and results in killing of defined neoplastic cell populations [78].

Denileukin difitox is administered intravenously for 5 consecutive days and repeated every 3 weeks at daily doses of 9 or 18 μg/kg over 1 h. Ontak has undergone a multicenter phase III trial in patients with IL-2 receptor (CD25$^+$)-expressing mycosis fungoides [75]. Patients with intermediate or advanced stages of disease were included in the phase III trial. The overall response rate was 30%, with complete-response and partial-response rates of 10% and 20%, respectively. Toxicities include fever, chills, nausea, a "capillary leak" syndrome, which may be ameliorated by pre- and post-treatment hydration, and a hypersensitivity reaction, which can be countered with premedication with corticosteroids [77, 78].

Bexarotene upregulates IL-2 receptors expression on T-cells. Hence, the use of bexarotene may lead to more enhanced binding of denileukin difitox and greater effectiveness [79].

Histone Deacetylase Inhibitors

HDAC-i are a novel class of agents. HDAC inhibition results in acetylation of histone and non-histone proteins leading to a transcriptionally active chromatin and activation of gene expression [80]. Defective histone-acetylation enzymes have been identified in malignant cells [81, 82]; hence, HDAC-i may have anticancer properties through the restoration of normal acetylation.

There are two HDAC-i used in advanced, refractory, and relapsed MF and SS. The first is vorinostat. It is generally used as monotherapy, but it can be used in combination with other skin directed and systemic agents. However, there is no data for the use of combination therapy involving HDAC-i, and caution is needed with regards to safety and efficacy. Vorinostat is an oral agent that is dosed orally at 400 mg daily. The clinical efficacy and safety was studied in a multicenter trial followed by United States FDA approval for the treatment of cutaneous manifestations of cutaneous T-cell lymphoma in patients with refractory disease [83, 84]. The overall response rate was 30% with no complete responses.

The most common side effects are gastrointestinal (nausea, vomiting, diarrhea), constitutional, hematologic, and taste disorders [83]. HDAC-i can potentially prolong QTc; thus, any electrolyte abnormalities should be corrected to minimize complications. This is especially relevant in patients with a history of heart disease. Other serious side effects to monitor include thromboembolic events, gastrointestinal hemorrhage, ischemic stroke, and thrombocytopenia [83].

A second HDAC-i, romidepsin, is FDA-approved for use in CTCL. It is an intravenous drug used which is primarily used as monotherapy. It is given on days 1, 8, and 15 of a 28-day cycle at a dose of 14 mg/m^2. Toxicities are similar to those in seen in vorinostat [85]. The same monitoring recommendations are applicable to vorinostat and romidepsin. A clinically meaningful response is seen in up to one-third of patients. In advanced disease, global response rates were higher with romidepsin than vorinostat [83, 84, 86].

Monoclonal Antibody Therapy

One of the most effective monoclonal antibodies used in the treatment of advanced disease such as erythrodermic (T4) MF and SS is alemtuzumab. It is reserved for those patients with advanced disease in whom other traditional therapies have failed. It is a humanized IgG antibody directed against CD52 [78]. CD52 is expressed on T-lymphocytes, B-lymphocytes, natural killer cells, monocyte, and malignant T-cells in CTCL [87, 88]. The mechanism through which alemtuzumab exerts its clinical effect is not well known, but likely includes apoptosis [89], antibody-dependent cellular cytotoxicity [90, 91], and complement mediated cell lysis [92, 93].

In the standard therapeutic schedule used in other lymphomas, such as chronic lymphocytic leukemia, T-cell prolymphocytic leukemia, and peripheral T-cell lymphoma, escalating doses from 3 to 10 mg and then to 30 mg are administered on alternating days followed by 30 mg three times per week for 12 weeks [94–97]. However, evidence suggests that low dose intermittent alemtuzumab (3 mg on day 1 with 10 mg on days administered subcutaneously thereafter), has equal efficacy and durable remissions with less toxicity [98]. Alemtuzumab is more efficacious in patients with SS. One of the goals of therapy is to keep the Sézary cell count <1,000 mm^3. The overall response rate for advanced disease is 28% and the duration of response is less than 3 months [99].

Complications of alemtuzumab include serious infections such as cytomegalovirus, generalized herpes simplex virus, fatal fungal and mycobacterial infections. Thus, prophylactic regimen of antivirals, antifungals, and antibacterials are typically utilized with alemtuzumab therapy [99]. In addition, other hematologic toxicities occur, such as severe neutropenia, thrombocytopenia, and anemia [99].

Systemic Cytotoxic Therapy (Chemotherapy)

Systemic chemotherapy is appropriate for patients with large cell transformed stage IIB MF and stage IV MF with extracutaneous involvement. Most chemotherapeutic regimens, however, result in only temporary palliative responses. Multiple single-agent and combination chemotherapies have been tried in advanced MF and SS. For single-agent chemotherapy, no particular drug has been shown to be superior and no large, randomized studies comparing agents have been reported. Single agent chemotherapy is more widely utilized in MF/SS. Combination regimens are largely reserved as salvage after single agent therapy has failed or if there is solid organ involvement.

While typically used in advanced MF and SS, methotrexate has been used in lower doses for extensive stage IB disease. Methotrexate inhibits dihydrofolate reductase (DHFR), leading to the subsequent inhibition of DNA synthesis [100]. Multiple dose ranges and schedules have been used as therapy in erythrodermic MF (T4) and SS. No clear benefit has been demonstrated for higher doses compared to lower doses of methotrexate. Side effects observed with the use of methotrexate include elevated serum aminotransferase levels (which are usually reversible after dose reduction or withdrawal), oral mucositis, pharyngeal mucositis, gastrointestinal complications such as nausea and diarrhea, interstitial pulmonary fibrosis, and uncommonly, reversible leucopenia [101]. More recently, newer antifolate prolatrexate has been shown to have clinical activity is relapsed on refractory MF or SS with less intensive dose regimen than systemic peripheral T- cell lymphoma.

Gemcitabine, a novel nucleoside analog, is activated by deoxycytidine kinase to its triphosphate form, gemcitabine triphosphate, which is then incorporated into RNA and DNA. The latter causes chain termination and inhibition of DNA repair, which is responsible for antitumor effect of the medication. Response rates as high as 70% have been reported, but the complete remission rate is low with a median duration of complete remission of 10 months (range 4–22 months) [102]. Recently this agent has been used as front-line therapy for patients in whom control is needed of massive lymph node disease. Gemcitabine is generally well tolerated, even in the elderly population. Myelosuppression with resulting anemia, thrombocytopenia, or leukopenia are the most common adverse events [102]. Cutaneous adverse events include flares of lesional erythema within 1 week of treatment as well as generalized hyperpigmentation [102]. Serious adverse events are rare.

Doxorubicin is an anthracycline agent used in advanced stages of MF and SS. Pegylated liposomal doxorubicin is a formulation of doxorubicin that is encapsulated into liposomes. The liposomes serve as stable, long-circulating carriers useful for delivering doxorubicin to tumor sites with a lower toxicity than the free drug. The most frequent side effects are mild anemia and lymphopenia. Another significant toxicity with this class of drugs is palmoplantar erythrodysesthesia [103].

Another cytotoxic agent is temozolomide, which has shown encouraging activity in advanced MF. It is an imidazotetrazine derivative and oral alkylating agent that has excellent oral bioavailability [104]. Its mechanism of action is similar to that of other alkylating agents, which induce DNA damage by cross-linking. Resistance has been associated with high levels of the scavenger protein O6-alkylguanine-DNA alkyltransferase in tumor cells. Response rates of 30% have been reported in stage IIB and III patients. In a phase II study, the most frequent adverse effects were nausea, vomiting, neutropenia, and thrombocytopenia [104].

In addition, other mechanisms to inhibit growth and encourage apoptosis of tumor cells are being developed. Bortezomib, which inhibits the proteasome, leads to the down-regulation of NF-KB activation and induction of CTCL cell apoptosis [105]. In a phase II trial, the response rate was 67% in all stages; however, the complete response rate was much lower at 10% [106]. With regard to hematologic adverse effects, neutropenia and thrombocytopenia were observed. The most significant non-hematologic toxicity was sensory neuropathy [106].

The purine analogs are a class of drugs that have demonstrated activity in MF and a variety of other NHL. T-cells have a high level of adenosine deaminase (ADA), a key enzyme in the purine degradation pathway. The purine analogs pentostatin, fludarabine, and 2-chloro-deoxyadenosine are a group of structurally similar agents, which were developed to target ADA. They have different interactions with ADA, but all result in DNA damage. Hematologic toxicity and opportunistic infections are the most common complications associated with this class of drugs. Prophylactic antibiotics against *Pneumocystis carinii* and antivirals to prevent herpes virus infection are routinely indicated [107].

Most of the patients treated with combination chemotherapy have failed single agent chemotherapy or have solid organ involvement (IIB to IV). There are no randomized trials comparing combination chemotherapy with single-agent regimens. The largest experience is with combinations such as cyclophosphamide, vincristine, and prednisone, with or without doxorubicin [108, 109]. Complete response rates are generally about 25% (range 11–57%) and response duration is 3–20 months.

Hematopoietic Stem Cell Transplantation

There has been recent interest in using hematopoietic stem cell transplantation (HSCT) in MF. Given the small number of patients treated thus far, there are no well-defined prognostic factors to identify patients suitable for this therapy. Bigler and associates reported that five of six patients achieved a complete response with an autologous transplant [110]. In another study, eight of nine patients achieved a complete response [111]. However, all of the patients in these studies ultimately relapsed, suggesting that autologous transplantation is not a curative approach.

The concept of allogeneic HSCT is promising. Even in the absence of a complete response, an allogeneic graft-versus-tumor effect may provide an immune mechanism to control the malignant T-cell process associated with mycosis fungoides. Molina and associates reported a complete response in all eight patients transplanted for refractory MF or SS. With a median follow-up of 56 months, six patients remained alive and without evidence of lymphoma [112]. Mild acute and chronic GVHD developed in all patients who survived. A non-myeloablative approach has also been reported in which all three patients who achieved a durable complete response [113].

It appears that compared to autologous HSCT, allogeneic HSCT may result in durable long-term remissions [114]. With better understanding of the disease biology, it may be possible to develop prognostic factors so that these aggressive approaches can be offered to suitable patients. Larger studies will be required to identify the best conditioning regimen, efficacy, safety, and impact on quality of life.

References

1. Chinn D, Chow S, Kim Y, Hoppe R. Total skin electron beam therapy with or without adjuvant topical nitrogen mustard or nitrogen mustard alone as initial treatment of T2 and T3 mycosis fungoides. Int J Radiat Oncol Biol Phys. 1999;43:951–8.
2. Criscione VD, Weinstock MA. Incidence of cutaneous T-cell lymphoma in the United States, 1973–2002. Arch Dermatol. 2007;143(7):854–9.
3. Crowley J, Nikko A, Varghese A, et al. Mycosis fungoides in young patients: clinical characteristics and outcome. J Am Acad Dermatol. 1998;38:696–701.
4. Kim Y, Liu H, Mraz-Gernhard S. Long-term outcome of 525 patients with mycosis fungoides and Sezary syndrome. Arch Dermatol. 2003;139:857–66.
5. Olsen A, Vonderheid E, Pimpinelli N. Revisions to the staging and classification of mycosis fungoides and Sezary syndrome: a proposal of the International Society for Cutaneous Lymphomas (ISCL) and the cutaneous lymphoma task force of the European Organization of Research and Treatment of Cancer (EORTC). Blood. 2007;110:1713–22.
6. Vonderheid E, Bernengo M, Burg G. Update on erythrodermic cutaneous T-cell lymphoma: report of the International Society for Cutaneous Lymphomas. J Am Acad Dermatol. 2002;46:95–106.
7. Willemze R, Jaffe E, Burg G, et al. WHO-EORTC classification for cutaneous lymphomas. Blood. 2005;105(10):3768–85.
8. Kim Y, Hoppe R. Mycosis fungoides and the Sezary syndrome. Semin Oncol. 1999;26:276–89.
9. Kim E, Hess S, Richardson S. Immunopathogenesis and therapy of cutaneous T-cell lymphoma. J Clin Invest. 2005;115:798–812.
10. Scarisbrick J, Woolford A, Russell-Jones R. Loss of heterozygosity on 10q and microsatellite instability in advanced stages of primary cutaneous T-cell lymphoma and possible association with homozygous deletion of PTEN. Blood. 2000;95:2937–42.
11. Immaculada C, Algara P, Mateo M. p16(INK4a) is selectively silenced in the tumoral progression of MF. Lab Invest. 2002;82:123–32.
12. Vermeer M, van Doorn R, Dijkman R, et al. Novel and highly recurrent chomosomal alterations in Sezary syndrome. Cancer Res. 2008;68(8):2689–98.
13. Shin J, Monti S, Aires D, et al. Lesional gene expression profiling in cutaneous T-cell lymphoma reveals natural clusters associated with disease outcome. Blood. 2007;110(8):3015–27.
14. Trotter M, Whittacker S, Orchard G, Smith N. Cutaneous histopathology of Sezary syndrome: a study of 41 cases with a proven circulating T-cell clone. J Cutan Pathol. 1997;24(5):286–91.
15. Zhang B, Beck A, Taube J, et al. Combined use of PCR-based TCRG and TCRB clonality tests on paraffin-embedded skin tissue in the differential diagnosis of mycosis fungoides and inflammatory dermatoses. J Mol Diagn. 2010;12(3):320–7.
16. Kohler S, Jones C, Warnke R. PCR-heteroduplex analysis of T-cell receptor gamma gene rearrangement in paraffin-embedded skin biopsies. Am J Dermatopathol. 2000;22:321–7.
17. Thurber S, Zhang B, Kim Y, Schrijver I, Zehnder J, Kohler S. T-cell clonality analysis in biopsy specimens from two different skin sites shows high specificity in the diagnosis of patients with suggested mycosis fungoides. J Am Acad Dermatol. 2007;57(5):782–90.
18. Sirois D, Miller A, Harwick R, Vonderheid E. Oral manifestations of cutaneous T-cell lymphoma. A report of eight cases. Oral Surg Oral Med Oral Pathol. 1993;75:700–5.
19. Zackheim H, Amin S, Kashani-Sabet M. Prognosis in cutaneous T-cell lymphoma by skins stage: long-term survival in 489 patients. J Am Acad Dermatol. 1999;40:418–25.
20. de Coninck E, Kim Y, Varghese A, Hoppe R. Clinical characteristics and outcome of patients with extracutaneous mycosis fungoides. J Clin Oncol. 2001;19:779–84.
21. Kim Y, Jensen R, Watanabe G. Clinical stage IA (limited patch and plaque) mycosis fungoides. A long-term outcome analysis. Arch Dermatol. 1996;132:1309–13.
22. van Doorn D, van Haselen C, van Voorst Vader P. Mycosis fungoides: disease evolution and prognosis of 309 Dutch patients. Arch Dermatol. 2000;136:504–10.
23. Tsai E, Taur A, Espinosa L, et al. Staging accuracy in mycosis fungoides and sezary syndrome using integraed positron emission tomography and computed tomography. Arch Dermatol. 2006;142(5):577–84.
24. Salhany S, Greer J, Cousar J. Marrow involvement in cutaneous T-cell lymphoma. A clinicopathologic study of 60 cases. Am J Clin Pathol. 1989;92:747–54.
25. Sausville E, Eddy J, Makuch R. Histopathologic staging at initial diagnosis of mycosis fungoides and

the Sezary syndrome. Definition of three distinctive prognostic groups. Ann Intern Med. 1988;109:372–82.
26. Kim Y, Bishop K, Varghese A. Prognostic factors in erythrodermic mycosis fungoides and the Sezary syndrome. Arch Dermatol. 1995;1995(131):1003–8.
27. Vergier B, de Muret N, Beylot-Barry M, et al. Transformation of mycosis fungoides: clinicopathological and prognostic features of 45 cases. Blood. 2000;95(7):2212–8.
28. Cerroni L, Rieger E, Hodl S. Clinicopathologic and immunologic features associated with transformation of mycosis fungoides to large-cell lymphoma. Am J Surg Pathol. 1992;16:543–52.
29. Salhany S, Cousar J, Greer J. Transformation of cutaneous T cell lymphoma to large cell lymphoma: a clinicopathologic and immunologic study. Am J Pathol. 1988;132:265–77.
30. Trautinger F, Knobler R, Willemze R. EORTC consensus recommendations for the treatment of mycosis fungoides/Sezary syndrome. Eur J Cancer. 2006;42:1014–30.
31. Harris R, Helfand M, Woolf S, Lohr K, Mulrow C, Teutsch S. Current methods of the US Preventative Services Task Force: a review of process. Am J Prev Med. 2001;20(3):21–35.
32. Demierre M, Taverna J. Mirtazapine and gabapentin for reducing pruritus in cutaneous T-cell lymphoma. J Am Acad Dermatol. 2006;55(3):543–4.
33. Pitzalis C, Pipitone N, Bajocchi G. Corticosteroids inhibit lymphocyte binding to endothelium and intercellular adhesion: an additional mechanism for their anti-inflammatory and immunosuppressive effect. J Immunol. 1997;158:5007–16.
34. Schwartzman R, Cidlowski J. Glucocorticoid-induced apoptosis of lymphoid cells. Int Arch Allergy Immunol. 1994;105:347–54.
35. Zackheim H, Kashani Sabet M, Amin S. Topical corticosteroids for mycosis fungoides: experience in 79 patients. Arch Dermatol. 1998;134:949–54.
36. Kim Y, Martinez G, Varghese A, Hoppe R. Topical nitrogen mustard in the management of mycosis fungoides: update of the Stanford experience. Arch Dermatol. 2003;139:165–73.
37. Zackheim H, Amin S, Kashani-Sabet M. Topical carmustine (BCNU) for cutaneous T-cell lymphoma: a 15-year experience in 143 patients. J Am Acad Dermatol. 1990;22:802–10.
38. Ramsay D, Halperin P, Zeleniuch-Jacquotte A. Topical mechlorethamine therapy for early stage mycosis fungoides. J Am Acad Dermatol. 1988;19:684–91.
39. Ramsay D, Meller J, Zackheim H. Topical treatment of early cutaneous T-cell lymphoma. Hematol Oncol Clin North Am. 1995;9:1031–56.
40. Vonderheid E, Tan E, Kantor AF. Long-term efficacy, curative potential, and carcinogenicity of topical mechlorethamine chemotherapy in cutaneous T cell lymphoma. J Am Acad Dermatol. 1989;20:416–28.
41. Smoller B, Marcus R. Risk of secondary cutaneous malignancies in patients with long-standing mycosis fungoides. J Am Acad Dermatol. 1994;30:201–4.
42. Zackheim H. Topical carmustine (BCNU) in the treatment of mycosis fungoides. Dermatol Ther. 2003;16:299–302.
43. Gupta A, Anderson T. Psoralen photochemotherapy. J Am Acad Dermatol. 1987;17:703–24.
44. Herrmann J, Roenigk H, Honigsmann H. Ultraviolet radiation for treatment of cutaneous T-cell lymphoma. Hematol Oncol Clin North Am. 1995;9:1077–88.
45. Querfeld C, Rosen S, Kuzel T. Long-term follow-up of patients with early-stage cutaneous T-cell lymphoma who achieved complete remisson with psoralen plus UV-A monotherapy. Arch Dermatol. 2005;141:305–11.
46. Stern R, Laird N, Melski J. Cutaneous squamous cell carcinoma in patients treated with PUVA. N Engl J Med. 1984;310:1156–61.
47. Rhodes A, Harrist T, Momtaz T. The PUVA-induced pigmented macule: a lentiginous proliferation of large, sometimes cytologically atypical, melanocytes. J Am Acad Dermatol. 1983;9:47–58.
48. Diederen P, van Weelden H, Sanders C, Toonstra J, van Vloten W. Narrowband UVB and psoralen-UVA in the treatment of early-stage mycosis fungoides: a retrospective study. J Am Acad Dermatol. 2003;48:215–9.
49. Boehm M, Heyman R, Nagpal S. A new generation of retinoid drugs for the treatment of dermatological diseases. Expert Opin Emerg Drugs. 1997;2:287–303.
50. Zhang C, Hazarika P, Xioa N, Duvic M. Induction of apoptosis by bexarotene in cutaneous T-cell lymphoma cells: relevance to mechanism of therapeutic action. Clin Cancer Res. 2002;2:1234–40.
51. Heald P, Mehlmauer M, Martin A, Crowley C, Yocum R, Reich S. Topical bexarotene for patients with refractory or persistent early-stage cutaneous T cell lymphoma: results of the phase III clinical trial. J Am Acad Dermatol. 2003;49:801–15.
52. Duvic M, Hymes K, Heald P, et al. Bexartoene is effective and safe for the treatment of refractory advanced-stage cutaneous T-celly lymphoma: multinational phase II–III trial results. J Clin Oncol. 2001;19:2456–71.
53. Apisamthanarax N, Talpur R, Ward S, Ni X, Kim H, Duvic M. Tazarotene 0.1% gel for refractory mycosis fungoides lesions: an open-label pilot study. J Am Acad Dermatol. 2004;50(4):600–7.
54. Imbertson L, Beaurline J, Couture A, Gibson S, Smith R, Miller R. Cytokine induction in hairless mouse and rat skin after topical application of the immune response modifiers imiquimod and S-28463. J Invest Dermatol. 1998;110:734–9.
55. Deeths M, Chapman J, Dellavalle R, Zeng C, Aeling JL. Treatment of patch and plaque stage mycosis fungoides with imiquimod 5% cream. J Am Acad Dermatol. 2005;52:275–80.

56. Jones G, Hoppe R, Glatstein E. Electron beam treatment for cutaneous T-cell lymphoma. Hematol Oncol Clin North Am. 1995;9:1057–76.
57. Jones G. Total skin electron beam radiotherapy for patients who have mycosis fungoides. Hematol Oncol Clin North Am. 2003;17(2003):1421–34.
58. Becker M, Hoppe R, Knox S. Multiple courses of high-dose total skin electron beam therapy in the management of mycosis fungoides. Int J Radiat Oncol Biol Phys. 1995;32:1445–9.
59. Edelson R. Photopheresis update. Prog Dermatol. 1991;25:1–6.
60. Edelson R. Cutaneous T-cell lymphoma: the helping hand of dendritic cells. Ann N Y Acad Sci. 2001;941:1–11.
61. Edelson R, Berger C, Gasparro F, et al. Treatment of cutaneous T-cell lymphoma by extracorporeal photochemotherapy: preliminary results. N Engl J Med. 1987;316:297–303.
62. Gottlieb S, Wolfe J, Fox F, et al. Treatment of cutaneous T-cell lymphoma with extracorporeal photopheresis monotherapy and in combination with recombinant interferon alfa: a 10-year experience at a single institution. J Am Acad Dermatol. 1996;35:946–57.
63. Evans A, Wood B, Scarisbrick J, et al. Extracorporeal photopheresis in Sezary syndrome: hematologic parameters as predictors of response. Blood. 2001; 98:1298–301.
64. Isaacs A, Lindenmann J. Virus interference I. The interferon. Proc R Soc Lond B Biol Sci. 1957; 147:258–63.
65. Trent J, Olson S, Lawn R. Chromosomal localization of human leucocyte, fibroblast and immune interferon genes by means of in situ hybridization. Proc Natl Acad Sci. 1982;79:7809–13.
66. Ross C, Tingsgaard P, Jorgensen H, Vejlsgaard G. Interferon treatment of cutaneous T-cell lymphoma. Eur J Haematol. 1993;51:63–72.
67. Olsen E, Rosen S, Vollmer R, et al. Interferon alfa-2a in the treatment of cutaneous T-cell lymphoma. J Am Acad Dermatol. 1989;20:395–407.
68. Vegna M, Papa G, Defazio D. Interferon alfa-2a in cutaneous T-cell lymphoma. Eur J Haematol Suppl. 1990;52:32–5.
69. Quesada J, Talpaz M, Rios A, Kurzrock R, Gutterman J. Clinical toxicity of interferons in cancer patients: a review. J Clin Oncol. 1986;4:234–43.
70. Querfeld C, Rose S, Guitart J. Comparison of selective retinoic acid receptor- and retinoic X receptor-mediated efficacy, tolerance, and survival in cutaneous T-cell lymphoma. J Am Acad Dermatol. 2004;51:25–32.
71. Budgin J, Richardson S, Newton S, et al. Biological effects of bexarotene in cutaneous T-cell lymphoma. Arch Dermatol. 2005;141:315–21.
72. Porcu P, Baiocchi R, Buckner M. Bexarotene-induced T-cell immunomodulation and response in CTCL. Blood. 2004;104:744.
73. Duvic M, Martin A, Kim Y, et al. Phase 2 and 3 clinical trial of oral bexarotene (targretin capsules) for the treatment of refractory or persistent early-stage cutaneous T-cell lymphoma. Arch Dermatol. 2001; 137:581–93.
74. Talpur R, Ward S, Apisamthanarax N. Optimizing bexarotene therapy for cutaneous T-cell lymphoma. J Am Acad Dermatol. 2002;47:672–84.
75. Olsen E, Duvic M, Frankel A, et al. Pivotal phase III trial of two dose levels of denileukin difitox for the treatment of CTCL. J Clin Oncol. 2001;19(2): 376–88.
76. Chin K, Foss F. Biologic correlates of response and survival in patients with cutaneous T-cell lymphoma treated with denileukin difitox. Clin Lymphoma Myeloma. 2006;7(3):199–204.
77. Foss F, Bacha P, Osann K, Demierre M, Bell T, Kuzel T. Biological correlates of acute hypersensitivity events with DAB389-IL-2 (denileukin difitox, ontak) in cutaneous T-cell lymphoma: decreased frequency and severity with steroid premedication. Clin Lymphoma Myeloma. 2001;1(4):298–302.
78. Rook A, McGinnis K, Richardson S, et al. The use of cytokines, fusion proteins and antibodies to treat cutaneous T-cell lymphoma. Dermatol Ther. 2003;16:331–6.
79. Gorgun G, Foss F. Immunomodulatory effects of RXR rexinoids: modulation of high-affinity IL-2R expression enhances susceptibility to denileukin difitox. Blood. 2002;100:1399–403.
80. O'Connor O. Developing new drugs for the treatment of lymphoma. Eur J Haematol. 2005;75: 150–8.
81. Marks P, Rifkind R, Richon V. Histone deacetylases and cancer: causes and therapies. Nat Rev Cancer. 2001;1:194–202.
82. Timmermann S, Lehrmann H, Polesskaya A. Histone acetylation and disease. Cell Mol Life Sci. 2001;58:728–36.
83. Olsen E, Kim Y, Kuzel T, et al. Phase IIB multicenter trial of vorinostat in patients with persistent, progressive, or treatment refractory cutaneous T-cell lymphoma. J Clin Oncol. 2007;25:3109–15.
84. Duvic M, Talpur R, Ni X, et al. Phase 2 trial of oral vorinostat (suberoylanilide hydroxamic acid, SAHA) for refractory cutaneous T-cell lymphoma (CTCL). Blood. 2007;109:31–9.
85. Piekarz R, Bates S. A review of depsipeptide and other histone deacetylase inhibitors in clinical trials. Curr Pharm Des. 2004;10:2289–98.
86. Piekarz R, Frye R, Turner M, et al. Phase II multi-institutinal trial of the histone deacetylase inhibitor romidepsin as monotherapy for patients with cutaneous T-cell lymphoma. J Clin Oncol. 2009;27(32): 5410–7.
87. Hale G, Zia M, Tighe H, Dyer M, Waldmann H. The CAMPATH-1 antigen (CDw52). Tissue Antigens. 1990;35:118–27.
88. Buggins A, Mufti G, Salisbury J, et al. Peripheral blood but not tissue dendritic cells express CD52 and are depleted by treatment with alemtuzumab. Blood. 2002;100:1715–20.

89. Rowan W, Tite J, Topley P, Brett S. Cross-linking of the CAMPATH-1 antigen (CD52) mediates growth inhibition in human B- and T-lymphoma cells lines, and subsequent emergence of CD52-deficient cells. Immunology. 1998;95:427–36.
90. Dyer M, Hale G, Hayhoe F, Waldmann H. Effects of CAMPATH-1 antibodies in vivo in patients with lymphoid malignancies: influence of antibody isotype. Blood. 1989;73:1431–9.
91. Greenwood J, Clark M, Waldmann H. Structural motifs involved in human IgG antibody effector functions. Eur J Immunol. 1993;23:1098–104.
92. Riechmann L, Clark M, Waldmann H, Winter G. Reshaping human antibodies for therapy. Nature. 1998;332:323–7.
93. Heit W, Bunjes D, Wiesneth M, et al. Ex vivo T-cell depletion with the monoclonal antibody Campath-1 plus human complement effectively prevents acute graft-versus-host disease in allogeneic bone marrow transplantation. Br J Haematol. 1986;64:479–86.
94. Dearden C. The role of alemtuzumab in the management of T-cell malignancies. Semin Oncol. 2006;33:S44–52.
95. Dearden C, Matutes E, Cazin B, et al. High remission rate in T cell prolymphocytic leukemia with CAMPATH-1H. Blood. 2001;98:1721–6.
96. Ravandi F, O'Brien S, Jones D, Lerner S, Faderl S, Ferrajoli A. T-cell prolymphocytic leukemia: a single-institution experience. Clin Lymphoma Myeloma. 2005;2005(6):234–9.
97. Enblad G, Hagberg H, Erlanson M, et al. A pilot study of alemtuzumab (anti-CD52 monoclonal antibody) therapy for patients with relapsed or chemotherapy-refractory peripheral T-cell lymphomas. Blood. 2004;103:2920–4.
98. Bernengo M, Quaglino P, Comessatti A, et al. Low-dose intermittent alemtuzumab in the treatment of Sezary syndrome: clinical and immunologic findings in 14 patients. Haematologica. 2007;92:784–94.
99. Kennedy G, Seymour J, Wolf M, et al. Treatment of patients with advanced mycosis fungoides and Sezary syndrome with alemtuzumab. Eur J Haematol. 2003;71:250–6.
100. Bender R, Makula D. Effect of interaction between methotrexate and dihydrofolate reductase on DNA synthesis in L1210 cells in vitro. Br J Cancer. 1978;37:403–10.
101. Zackheim H, Kashani-Sabet M, Hwang S. Low-dose methotrexate to treat erythrodermic cutaneous T-cell lymphoma: results in twenty-nine patients. J Am Acad Dermatol. 1996;34:626–31.
102. Zinzani P, Baliva G, Magagnoli M, et al. Gemcitabine treatment in pretreated cutaneous T-cell lymphoma: experience in 44 patients. J Clin Oncol. 2000; 18:2603–6.
103. Quererux G, Marques S, Nguyen J. Prospective multicenter study of pegylated liposomal doxorubicin treatment in patients with advanced or refractory mycosis fungoides or Sezary syndrome. Arch Dermatol. 2008;144(6):727–33.
104. Tani M, Fina M, Alinari L, Stefoni V, Baccarani M, Zinzina P. Phase II trial of temozolomide in patients with pretreated cutaneous T-cell lymphoma. Haematologica. 2005;90(9):1283–4.
105. Sors A, Jean-Louis F, Pellet C. Down-regulation constitutive activationof the NF-kappaB canonical pathway overcomes the resistance of cutnaeous T-cell lymphoma to apoptosis. Blood. 2006;107: 2354–63.
106. Zinzini P, Musuraca G, Tani M, et al. Phase II trial of proteasome inhibitor bortezomib in patients with relapsed or refractory cutaneous T-cell lymphoma. J Clin Oncol. 2007;25:4293–7.
107. Kim Y, Advani R, Hoppe R. Mycosis fungoides and Sezary syndrome. In: Magrith I, Boffetta P, Potter M, Stein H, Gascoynes R, Dearden C, Diehi V, Rohatiner A, Bhatia K, editors. The lymphoid neoplasms. 3rd ed. London: Hodder Arnold; 2009.
108. Molin L, Thomsen K, Volden G. Combination chemotherapy in the tumor stage of mycosis fungoides with cyclophosphamide, vincristine, VP-16, adriamycin, and prednisolone (COP, CHOP, CAVOP): a report from the Scandinavian Mycosis Fungoides Study Group. Acta Derm Venereol. 1980;60:542–4.
109. Tirelli U, Carbone A, Zagonel V. Staging and treatment with cyclophosphamide, vincristine, and prednisone (CVP) in advanced cutaneous T-cell lymphoma. Hematol Oncol Clin North Am. 1986;4:83–90.
110. Bigler R, Crilley P, Micaily B, et al. Autologous bone marrow transplantation for advanced stage mycosis fungoides. Bone Marrow Transplant. 1991;7:133–7.
111. Russell-Jones R, Child F, Olavarria E. Autologous peripheral blood stem cell transplantation in tumor-stage mycosis fungoides: predictors of disease-free survival. Ann N Y Acad Sci. 2001;941:147–54.
112. Molina A, Zain J, Arber D. Durable clinical, cytogenetic, and molecular remissions after allogeneic hematopoietic cell transplantation for refractory Sezary syndrome and mycosis fungoides. J Clin Oncol. 2005;23:6163–7.
113. Soligo D, Ibatici A, Berti E. Treatment of advanced mycosis fungoides by allogeneic stem-cell transplantation with a nonmyeloablative regimen. Bone Marrow Transplant. 2003;31:663–6.
114. Wu P, Kim Y, Lavori P, Hoppe R, Stockeri-Goldstein K. A meta-analysis of patients receiving allogeneic or autologous hematopoietic stem cell transplant in mycosis fungoides and Sezary syndrome. Biol Blood Marrow Transplant. 2009;15(8):982–90.

T-Cell Malignancies in Children and Adolescents: State of the Clinical and Biological Science

11

Nader Kim El-Mallawany, Pieter Van Vlierberghe, Adolfo A. Ferrando, Megan S. Lim, and Mitchell S. Cairo

Introduction

T-cell malignancies arise from cells of the innate and adaptive immune system. The current World Health Organization (WHO) [1, 2] classification recognizes over 20 distinct entities within the T/natural killer (NK) cell neoplasms. The more common subtypes that occur in children and young adolescents are the precursor T lymphoblastic leukemia/lymphoma and anaplastic large cell lymphoma (ALCL), anaplastic lymphoma kinase (ALK) positive. The rest are rarely observed in children. The majority of T-cell malignancies are aggressive neoplasms [3] and although rare relative to the adult population they present a formidable challenge from diagnostic and therapeutic perspectives. In this chapter, we provide an update of the clinical and biologic features of the common T-cell malignancies that occur in children and adolescents with a focus on molecular perspectives and implications for novel therapeutics.

N.K. El-Mallawany
Departments of Pediatric Hematology, Oncology, Blood and Marrow Transplantation, Columbia University, New York, NY, USA

P. Van Vlierberghe
Institute for Cancer Genetics, Columbia University Medical Center, New York, NY, USA

A.A. Ferrando
Institute for Cancer Genetics, Departments of Pediatrics and Pathology, Columbia University Medical Center, New York, NY, USA

M.S. Lim
Department of Pathology, University of Michigan Medical School, Ann Arbor, MI, USA

M.S. Cairo (✉)
Pediatric Hematology/Oncology/Stem Cell Transplantation, New York Medical College, 50 Plaza West, Munger Pavilion, Room 110A, Valhalla, NY 10595, USA
e-mail: mitchell_cairo@nymc.edu

T-Cell Acute Lymphoblastic Leukemia in Children and Adolescents

Acute lymphoblastic leukemia (ALL) is the most prevalent type of cancer occurring in children and adolescents in the Western World. A lymphoid malignancy derived from early progenitor cells in the bone marrow, it represents a heterogeneous group of diseases comprising multiple subtypes with biologically different behaviors. T-cell lineage ALL is a less common subtype, accounting for approximately 15% of cases [4]. T-cell acute lymphoblastic leukemia (T-ALL) is associated with numerous unfavorable clinical factors and carries a worse prognosis than its counterpart precursor B-cell ALL (B-ALL) [4]. Children with T-ALL are more likely to manifest with National Cancer Institute (NCI) high-risk features such as WBC >50,000 at diagnosis, older age, and central nervous system (CNS) involvement. They are also more likely to have bulky disease with enlargement of the liver, spleen, lymph nodes, and to have a mediastinal mass [4].

F. Foss (ed.), *T-Cell Lymphomas*, Contemporary Hematology,
DOI 10.1007/978-1-62703-170-7_11,

Table 11.1 Outcome in childhood T lymphoblastic leukemia: twenty-first century results

References	Goldberg et al. [7]	Moghrabi et al. [8]	Ballerini et al. [6]	Moricke et al. [9]	Pui et al. [10]
Institution/group	DFCI	DFCI	FRALLE	BFM	St. Judes
Protocol/treatment	87-01, 91-01, 95-01	95-01	FRALLE-93	ALL BFM-95	Total therapy XV
Number of patients	125	52	200	275	76
EFS (%)	75±4	85±6	58±3	70±3.3	80±8.7

Although improvements have been achieved in outcomes with conventional chemotherapy regimens, event-free survival (EFS) rates for children with T-ALL in some series may be inferior to those for children with precursor B-cell ALL. As discussed in the following section on T-cell lymphoblastic lymphoma (T-LBL), there are important biological and clinical differences between T-LBL and T-ALL despite the overarching similarities. The same is to be said in comparing B-ALL and T-ALL. Inasmuch, with continued advances in the understanding of the unique characteristics of T-ALL, there is hope for even further improvement of outcomes with development of new treatment strategies.

Unlike T-LBL, which often presents with systemic B-symptoms and complications of supradiaphragmatic lymphadenopathy, T-ALL is more likely to present with fever, bone pain, and the typical symptoms associated with cytopenias-petechiae and/or easy bruising, fatigue and pallor, and infection [5]. However, since T-ALL is more likely than precursor B-cell ALL to present with significant lymphadenopathy, hepatosplenomegaly, and a mediastinal mass, the clinical symptoms associated with T-ALL can overlap with those of T-LBL [5]. The distinction would therein be that ALL is defined by having more than 25% involvement of the bone marrow with lymphoblasts. Flow cytometry studies are critically important in making an accurate distinction between the immunophenotypes of B and T lymphoblasts.

Treatment regimens for T-ALL have achieved significant improvements over the past 25 years through the introduction of intensive, high-dose, multi-agent chemotherapy regimens. Most contemporary protocols treat pediatric T-ALL with the same regimens given to children with high-risk B-ALL. Using multi-agent intensive regimens, several pediatric oncology cooperative groups including the Children's Oncology Group (COG [formerly Children's Cancer Group (CCG)]), Dana Farber Cancer Institute (DFCI), Berlin-Frankfurt-Munster (BFM), French ALL Cooperative Group (FRALLE), and St. Jude's ALL protocols over the past decade have consistently reported EFS rates ranging from 58 to 85% for children with T-ALL (Table 11.1 and Fig. 11.1) [6–13]. These regimens are similar in execution, utilizing treatment programs of greater than 2 years in duration, employing phases focused on remission induction, consolidation, intensification, CNS-directed therapy, and maintenance, as well as combining multiple chemotherapeutic agents. Chemotherapy frequently used across protocols includes glucocorticoids (prednisone and/or dexamethasone), anthracyclines, methotrexate (MTX) (at high and low doses), vincristine, asparaginase, 6-mercaptopurine, and cyclophosphamide. Many high-risk regimens will also incorporate cytarabine and etoposide into the combination. Intrathecal (IT) chemotherapy is given universally utilizing MTX, cytarabine, and hydrocortisone. Until recently, all treatment protocols utilized cranial radiation therapy (CRT) for patients with CNS disease, as well as those with high-risk for CNS relapse, which includes children with T-ALL.

The St. Jude's group just completed their analysis of 498 ALL patients treated without the use of CRT. It was a landmark protocol in that even those patients who were CNS positive at diagnosis did not receive radiation. Based upon the rate of CNS relapse in comparison with historical controls that received CRT, the results demonstrated that omission of CRT was safe and associated with EFS and overall survival (OS) rates

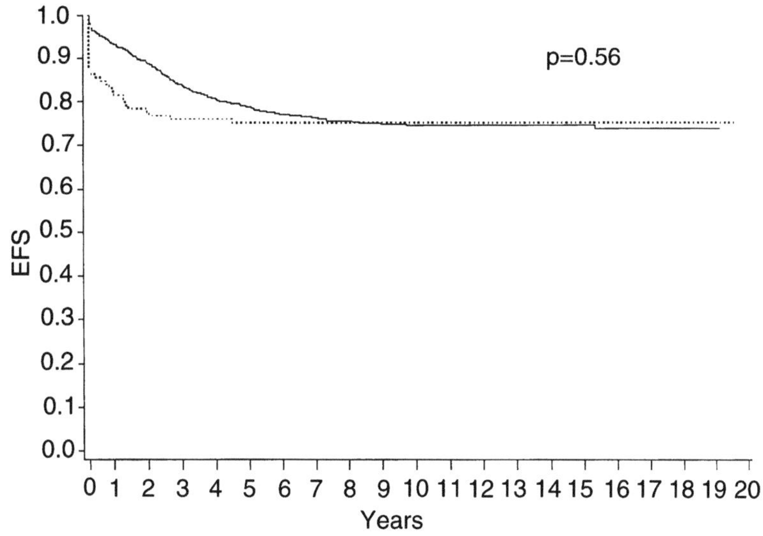

Phenotype	0–5	5–10	10–15	15–20	20–25
——— B-ALL	237/1130	33/777	0/364	1/103	0/0
·········· T-ALL	31/125	0/81	0/45	0/18	0/0

(# events/ # at risk)

Fig. 11.1 Event-free survival (EFS) by immunophenotype. Children with B-progenitor acute lymphoblastic leukemia (B-ALL, ______) had an EFS rate of 79%±1%. Children with T-cell acute lymphoblastic leukemia ALL (T-ALL, - - -) had an EFS rate of 75%±4% (P=0.56). Early events are more common in T-ALL (reprinted from Goldberg et al. [7], with permission from American Society of Clinical Oncology)

comparable to prior protocols that utilized CRT. However, patients with T-ALL (in addition to those that were CNS positive at diagnosis and children with the t1;19 translocation) had a remarkably high hazard ratio for risk of CNS relapse, despite having received higher doses of MTX than in standard regimens (it has been shown that T-lineage lymphoblasts have a decreased affinity for uptake of MTX substrates and that higher doses are required to overcome this pharmacodynamic challenge) [14]. The authors make the argument that these patients nonetheless, should be treated without CRT regardless of the CNS relapse risk. Their rationale is that otherwise nearly 90% of this risk group of patients will thereby receive CRT that could have been avoided. Certainly the counterpoint can be made that until we are able to more accurately predict which subgroup of children with T-ALL are at an especially high risk for CNS relapse, they should all uniformly receive CRT. Overall, T-ALL patients on this protocol had an EFS of 78% which is comparable with prior treatment regimens [10].

The best EFS rate to date for patients with T-ALL was reported on the DFCI 95-001 treatment regimen (Table 11.1). They also treated T-ALL patients similar to the therapy for the high-risk B-ALL subgroup. However, their high-risk treatment regimen was notable for an increased overall dose of asparaginase and additional doxorubicin. This treatment regimen did include CRT for T-ALL patients. The 5-year EFS was 85%, which is remarkably favorable compared to all other large series of patients with T-ALL. In fact, children with T-ALL fared better on this protocol than those with pre-B ALL. The authors attributed the favorable outcome to the efficacy of the high-risk treatment regimen, but it is perplexing that the high-risk pre-B ALL patients did not fare better as well [8].

Relapsed ALL of both B and T-cell lineages presents an enormous challenge to the goal of achieving long-term cure. Only about one-third of patients with relapsed ALL will experience long-term survival despite intensive re-induction regimens including the utilization of allogeneic stem cell transplantation (alloSCT) [15]. Patients with early relapse are defined as occurring less than 36 months after initial diagnosis; early relapse portends a particularly dismal prognosis with less than 20% 3-year EFS [16]. It is difficult to comment on the prognosis of relapsed T-ALL as results are only occasionally reported as subsets within already small numbers of patients of relapsed ALL in general. In a recent COG analysis of children with ALL in first relapse, 7/124 patients had T-ALL, only 2 out of those 7 achieved a second remission, and no T-ALL patient lived longer than 10 months [17]. Another COG analysis of children with early relapse of ALL had 28 patients with T-ALL and an EFS of <5% for that subgroup of patients [16]. New developments in treatment strategies for relapsed T-ALL are desperately needed.

Nelarabine is a novel agent that has shown promise in relapsed and refractory T-ALL but not T-LL. It is a purine analog whose mechanism of action delivers markedly specific toxicity to T lymphocytes. The use of Nelarabine in T-cell malignancies was first investigated based upon the observation that patients with purine nucleoside phosphorylase (PNP) deficiency suffer from T-cell immune deficiency due to the abnormal and toxic accumulation of deoxyguanosine triphosphate (dGTP) in T cells. Nelarabine is a derivative of dGTP and is resistant to degradation by PNP. In a phase II COG study, patients with T-ALL in first relapse (not involving the CNS) had a response rate of 55% (with 16 of 33 patients achieving a complete remission [CR]). CNS toxicity ≥grade 3 was experienced in 18% of patients, manifesting as peripheral neuropathy, seizure, and hallucinations. The promise of such extraordinary results in a historically extremely high-risk group of patients has led to the investigation of Nelarabine's utility in front-line therapy for children with high-risk T-ALL [18].

Two groups of T-ALL patients that demonstrated an especially high-risk for treatment failure are those who are poor initial responders to prednisone and those with minimal residual disease (MRD) at the end of induction therapy. The BFM cooperative group demonstrated that children with T-ALL that exhibit a poor response to 1 week of prednisone plus IT MTX on day 1 have an EFS of 32% compared to 78% in good responders. Poor response was demonstrated as having ≥1,000 leukemic blasts/μL peripheral blood on day 8 of induction [19]. The presence of MRD at the end of induction in patients with ALL has been an ominous prognostic sign for both pre-B and T-ALL, with as high as a 70% chance for early relapse. Patients with T-ALL have demonstrated an even higher risk of being MRD positive than their B-ALL counterparts [20–22]. These risk factors have thereby served as a platform for building clinical trials investigating the role of new drugs in improving overall EFS for patients with T-ALL.

The current COG study (AALL-0434) is one of the few ALL protocols designed specifically for patients with T-ALL. Utilizing a BFM ALL treatment backbone, it is investigating the use of Nelarabine and high-dose MTX in the treatment of intermediate and high-risk T-ALL. Risk stratification is based upon the aforementioned prognostic factors. High-risk patients are those with positive MRD (or gross induction failure) at end of induction. Low-risk patients are CNS negative, low-risk by NCI standards for age and initial WBC, exhibit good response to initial 1 week of prednisone, and are MRD negative. Intermediate-risk patients do not fit the low-risk category, but are MRD negative at the end of induction. In preliminary pilot data from COG study AALL-02P2, higher-risk patients receiving Nelarabine fared as well as their low-risk counterparts not receiving the drug. More specifically, patients with a poor response to prednisone that received Nelarabine in combination therapy achieved an equivalent 3-year EFS of 75% in comparison to those with a good response that did not receive Nelarabine. Moreover, this was achieved without the Nelarabine group experiencing excess toxicity [23]. Improvement of the cure rates for patients with high-risk T-ALL offers significant opportunity to improve on the EFS for patients with T-cell lineage ALL overall.

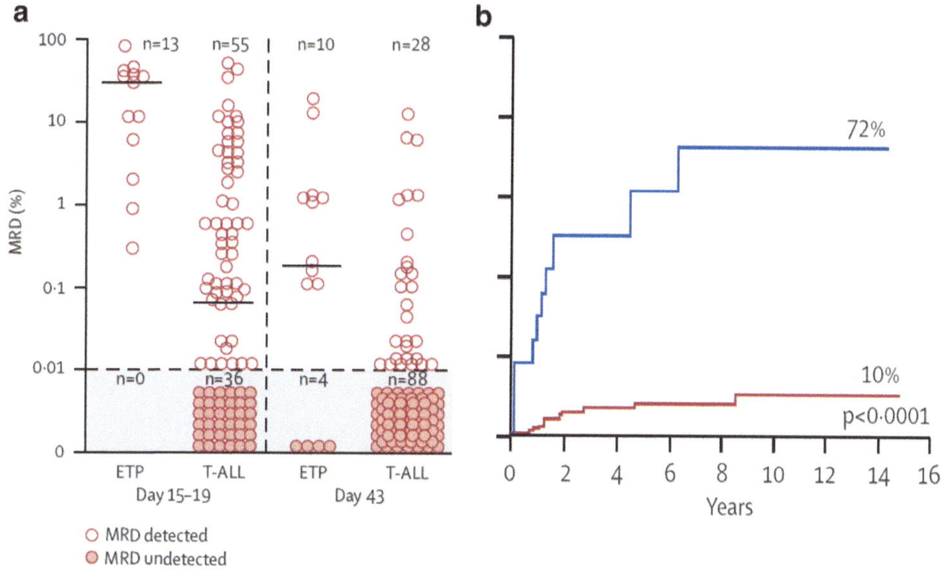

Fig. 11.2 (**a**) Prevalence of minimal residual disease (MRD) during the early phases of therapy for patients with early T-precursor (ETP) or typical T-ALL. MRD levels were measured by flow cytometry (**a**). *Horizontal bars* indicate median values, if above 0.01%. (**b**) Kaplan–Meier plots of the cumulative incidence of remission failure or hematological relapse in patients with typical T lymphoblastic leukemia (T-ALL; *red*) vs. early T-cell precursor (ETP)-ALL (*blue*) treated on St. Jude protocols. The curves start at the time of diagnosis. Outcome estimates at 10 years of follow-up are shown; *P* values are from the log-rank test (reprinted from Coustan-Smith et al. [24], with permission from Elsevier)

Recently, another smaller subset of patients with T-ALL has also demonstrated a markedly poor prognosis [24]. Lymphoblasts characterized by an immunophenotype of early T-cell precursors (ETP-ALL) seem to have a distinct biology in comparison to typical precursor T lymphoblasts. The early precursors tend to retain stem-cell-like features and exhibit genomic instability. Of 239 patients investigated with T-ALL, 30 were found to have the ETP-ALL subtype. Of patients with ETP-ALL, there was a significant increase in MRD at day 18 and day 43, resulting in a significant increase in the risk of remission failure and/or hematologic relapses [24]. There was a 72% risk for failure or relapse at 10 years in patients with ETP-ALL vs. 10% for patients with typical T-ALL treated at St. Jude's Children's Research Hospital (Fig. 11.2a, b). Currently the St. Jude's treatment protocols have been adjusted to modify therapy by introducing alloSCT in CR1 for patients with ETP-ALL [24].

The BFM and CCG cooperative groups have previously examined the role of alloSCT in CR1 for patients with high-risk disease [25, 26]. The BFM group defined high risk as those having a poor response to prednisone and/or the inability to achieve remission with induction chemotherapy [26]. The BFM group compared outcomes of 179 patients that achieved CR1, 23 of whom received an alloSCT (8 from matched unrelated donors, 15 from sibling donors). The 5-year OS for patients who received an alloSCT was 67% vs. 47% for those who received only chemotherapy (Fig. 11.3) [26]. While the utility of alloSCT represents a reasonable treatment escalation strategy for the high-risk group of T-ALL patients, it remains to be seen whether the encouraging results from the Nelarabine trials in front-line therapy may offset the survival advantage seen in patients treated with alloSCT in CR1.

Another developmental therapeutic strategy is based upon the unraveling of the Notch pathway involvement in the pathogenesis of T-ALL. The Notch family of transmembrane receptors is critically involved in cell differentiation, proliferation, and apoptosis pathways (see section on

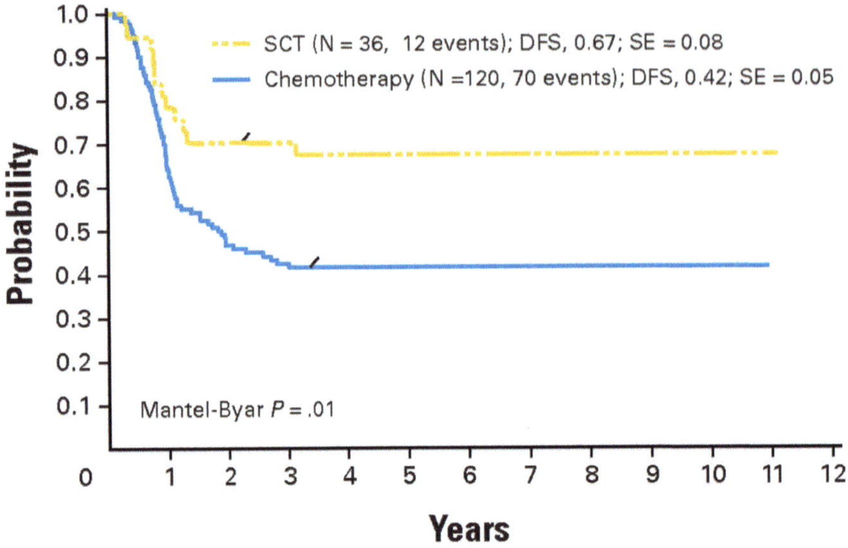

Fig. 11.3 Kaplan–Meier estimate of disease-free survival (DFS) at 5 years in stem-cell transplantation (SCT) patients vs. patients treated with chemotherapy alone (Acute Lymphoblastic Leukemia-Berlin-Frankfurt-Munster trials 90 and 95; analysis as treated). From the group of patients treated with chemotherapy alone, patients with an event before 0.43 years (medium time to transplantation) were excluded (reprinted from Schrauder et al. [26], with permission from American Society of Clinical Oncology)

molecular basis of pediatric T-ALL) [27]. Activating Notch mutations have been found in 50–60% of human T-ALL samples [28]. Gamma-secretase inhibitors (GSIs) are a family of drugs that inhibit the activation of Notch1 and their utility in the treatment of T-ALL has been under investigation. GSIs in combination with glucocorticoids can exhibit potent anti-leukemic effects *in vivo*, while combination of the two medicines results in a decrease of the dose-limiting gastrointestinal toxicities seen with GSIs. The effect of this combination also revealed the ability to induce apoptotic cell death in leukemic cells that were prior considered glucocorticoid-resistant [29]. It has also been shown that Notch positively regulates the mTOR pathway with c-Myc as a potential intermediary. Combination treatment with GSIs plus an mTOR inhibitor has shown synergistic effects against T-ALL cells in both *in vitro* and *in vivo* models [30, 31]. In addition, GSIs have also been combined in preclinical models with the proteasome inhibitor bortezomib and P13K-AKT inhibitors [32, 33]. Ultimately, after it seemed curative effects in T-ALL had plateaued after many years of unwavering EFS rates, promising new therapies targeting specific characteristics of T-cell pathology are offering exciting new hope for physicians, scientists, and patients alike.

T-Cell Lymphoblastic Lymphoma in Children and Adolescents

Lymphoblastic lymphoma (LBL) is the second most common type of childhood non-Hodgkin lymphoma (NHL) after Burkitt lymphoma (BL). The vast majority (80–90%) of cases of LBL are derived from the T-cell lineage, in contrast to ALL, in which most cases are precursor B-cell in origin. This renders T-LBL the most common type of T-cell lymphoma occurring in children [34–36]. For many years T-LBL and T-ALL were thought to be diseases on different ends of a single spectrum of pathology, but recent advances in the understanding of the biology of lymphoblastic disease have shed light on some important differences amidst the many shared commonalities [37, 38]. Furthermore, there are some important clinical distinctions between T-LBL and T-ALL.

Table 11.2 Advanced disease lymphoblastic lymphoma in children

	BFM [218]	St. Jude [219]	EORTC-CLCG [220]	DFCI [221]	UKCCSG [222]	CCG [223]
Patients (*N*)	101	24	60	21	95	102
Protocol	NHL-BFM-90	Total therapy-X	EORTC 58881	APO	UKCCSG 8503	CCG 5941
Duration (months)	24	32	24	24	24	12
EFS (Est) 3–6 years	90%	73%	76%	58%	65%	79%

Reprinted from Cairo [34], www.jbpub.com, with permission from Jones and Bartlett
EFS event-free survival; *Est* estimate

While T-LBL tends to have localized and earlier relapse than its counterpart, T-ALL tends to have more frequent CNS involvement at initial diagnosis [39–41].

Childhood T-LBL commonly presents with a supradiaphragmatic mass and as advanced stage III/IV disease, while B-cell LBL tends to present with limited disease in sites including the skin, bone, and peripheral lymph nodes. Typically, T-LBL may present as an adolescent male with respiratory distress found to have an anterior mediastinal mass. Severe complications can potentially arise from a supradiaphragmatic mass including respiratory failure and superior vena cava (SVC) syndrome warranting emergent intervention with steroids and/or radiation therapy. Disease may also involve the bone marrow and CNS; however, one must keep in mind that greater than 25% involvement of the bone marrow with lymphoblasts is referred to as lymphoblastic leukemia, while >5% but <25% involvement of the bone marrow would be termed stage IV LBL [42].

Children with limited disease T-LBL have a favorable prognosis with long-term OS of 85–90% [34–36, 42]. Although disease free survival (DFS) rates are only 63–73%, children with limited disease (Murphy stages I and II) have favorable responses to salvage therapies. ALL-based treatment protocols have been the mainstay of therapy for this group of children with T-LBL [43, 44]. Patients with localized disease are currently being treated without local surgical intervention, local radiation therapy, and CRT. However, most cases of T-LBL are advanced stage, so the focus of the treatment discussion will be on therapeutic approaches for children with advanced stage III/IV disease.

The prognosis for children with advanced stage T-LBL improved significantly after the introduction of the 10-drug LSA_2L_2 regimen in the 1970s [45]. From that point forward, most treatment protocols for LBL have been based upon the combination of corticosteroids, vincristine, anthracyclines, L-asparaginase, cyclophosphamide, MTX, cytarabine, 6-mercaptopurine, and 6-thioguanine. The BFM regimens employ an ALL backbone therapy with some adjustments, while many other regimens have been based on the LSA_2L_2 regimen with various modifications. Nearly all contemporary strategies are divided into stages that include induction, consolidation, re-intensification, and maintenance chemotherapy. The timing and dosing of some specific medicines may vary, but overall most protocols reported since the year 2000 have been able to achieve a 75–90% EFS with regimens ranging from 12 to 24 months duration (Table 11.2).

The highest EFS reported to date was from the BFM-90 protocol in which patients with advanced stage disease all received CRT, regardless of whether or not they had CNS involvement. The EFS was 90% for stage III/IV patients; however due to the deleterious long-term effects of CRT, subsequent studies have focused on the safety and efficacy of omitting CRT (Fig. 11.4a) [40]. Multiple studies have investigated protocols in which CRT was only utilized in patients with CNS positive disease. The Italian AIEOP LNH-92 protocol reported an EFS of 65% in advanced stage T-LBL; however they notably did not implement a re-intensification phase after induction and consolidation therapy [46]. The BFM-95 protocol also administered CRT to patients with

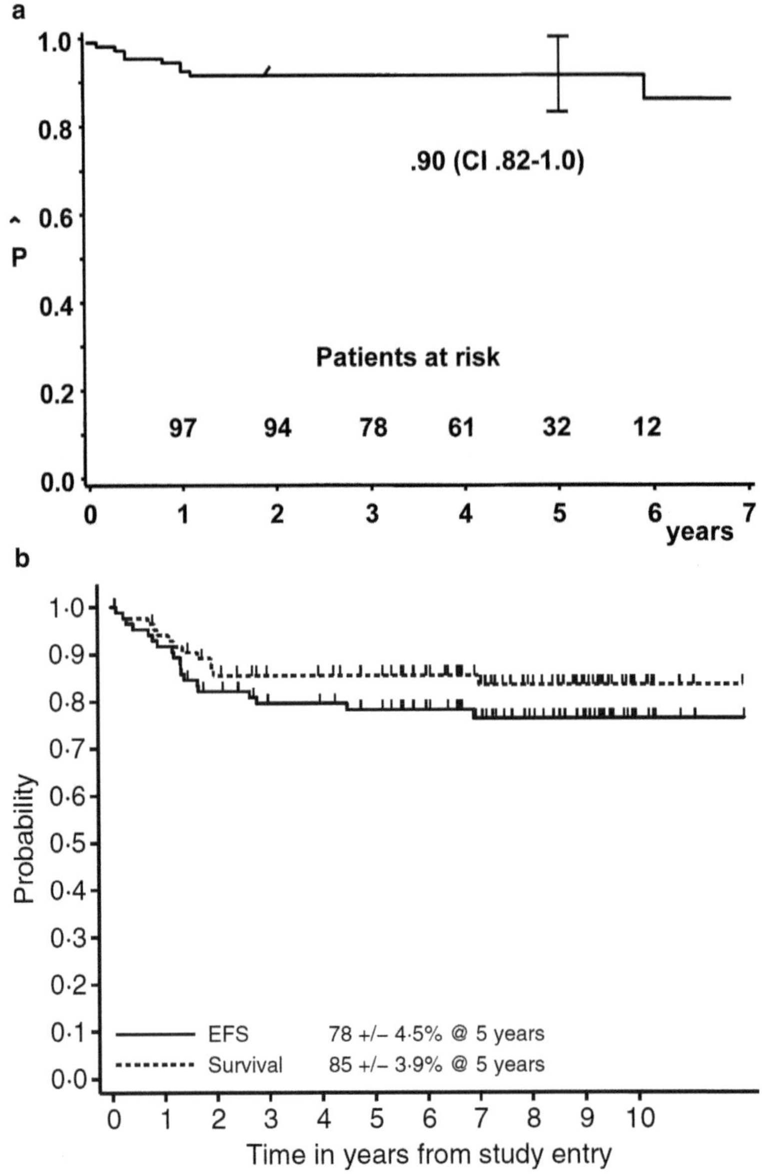

Fig. 11.4 (**a**) Probability of duration of EFS and 95% confidence bands. This research was originally published in *Blood* [40]. © American Society of Hematology. (**b**) Probability of EFS and overall survival (survival) of all patients from diagnosis (reprinted from Abromowitch et al. [48], with permission from Wiley-Blackwell Publishing)

CNS positive disease only, choosing to optimize delivery of high-dose MTX and IT chemotherapy. In a historical comparison to their earlier protocols including BFM-90 and 86, they determined that omitting CRT may be non-inferior to treatment including CRT in CNS negative patients. However, the EFS for advanced stage LBL in the BFM-95 protocol was 82%, lower than that of the BFM-90 study [47]. The COG reported on a shortened (12-month) intensified multi-agent chemotherapy regimen for advanced stage disease, also only administering CRT to patients that were CNS positive. This strategy yielded a 5-year EFS of 78% concluding that the shortened approach was safe and achieved similar results as more prolonged ALL-based regimens

(Fig. 11.4b) [48]. The most recent COG study for T-LBL examined whether the effects of high-dose MTX and early intensification of therapy with anthracycline and cyclophosphamide would further improve DFS. Preliminary data shows that neither high-dose MTX nor early intensification in BFM-type ALL therapy resulted in improvement in EFS for T-LBL [49].

Recently, the European Organisation for Research and Treatment of Cancer (EORTC) and St. Jude's have employed treatment protocols entirely omitting CRT, even in patients who are CNS positive. The EORTC CLG 58881 trial utilized a BFM-based regimen and achieved a 6-year EFS of 78% for advanced stage disease. They successfully demonstrated that omission of CRT did not influence the rate of CNS relapse. And notably, they also established treatment response to the 7-day prednisone-only prephase as a significant prognostic factor. Patients with a CR after the prephase (16 out of 121) had an EFS of 100%, contrasting with an EFS of 14% for those with no response to the prephase [50]. The NHL13 protocol utilized by the group at St. Jude's was based on their institutional ALL therapy including a maintenance phase with alternating pairs of therapeutic agents and incorporating high-dose MTX every 8 weeks in addition to a re-induction regimen 16 weeks into the maintenance phase. They were able to demonstrate an excellent EFS rate of 83% for advanced stage T-LBL despite omission of CRT as well. The study however only analyzed 41 patients, in comparison to the other studies discussed above in which the number of patients ranged from 85 to 156 [51].

The majority of children who relapse/progress do so within 24 months of diagnosis and the prognosis for children who develop recurrent disease is poor, with less than a 10% 5-year OS (Fig. 11.5a) [39, 52]. In an effort to improve outcome for patients with relapsed disease, intensive re-induction chemotherapy followed by either autologous (auto) or alloSCT improved DFS to between 23 and 58% [53–55]. Retrieval chemotherapy has included NHL regimens such as DECAL (dexamethasone, etoposide, cisplatin, high-dose cytarabine and L-asparaginase) [56] and ICE (ifosfamide, carboplatin, and etoposide) [57]. Patients with disease that is chemosensitive to the retrieval regimen have better outcomes following either auto or alloSCT [57, 58]. In a retrospective comparison of auto vs. alloSCT, significantly lower relapse rates were observed following alloSCT vs. autoSCT; however higher treatment-related mortality offset any survival benefit [59, 60]. In a more recent analysis from the BFM, OS was 14% among 28 patients with relapsed T-LBL (Fig. 11.5b). They all went on to receive salvage therapy, while 9 patients went on to receive an alloSCT. Of those who received an alloSCT, 4 were still alive >4 years post-alloSCT. The two patients that received autoSCT succumbed to their disease [39]. Although these numbers are too low to derive any statistically significant conclusions, it remains that any chance for survival in this group of patients with relapsed or progressive T-LBL depends upon a sufficient response to salvage chemotherapy and a successful alloSCT. The development of newer therapies for T-LBL has not met much success. Nelarabine has been shown to have a significantly more substantial effect on refractory T-ALL than T-LBL [18]. In terms of targeted therapies, the upregulation of Notch and the associated mTOR protein kinase pathway has stimulated investigation to the effects of mTOR and/or Notch inhibition *in vitro* [61]. And finally, phase I studies have been undertaken examining the role of Forodesin in T-cell malignancies, although mostly in adults with peripheral T-cell lymphoma (PTCL). Forodesin is a PNP which was recognized more than 30 years ago as a potential target for the treatment of patients with T-cell malignancies when an inherited deficiency of PNP was reported to be associated with a profound T-cell lymphopenia [62].

With such dismal salvage rates in LBL, accurate delineation of prognostic factors to identify patients at high risk of relapse is vitally important. Unfortunately though, definitive prognostic factors in childhood T-LBL have yet to be well established. Aside from the striking results of the EORTC CLG trial in which treatment response to the 7-day prednisone prephase demonstrated polar extremes of eventual EFS rates, clinical

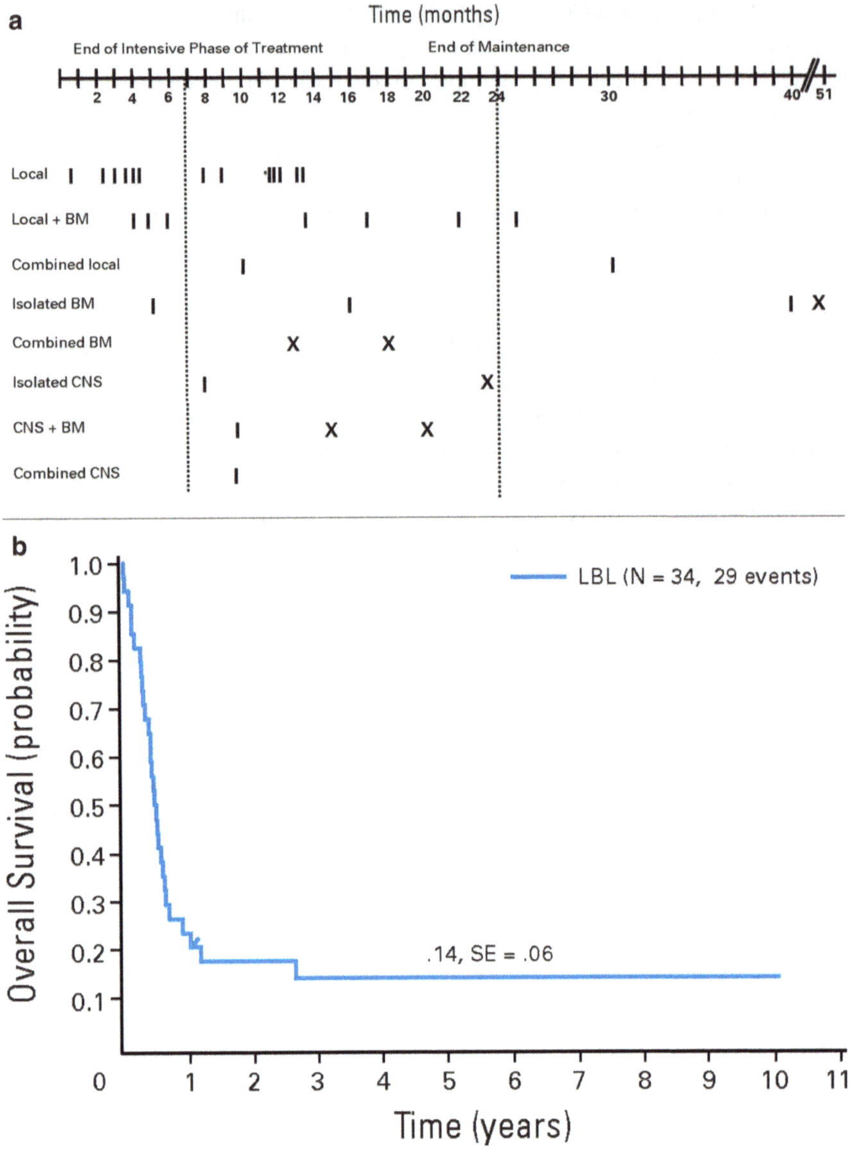

Fig. 11.5 (**a**) Time and site of disease progression or relapse in children with relapse of a lymphoblastic lymphoma (LBL). *I*, patients with T-cell lymphoblastic lymphoma; *X*, patients with precursor B-cell lymphoblastic lymphoma; *BM* bone marrow. (*)This patient was treated according to high-risk arm and experienced relapse during intensive phase of treatment 11 months after start of therapy. (**b**) Probability of survival at 5 years for children with disease progression or relapse of LBL (reprinted from Burkhardt et al. [39], with permission from American Society of Clinical Oncology)

prognostic factors have not been elucidated. The assessment of treatment response, either by laboratory or radiographic monitoring (including 2-Deoxy-2-[18F]fluoro-D-Glucose positron emission tomography [FDG PET]), is a potential method of identifying high-risk patients and determining prognostic parameters to guide therapeutic adjustments for patients that require intensification of up-front therapy [63].

T-LBL has a scarcity of cytogenetic and molecular factors associated with poor response to therapy. Recently, however, there have been

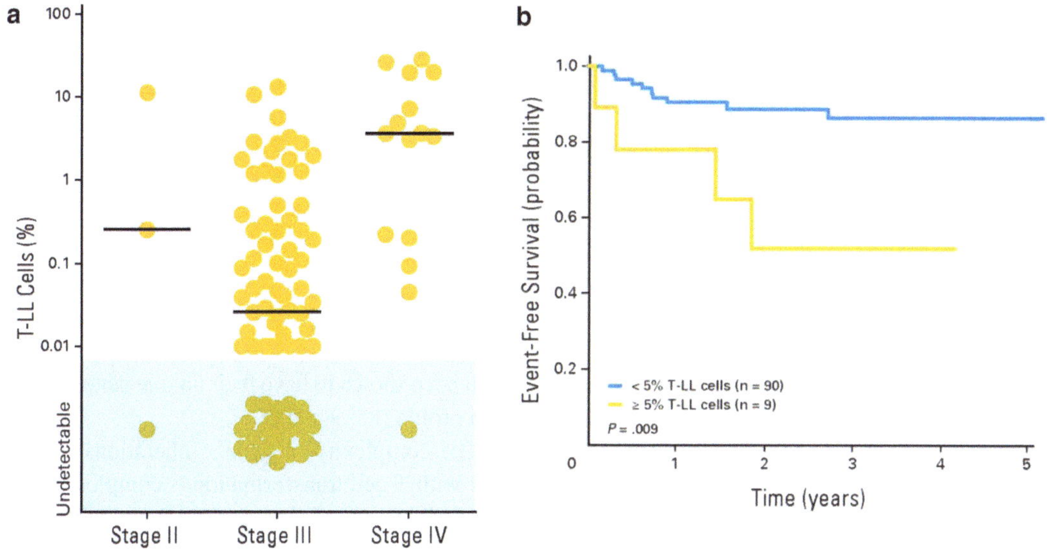

Fig. 11.6 (**a**) Percentage of T-cell lymphoblastic lymphoma (T-LL) cells in bone marrow at diagnosis as detected by flow cytometry according to disease stage based on conventional criteria. *Horizontal bars* indicate the median value in each group. (**b**) EFS according to levels of T-LL cells in bone marrow at diagnosis measured by flow cytometry: (**a**) <5% and ≥5% T-LL cells (reprinted from Coustan-Smith et al. [65], with permission from American Society of Clinical Oncology)

some interesting studies shedding light on potentially important prognostic factors. Loss of heterozygosity at chromosome 6q was associated with an increased risk of relapse in T-LBL [37]. Meanwhile, substantial advances have been established in the ability to detect levels of minimal disseminated disease (MDD) and MRD. T-cell receptor (TCR) real-time quantitative polymerase chain reaction (PCR) assays have been successfully utilized as a technique to assess and monitor MDD and MRD in T-LBL [64]. In a recent analysis of flow cytometry methods of detecting disease at molecular levels in 99 patients, two-thirds were found to have MDD in the bone marrow at diagnosis, and of those with ≥5% T-LBL cells in the marrow, the 2-year EFS was 51.9% vs. 88.7% for those patients with lower levels (Fig. 11.6a, b). The analysis reveals a very striking trend towards poor response to therapy and the presence of MDD and provides a foundation for further studies to examine the relationship between MDD and risk for relapse [65]. Having encountered a relative ceiling in the inability to significantly improve EFS in the treatment of advanced stage LL over the past decade, development of accurate prognostic factors will likely serve as the key to future improvements in outcome. Ultimately, it will be crucial to determine subgroups of high-risk patients that will benefit from alternative and intensified modalities of treatment including alloSCT as first line strategies.

Molecular Basis of T-ALL/T-LBL in Children and Adolescents

T-ALL and T-LBL represent 15% of childhood ALL and one-third of childhood and adolescent NHLs, respectively. T-ALL is characterized by prominent (>30%) bone marrow infiltration by T-cell lymphoblasts, whereas T-LBL demonstrate mediastinal masses in the context of limited or no bone marrow involvement [66]. Both clinical entities share a similar spectrum of molecular and cytogenetic abnormalities and most probably represent different clinical manifestations of the same thymocytic neoplasm, commonly referred to as T-ALL [66]. Current treatment, mainly consisting of multi-agent combination chemotherapy, provides an OS rate of approximately 70–90% in children and adolescents [67, 68]. Despite recent progress in the treatment of these diseases, the prognosis of T-ALL/T-LBL patients with primary resistant or relapsed leukemia is very poor, underscoring the need to develop more effective antileukemic drugs [67, 68].

Over the last 20 years, great progress has been made in unraveling molecular-genetic defects that are involved in the pathogenesis of T-ALL [69, 70]. It is now generally accepted that the leukemic transformation of immature thymocytes is caused by a multistep pathogenesis involving numerous genetic abnormalities that permit uncontrolled cell growth [66, 71].

In T-ALL, transcription factors are frequently activated due to disturbances in the rearrangement process of the TCR genes, juxtaposing the proto-oncogenes to the enhancers of *TCR*β (7q34) or *TCR*$\alpha\delta$ (14q11) [72]. These TCR-mediated translocations occur in approximately 33% of T-ALL cases [73] and cause deregulation of (1) basic helix-loop-helix (bHLH) family members such as *TAL1* [74–76], *TAL2* [77], *LYL1* [78], and *BHLHB1* [79]; (2) LIM-only domain (LMO) factors such as *LMO1* and *LMO2* [80–82]; and (3) the *TLX1/HOX11* [83–86], *TLX3/HOX11L2* [87, 88], *NKX2.5* [89], and *HOXA9* [90, 91] homeobox genes; *MYC* [92, 93], *MYB* [94, 95], and *TAN1*, a truncated and constitutively activated form of the NOTCH1 receptor [96]. In addition, a number of non-TCR-mediated translocations generate specific fusion products including *MLL-ENL* [97], *CALM-AF10* [98], and *SET-NUP214* [99].

From gene expression profiling studies and the analysis of T-ALL mouse models, the concept emerged that aberrant expression of these oncogenic transcription factors cause disruption of the normal circuitry that controls cell proliferation, differentiation, and survival during T-cell development [88, 90, 100]. Since these microarray studies also suggested that the transcription factor deregulations are associated with specific patterns of gene expression and a differentiation arrest at specific stages of T-cell development, these genetic lesions are thought to define different molecular-genetic subgroups in T-ALL. For example, T-ALL patients that show rearrangements of the *TAL1*, *TAL2*, *LMO1*, or *LMO2* genes are characterized by a highly similar gene expression signature, probably due to the fact that these transcription factors normally participate in the same transcriptional complex [101]. Also, *CALM-AF10*, *MLL*-rearrangements, inversion 7 positive patients, and *SET-NUP214* positive T-ALL patients share a common expression profile that is characterized by the activation of the cluster of *HOXA* transcription factors [90, 99]. Activation of other transcription factors including *TLX1*, *TLX3*, and *MYB* has each been shown to have their unique gene expression profile [88, 94, 100].

The complexity of genetic alterations associated with T-cell transformation is completed with a few highly prevalent cytogenetic and molecular alterations that occur throughout all molecular subtypes of T-ALL. The most prominent T-cell-specific abnormality is the presence of activating mutations in *NOTCH1*, which are detected in over 55% of T-ALL cases [28]. However, the most prevalent genetic lesion in T-ALL is the homozygous or heterozygous inactivation of the genomic *CDKN2A* and *CDKN2B* loci, located in tandem at chromosome 9p21, occurring in more than 70% of T-ALL cases [102]. T-ALL is further characterized by a wide variety of rare but recurrent genetic lesions which result in (1) activation of genes involved in cell proliferation such as *LCK* [103], *CCND2* [104], *JAK1* [105], *ETV6-JAK2* [106], *ETV6-ABL1* [107], *NUP214-ABL1* [108], *EML1-ABL1* [109], *FLT3* [110, 111], and *RAS* [112] and (2) inactivation of tumor suppressor genes responsible for control of cell growth including *NF1* [113], *SHIP1* [114], and *PTEN* [115]. Some other genetic defects are more restricted to specific molecular-genetic subtypes, including *WT1* mutations that are most prominently found in T-ALL cases with aberrant rearrangements of the oncogenic *TLX1*, *TLX3*, and *HOXA* transcription factor oncogenes [116].

Activation of NOTCH1 Signaling

NOTCH1 is a transmembrane receptor that plays a major role in normal hematopoiesis driving lineage commitment of lymphoid progenitor cells towards T-cell development [117]. Thus, inactivation of NOTCH1 signaling in lymphoid progenitors in mice blocks T-cell development and promotes differentiation towards the B-cell lineage [118–120]. In the reciprocal setting, constitutive activation of NOTCH1 inhibits B-cell development and promotes extrathymic T-cell development [121].

NOTCH1 is synthesized as a single precursor protein (pre-NOTCH), which is processed by a furin protease to generate a heterodimeric protein consisting of an extracellular subunit and a transmembrane/intracellular subunit. Upon binding to the Jagged and Delta-like family of receptors, NOTCH1 undergoes two additional proteolytic cleavages which ultimately release the intracellular domains of the receptor (ICN1) in the cytosol [119, 120]. ICN1 is then transported to the nucleus where it mediates the expression of target genes such as *HES1*, *HEY1*, *MYC*, *PTCRA*, and *DTX1* [122–124].

A specific role for *NOTCH1* in human T-ALL was originally postulated due to its involvement in the rare chromosomal translocation, t(7;9)(q34;q34.3), which couples the intracellular part of *NOTCH1* to the *TCRβ* locus and leads to the aberrant expression of an intracellular constitutively active form of NOTCH1 [96]. The involvement of activated NOTCH1 in the pathogenesis of T-ALL was further demonstrated by animal models, in which expression of constitutively active forms of NOTCH1 were shown to induce T-cell tumorigenesis *in vivo* [125].

A broader role for NOTCH1 in T-cell leukemogenesis emerged when activating *NOTCH1* mutations were identified in more than 50% of T-ALL samples resulting in constitutive NOTCH signaling [28]. *NOTCH1* mutations mainly affect the heterodimerization (HD) domain and the C-terminal PEST domain. In addition, about 20% of T-ALL patients harbor mutations in both the HD and PEST domain of *NOTCH1* [28]. Finally, a rare but highly active group of alleles, the so-called juxtamembrane expansion (JME) mutations, result from internal duplication insertions in the extracellular juxtamembrane region of the receptor [126].

It was postulated that point mutations in the HD domain and JME alleles enhance the accessibility for proteolytic cleavage by γ-secretase, leading to ligand independent cleavage of NOTCH1 and release of ICN [28, 126]. Truncating mutations, as predominantly identified in the PEST domain, result in the removal of so-called Cdc phosphodegron domains (CPDs), which are normally involved in the degradation of ICN1 by the proteasome complex. PEST domain mutations therefore lead to the stabilization of ICN1. One of the proteins that bind to CPDs, thereby priming ICN for degradation, is the F-box protein FBXW7. FBXW7 is an E3-ubiquitin ligase that also regulates the half-life of other proteins including Cyclin E, cMYC, and cJUN [127].

Not surprisingly, mutations in this *FBXW7* gene were also identified as alternative or additional mechanism of NOTCH1 activation/stabilization in human T-ALL. Indeed, *FBXW7* point mutations were identified in 8–30% of T-ALL patients [128–130], frequently in association with NOTCH1 HD mutations [128–130].

Great interest exists in the inhibition of NOTCH1 signaling by GSIs as a potential therapeutic strategy in T-ALL. These small molecules interfere with the proteolytic cleavage of the receptor, inhibiting the release of ICN1 to the nucleus. GSIs induce growth arrest in some T-ALL cell lines and cause prolonged cell cycle arrest and apoptosis in primary T-ALL cells [28, 131]. However, despite the high prevalence of *NOTCH1* mutations and the presence of high levels of ICN1 in these tumors, some of these T-ALL cell lines failed to respond to NOTCH1 inhibition, suggesting primary resistance to GSI treatment [28]. Recently, it was shown that mutational loss of the tumor suppressor *PTEN* was associated with resistance towards NOTCH inhibition in T-ALL cell lines [115]. Importantly, although resistant for GSI treatment, PTEN mutant T-cell lines were highly sensitive for AKT inhibition, providing a rational for combined NOTCH1- and PI3K-AKT-directed therapeutic approaches in human T-ALL [32, 115]. Similarly, NOTCH1 regulates the NF-κB signaling pathway and inhibition of NOTCH signaling with GSIs can be synergistic with blocking the NF-κB with bortezomib [33].

However, the clinical development of GSIs has been hampered by the emergence of serious side effects, including severe gastrointestinal toxicity that results from conversion of intestinal

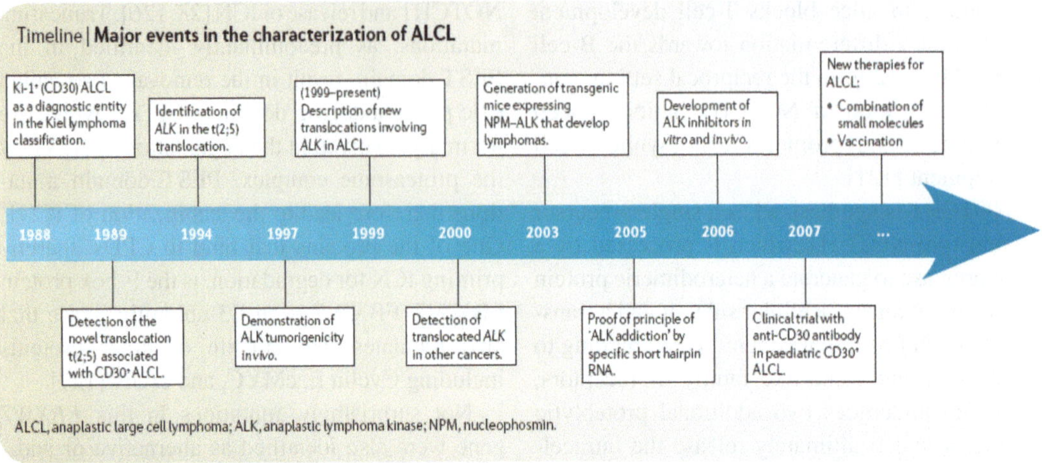

Fig. 11.7 Timeline of major events in the characterization of ALCL (reprinted from Chiarle et al. [138], with permission from Macmillan Publishers Ltd.)

crypt cells into goblet cells in the gut [132–134]. Notably, recent data suggested that inhibition of NOTCH1 signaling may reverse glucocorticoid resistance in some T-ALLs and that the combination of dexamethasone, a glucocorticoid extensively used in T-ALL treatment, and GSIs may ameliorate GSI-induced gut toxicity and provide a useful combination in the treatment of T-cell leukemias [29, 135]. Thus, NOTCH1 inhibition enhanced the effects of dexamethasone in glucocorticoid receptor autoupregulation and the activation of BIM-induced apoptosis [29].

Another clinically relevant downstream target of *NOTCH1* is the chemokine receptor *CCR7* which mediates the infiltration of CNS by leukemic lymphoblasts [136]. Therefore, pharmacological targeting of this chemokine receptor might reduce the risk of CNS relapse in T-ALL/T-LBL [136].

Overall, the identification of a multiplicity of molecular abnormalities in T-ALL has significantly improved our understanding of the mechanisms that contribute to the malignant transformation of T-cell precursors and opened the field for the development of specific targeted therapies blocking the activity of key genes and pathways required for the aberrant cell growth, proliferation, and survival of T-ALL/T-LBL lymphoblasts. In addition, further insights in the transcriptional networks regulated by the major T-cell oncogene *NOTCH1* revealed a variety of novel targets or treatment approaches that might be explored for T-ALL/T-LBL therapy, including the combined use of NOTCH inhibitors with PI3K-AKT pathway inhibitors [32, 115], anti-NF-κB drugs [33], and/or glucocorticoids [29, 135] or the targeting of the CCR7 receptor to prevent CNS relapse [136]. Hopefully, these novel treatment strategies will further improve T-ALL/T-LBL treatment outcome and reduce the therapy-related toxicities associated with intensive chemotherapy in T-ALL/T-LBL.

Anaplastic Large Cell Lymphoma in Children and Adolescents

Approximately 10% of NHLs that occur in children and adolescents are ALCL. First recognized in the 1980s [137], there have been significant advances in elucidating the distinct biological features of ALCL over the past 20 years (Fig. 11.7) [138]. There are two clinically distinct presentations of ALCL: a primary cutaneous form that presents exclusively in the skin and systemic ALCL [139]. Most cases of ALCL demonstrate TCR gene rearrangements, even when immunophenotypic analysis fails to demonstrate expression of T-cell antigens [140]. The systemic form of ALCL is most often characterized by

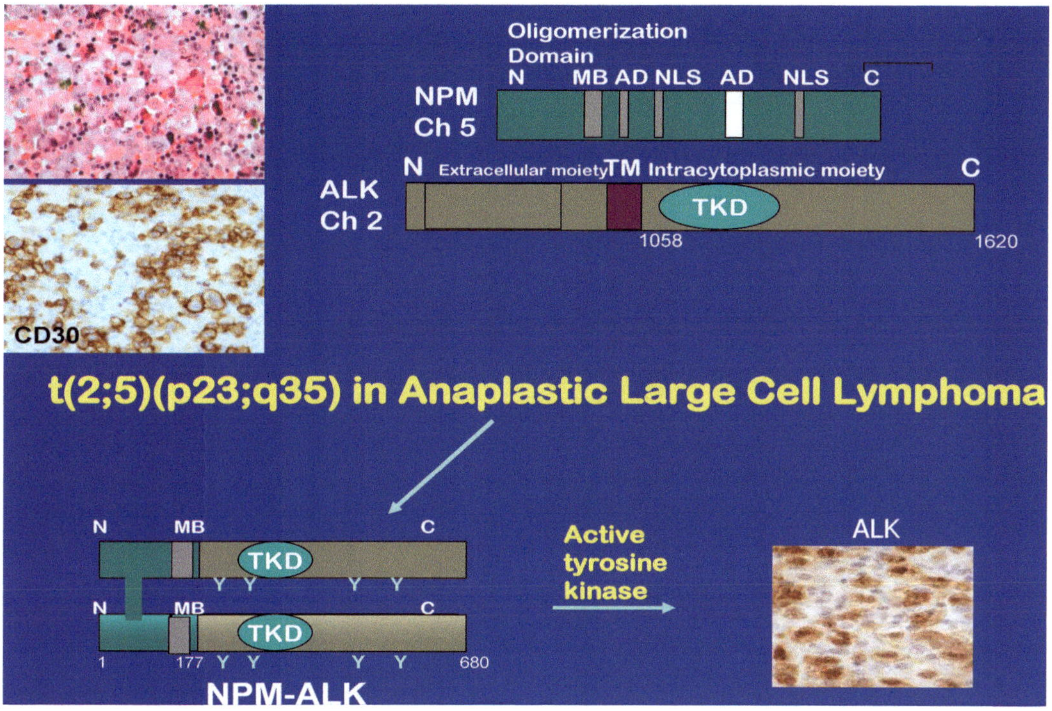

Fig. 11.8 Translocation of ALK gene on chromosome 2 with NPM gene on chromosome 5 in ALCL (adapted from Lim and Elenitoba-Johnson [180], with permission from The American Society for Biochemistry and Molecular Biology)

translocations of the *ALK* gene. Translocation of the *ALK* gene on chromosome 2q23 renders the disease *ALK*+ (Fig. 11.8). The most common translocation in ALCL partners *ALK* with the nucleophosmin (*NPM*) gene on chromosome 5q35. Less common findings include translocation of *ALK* to partner genes on chromosomes 1, 2, 3, and 17 that also result in upregulation of *ALK* expression (Table 11.3) [141]. *ALK*+ ALCL carries a significantly better prognosis than the *ALK*− ALCL counterpart. These categorizations help determine risk stratification parameters and enable the implementation of appropriately different therapeutic approaches.

ALCLs are characterized by large, pleomorphic, multinucleated cells with eccentric horseshoe-shaped nuclei and abundant clear to basophilic cytoplasm with an area of eosinophilia near the nucleus (termed "hallmark cells") [142]. These "hallmark cells" may resemble Reed–Sternberg cells found in Hodgkin lymphoma (HL), although they tend to have less conspicuous nucleoli compared to Reed–Sternberg cells. Several morphologic variants of ALCL have been identified in the revised European American lymphoma (REAL) and WHO classifications [143]. These include the common variant (75%) composed primarily of hallmark cells, the lymphohistiocytic variant (10%) that has a large number of benign histiocytes admixed with neoplastic cells, and the small cell variant (10%) where small neoplastic cells predominate and only scattered hallmark cells are visualized. Other (<5%) less well-described variants include a sarcomatoid variant, signet ring variant, neutrophil rich variant, and giant cell variant [140].

The distribution of ALCL subtypes in children is different than in adults. More than 90% of childhood ALCL cases are *ALK*+ [140], while approximately 60% of ALCL cases overall express *ALK* [144]. Primary cutaneous cases of ALCL are nearly always *ALK*− and are quite uncommon in children [141]. Expression of *ALK* is not entirely unique to ALCL, as it is a gene

Table 11.3 Recurrent chromosomal translocations involving ALK in cancers

Chromosomal translocation	Partner protein	Frequency (%)	Fusion protein (KDa)	Cellular localization	Type of tumor	References
t(2;5)(p23;q35)	Nucleophosmin (MPM)	75–80	NPM-ALK (80)	Nucleus, nucleolus, and cytoplasm	ALK^+ ALCL and ALK^+ DLBCL	[224–227]
t(1;2)(q25;p23)	Tropomyosin 3 (TPM3)	12–18	TPM3-ALK (104)	Cytoplasm	ALK^+ ALCL and IMT	[228–230]
t(2;3)(p23;q21)	TRK-fused gene (TFG)	2	TFG-ALK (113, 97, 85)	Cytoplasm	ALK^+ ALCL	[231, 232]
inv(2)(p23;q35)	ATIC	2	ATIC-ALK (96)	Cytoplasm	ALK^+ ALCL and IMT	[233–235]
t(2;17)(p23;q23)	Clathrin heavy chain-like 1 (CLTC1)	2	CLTC1-AKL (250)	Granular cytoplasmic	ALK^+ ALCL, IMT and ALK^+ DLBCL	[236–238]
t(2;X)(p23;q11-12)	Moesin (MSN)	<1	MSN-ALK (125)	Cell membrane associated	ALK^+ ALCL	[239, 240]
t(2;19)(p23;p13)	Tropomyosin 4 (TPM4)	<1	TPM4-ALK (95–105)	Cytoplasm	ALK^+ ALCL and IMT	[229, 241]
t(2;17)(p23;q25)	ALO17	<1	ALO17-ALK (ND)	Cytoplasm	ALK^+ ALCL	[242]
t(2l2)(p23;q13) or inv(2)(p23;q11-13)	RAN binding protein 2 (RANBP2)	<1	RANBP2-ALK (160)	Periphery of the nucleus	IMT	[243]
t(2;22)(p23;q11.2)	Non-muscle myosin heavy chain (MYH9)	<1	MYH9-ALK (220)	Cytoplasm	ALK^+ ALCL	[244]
t(2;11;2)(p23;p15;q31)	Cysteinyl-tRNA synthetase (CARS)	<1	CARS-ALK (130)	Unknown	IMT	[242, 245]
ins(3′ALK)(4q22-24)	Unknown	<1	Unknown	Granular cytoplasmic	ALK^+ DLBCL	[246]
t(2;4)(p23;q21)	SEC31 homologue A (*S. cerevisiae*) (SEC31L1)	<1	SEC31L1-ALK (ND)	Cytoplasm	IMT	[247]
inv(2)(p21;p23)	Echinoderm microtubule-associated protein-like 4 (EML4)	6	EML4-ALK (ND)	Unknown	NSCLC	[248]

Reprinted from Chiarle et al. [138], with permission from Macmillan Publishers Ltd.

ALCL anaplastic large cell lymphoma; *ALK* anaplastic lymphoma kinase; *ALO17* ALK lymphoma oligomerization partner on chromosome 17; *ATIC* 5-aminoimidazole-4-carboxamide ribonucleotide formyltransferase/IMP cyclohydrolase; *DLBCL* diffuse large B-cell lymphoma; *IMT* inflammatory myofibroblastic tumors; *ND* not determined; *NSCLC* non-small-cell lung cancer

normally involved in neuronal development and is rarely seen in cases of diffuse large B-cell lymphoma (DLBCL) and also in inflammatory myofibroblastic tumors [145].

Children tend to present with advanced stage III/IV ALCL at diagnosis [146]. Around 40–60% of patients with systemic ALCL present with B symptoms and have extranodal disease, most commonly involving the skin (20–25%), bone, and soft tissue, and commonly in association with nodal disease [147]. This contrasts with primary cutaneous ALCL, which although extranodal, is limited solely to the skin. Skin lesions usually present as solitary or localized nodules; however multifocal skin involvement occurs in 15–20% of patients [1, 2]. Involvement of the bone marrow occurs in less than 10% of patients [144], and CNS involvement is less common in ALCL than in other forms of childhood NHL such as BL and LBL, occurring in less than 5% of patients [148].

Risk stratification is ultimately important in the determination of the treatment of ALCL. Optimal therapeutic approaches for limited disease ALCL has yet to be established, as both B-NHL intensive therapy and T-ALL protocols have been used with similar efficacies. EFS has been reported to be as high as 100% for children with localized ALCL (stage I/stage II resected) in the NHL-BFM90 trial with 2 months of chemotherapy including dexamethasone, ifosfamide, MTX, cytarabine, etoposide, and prophylactic IT therapy [149]. St. Jude Children's Research Hospital reported a 75% EFS on a small number of children with localized CD30 positive large cell lymphoma (presumably ALCL) treated with three courses of CHOP (cyclophosphamide, doxorubicin, vincristine, and prednisone), either with or without maintenance therapy (6-mercaptopurine plus MTX) [150].

Treatment of advanced stage ALCL in children has evolved over the past two decades. Different strategies, including B-NHL intensive protocols and LSA_2-L_2-type therapies, have achieved EFS rates ranging between 65 and 75% (Table 11.4) [149, 151–155]. The backbone of combination doxorubcin, prednisone, and vincristine (APO) has been investigated in multiple trials over the past 15 years. Pediatric Oncology Group (POG)-9315 examined the utility of adding intermediate-dose MTX and high-dose cytarabine to the backbone APO regimen vs. standard APO alone; however there was insufficient power in the study to detect a difference between the two arms and those patients receiving MTX and cytarabine experienced greater toxicity. Children treated on the backbone APO arm had a 2-year EFS of 75.1% [152]. More recently, the COG has examined the addition of weekly vinblastine to the APO regimen based upon French data showing the remarkable overall response rate (ORR) of patients (10 out of 12) with relapsed ALCL to weekly vinblastine [156]. However in a recent report of the results from the COG study, the addition of vinblastine had no statistically significant improvement on the EFS or OS and was associated with increased myelosuppression. The overall 2-year EFS for the study was 77% [157]. Results from the international trial ALCL99 based upon the European approach of utilizing multi-agent intensive B-NHL-like therapy (built upon the BFM90 protocol) were recently reported. The study revealed an improvement in safety in utilizing a less toxic regimen including administration of high-dose MTX without IT chemotherapy and reported a 2-year EFS of 74% [158].

Until the ALCL99 trial, cases of CNS negative ALCL had been treated with prophylactic IT chemotherapy. With the recent success in preventing CNS relapse without the use of IT chemotherapy, the question arises whether a reduction in the number of high-dose MTX administrations can be employed. CRT in doses of 18–24 Gy in addition to high-dose MTX and/or Cytarabine and IT medicines has been reserved for cases of those rare patients with overt CNS disease [149, 151].

Several prognostic parameters have been identified in children with advanced disease ALCL. Some of the poor-risk clinical prognostic factors that have been identified include visceral organ involvement (liver, lung, spleen), mediastinal involvement, elevated lactate dehydrogenase (LDH), and disseminated skin disease (Fig. 11.9) [151, 159, 160]. More recently, correlation between tumor biology and treatment failure has become extremely important. Presence of MRD

Table 11.4 Advanced anaplastic large cell lymphoma in children

	BFM [149]	POG [152]	SFOP [151]	St. Jude [150]	MSKCC [166]	CCG [153]	EICNHL [159]	EICNHL [158]
Patients (*N*)	89	67	82	18	19	86	225	352
Protocol	NHL-BFM 90	POG 9315	HM89-91	CHOP-based	LSA_2L_2, LSA_4	CCG-5941	BFM, SFOP, UKCCSG	Modified NHL-BFM 90
Duration (months)	2–5	12	7–8	6–18	14–36	12	2–8	4–12
EFS (Est) 2–5 year	76%	73%	66%	57%	56%	68%	69%	75%
OS 2–5 years	NR	93%	83%	84%	84%	80%	81%	94%

Reprinted from Cairo [34], www.jbpub.com, with permission from Jones and Bartlett
EFS event-free survival; *Est* estimate; *OS* overall survival

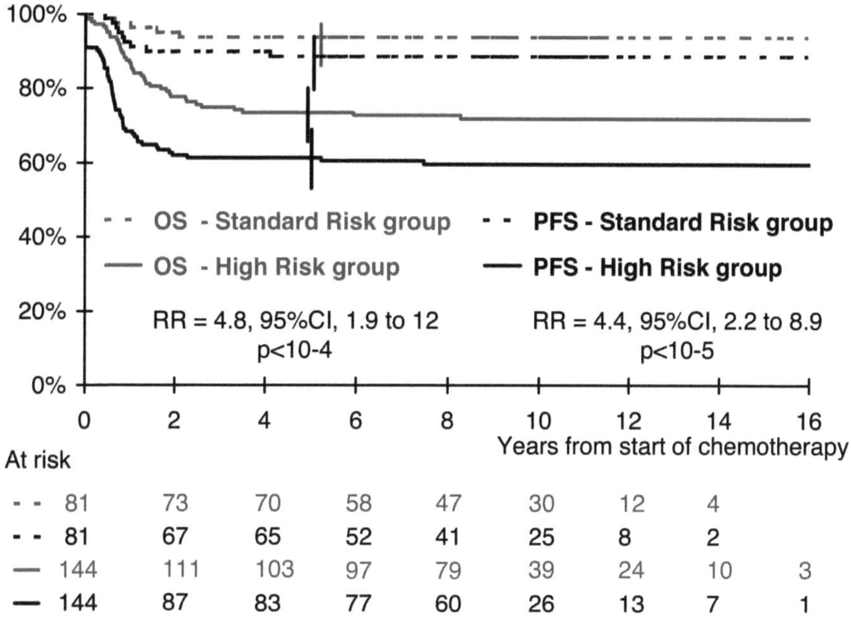

Fig. 11.9 OS and PFS according to risk group. Standard risk group indicates no risk factor (i.e., no mediastinal involvement and no lung, spleen, or liver involvement, and no skin lesion). High-risk group, at least 1 risk factor, mediastinal involvement, visceral involvement, or skin lesion. This research was originally published in *Blood* [159]. © American Society of Hematology

as detected by PCR analysis of the *NPM-ALK* transcript in the bone marrow and peripheral blood was associated with a significant increase in cumulative incidence of relapse in ALCL, 50% for PCR positive vs. 15% for negative (Fig. 11.10) [161]. Meanwhile, the presence of anti-*ALK* antibodies is inversely correlated to tumor dissemination and the risk of relapse in ALK^{+} ALCL and supports the use of *ALK* as an important potential immunotherapeutic target [162]. Additionally, analysis of the recent ALCL99 international trial revealed that two of the less common morphologic subtypes of ALCL, small cell and lymphohistiocytic, were significantly associated with a high risk of treatment failure, independent of clinical risk factors [163]. Ultimately, the continued development in the ability to predict those patients at higher risk for relapse will enable an intensification of front-line therapy and potentially improve outcomes.

Chemosensitivity at the time of relapse is a hallmark feature of childhood ALCL and has rendered salvage strategies for ALCL generally effective [164, 165]. Relapses in ALCL tend to occur later than in other histologic subtypes of childhood NHL [166]. The clinical behavior after relapse has been variable with some patients developing rapidly progressive disease and others having an indolent, waxing and waning course [167]. These differences have made uniform treatment approaches difficult to establish. In analyzing a series of three clinical trials in France over two decades, therapeutic intervention for relapse varied widely from single agent Vinblastine, to multi-agent chemotherapy, to fully ablative chemotherapy with both autoSCT and alloSCT. Higher risk for treatment failure included earlier relapse and more intensive initial treatment. Three-year risk DFS was not significantly different in patients who underwent ablative SCT in CR2 vs. those treated with chemotherapy alone [156]. However, more recent reports of alloSCT for relapsed and refractory ALCL have demonstrated encouraging results including a 3-year EFS of 75% for the larger series of 20 patients (Fig. 11.11) [168, 169].

Currently, new treatment strategies are focusing on determining the utility of targeted agents

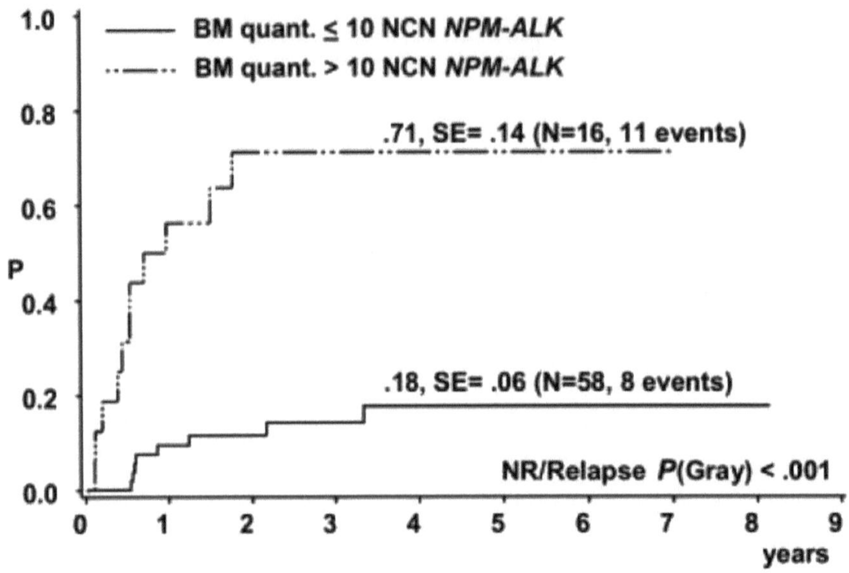

Fig. 11.10 Outcome of ALCL patients according to quantitative PCR results for *NPM-ALK* in bone marrow. Cumulative incidence of relapse of the 74 patients with either a negative qualitative BM PCR or a positive qualitative BM PCR using quantitative PCR results and a *NPM-ALK* cutoff copy number of 10/10^4 copies *ABL* (NCN). This research was originally published in *Blood* [161]. © American Society of Hematology

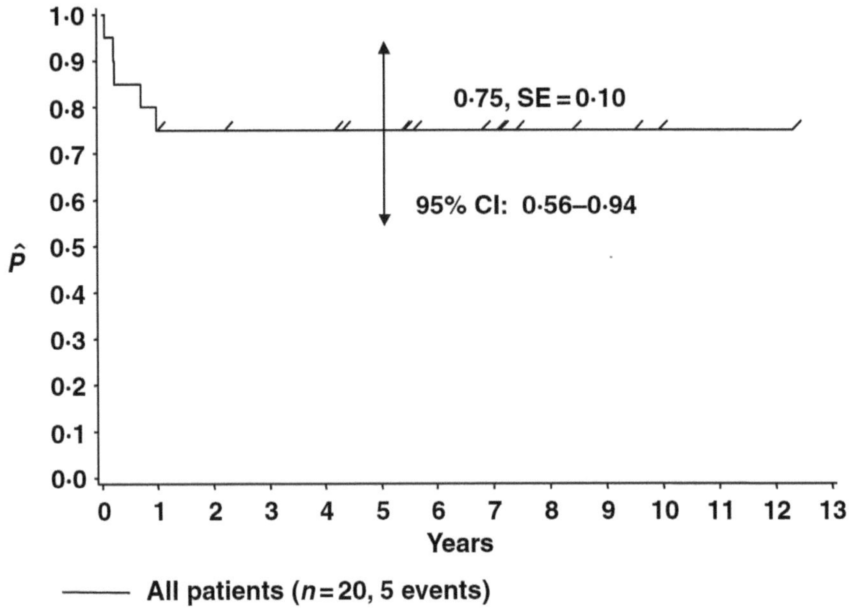

Fig. 11.11 EFS estimate for the 20 patients with anaplastic large cell lymphoma-relapse treated by allogeneic hematopoietic stem cell transplantation (reprinted from Woessmann et al. [169], with permission from Wiley-Blackwell Publishing)

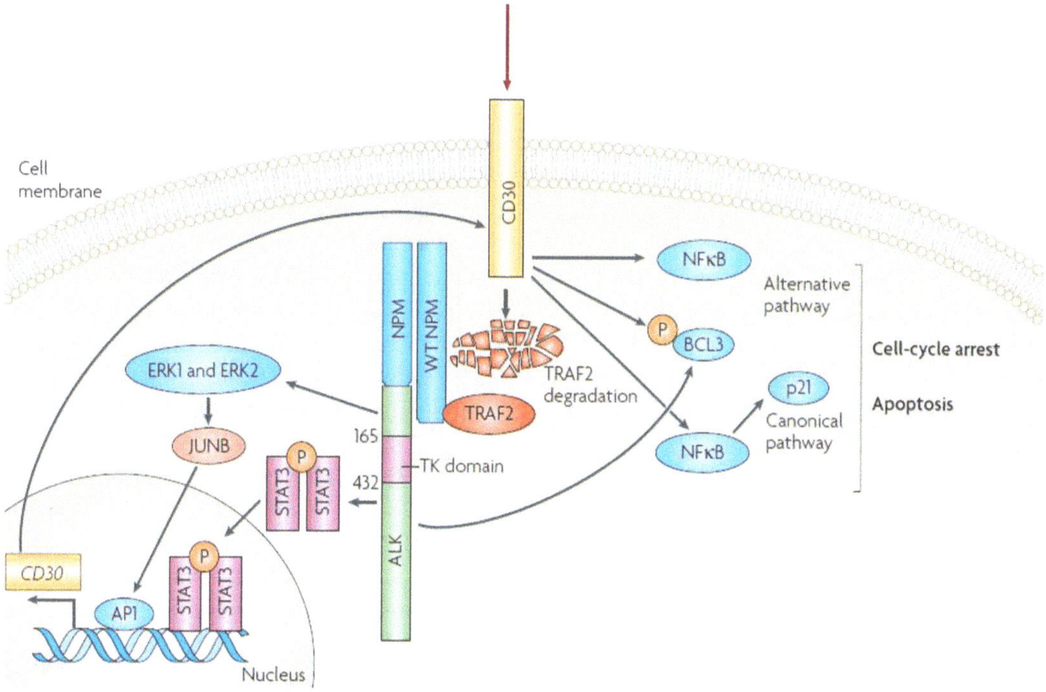

Fig. 11.12 ALK and CD30 signaling. In anaplastic large cell lymphoma (ALCL), CD30 expression is controlled by anaplastic lymphoma kinase (ALK) activity through the phosphorylation of signal transducer and activator of transcription 3 (STAT3) and the extracellular signal-regulated kinase 1 (ERK1)- and ERK2-mediated upregulation of JUNB protein levels. Phosphorylated STAT3 and activated AP1 complexes containing JUNB cooperate to enhance *CD30* transcription. The nucleophosmin (NPM)–ALK fusion protein impedes full CD30 signaling and nuclear factor κB (NFκB) activation by titrating tumor necrosis factor receptor-associated factor 2 (TRAF2) away from CD30 through dimerization with wild-type (WT) NPM. CD30 engagement results in TRAF2 degradation and BCL3 phosphorylation. The effect of CD30 engagement in ALCL cells is the activation of both the canonical and alternative NFκB pathways, which result in apoptosis and p21-mediated cell-cycle arrest. Clinical trials are currently using specific antibodies directed against CD30 (*red arrow*) in ALCL109. *TK* tyrosine kinase (reprinted from Chiarle et al. [138], with permission from Macmillan Publishers Ltd.)

as well as the optimal risk stratification that would determine using alloSCT in frontline therapy. CD30 antigen is expressed in close to 100% of all childhood and adolescent ALCL; this expression is controlled by *ALK* (Fig. 11.12). In phase I/II trials, one partial response and one CR have been achieved with SGN-30 monotherapy in heavily pretreated patients with relapsed and refractory ALCL [170, 171]. More recently, SGN-35, another monoclonal antibody targeting the CD30 antigen, has met even greater success than its predecessor. Two separate phase I trials have examined the role of SGN-35 monotherapy in patients with refractory/recurrent CD30⁺ lymphomas including cases of both ALCL and HL. At higher dose ranges of drug, preliminary data in one trial revealed that 7 of 8 evaluable patients achieved CR. In the other trial, also at the higher dose ranges of drug, 7 of 28 evaluable patients achieved CR with an ORR of 46% [172, 173]. The impressive response to monotherapy in heavily pretreated patients offers exciting hope that incorporating SGN-35 into combination therapy will provide promise for better results with frontline therapy.

Advances in the study of the biological characteristics of ALCL have also led to the development of novel therapeutic agents. Potential developmental therapeutic strategies include targeting the *ALK* protein with both small molecule inhibition as well as directed antibodies. The *ALK* inhibitor TAE684 has proven effective with *in vitro* and *in vivo* inhibition of *ALK*⁺ ALCL. In separate mouse models the drug was able to achieve prevention of tumor development as well as regression of pre-induced tumor [174]. The aforementioned evidence showing a strong correlation with circulating anti-*ALK* antibodies and a lower risk for relapse has led to investigations in vaccination strategies stimulated by the *ALK* antigen [175]. Somatic mutations in ALCL are rare. Monoallelic and biallelic mutations of the perforin (*PRF1*) gene and sonic hedgehog (*SHH*) have been reported in some cases of childhood lymphomas. Direct sequencing identified 6 different mutations in 12 patients (27.3%) of 44 patients with t(2;5)+ALCL. The incidence of *PRF1* mutations was found to be significantly higher in patients with ALCL compared with 400 control subjects, among whom only heterozygous A91V was observed in 41 subjects (10.2%) (chi-square test, 10.9; $P<0.01$) [176]. *PRF1* mutations have been described in other NHLs and are thought to result in defective perforin-mediated cytotoxicity due to abnormal conformational changes induced by the A91V mutation [177]. Amplification of *SHH* gene in a subset of *ALK* positive ALCL [178] has been shown to lead to deregulation of the *SHH* signaling pathway. While genomic studies were essential in identifying the characteristic upregulation of the *ALK* protein in ALCL, proteomic studies of ALCL have been instrumental in understanding the importance of the *ALK* gene and its associated network of proteins (Fig. 11.13a, b) [179, 180]. Most recently, unraveling of the proteomic signature of the *NPM/ALK* fusion gene identified cellular changes affecting cell proliferation, ribosome synthesis, survival, apoptosis evasion, angiogenesis, and cytoarchitectural organization [179]. Further investigation showed loss of cell adhesion as a consequence of *NPM/ALK* expression in a kinase-dependent manner, and sensitivity of *NPM/ALK*-positive ALCLs to inhibition of the *RAS*, p42/44ERK, and FRAP/mTOR signaling pathways [179]. Understanding the effects of *NPM/ALK* alteration on a diverse array of cellular pathways offers novel insights into *NPM/ALK*-positive ALCL pathobiology. Other proteomic studies have demonstrated the constitutive expression of CD25 in pediatric ALCL and have led to *in vitro* investigations of the anti-CD25 agent, denileukin diftitox, as a novel therapeutic approach [181, 182]. Furthermore, the identification of other important downstream cellular pathways interconnected with *ALK* has led to studies examining the utility of disrupting *ALK*-associated pathways in an attempt to prevent tumorigenesis. Heat shock protein 90 (*Hsp-90*) and the PI3K/Akt apoptosis pathway have both demonstrated interactions with the *ALK* protein network. *In vitro* studies targeting *Hsp-90* resulted in increased degradation of *NPM-ALK* and subsequent apoptosis in ALCL cell lines [183], while PI3K/Akt negative mice injected with *NPM/ALK*⁺ cells showed significantly impaired tumor forming capacity [184]. Altogether, advances in our understanding of the genomic and proteomic characteristics of ALCL have enabled an expanded approach to therapeutic targeting of developmental strategies. Combining new and less toxic therapies offers an exciting opportunity to enhance both the efficacy and safety of therapies for future patients.

Other Peripheral T-Cell Lymphomas in Children and Adolescents

PTCLs other than ALCLs are composed of a diverse group of rare disease entities. After ALCL, PTCL-not otherwise specified (nos) makes up the second largest type of PTCL. In children, PTCL-nos accounts for only approximately 1% of all cases of NHL [185]. In contrast, it represents around 4% of NHL in adults [186]. It is important to remember though, that the incidence of PTCL varies based on geographical and ethnic differences; for example, there is a distinctly higher prevalence of PTCL in Asia [186]. While the etiology of certain subtypes of PTCL is well described (i.e., human T-cell lymphotropic virus [HTLV] in adult T-cell leukemia/lymphoma and Epstein–Barr virus [EBV] in the EBV T-cell lymphoproliferative [LPD]), for the most part the etiology of this diverse group of diseases has yet to be determined [3].

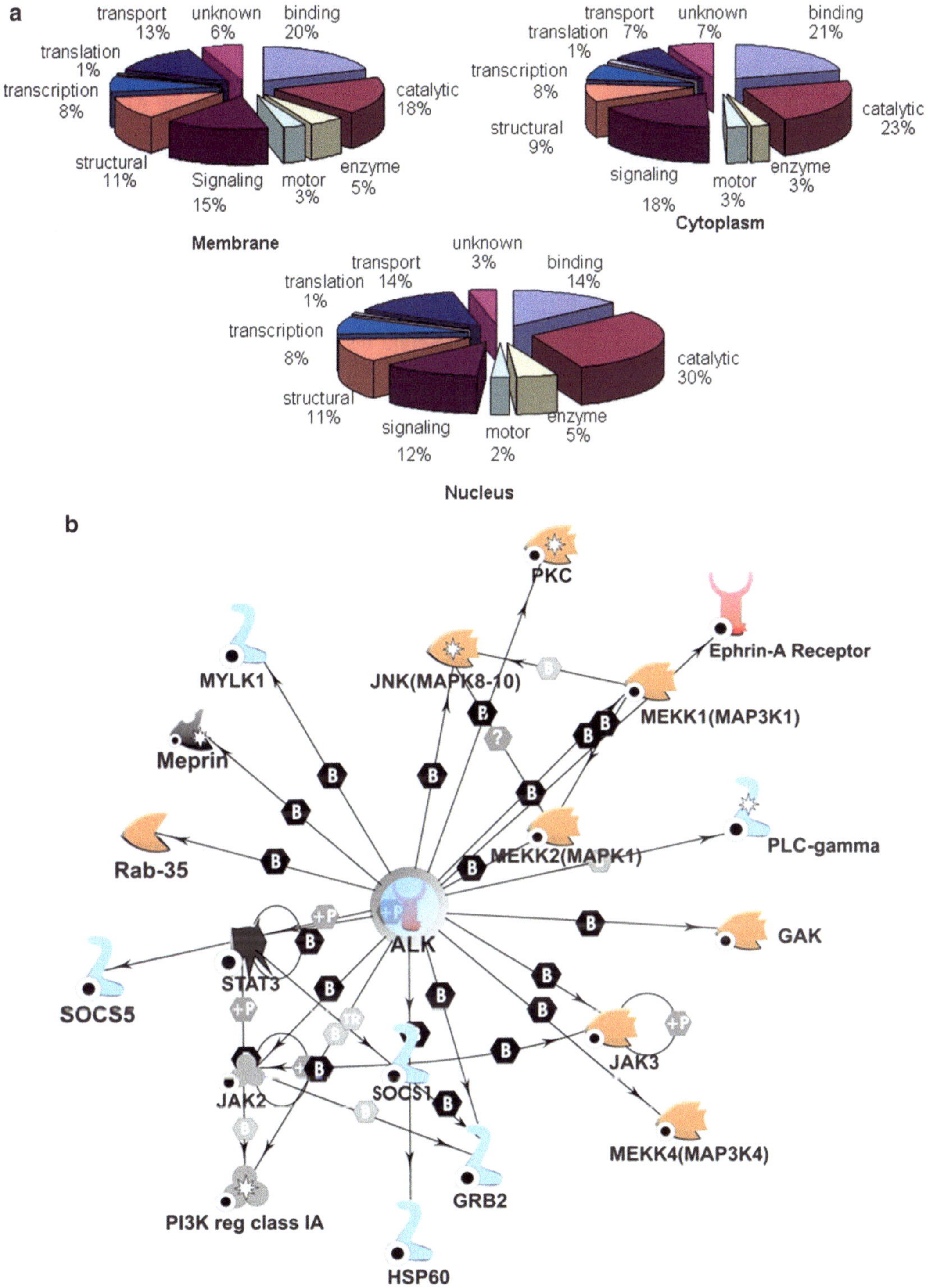

Fig. 11.13 (**a**) Functional categories of proteins expressed in the membrane, cytoplasmic, and nuclear fraction of ALCL. GoMiner analysis of proteins identified in the membrane, cytoplasmic, and nuclear fractions reveals proteins from diverse functional categories. (**b**) Proteins identified within the NPM/ALK protein network. The proteins identified within the NPM/ALK immunocomplex are visualized using GeneGO software analysis. *reg* regulated; *PKC* protein kinase C; *GAK* cyclin G-associated kinase (reprinted from Lim and Elenitoba-Johnson [180], with permission from The American Society for Biochemistry and Molecular Biology)

Table 11.5 WHO 2008 classification of precursor and mature T/NK-cell neoplasms

Leukemic or disseminated
T lymphoblastic leukemia/lymphoma
T-cell prolymphocytic leukemia
T-cell large granular lymphocytic leukemia
Chronic lymphoproliferative disorders of NK cells
Aggressive NK-cell leukemia
Adult T-cell lymphoma/leukemia (HTLV1-positive)
Systemic Epstein–Barr virus (EBV)-positive T-cell lymphoproliferative disorders of childhood
Extranodal
Extranodal NK/T-cell lymphoma, nasal type
Enteropathy-associated T-cell lymphoma
Hepatosplenic T-cell lymphoma
Extranodal-cutaneous
Mycosis fungoides
Sezary syndrome
Primary cutaneous $CD30^{+}$ lymphoproliferative disorders
Primary cutaneous anaplastic large cell lymphoma
Lymphomatoid papulosis
Subcutaneous panniculitis-like T-cell lymphoma
Primary cutaneous gamma-delta T-cell lymphoma
Primary cutaneous aggressive epidermotropic $CD8^{+}$ cytotoxic lymphoma
Nodal
Angioimmunoblastic T-cell lymphoma
Anaplastic large cell lymphoma, ALK-positive
Anaplastic large cell lymphoma, ALK-negative
Primary cutaneous small/medium $CD4^{+}$ T-cell lymphoma

Based on data from refs. [1, 2]

The other entities of PTCL are too numerous to discuss each in great detail, but are listed in Table 11.5. The 2008 WHO Classification of Lymphoid Neoplasms has subdivided PTCLs into four groups based upon their mode of clinical presentation: leukemic/disseminated, extranodal, extranodal-cutaneous, and nodal. Examples of the leukemic/disseminated types include the HTLV-1 positive adult T-cell lymphoma/leukemia and systemic EBV positive T-cell LPD of childhood. The extranodal variety of PTCL includes extranodal NK/T-cell lymphoma, enteropathy-associated T-cell lymphoma, and hepatosplenic lymphoma. The extranodal-cutaneous forms include Mycosis Fungoides/Sezary syndrome, primary cutaneous $CD30^{+}$ LPD (discussed in more detail in the ALCL section), subcutaneous panniculitis-like T-cell lymphoma, and primary cutaneous $\gamma\delta$ T-cell lymphoma. The nodal sub group includes ALCL, angioimmunoblastic T-cell lymphoma, and PTCL-nos, previously referred to as PTCL-u [139].

The biological characteristics of PTCL-nos also exhibit diversity. It has been challenging to identify the normal counterpart T cells that correlate with the cellular origin of disease for PTCL-nos. A variety of immunophenotypic changes have been observed across different stages of T-cell differentiation with cells expressing different combinations of pan-T-cell antigens as well as markers of both cytotoxic and activated T-cell subtypes [187]. Similarly, although several different cytogenetic changes have been observed in cases of PTCL-u, a specific pattern that correlates to clinically meaningful consequences has yet to be established [188]. In fact, ALCL is the only T-cell lymphoma that is characterized by a consistently recurring genetic abnormality in the t2;5 translocation [189]. Furthermore, although clonal gene rearrangements of the TCR are often seen in cases of PTCL-u, these molecular changes vary and none serve to represent a characteristic pattern [3].

Some recent observations in the biological behavior of PTCL have opened the door to some exciting scientific investigations. Gene array analysis of PTCL-u specimens has linked the reduced expression of *NF-κB* genes with shorter survival [190]. While further studies are required to understand the precise relationship between the *NF-κB* pathway and PTCL-u tumorigenesis, this data offers an excellent opportunity to improve our understanding of disease progression as well as discover a target for developmental therapeutics. Similarly, another study was able to separate PTCL-u into three subgroups based upon microarray-based genomic findings. These three groups included one characterized by the expression of cyclin D2, another with the overexpression of *NF-κB1* and *Bcl-2* genes, and the third marked by overexpression of genes involved in the interferon/JAK/STAT pathway [191]. Again, while further investigations are required to unravel a deeper understanding of these pathways and how they are involved in lymphomagenesis, these studies have identified novel and potentially important biological observations in PTCL.

The clinical presentations of PTCL are as varied as the biological characteristics. Most patients present with either generalized lymphadenopathy (commonly in the cervical region) or extranodal disease. The extranodal presentation often involves the liver, spleen, skin, and bone marrow. The majority of patients have advanced stage disease at diagnosis and exhibit systemic constitutional B symptoms such as fevers, night sweats, and/or weight loss. LDH is often elevated and there may or may not be abnormalities appreciated on the CBC. Often times patients are found to have symptoms associated with increased cytokine production from the abnormal T cells and can even present with the overt hyperinflammatory signs of a hemophagocytic syndrome [3].

Unfortunately, treatment strategies employed over the years for PTCL have been as varied as their clinical and pathological findings. It has been extremely challenging to develop and establish effective treatment regimens because the clinical experience in pediatric PTCL has been sparse and individual studies have been hampered by too few patients. The largest cohorts of pediatric PTCL patients have recently been reported from the United States of America (USA) and the United Kingdom (UK).

The COG analyzed 20 pediatric patients identified over a 9-year period. The cohort included mostly patients with PTCL-u; however there were also patients with extranodal NK/T-cell lymphoma nasal type, subcutaneous panniculitis-like T-cell lymphoma, and enteropathy-type T-cell lymphoma. Treatment choice was differentiated based upon clinical staging. Patients with advanced stage III/IV disease were treated with a regimen of doxorubicin, prednisone, vincristine, mercaptopurine, and MTX ± alternating therapy with high-dose cytarabine and intermediate-dose MTX. Patients with localized stage I/II disease were treated with CHOP. Of patients with localized disease, 2 relapsed and 9 of 10 survived. Of patients with advanced stage disease, 6 relapsed and 5 of 10 survived. These results are markedly better than most studies analyzing adults with PTCL. However, while CHOP-like therapy seems adequate for patients with localized disease, the OS for patients with advanced stage disease was only 50%, leaving plenty of room for improvement [192].

The experience in the UK was quite similar to that of the COG in the USA. The UK study analyzed 25 cases of PTCL in children and adolescents over a 20-year period. They observed a similar distribution of PTCL subtypes with 68% of patients having PTCL-u, the remainder of cases were angiocentric PTCL, angioimmunoblastic T-cell lymphoma, and subcutaneous panniculitis-like T-cell lymphoma. In this retrospective analysis, patients were treated either with B-NHL CHOP-like regimens or with T-ALL type of treatment strategies. Among children with PTCL-u, 9 of 12 survived with T-ALL therapy, while only 1 of 5 that received B-NHL therapy survived. Similar to the COG results, when analyzed based upon extent of disease, the majority of patients (9 of 12) with localized stage I/II disease survived, while only 6 of 12 children with advanced stage disease survived. The authors concluded that children with PTCL-u should be treated with T-ALL-like therapy; however it is still apparent that a large percentage of children with advanced stage disease do not survive [185].

Outcomes for adults with PTCL have been even worse. Treatment strategies have varied widely, yet 5-year OS in adult studies has ranged from 25 to 45% [3, 193–195]. Conventional chemotherapy combinations used in adults have most frequently included CHOP-like therapy; however there have also been attempts to incorporate cytarabine, cisplatin, and etoposide without any improvement in survival rates. With the poor outcomes from conventional chemotherapy, the use of high-dose chemotherapy with both autoSCT and alloSCT has also been explored.

High-dose chemotherapy with autoSCT has been attempted as both salvage and front-line therapy in PTCL. In the setting of refractory or recurrent disease, OS after autoSCT has been reported around 33% [196]. Some studies report higher OS rates ranging between 39 and 48%; however their cohorts included cases of ALCL which typically do well with autoSCT for salvage therapy. When analyzed based upon histologic subtype, the cases of PTCL had OS closer to 30% in those same studies [197]. Attempts to treat PTCL with front-line autoSCT have yielded slightly better results; however the biggest obstacle to achieving better outcomes was the inability to attain remission in significant numbers of patients. A large study performed in Italy for patients with high-risk PTCL receiving autoSCT as up-front therapy reported long-term OS rates of 39%. However, a number of patients progressed before autoSCT and never received the therapy. Of the patients that did get high-dose chemo and autoSCT, 12-year DFS rate was 55% [198].

Many groups have also attempted alloSCT for PTCL. This strategy provides the advantage of infusing lymphoma-free grafts and potential for a graft vs. lymphoma effect. Studies have demonstrated a lower risk of relapse in patients receiving alloSCT (in comparison to autoSCT); however the high rates of transplant-related mortality with fully ablative conditioning regimens have offset any survival advantages [199]. The Italian group has recently reported on the role of alloSCT with reduced intensity conditioning regimens. In a pilot study of 17 patients with refractory and recurrent disease (8 of whom relapsed after prior autoSCT), a 3-year progression-free survival of 64% was achieved, with only 1 of 17 patients suffering from transplant-related mortality [200]. This study offers promising data for a disease that has been notoriously difficult to treat for many years.

Pediatric studies have shown that patients with advanced stage III/IV disease have markedly worse outcomes than those with localized stage I/II disease [185, 192]. In adults, the International Prognostic Index (IPI) has commonly been used for risk stratification. The IPI incorporates high-risk features such as advanced stage disease, LDH level greater than twice normal, elderly patient age, multifocal extranodal involvement of disease, and poor performance status. A Canadian study demonstrated the validity of the IPI in adult patients with PTCL-u, showing that of 117 patients, those with an IPI score of 0–1 (30% of the cohort) had a 5-year OS of 64%, while those with an IPI score >2 (70% of the cohort) had an OS of 30% [195]. The Italian group has established the Prognostic Index for PTCL-u (PIT) model based upon principles from the IPI and results from a series of nearly 400 patients. Using four clinical variables, age, performance status, LDH level, and bone marrow involvement, they were able to identify prognostic groups. Groups 1 and 2 had zero or one adverse factor and 5-year OS rates of 62% and 53%, respectively. Groups 3 and 4 had two or more than two adverse factors and OS rates of 33% and 18%, respectively [201]. In application to pediatric patients, certainly they will not carry the adverse factor of elderly age status, but indicators of advanced stage disease like elevated LDH and bone marrow involvement will portend for a worse prognosis.

With the overall poor outcomes in adult patients with PTCL and pediatric patients with advanced stage PTCL, advances in therapeutic strategies are desperately needed. New agents in investigation for PTCL include a wide array of agents from the following pharmacologic categories: nucleoside analogs, histone deacetylase inhibitors, anti-angiogenesis agents, folate inhibitors, proteasome inhibitors, and monoclonal antibodies. Of the nucleoside analogs, pentostatin and gemcitabine have shown the most promise. A single institution study demonstrated an ORR to gemcitabine in refractory/recurrent disease to be 60%; however there were only ten patients evaluated [202]. Currently gemcitabine is being investigated in combination with other agents against a variety of lymphomas. Nelarabine, on the other hand, achieved an ORR of only 10.5% and also exhibited marked toxicity [203]. The histone deacetylase inhibitor, depsipeptide, induced an ORR of 26% in data from a phase II trial [204]. Anti-angiogenesis agents like bevacizumab have been utilized specifically in angioimmunoblastic T-cell lymphoma and there are some case reports of achieving CR in refractory/recurrent cases [205, 206]. The new anti-folate agent Pralatrexate has shown promise in phase I/II trials with an ORR of 47% in 26 patients with T-cell lymphoma, many of whom had PTCL [207]. Investigations were expanded to a multicenter trial enrolling over 100 patients with PTCL, with interim data showing ORR of 29% in 65 patients, with 11% of total patients achieving CR [208]. Combining proteasome inhibitor, bortezomib, with liposomal doxorubicin has proven safe and effective for advanced stage hematologic malignancies [209]. Proteasome inhibitors are known to promote apoptosis and the anti-proliferative properties via inhibition of the NF-κB pathway. Bortezomib thus provides an attractive mechanism of action in PTCL with recent biology studies demonstrating an overexpression of *NF-κB1* genes in certain subgroups of PTCL. It has been investigated in refractory and relapsed cutaneous T-cell lymphomas, achieving an ORR of 67% as single-agent therapy. Although the majority of cases in that trial were *Mycoses Fungoides*, which is characteristically unique in comparison to other forms of PTCL, there were two patients with PTCL-u in that study, one of whom achieved response [210]. Currently there are studies examining the role of bortezomib in combination with other therapies for PTCL as front-line therapy [211].

The development of monoclonal antibodies has fostered much progress in the treatment of pediatric lymphomas in the past decade. In PTCL there has been much interest in incorporating monoclonal antibodies into combination therapeutic regimens. Alemtuzumab is a humanized monoclonal antibody that targets CD52, an antigen expressed on nearly all lymphocytes. It has been studied as a single agent in refractory/recurrent cases of PTCL, achieving a 36% ORR in a pilot study of 14 patients. However, there were excessive infectious complications experienced in the study with five patients suffering from treatment-related mortality [212]. A more recent study examined the role of alemtuzumab in combination with CHOP chemotherapy as front-line therapy. This experience revealed tolerable rates of toxicity and 1-year EFS of 41% [213]. Other monoclonal antibodies have been explored in the setting of cutaneous T-cell lymphomas and their utility in other forms of PTCL remains to be elucidated. They include the anti-CD4 antibody zanolimumab, as well as daclizumab and denileukin diftitox, two antibodies targeting the CD25 antigen, which is a form of the human IL-2 receptor [214, 215].

Rare T-Cell Lymphomas in Children and Young Adolescents

Hepatosplenic Gamma Delta T-Cell Lymphoma

This is a very rare and aggressive peripheral T-cell neoplasm that is characterized by involvement of the liver, spleen, and bone marrow. It is a disease of young adults with a distinct male predominance. Patients present with marked hepatosplenomegaly without lymphadenopathy. Up to 20% of cases arise in the setting of chronic immune suppression, most commonly in the setting of solid organ transplantation or prolonged antigenic stimulation as in inflammatory bowel disease after exposure to azathioprine and infliximab. More recently, EBV-negative T-cell lymphomas with features consistent with hepatosplenic T-cell lymphomas have been reported in patients receiving infliximab for inflammatory bowel disease [216]. Molecular studies consistently show isochromosome 7q often in conjunction with trisomy 8. The cells have rearranged TCR genes. Gene expression profiling of γ/δ T-cell lymphoma [217] revealed that genes of NK-cell associated molecules such as killer cell immunoglobulin-like receptor genes and killer cell lectin-like receptors were found to be overexpressed relative to other PTCL with α/β phenotype. Gene ontology analysis of differentially expressed genes show enrichment of those involved in cellular defense response, signal transduction activity, receptor activity, transmembrane receptor activity, and immunoglobulin-G binding.

EBV Positive T-Cell Lymphoproliferative Disorders

In the 2008 WHO classification two new major types of EBV-associated T-cell LPDs affecting the pediatric population have been incorporated:

systemic EBV-positive T-cell LPD of childhood and Hydroa vacciniforme-like lymphoma. Both of them occur predominantly in Asians and in Native Americans from Central and South America and Mexico.

Systemic EBV-Positive T-Cell Lymphoproliferative Disease of Childhood

Most patients present with acute onset of fever and general malaise after which patients develop hepatosplenomegaly and liver failure with or without lymphadenopathy. The disease has a rapid progression to multiple organ failure, sepsis, hemophagocytic syndrome, and death. Chronic EBV infection has been documented in some patients prior to the development of disease. Most cases secondary to acute primary EBV infection are $CD8^+$ whereas those in the setting of severe chronic active EBV infection (CAEBV) are $CD4^+$. EBER-1 is positive in the neoplastic T cells. The neoplastic cells exhibit clonal TCR gene rearrangement and harbor EBV in a clonal episomal form. All cases carry type A EBV, either with wild-type or the 30 base pair deleted product of *LMP1* gene. This is a life-threatening illness of children and young adults characterized by a clonal proliferation of EBV-infected T cells with an activated cytotoxic phenotype. It usually occurs shortly after primary acute EBV infection in previously healthy patients or in the setting of CAEBV. It has a rapid progression with multiple organ failure, sepsis, and death, usually from days to weeks. The most frequent sites of involvements are liver and spleen followed by lymph nodes, bone marrow, skin, and lung. The most typical phenotype of the tumor cells is $CD2^+CD3^+CD56^-$ and positive for cytotoxic proteins. Most cases secondary to acute primary EBV infection are $CD8^+$, whereas cases in the setting of severe CAEBV are $CD4^+$. EBV is always positive. The tumor cells have monoclonally rearranged TCR genes.

Hydroa Vacciniforme-Like Lymphoma

This is an EBV-positive cutaneous T-cell lymphoma occurring in children and associated with sun sensitivity. This condition affects primarily sun-exposed skin, in particular the face. The lesions present as papulovesicular eruptions that precede ulcerations and scarring. The clinical course is variable and some may have recurrent skin lesions. Late in the disease course, there is development of systemic symptoms such as fever, wasting, lymphadenopathy, and hepatosplenomegaly. The neoplastic cells exhibit clonal TCR gene rearrangement and harbor EBV in a clonal episomal form. It is still not clear whether severe mosquito-bite allergy, which is of NK derivation and EBV-associated, is part of Hydroa vacciniforme-like lymphoma or a distinctive entity within the spectrum of EBV-associated disorders. Both disorders are considered part of the spectrum of severe CAEBV, with a broad spectrum of clinical aggressiveness.

Ultimately, despite its rare occurrence in children and adolescents, PTCL remains a diagnostic and therapeutic challenge for this age group. While there continues to be progress in the identification of specific disease entities, improvements in the outcomes with treatment strategies have been slow to improve. A large number of developmental therapeutic agents are continually being examined in adults, where the numbers of patients enable such investigations. However, with the paucity of pediatric cases of PTCL, there will have to be extrapolation of adult data to improve on the outcomes of cases with advanced stage disease. As we learn more about the biology of these diseases and the potential benefits of specific targeted agents, decisions in treatment strategies will become more enlightened. Until a tried and true therapeutic regimen is discovered, it seems that children with advanced stage and/or refractory/recurrent PTCL may benefit from induction therapy followed by an alloSCT with reduced-intensity conditioning regimens.

Summary

T-cell malignancies in children and adolescents represent a heterogeneous group of neoplasms that arise from precursor T lymphocytes and a variety of mature T subsets. Most T-cell malignancies exhibit aggressive clinical behavior.

T-ALL and T-LBL represent 15% of childhood ALL and one-third of childhood and adolescent NHL respectively. Although the molecular genetics of T-ALL has been well studied, relatively little is known regarding the molecular pathogenetic mechanism involved in T-LBLs. It has been widely accepted that T-ALL and T-LBL likely represent different clinical manifestations of the same disease. Recent molecular analyses of T-LBLs however provide some evidence that they may exhibit distinct molecular genetic aberrations. Furthermore, many clinical trials have considered these diseases as one entity. The prevalence of *NOTCH* activation in T-ALLs has generated significant interest in the use of GSIs as a therapeutic strategy in T-ALLs. The results of clinical trials which are currently underway would be of interest. Within the mature T-cell malignancies, the *ALK* positive ALCLs are the most prevalent. Logically, the molecular aberration that defines this group of T-cell malignancies has led to the generation of a panel of potential tyrosine kinase inhibitors. Small molecule inhibitors to the *ALK* tyrosine kinase are currently under clinical investigation for relapsed ALCLs. Clearly, the number of developmental therapeutic agents available for children and adolescents is significantly lower than that for adults, where the numbers of patients enable such investigations. However, with the paucity of pediatric cases of PTCL, there will have to be extrapolation of adult data to improve on the outcomes of cases with advanced stage disease. As we learn more about the biology of these diseases and the potential benefits of specific targeted agents, decisions in treatment strategies will become more enlightened. Until a tried and true therapeutic regimen is discovered, it seems that children with advanced stage and/or refractory/recurrent PTCL may benefit from induction therapy followed by an alloSCT with reduced-intensity conditioning regimens. With improved diagnostic criteria for subclassification of T-cell neoplasms and better understanding of the molecular pathogenetic mechanisms, there is increasing optimism for greater availability of therapeutic agents for T-cell malignancies in children and adolescents.

References

1. Borowitz MJ, Chan JKC. T lymphoblastic leukaemia/lymphoma. In: Swerdlow SH, Campo E, Harris NL, et al., editors. WHO classification of tumours of haematopoietic and lymphoid tissues. Lyon: IARC Press; 2008. p. 176–8.
2. Mature T- and NK-cell neoplasms. In: Swerdlow SH, Campo E, Harris NL, et al., editors. WHO classification of tumours of haematopoietic and lymphoid tissues. Lyon: IARC Press; 2008. p. 270–319.
3. Rodriguez-Abreu D, Filho VB, Zucca E. Peripheral T-cell lymphomas, unspecified (or not otherwise specified): a review. Hematol Oncol. 2008;26: 8–20.
4. Uckun FM, Sensel MG, Sun L, et al. Biology and treatment of childhood T-lineage acute lymphoblastic leukemia. Blood. 1998;91:735–46.
5. Margolin JF, Steuber CP, Poplack DG. Acute lymphoblastic leukemia. In: Pizzo PA, Poplack DG, editors. Principles and practice of pediatric oncology. 5th ed. Philadelphia: Lippincott, Williams and Wilkins; 2006. p. 538–90.
6. Ballerini P, Landman-Parker J, Cayuela JM, et al. Impact of genotype on survival of children with T-cell acute lymphoblastic leukemia treated according to the French protocol FRALLE-93: the effect of TLX3/HOX11L2 gene expression on outcome. Haematologica. 2008;93:1658–65.
7. Goldberg JM, Silverman LB, Levy DE, et al. Childhood T-cell acute lymphoblastic leukemia: the Dana-Farber Cancer Institute acute lymphoblastic leukemia consortium experience. J Clin Oncol. 2003;21:3616–22.
8. Moghrabi A, Levy DE, Asselin B, et al. Results of the Dana-Farber Cancer Institute ALL Consortium Protocol 95-01 for children with acute lymphoblastic leukemia. Blood. 2007;109:896–904.
9. Moricke A, Reiter A, Zimmermann M, et al. Risk-adjusted therapy of acute lymphoblastic leukemia can decrease treatment burden and improve survival: treatment results of 2169 unselected pediatric and adolescent patients enrolled in the trial ALL-BFM 95. Blood. 2008;111:4477–89.
10. Pui CH, Campana D, Pei D, et al. Treating childhood acute lymphoblastic leukemia without cranial irradiation. N Engl J Med. 2009;360:2730–41.
11. Pui CH, Sandlund JT, Pei D, et al. Improved outcome for children with acute lymphoblastic leukemia: results of Total Therapy Study XIIIB at St Jude Children's Research Hospital. Blood. 2004;104:2690–6.
12. Reiter A, Schrappe M, Ludwig WD, et al. Chemotherapy in 998 unselected childhood acute lymphoblastic leukemia patients. Results and conclusions of the multicenter trial ALL-BFM 86. Blood. 1994;84:3122–33.
13. Uckun FM, Reaman G, Steinherez PG, et al. Improved clinical outcome for children with T-lineage acute lymphoblastic leukemia after

contemporary chemotherapy: a Children's Cancer Group Study. Leuk Lymphoma. 1996;24:57–70.
14. Kager L, Cheok M, Yang W, et al. Folate pathway gene expression differs in subtypes of acute lymphoblastic leukemia and influences methotrexate pharmacodynamics. J Clin Invest. 2005;115:110–7.
15. Saarinen-Pihkala UM, Heilmann C, Winiarski J, et al. Pathways through relapses and deaths of children with acute lymphoblastic leukemia: role of allogeneic stem-cell transplantation in Nordic data. J Clin Oncol. 2006;24:5750–62.
16. Gaynon PS, Harris RE, Altman AJ, et al. Bone marrow transplantation versus prolonged intensive chemotherapy for children with acute lymphoblastic leukemia and an initial bone marrow relapse within 12 months of the completion of primary therapy: Children's Oncology Group study CCG-1941. J Clin Oncol. 2006;24:3150–6.
17. Raetz EA, Borowitz MJ, Devidas M, et al. Reinduction platform for children with first marrow relapse of acute lymphoblastic leukemia: a Children's Oncology Group Study [corrected]. J Clin Oncol. 2008;26:3971–8.
18. Berg SL, Blaney SM, Devidas M, et al. Phase II study of nelarabine (compound 506U78) in children and young adults with refractory T-cell malignancies: a report from the Children's Oncology Group. J Clin Oncol. 2005;23:3376–82.
19. Schrappe M, Reiter A, Ludwig WD, et al. Improved outcome in childhood acute lymphoblastic leukemia despite reduced use of anthracyclines and cranial radiotherapy: results of trial ALL-BFM 90. German-Austrian-Swiss ALL-BFM Study Group. Blood. 2000;95:3310–22.
20. Cave H, van der Werff ten Bosch J, Suciu S, et al. Clinical significance of minimal residual disease in childhood acute lymphoblastic leukemia. European Organization for Research and Treatment of Cancer—Childhood Leukemia Cooperative Group. N Engl J Med. 1998;339:591–8.
21. Coustan-Smith E, Sancho J, Behm FG, et al. Prognostic importance of measuring early clearance of leukemic cells by flow cytometry in childhood acute lymphoblastic leukemia. Blood. 2002; 100:52–8.
22. van Dongen JJ, Seriu T, Panzer-Grumayer ER, et al. Prognostic value of minimal residual disease in acute lymphoblastic leukaemia in childhood. Lancet. 1998;352:1731–8.
23. Dunsmore K, Devidas M, Borowitz MJ, et al. Nelarabine in combination with intensive modified BFM AALL00P2: a pilot study for the treatment of high risk T-ALL a report from the Children's Oncology Group. J Clin Oncol. 2008;26:10002.
24. Coustan-Smith E, Mullighan CG, Onciu M, et al. Early T-cell precursor leukaemia: a subtype of very high-risk acute lymphoblastic leukaemia. Lancet Oncol. 2009;10:147–56.
25. Satwani P, Sather H, Ozkaynak F, et al. Allogeneic bone marrow transplantation in first remission for children with ultra-high-risk features of acute lymphoblastic leukemia: a children's oncology group study report. Biol Blood Marrow Transplant. 2007;13:218–27.
26. Schrauder A, Reiter A, Gadner H, et al. Superiority of allogeneic hematopoietic stem-cell transplantation compared with chemotherapy alone in high-risk childhood T-cell acute lymphoblastic leukemia: results from ALL-BFM 90 and 95. J Clin Oncol. 2006;24:5742–9.
27. Artavanis-Tsakonas S, Rand MD, Lake RJ. Notch signaling: cell fate control and signal integration in development. Science. 1999;284:770–6.
28. Weng AP, Ferrando AA, Lee W, et al. Activating mutations of NOTCH1 in human T cell acute lymphoblastic leukemia. Science. 2004;306:269–71.
29. Real PJ, Tosello V, Palomero T, et al. Gamma-secretase inhibitors reverse glucocorticoid resistance in T cell acute lymphoblastic leukemia. Nat Med. 2009;15:50–8.
30. Chan SM, Weng AP, Tibshirani R, Aster JC, Utz PJ. Notch signals positively regulate activity of the mTOR pathway in T-cell acute lymphoblastic leukemia. Blood. 2007;110:278–86.
31. Cullion K, Draheim KM, Hermance N, et al. Targeting the Notch1 and mTOR pathways in a mouse T-ALL model. Blood. 2009;113:6172–81.
32. Palomero T, Dominguez M, Ferrando AA. The role of the PTEN/AKT pathway in NOTCH1-induced leukemia. Cell Cycle. 2008;7:965–70.
33. Vilimas T, Mascarenhas J, Palomero T, et al. Targeting the NF-kappaB signaling pathway in Notch1-induced T-cell leukemia. Nat Med. 2007; 13:70–7.
34. Cairo MS. Non-Hodgkin's lymphoma and lymphoproliferative disorders in children. In: Carroll WL, Finlay J, editors. Cancer in children and adolescents. Sudbury: Jones and Bartlett Publishers; 2010. p. 217–34.
35. Cairo MS, Bradley MB. Lymphoma. In: Kliegman RM, Behrman RE, Jenson HB, Stanton BF, editors. Nelson textbook of pediatrics. 18th ed. Philadelphia: Elsevier; 2007. p. 2123–6.
36. Cairo MS, Raetz E, Perkins SL. Non-Hodgkin's lymphoma in children. In: Kufe DW, Bast RC, Hait WN, et al., editors. Cancer medicine. 7th ed. Hamilton, ON: BC Decker Inc.; 2005. p. 1962–76.
37. Burkhardt B, Moericke A, Klapper W, et al. Pediatric precursor T lymphoblastic leukemia and lymphoblastic lymphoma: differences in the common regions with loss of heterozygosity at chromosome 6q and their prognostic impact. Leuk Lymphoma. 2008;49:451–61.
38. Raetz EA, Perkins SL, Bhojwani D, et al. Gene expression profiling reveals intrinsic differences between T-cell acute lymphoblastic leukemia and T-cell lymphoblastic lymphoma. Pediatr Blood Cancer. 2006;47:130–40.
39. Burkhardt B, Reiter A, Landmann E, et al. Poor outcome for children and adolescents with progressive

disease or relapse of lymphoblastic lymphoma: a report from the Berlin-Frankfurt-Muenster Group. J Clin Oncol. 2009;27:3363–9.
40. Reiter A, Schrappe M, Ludwig WD, et al. Intensive ALL-type therapy without local radiotherapy provides a 90% event-free survival for children with T-cell lymphoblastic lymphoma: a BFM group report. Blood. 2000;95:416–21.
41. Schrappe M, Reiter A, Zimmermann M, et al. Long-term results of four consecutive trials in childhood ALL performed by the ALL-BFM study group from 1981 to 1995. Berlin-Frankfurt-Munster. Leukemia. 2000;14:2205–22.
42. Link MP, Weinstein HJ. Malignant non-Hodgkin lymphomas in children. In: Pizzo PA, Poplack DG, editors. Principles and practice of pediatric oncology. 5th ed. Philadelphia: Lippincott, Williams and Wilkins; 2006. p. 722–47.
43. Link MP, Shuster JJ, Donaldson SS, Berard CW, Murphy SB. Treatment of children and young adults with early-stage non-Hodgkin's lymphoma. N Engl J Med. 1997;337:1259–66.
44. Patte C, Kalifa C, Flamant F, et al. Results of the LMT81 protocol, a modified LSA2L2 protocol with high dose methotrexate, on 84 children with non-B-cell (lymphoblastic) lymphoma. Med Pediatr Oncol. 1992;20:105–13.
45. Wollner N, Burchenal JH, Lieberman PH, Exelby P, D'Angio G, Murphy ML. Non-Hodgkin's lymphoma in children. A comparative study of two modalities of therapy. Cancer. 1976;37:123–34.
46. Pillon M, Piglione M, Garaventa A, et al. Long-term results of AIEOP LNH-92 protocol for the treatment of pediatric lymphoblastic lymphoma: a report of the Italian Association of pediatric hematology and oncology. Pediatr Blood Cancer. 2009;53:953–9.
47. Burkhardt B, Woessmann W, Zimmermann M, et al. Impact of cranial radiotherapy on central nervous system prophylaxis in children and adolescents with central nervous system-negative stage III or IV lymphoblastic lymphoma. J Clin Oncol. 2006;24: 491–9.
48. Abromowitch M, Sposto R, Perkins S, et al. Shortened intensified multi-agent chemotherapy and non-cross resistant maintenance therapy for advanced lymphoblastic lymphoma in children and adolescents: report from the Children's Oncology Group. Br J Haematol. 2008;143:261–7.
49. Abromowitch M, Termuhlen A, Lynch J, et al. High-dose methotrexate and early intensification of therapy do not improve 3 year EFS in children and adolescents with disseminated lymphoblastic lymphoma. Results of the randomized arms of COG A5971. Hematol Meeting Rep. 2009;3:33.
50. Uyttebroeck A, Suciu S, Laureys G, et al. Treatment of childhood T-cell lymphoblastic lymphoma according to the strategy for acute lymphoblastic leukaemia, without radiotherapy: long term results of the EORTC CLG 58881 trial. Eur J Cancer. 2008; 44:840–6.
51. Sandlund JT, Pui CH, Zhou Y, et al. Effective treatment of advanced-stage childhood lymphoblastic lymphoma without prophylactic cranial irradiation: results of St Jude NHL13 study. Leukemia. 2009;23:1127–30.
52. Anderson JR, Jenkin RD, Wilson JF, et al. Long-term follow-up of patients treated with COMP or LSA2L2 therapy for childhood non-Hodgkin's lymphoma: a report of CCG-551 from the Childrens Cancer Group. J Clin Oncol. 1993;11:1024–32.
53. Hartmann O, Pein F, Beaujean F, et al. High-dose polychemotherapy with autologous bone marrow transplantation in children with relapsed lymphomas. J Clin Oncol. 1984;2:979–85.
54. Mills W, Chopra R, McMillan A, Pearce R, Linch DC, Goldstone AH. BEAM chemotherapy and autologous bone marrow transplantation for patients with relapsed or refractory non-Hodgkin's lymphoma. J Clin Oncol. 1995;13:588–95.
55. Won SC, Han JW, Kwon SY, et al. Autologous peripheral blood stem cell transplantation in children with non-Hodgkin's lymphoma: a report from the Korean society of pediatric hematology-oncology. Ann Hematol. 2006;85:787–94.
56. Kobrinsky NL, Sposto R, Shah NR, et al. Outcomes of treatment of children and adolescents with recurrent non-Hodgkin's lymphoma and Hodgkin's disease with dexamethasone, etoposide, cisplatin, cytarabine, and l-asparaginase, maintenance chemotherapy, and transplantation: Children's Cancer Group Study CCG-5912. J Clin Oncol. 2001;19:2390–6.
57. Kleiner S, Kirsch A, Schwaner I, et al. High-dose chemotherapy with carboplatin, etoposide and ifosfamide followed by autologous stem cell rescue in patients with relapsed or refractory malignant lymphomas: a phase I/II study. Bone Marrow Transplant. 1997;20:953–9.
58. Bureo E, Ortega JJ, Munoz A, et al. Bone marrow transplantation in 46 pediatric patients with non-Hodgkin's lymphoma. Spanish Working Party for bone marrow transplantation in children. Bone Marrow Transplant. 1995;15:353–9.
59. Jones RJ, Ambinder RF, Piantadosi S, Santos GW. Evidence of a graft-versus-lymphoma effect associated with allogeneic bone marrow transplantation. Blood. 1991;77:649–53.
60. Levine JE, Harris RE, Loberiza Jr FR, et al. A comparison of allogeneic and autologous bone marrow transplantation for lymphoblastic lymphoma. Blood. 2003;101:2476–82.
61. Smock KJ, Lim MS, Agarwal AM, et al. Expression of mTOR pathway proteins and notch1 in pediatric lymphoblastic lymphoma (LBL): a Children's Oncology Group Report. Hematol Meeting Rep. 2009;3:38.
62. Balakrishnan K, Nimmanapalli R, Ravandi F, Keating MJ, Gandhi V. Forodesine, an inhibitor of purine nucleoside phosphorylase, induces apoptosis in chronic lymphocytic leukemia cells. Blood. 2006;108:2392–8.

63. Haioun C, Itti E, Rahmouni A, et al. [18 F]fluoro-2-deoxy-D-glucose positron emission tomography (FDG-PET) in aggressive lymphoma: an early prognostic tool for predicting patient outcome. Blood. 2005;106:1376–81.
64. Lovisa F, Mussolin L, Corral L, et al. TCR-based RQ-PCR assay for MDD and MRD assessment in T-cell lymphoblastic lymphoma of childhood. Hematol Meeting Rep. 2009;3:37.
65. Coustan-Smith E, Sandlund JT, Perkins SL, et al. Minimal disseminated disease in childhood T-cell lymphoblastic lymphoma: a report from the children's oncology group. J Clin Oncol. 2009;27:3533–9.
66. Aifantis I, Raetz E, Buonamici S. Molecular pathogenesis of T-cell leukaemia and lymphoma. Nat Rev. 2008;8:380–90.
67. Pui CH, Evans WE. Treatment of acute lymphoblastic leukemia. N Engl J Med. 2006;354:166–78.
68. Pui CH, Robison LL, Look AT. Acute lymphoblastic leukaemia. Lancet. 2008;371:1030–43.
69. De Keersmaecker K, Marynen P, Cools J. Genetic insights in the pathogenesis of T-cell acute lymphoblastic leukemia. Haematologica. 2005;90:1116–27.
70. Van Vlierberghe P, Pieters R, Beverloo HB, Meijerink JP. Molecular-genetic insights in paediatric T-cell acute lymphoblastic leukaemia. Br J Haematol. 2008;143:153–68.
71. Armstrong SA, Look AT. Molecular genetics of acute lymphoblastic leukemia. J Clin Oncol. 2005; 23:6306–15.
72. Look AT. Oncogenic transcription factors in the human acute leukemias. Science. 1997; 278:1059–64.
73. Teitell MA, Pandolfi PP. Molecular genetics of acute lymphoblastic leukemia. Annu Rev Pathol. 2009;4:175–98.
74. Begley CG, Aplan PD, Davey MP, et al. Chromosomal translocation in a human leukemic stem-cell line disrupts the T-cell antigen receptor delta-chain diversity region and results in a previously unreported fusion transcript. Proc Natl Acad Sci U S A. 1989;86:2031–5.
75. Bernard O, Guglielmi P, Jonveaux P, et al. Two distinct mechanisms for the SCL gene activation in the t(1;14) translocation of T-cell leukemias. Genes Chromosomes Cancer. 1990;1:194–208.
76. Chen Q, Cheng JT, Tasi LH, et al. The tal gene undergoes chromosome translocation in T cell leukemia and potentially encodes a helix-loop-helix protein. EMBO J. 1990;9:415–24.
77. Xia Y, Brown L, Yang CY, et al. TAL2, a helix-loop-helix gene activated by the (7;9)(q34;q32) translocation in human T-cell leukemia. Proc Natl Acad Sci U S A. 1991;88:11416–20.
78. Mellentin JD, Smith SD, Cleary ML. lyl-1, a novel gene altered by chromosomal translocation in T cell leukemia, codes for a protein with a helix-loop-helix DNA binding motif. Cell. 1989;58:77–83.
79. Wang J, Jani-Sait SN, Escalon EA, et al. The t(14;21)(q11.2;q22) chromosomal translocation associated with T-cell acute lymphoblastic leukemia activates the BHLHB1 gene. Proc Natl Acad Sci U S A. 2000;97:3497–502.
80. Boehm T, Foroni L, Kaneko Y, Perutz MF, Rabbitts TH. The rhombotin family of cysteine-rich LIM-domain oncogenes: distinct members are involved in T-cell translocations to human chromosomes 11p15 and 11p13. Proc Natl Acad Sci U S A. 1991; 88:4367–71.
81. McGuire EA, Hockett RD, Pollock KM, Bartholdi MF, O'Brien SJ, Korsmeyer SJ. The t(11;14)(p15;q11) in a T-cell acute lymphoblastic leukemia cell line activates multiple transcripts, including Ttg-1, a gene encoding a potential zinc finger protein. Mol Cell Biol. 1989;9:2124–32.
82. Royer-Pokora B, Loos U, Ludwig WD. TTG-2, a new gene encoding a cysteine-rich protein with the LIM motif, is overexpressed in acute T-cell leukaemia with the t(11;14)(p13;q11). Oncogene. 1991;6:1887–93.
83. Dube ID, Kamel-Reid S, Yuan CC, et al. A novel human homeobox gene lies at the chromosome 10 breakpoint in lymphoid neoplasias with chromosomal translocation t(10;14). Blood. 1991;78:2996–3003.
84. Hatano M, Roberts CW, Minden M, Crist WM, Korsmeyer SJ. Deregulation of a homeobox gene, HOX11, by the t(10;14) in T cell leukemia. Science. 1991;253:79–82.
85. Kennedy MA, Gonzalez-Sarmiento R, Kees UR, et al. HOX11, a homeobox-containing T-cell oncogene on human chromosome 10q24. Proc Natl Acad Sci U S A. 1991;88:8900–4.
86. Lu M, Gong ZY, Shen WF, Ho AD. The tcl-3 proto-oncogene altered by chromosomal translocation in T-cell leukemia codes for a homeobox protein. EMBO J. 1991;10:2905–10.
87. Bernard OA, Busson-LeConiat M, Ballerini P, et al. A new recurrent and specific cryptic translocation, t(5;14)(q35;q32), is associated with expression of the Hox11L2 gene in T acute lymphoblastic leukemia. Leukemia. 2001;15:1495–504.
88. Ferrando AA, Neuberg DS, Staunton J, et al. Gene expression signatures define novel oncogenic pathways in T cell acute lymphoblastic leukemia. Cancer Cell. 2002;1:75–87.
89. Przybylski GK, Dik WA, Grabarczyk P, et al. The effect of a novel recombination between the homeobox gene NKX2-5 and the TRD locus in T-cell acute lymphoblastic leukemia on activation of the NKX2-5 gene. Haematologica. 2006;91:317–21.
90. Soulier J, Clappier E, Cayuela JM, et al. HOXA genes are included in genetic and biologic networks defining human acute T-cell leukemia (T-ALL). Blood. 2005;106:274–86.
91. Speleman F, Cauwelier B, Dastugue N, et al. A new recurrent inversion, inv(7)(p15q34), leads to

transcriptional activation of HOXA10 and HOXA11 in a subset of T-cell acute lymphoblastic leukemias. Leukemia. 2005;19:358–66.
92. Erikson J, Finger L, Sun L, et al. Deregulation of c-myc by translocation of the alpha-locus of the T-cell receptor in T-cell leukemias. Science. 1986;232:884–6.
93. Shima EA, Le Beau MM, McKeithan TW, et al. Gene encoding the alpha chain of the T-cell receptor is moved immediately downstream of c-myc in a chromosomal 8;14 translocation in a cell line from a human T-cell leukemia. Proc Natl Acad Sci U S A. 1986;83:3439–43.
94. Clappier E, Cuccuini W, Kalota A, et al. The C-MYB locus is involved in chromosomal translocation and genomic duplications in human T-cell acute leukemia (T-ALL), the translocation defining a new T-ALL subtype in very young children. Blood. 2007;110:1251–61.
95. Lahortiga I, De Keersmaecker K, Van Vlierberghe P, et al. Duplication of the MYB oncogene in T cell acute lymphoblastic leukemia. Nat Genet. 2007;39:593–5.
96. Ellisen LW, Bird J, West DC, et al. TAN-1, the human homolog of the Drosophila notch gene, is broken by chromosomal translocations in T lymphoblastic neoplasms. Cell. 1991;66:649–61.
97. Rubnitz JE, Camitta BM, Mahmoud H, et al. Childhood acute lymphoblastic leukemia with the MLL-ENL fusion and t(11;19)(q23;p13.3) translocation. J Clin Oncol. 1999;17:191–6.
98. Bohlander SK, Muschinsky V, Schrader K, et al. Molecular analysis of the CALM/AF10 fusion: identical rearrangements in acute myeloid leukemia, acute lymphoblastic leukemia and malignant lymphoma patients. Leukemia. 2000;14:93–9.
99. Van Vlierberghe P, van Grotel M, Tchinda J, et al. The recurrent SET-NUP214 fusion as a new HOXA activation mechanism in pediatric T-cell acute lymphoblastic leukemia. Blood. 2008;111:4668–80.
100. Ferrando AA, Look AT. Gene expression profiling in T-cell acute lymphoblastic leukemia. Semin Hematol. 2003;40:274–80.
101. Herblot S, Steff AM, Hugo P, Aplan PD, Hoang T. SCL and LMO1 alter thymocyte differentiation: inhibition of E2A-HEB function and pre-T alpha chain expression. Nat Immunol. 2000;1:138–44.
102. Hebert J, Cayuela JM, Berkeley J, Sigaux F. Candidate tumor-suppressor genes MTS1 (p16INK4A) and MTS2 (p15INK4B) display frequent homozygous deletions in primary cells from T- but not from B-cell lineage acute lymphoblastic leukemias. Blood. 1994;84:4038–44.
103. Tycko B, Smith SD, Sklar J. Chromosomal translocations joining LCK and TCRB loci in human T cell leukemia. J Exp Med. 1991;174:867–73.
104. Clappier E, Cuccuini W, Cayuela JM, et al. Cyclin D2 dysregulation by chromosomal translocations to TCR loci in T-cell acute lymphoblastic leukemias. Leukemia. 2006;20:82–6.
105. Flex E, Petrangeli V, Stella L, et al. Somatically acquired JAK1 mutations in adult acute lymphoblastic leukemia. J Exp Med. 2008;205:751–8.
106. Lacronique V, Boureux A, Valle VD, et al. A TEL-JAK2 fusion protein with constitutive kinase activity in human leukemia. Science. 1997;278:1309–12.
107. Van Limbergen H, Beverloo HB, van Drunen E, et al. Molecular cytogenetic and clinical findings in ETV6/ABL1-positive leukemia. Genes Chromosomes Cancer. 2001;30:274–82.
108. Graux C, Cools J, Melotte C, et al. Fusion of NUP214 to ABL1 on amplified episomes in T-cell acute lymphoblastic leukemia. Nat Genet. 2004;36:1084–9.
109. De Keersmaecker K, Graux C, Odero MD, et al. Fusion of EML1 to ABL1 in T-cell acute lymphoblastic leukemia with cryptic t(9;14)(q34;q32). Blood. 2005;105:4849–52.
110. Paietta E, Ferrando AA, Neuberg D, et al. Activating FLT3 mutations in CD117/KIT(+) T-cell acute lymphoblastic leukemias. Blood. 2004;104:558–60.
111. Van Vlierberghe P, Meijerink JP, Stam RW, et al. Activating FLT3 mutations in CD4+/CD8- pediatric T-cell acute lymphoblastic leukemias. Blood. 2005;106:4414–5.
112. Bar-Eli M, Ahuja H, Foti A, Cline MJ. N-RAS mutations in T-cell acute lymphocytic leukaemia: analysis by direct sequencing detects a novel mutation. Br J Haematol. 1989;72:36–9.
113. Balgobind BV, Van Vlierberghe P, van den Ouweland AM, et al. Leukemia-associated NF1 inactivation in patients with pediatric T-ALL and AML lacking evidence for neurofibromatosis. Blood. 2008;111:4322–8.
114. Lo TC, Barnhill LM, Kim Y, Nakae EA, Yu AL, Diccianni MB. Inactivation of SHIP1 in T-cell acute lymphoblastic leukemia due to mutation and extensive alternative splicing. Leuk Res. 2009;33:1562–6.
115. Palomero T, Sulis ML, Cortina M, et al. Mutational loss of PTEN induces resistance to NOTCH1 inhibition in T cell leukemia. Nat Med. 2007;13:1203–10.
116. Tosello V, Mansour MR, Barnes K, et al. WT1 mutations in T-ALL. Blood. 2009;114:1038–45.
117. Sambandam A, Maillard I, Zediak VP, et al. Notch signaling controls the generation and differentiation of early T lineage progenitors. Nat Immunol. 2005;6:663–70.
118. Radtke F, Ferrero I, Wilson A, Lees R, Aguet M, MacDonald HR. Notch1 deficiency dissociates the intrathymic development of dendritic cells and T cells. J Exp Med. 2000;191:1085–94.
119. Radtke F, Wilson A, MacDonald HR. Notch signaling in T- and B-cell development. Curr Opin Immunol. 2004;16:174–9.
120. Radtke F, Wilson A, Mancini SJ, MacDonald HR. Notch regulation of lymphocyte development and function. Nat Immunol. 2004;5:247–53.
121. Schmitt TM, Zuniga-Pflucker JC. Induction of T cell development from hematopoietic progenitor cells by delta-like-1 in vitro. Immunity. 2002;17:749–56.

122. Grabher C, von Boehmer H, Look AT. Notch 1 activation in the molecular pathogenesis of T-cell acute lymphoblastic leukaemia. Nat Rev Cancer. 2006;6:347–59.
123. Palomero T, Lim WK, Odom DT, et al. NOTCH1 directly regulates c-MYC and activates a feed-forward-loop transcriptional network promoting leukemic cell growth. Proc Natl Acad Sci U S A. 2006;103:18261–6.
124. Weng AP, Millholland JM, Yashiro-Ohtani Y, et al. c-Myc is an important direct target of Notch1 in T-cell acute lymphoblastic leukemia/lymphoma. Genes Dev. 2006;20:2096–109.
125. Pear WS, Aster JC, Scott ML, et al. Exclusive development of T cell neoplasms in mice transplanted with bone marrow expressing activated Notch alleles. J Exp Med. 1996;183:2283–91.
126. Sulis ML, Williams O, Palomero T, et al. NOTCH1 extracellular juxtamembrane expansion mutations in T-ALL. Blood. 2008;112:733–40.
127. Welcker M, Clurman BE. FBW7 ubiquitin ligase: a tumour suppressor at the crossroads of cell division, growth and differentiation. Nat Rev Cancer. 2008;8:83–93.
128. Malyukova A, Dohda T, von der Lehr N, et al. The tumor suppressor gene hCDC4 is frequently mutated in human T-cell acute lymphoblastic leukemia with functional consequences for Notch signaling. Cancer Res. 2007;67:5611–6.
129. O'Neil J, Grim J, Strack P, et al. FBW7 mutations in leukemic cells mediate NOTCH pathway activation and resistance to gamma-secretase inhibitors. J Exp Med. 2007;204:1813–24.
130. Thompson BJ, Buonamici S, Sulis ML, et al. The SCFFBW7 ubiquitin ligase complex as a tumor suppressor in T cell leukemia. J Exp Med. 2007;204:1825–35.
131. Lewis HD, Leveridge M, Strack PR, et al. Apoptosis in T cell acute lymphoblastic leukemia cells after cell cycle arrest induced by pharmacological inhibition of notch signaling. Chem Biol. 2007;14:209–19.
132. Deangelo D, Stone R, Silverman L, et al. A phase I clinical trial of the notch inhibitor MK-0752 in patients with T-cell acute lymphoblastic leukemia/lymphoma (T-ALL) and other leukemias. J Clin Oncol. 2006;24:6585.
133. Milano J, McKay J, Dagenais C, et al. Modulation of notch processing by gamma-secretase inhibitors causes intestinal goblet cell metaplasia and induction of genes known to specify gut secretory lineage differentiation. Toxicol Sci. 2004;82:341–58.
134. van Es JH, van Gijn ME, Riccio O, et al. Notch/gamma-secretase inhibition turns proliferative cells in intestinal crypts and adenomas into goblet cells. Nature. 2005;435:959–63.
135. Real PJ, Ferrando AA. NOTCH inhibition and glucocorticoid therapy in T-cell acute lymphoblastic leukemia. Leukemia. 2009;23:1374–7.
136. Buonamici S, Trimarchi T, Ruocco MG, et al. CCR7 signalling as an essential regulator of CNS infiltration in T-cell leukaemia. Nature. 2009;459:1000–4.
137. Stein H, Mason DY, Gerdes J, et al. The expression of the Hodgkin's disease associated antigen Ki-1 in reactive and neoplastic lymphoid tissue: evidence that Reed-Sternberg cells and histiocytic malignancies are derived from activated lymphoid cells. Blood. 1985;66:848–58.
138. Chiarle R, Voena C, Ambrogio C, Piva R, Inghirami G. The anaplastic lymphoma kinase in the pathogenesis of cancer. Nat Rev Cancer. 2008;8:11–23.
139. Tumours of haematopoietic and lymphoid tissues. In: Jaffe E, Harris N, Stein H, Vardiman J, editors. World Health Organization Classification of Tumors. Washington, DC: IARC Press; 2000.
140. Stein H, Foss HD, Durkop H, et al. CD30(+) anaplastic large cell lymphoma: a review of its histopathologic, genetic, and clinical features. Blood. 2000;96:3681–95.
141. Duyster J, Bai RY, Morris SW. Translocations involving anaplastic lymphoma kinase (ALK). Oncogene. 2001;20:5623–37.
142. Benharroch D, Meguerian-Bedoyan Z, Lamant L, et al. ALK-positive lymphoma: a single disease with a broad spectrum of morphology. Blood. 1998;91:2076–84.
143. Harris NL, Jaffe ES, Stein H, et al. A revised European-American classification of lymphoid neoplasms: a proposal from the International Lymphoma Study Group. Blood. 1994;84:1361–92.
144. Falini B, Pileri S, Zinzani PL, et al. ALK+ lymphoma: clinico-pathological findings and outcome. Blood. 1999;93:2697–706.
145. Pulford K, Lamant L, Espinos E, et al. The emerging normal and disease-related roles of anaplastic lymphoma kinase. Cell Mol Life Sci. 2004;61:2939–53.
146. Murphy SB. Pediatric lymphomas: recent advances and commentary on Ki-1-positive anaplastic large-cell lymphomas of childhood. Ann Oncol. 1994;5 Suppl 1:31–3.
147. Jaffe ES. Anaplastic large cell lymphoma: the shifting sands of diagnostic hematopathology. Mod Pathol. 2001;14:219–28.
148. Salzburg J, Burkhardt B, Zimmermann M, et al. Prevalence, clinical pattern, and outcome of CNS involvement in childhood and adolescent non-Hodgkin's lymphoma differ by non-Hodgkin's lymphoma subtype: a Berlin-Frankfurt-Munster Group Report. J Clin Oncol. 2007;25:3915–22.
149. Seidemann K, Tiemann M, Schrappe M, et al. Short-pulse B-non-Hodgkin lymphoma-type chemotherapy is efficacious treatment for pediatric anaplastic large cell lymphoma: a report of the Berlin-Frankfurt-Munster Group Trial NHL-BFM 90. Blood. 2001;97:3699–706.
150. Sandlund JT, Pui CH, Santana VM, et al. Clinical features and treatment outcome for children with CD30+ large-cell non-Hodgkin's lymphoma. J Clin Oncol. 1994;12:895–8.
151. Brugieres L, Deley MC, Pacquement H, et al. CD30(+) anaplastic large-cell lymphoma in children: analysis of 82 patients enrolled in two consecutive

studies of the French Society of Pediatric Oncology. Blood. 1998;92:3591–8.

152. Laver JH, Kraveka JM, Hutchison RE, et al. Advanced-stage large-cell lymphoma in children and adolescents: results of a randomized trial incorporating intermediate-dose methotrexate and high-dose cytarabine in the maintenance phase of the APO regimen: a Pediatric Oncology Group phase III trial. J Clin Oncol. 2005;23:541–7.
153. Lowe EJ, Sposto R, Perkins SL, et al. Intensive chemotherapy for systemic anaplastic large cell lymphoma in children and adolescents: final results of Children's Cancer Group Study 5941. Pediatr Blood Cancer. 2009;52:335–9.
154. Rosolen A, Pillon M, Garaventa A, et al. Anaplastic large cell lymphoma treated with a leukemia-like therapy: report of the Italian Association of Pediatric Hematology and Oncology (AIEOP) LNH-92 protocol. Cancer. 2005;104:2133–40.
155. Williams DM, Hobson R, Imeson J, Gerrard M, McCarthy K, Pinkerton CR. Anaplastic large cell lymphoma in childhood: analysis of 72 patients treated on The United Kingdom Children's Cancer Study Group chemotherapy regimens. Br J Haematol. 2002;117:812–20.
156. Brugieres L, Quartier P, Le Deley MC, et al. Relapses of childhood anaplastic large-cell lymphoma: treatment results in a series of 41 children—a report from the French Society of Pediatric Oncology. Ann Oncol. 2000;11:53–8.
157. Kraveka JM, Weitzman S, Smith L, et al. Advanced-stage anaplastic large-cell lymphoma in children and adolescents: results of ANHL0131, a randomized phase III trial with standard APO (doxorubicin, prednisone, vincristine) versus consolidation with a regimen including vinblastine: a report from the Children's Oncology Group. Hematol Meeting Rep. 2009;3:41.
158. Brugieres L, Le Deley MC, Rosolen A, et al. Impact of the methotrexate administration dose on the need for intrathecal treatment in children and adolescents with anaplastic large-cell lymphoma: results of a randomized trial of the EICNHL Group. J Clin Oncol. 2009;27:897–903.
159. Le Deley MC, Reiter A, Williams D, et al. Prognostic factors in childhood anaplastic large cell lymphoma: results of a large European intergroup study. Blood. 2008;111:1560–6.
160. Massimino M, Spreafico F, Luksch R, Giardini R. Prognostic significance of p80 and visceral involvement in childhood CD30 anaplastic large cell lymphoma (ALCL). Med Pediatr Oncol. 2001;37:97–102.
161. Damm-Welk C, Busch K, Burkhardt B, et al. Prognostic significance of circulating tumor cells in bone marrow or peripheral blood as detected by qualitative and quantitative PCR in pediatric NPM-ALK-positive anaplastic large-cell lymphoma. Blood. 2007;110:670–7.
162. Mussolin L, Bonvini P, Ait-Tahar K, et al. Kinetics of humoral response to ALK and its relationship with minimal residual disease in pediatric ALCL. Leukemia. 2009;23:400–2.
163. Lamant L, McCarthy K, d'Amore ESG, et al. Prognostic impact of morphologic and phenotypic features of childhood ALK-positive anaplastic large cell lymphoma (ALCL): results of the ALCL99 study. Hematol Meeting Rep. 2009;3:42.
164. Sandlund JT, Pui CH, Roberts WM, et al. Clinicopathologic features and treatment outcome of children with large-cell lymphoma and the t(2;5)(p23;q35). Blood. 1994;84:2467–71.
165. Vecchi V, Burnelli R, Pileri S, et al. Anaplastic large cell lymphoma (Ki-1+/CD30+) in childhood. Med Pediatr Oncol. 1993;21:402–10.
166. Mora J, Filippa DA, Thaler HT, Polyak T, Cranor ML, Wollner N. Large cell non-Hodgkin lymphoma of childhood: analysis of 78 consecutive patients enrolled in 2 consecutive protocols at the Memorial Sloan-Kettering Cancer Center. Cancer. 2000;88:186–97.
167. Reiter A, Schrappe M, Tiemann M, et al. Successful treatment strategy for Ki-1 anaplastic large-cell lymphoma of childhood: a prospective analysis of 62 patients enrolled in three consecutive Berlin-Frankfurt-Munster group studies. J Clin Oncol. 1994;12:899–908.
168. Cesaro S, Pillon M, Visintin G, et al. Unrelated bone marrow transplantation for high-risk anaplastic large cell lymphoma in pediatric patients: a single center case series. Eur J Haematol. 2005;75:22–6.
169. Woessmann W, Peters C, Lenhard M, et al. Allogeneic haematopoietic stem cell transplantation in relapsed or refractory anaplastic large cell lymphoma of children and adolescents—a Berlin-Frankfurt-Munster group report. Br J Haematol. 2006;133:176–82.
170. Bartlett NL, Younes A, Carabasi MH, et al. A phase 1 multidose study of SGN-30 immunotherapy in patients with refractory or recurrent CD30+ hematologic malignancies. Blood. 2008;111:1848–54.
171. Forero-Torres A, Leonard JP, Younes A, et al. A phase II study of SGN-30 (anti-CD30 mAb) in Hodgkin lymphoma or systemic anaplastic large cell lymphoma. Br J Haematol. 2009;146:171–9.
172. Bartlett N, Forero-Torres A, Rosenblatt J, et al. Complete remissions with SGN-35 weekly dosing: a phase I dose-escalation study in relapsed/refractory Hodgkin lymphoma or systemic ALCL patients. J Clin Oncol. 2009;17:8500.
173. Younes A, Forero-Torres A, Bartlett NL, et al. Multiple complete responses in a phase 1 dose-escalation study of the antibody-drug conjugate SGN-35 in patients with relapsed or refractory CD30-positive lymphomas. Blood. 2008;112:1006.
174. Galkin AV, Melnick JS, Kim S, et al. Identification of NVP-TAE684, a potent, selective, and efficacious inhibitor of NPM-ALK. Proc Natl Acad Sci U S A. 2007;104:270–5.
175. Palmer RH, Vernersson E, Grabbe C, Hallberg B. Anaplastic lymphoma kinase: signalling in development and disease. Biochem J. 2009;420:345–61.

176. Cannella S, Santoro A, Bruno G, et al. Germline mutations of the perforin gene are a frequent occurrence in childhood anaplastic large cell lymphoma. Cancer. 2007;109:2566–71.
177. Clementi R, Locatelli F, Dupre L, et al. A proportion of patients with lymphoma may harbor mutations of the perforin gene. Blood. 2005;105:4424–8.
178. Singh RR, Cho-Vega JH, Davuluri Y, et al. Sonic hedgehog signaling pathway is activated in ALK-positive anaplastic large cell lymphoma. Cancer Res. 2009;69:2550–8.
179. Lim MS, Carlson ML, Crockett DK, et al. The proteomic signature of NPM/ALK reveals deregulation of multiple cellular pathways. Blood. 2009;114: 1585–95.
180. Lim MS, Elenitoba-Johnson KS. Mass spectrometry-based proteomic studies of human anaplastic large cell lymphoma. Mol Cell Proteomics. 2006;5:1787–98.
181. Lim M, Tygeson J, Seiler C, et al. Proteomic analysis of Denileukin Diftitox (Ontak) as a potential therapeutic agent for ALCL. Hematol Meeting Rep. 2009;3:44.
182. Miles RR, Cairo MS, Satwani P, et al. Immunophenotypic identification of possible therapeutic targets in paediatric non-Hodgkin lymphomas: a children's oncology group report. Br J Haematol. 2007;138:506–12.
183. Bonvini P, Gastaldi T, Falini B, Rosolen A. Nucleophosmin-anaplastic lymphoma kinase (NPM-ALK), a novel Hsp90-client tyrosine kinase: down-regulation of NPM-ALK expression and tyrosine phosphorylation in ALK(+) CD30(+) lymphoma cells by the Hsp90 antagonist 17-allylamino,17-demethoxygeldanamycin. Cancer Res. 2002;62:1559–66.
184. Slupianek A, Nieborowska-Skorska M, Hoser G, et al. Role of phosphatidylinositol 3-kinase-Akt pathway in nucleophosmin/anaplastic lymphoma kinase-mediated lymphomagenesis. Cancer Res. 2001;61:2194–9.
185. Windsor R, Stiller C, Webb D. Peripheral T-cell lymphoma in childhood: population-based experience in the United Kingdom over 20 years. Pediatr Blood Cancer. 2008;50:784–7.
186. The Non-Hodgkin's Lymphoma Classification Project. A clinical evaluation of the International Lymphoma Study Group classification of non-Hodgkin's lymphoma. Blood. 1997;89:3909–18.
187. Rudiger T, Geissinger E, Muller-Hermelink HK. 'Normal counterparts' of nodal peripheral T-cell lymphoma. Hematol Oncol. 2006;24:175–80.
188. Nelson M, Horsman DE, Weisenburger DD, et al. Cytogenetic abnormalities and clinical correlations in peripheral T-cell lymphoma. Br J Haematol. 2008;141:461–9.
189. Zettl A, Rudiger T, Konrad MA, et al. Genomic profiling of peripheral T-cell lymphoma, unspecified, and anaplastic large T-cell lymphoma delineates novel recurrent chromosomal alterations. Am J Pathol. 2004;164:1837–48.
190. Martinez-Delgado B, Cuadros M, Honrado E, et al. Differential expression of NF-kappaB pathway genes among peripheral T-cell lymphomas. Leukemia. 2005;19:2254–63.
191. Ballester B, Ramuz O, Gisselbrecht C, et al. Gene expression profiling identifies molecular subgroups among nodal peripheral T-cell lymphomas. Oncogene. 2006;25:1560–70.
192. Hutchison RE, Laver JH, Chang M, et al. Non-anaplastic peripheral T-cell lymphoma in childhood and adolescence: a Children's Oncology Group study. Pediatr Blood Cancer. 2008;51:29–33.
193. Gisselbrecht C, Gaulard P, Lepage E, et al. Prognostic significance of T-cell phenotype in aggressive non-Hodgkin's lymphomas. Groupe d'Etudes des Lymphomes de l'Adulte (GELA). Blood. 1998;92: 76–82.
194. Savage KJ. Peripheral T-cell lymphomas. Blood Rev. 2007;21:201–16.
195. Savage KJ, Chhanabhai M, Gascoyne RD, Connors JM. Characterization of peripheral T-cell lymphomas in a single North American institution by the WHO classification. Ann Oncol. 2004;15:1467–75.
196. Kewalramani T, Zelenetz AD, Teruya-Feldstein J, et al. Autologous transplantation for relapsed or primary refractory peripheral T-cell lymphoma. Br J Haematol. 2006;134:202–7.
197. Paolo C, Lucia F, Anna D. Hematopoietic stem cell transplantation in peripheral T-cell lymphomas. Leuk Lymphoma. 2007;48:1496–501.
198. Corradini P, Tarella C, Zallio F, et al. Long-term follow-up of patients with peripheral T-cell lymphomas treated up-front with high-dose chemotherapy followed by autologous stem cell transplantation. Leukemia. 2006;20:1533–8.
199. Mollee P, Lazarus HM, Lipton J. Why aren't we performing more allografts for aggressive non-Hodgkin's lymphoma? Bone Marrow Transplant. 2003; 31:953–60.
200. Corradini P, Dodero A, Zallio F, et al. Graft-versus-lymphoma effect in relapsed peripheral T-cell non-Hodgkin's lymphomas after reduced-intensity conditioning followed by allogeneic transplantation of hematopoietic cells. J Clin Oncol. 2004;22:2172–6.
201. Gallamini A, Stelitano C, Calvi R, et al. Peripheral T-cell lymphoma unspecified (PTCL-U): a new prognostic model from a retrospective multicentric clinical study. Blood. 2004;103:2474–9.
202. Sallah S, Wan JY, Nguyen NP. Treatment of refractory T-cell malignancies using gemcitabine. Br J Haematol. 2001;113:185–7.
203. Czuczman MS, Porcu P, Johnson J, Niedzwiecki D, Canellos GP, Cheson BD. CALGB 59901: results of a phase II study of 506U78 in CTCL and PTCL. Blood. 2004;104:2486.
204. Piekarz R, Wright J, Frye R, et al. Results of a phase 2 NCI multicenter study of romidepsin in patients with relapsed peripheral T-cell lymphoma (PTCL). Blood (ASH Annual Meeting Abstracts). 2008; 112:1567.

205. Aguiar Bujanda D. Complete response of relapsed angioimmunoblastic T-cell lymphoma following therapy with bevacizumab. Ann Oncol. 2008; 19:396–7.
206. Bruns I, Fox F, Reinecke P, et al. Complete remission in a patient with relapsed angioimmunoblastic T-cell lymphoma following treatment with bevacizumab. Leukemia. 2005;19:1993–5.
207. O'Connor OA, Horwitz S, Hamlin P, et al. Phase II-I-II study of two different doses and schedules of pralatrexate, a high-affinity substrate for the reduced folate carrier, in patients with relapsed or refractory lymphoma reveals marked activity in T-cell malignancies. J Clin Oncol. 2009;27:4357–64.
208. O'Connor OA, Pro B, Pinter-Brown L, et al. PROPEL: a multi-center phase 2 open-label study of pralatrexate (PDX) with vitamin B12 and folic acid supplementation in patients with relapsed or refractory peripheral T-cell lymphoma. Blood (ASH Annual Meeting Abstracts). 2008;112:261.
209. Orlowski RZ, Voorhees PM, Garcia RA, et al. Phase 1 trial of the proteasome inhibitor bortezomib and pegylated liposomal doxorubicin in patients with advanced hematologic malignancies. Blood. 2005;105:3058–65.
210. Zinzani PL, Musuraca G, Tani M, et al. Phase II trial of proteasome inhibitor bortezomib in patients with relapsed or refractory cutaneous T-cell lymphoma. J Clin Oncol. 2007;25:4293–7.
211. Lee J, Suh C, Kang HJ, et al. Phase I study of proteasome inhibitor bortezomib plus CHOP in patients with advanced, aggressive T-cell or NK/T-cell lymphoma. Ann Oncol. 2008;19:2079–83.
212. Enblad G, Hagberg H, Erlanson M, et al. A pilot study of alemtuzumab (anti-CD52 monoclonal antibody) therapy for patients with relapsed or chemotherapy-refractory peripheral T-cell lymphomas. Blood. 2004;103:2920–4.
213. Gallamini A, Zaja F, Patti C, et al. Alemtuzumab (Campath-1 H) and CHOP chemotherapy as first-line treatment of peripheral T-cell lymphoma: results of a GITIL (Gruppo Italiano Terapie Innovative nei Linfomi) prospective multicenter trial. Blood. 2007;110:2316–23.
214. Cheson BD. Novel therapies for peripheral T-cell non-Hodgkin's lymphomas. Curr Opin Hematol. 2009;16:299–305.
215. Horwitz SM. Novel therapies and role of transplant in the treatment of peripheral T-cell lymphomas. Hematology Am Soc Hematol Educ Program. 2008;2008:289–96.
216. Mackey AC, Green L, Liang LC, Dinndorf P, Avigan M. Hepatosplenic T cell lymphoma associated with infliximab use in young patients treated for inflammatory bowel disease. J Pediatr Gastroenterol Nutr. 2007;44:265–7.
217. Miyazaki K, Yamaguchi M, Imai H, et al. Gene expression profiling of peripheral T-cell lymphoma including gammadelta T-cell lymphoma. Blood. 2009;113:1071–4.
218. Reiter A, Schrappe M, Parwaresch R, et al. Non-Hodgkin's lymphomas of childhood and adolescence: results of a treatment stratified for biologic subtypes and stage—a report of the Berlin-Frankfurt-Munster Group. J Clin Oncol. 1995;13:359–72.
219. Dahl GV, Rivera G, Pui CH, et al. A novel treatment of childhood lymphoblastic non-Hodgkin's lymphoma: early and intermittent use of teniposide plus cytarabine. Blood. 1985;66:1110–4.
220. Millot F, Suciu S, Philippe N, et al. Value of high-dose cytarabine during interval therapy of a Berlin-Frankfurt-Munster-based protocol in increased-risk children with acute lymphoblastic leukemia and lymphoblastic lymphoma: results of the European Organization for Research and Treatment of Cancer 58881 randomized phase III trial. J Clin Oncol. 2001;19:1935–42.
221. Weinstein HJ, Cassady JR, Levey R. Long-term results of the APO protocol (vincristine, doxorubicin [adriamycin], and prednisone) for treatment of mediastinal lymphoblastic lymphoma. J Clin Oncol. 1983;1:537–41.
222. Eden OB, Hann I, Imeson J, Cotterill S, Gerrard M, Pinkerton CR. Treatment of advanced stage T cell lymphoblastic lymphoma: results of the United Kingdom Children's Cancer Study Group (UKCCSG) protocol 8503. Br J Haematol. 1992;82:310–6.
223. Abromowitch M, Sposto R, Perkins S, Finlay J, Cairo MS. Results of CCG-5941: intensified multi-agent chemotherapy and non-cross resistant maintenance therapy for advanced lymphoblastic lymphoma in children and adolescents. Blood. 2006;108:533.
224. Adam P, Katzenberger T, Seeberger H, et al. A case of a diffuse large B-cell lymphoma of plasmablastic type associated with the t(2;5)(p23;q35) chromosome translocation. Am J Surg Pathol. 2003; 27:1473–6.
225. Morris SW, Kirstein MN, Valentine MB, et al. Fusion of a kinase gene, ALK, to a nucleolar protein gene, NPM, in non-Hodgkin's lymphoma. Science. 1994;263:1281–4.
226. Onciu M, Behm FG, Downing JR, et al. ALK-positive plasmablastic B-cell lymphoma with expression of the NPM-ALK fusion transcript: report of 2 cases. Blood. 2003;102:2642–4.
227. Shiota M, Nakamura S, Ichinohasama R, et al. Anaplastic large cell lymphomas expressing the novel chimeric protein p80NPM/ALK: a distinct clinicopathologic entity. Blood. 1995;86:1954–60.
228. Lamant L, Dastugue N, Pulford K, Delsol G, Mariame B. A new fusion gene TPM3-ALK in anaplastic large cell lymphoma created by a (1;2) (q25;p23) translocation. Blood. 1999;93:3088–95.
229. Lawrence B, Perez-Atayde A, Hibbard MK, et al. TPM3-ALK and TPM4-ALK oncogenes in inflammatory myofibroblastic tumors. Am J Pathol. 2000;157:377–84.
230. Siebert R, Gesk S, Harder L, et al. Complex variant translocation t(1;2) with TPM3-ALK fusion due to

cryptic ALK gene rearrangement in anaplastic large-cell lymphoma. Blood. 1999;94:3614–7.
231. Hernandez L, Bea S, Bellosillo B, et al. Diversity of genomic breakpoints in TFG-ALK translocations in anaplastic large cell lymphomas: identification of a new TFG-ALK(XL) chimeric gene with transforming activity. Am J Pathol. 2002;160:1487–94.
232. Hernandez L, Pinyol M, Hernandez S, et al. TRK-fused gene (TFG) is a new partner of ALK in anaplastic large cell lymphoma producing two structurally different TFG-ALK translocations. Blood. 1999;94:3265–8.
233. Colleoni GW, Bridge JA, Garicochea B, Liu J, Filippa DA, Ladanyi M. ATIC-ALK: a novel variant ALK gene fusion in anaplastic large cell lymphoma resulting from the recurrent cryptic chromosomal inversion, inv(2)(p23q35). Am J Pathol. 2000; 156:781–9.
234. Ma Z, Cools J, Marynen P, et al. Inv(2)(p23q35) in anaplastic large-cell lymphoma induces constitutive anaplastic lymphoma kinase (ALK) tyrosine kinase activation by fusion to ATIC, an enzyme involved in purine nucleotide biosynthesis. Blood. 2000;95: 2144–9.
235. Trinei M, Lanfrancone L, Campo E, et al. A new variant anaplastic lymphoma kinase (ALK)-fusion protein (ATIC-ALK) in a case of ALK-positive anaplastic large cell lymphoma. Cancer Res. 2000; 60:793–8.
236. Bridge JA, Kanamori M, Ma Z, et al. Fusion of the ALK gene to the clathrin heavy chain gene, CLTC, in inflammatory myofibroblastic tumor. Am J Pathol. 2001;159:411–5.
237. Reichard KK, McKenna RW, Kroft SH. ALK-positive diffuse large B-cell lymphoma: report of four cases and review of the literature. Mod Pathol. 2007;20:310–9.
238. Touriol C, Greenland C, Lamant L, et al. Further demonstration of the diversity of chromosomal changes involving 2p23 in ALK-positive lymphoma: 2 cases expressing ALK kinase fused to CLTCL (clathrin chain polypeptide-like). Blood. 2000;95: 3204–7.
239. Tort F, Campo E, Pohlman B, Hsi E. Heterogeneity of genomic breakpoints in MSN-ALK translocations in anaplastic large cell lymphoma. Hum Pathol. 2004;35:1038–41.
240. Tort F, Pinyol M, Pulford K, et al. Molecular characterization of a new ALK translocation involving moesin (MSN-ALK) in anaplastic large cell lymphoma. Lab Invest. 2001;81:419–26.
241. Meech SJ, McGavran L, Odom LF, et al. Unusual childhood extramedullary hematologic malignancy with natural killer cell properties that contains tropomyosin 4—anaplastic lymphoma kinase gene fusion. Blood. 2001;98:1209–16.
242. Cools J, Wlodarska I, Somers R, et al. Identification of novel fusion partners of ALK, the anaplastic lymphoma kinase, in anaplastic large-cell lymphoma and inflammatory myofibroblastic tumor. Genes Chromosomes Cancer. 2002;34:354–62.
243. Ma Z, Hill DA, Collins MH, et al. Fusion of ALK to the Ran-binding protein 2 (RANBP2) gene in inflammatory myofibroblastic tumor. Genes Chromosomes Cancer. 2003;37:98–105.
244. Lamant L, Gascoyne RD, Duplantier MM, et al. Non-muscle myosin heavy chain (MYH9): a new partner fused to ALK in anaplastic large cell lymphoma. Genes Chromosomes Cancer. 2003;37:427–32.
245. Debelenko LV, Arthur DC, Pack SD, Helman LJ, Schrump DS, Tsokos M. Identification of CARS-ALK fusion in primary and metastatic lesions of an inflammatory myofibroblastic tumor. Lab Invest. 2003;83:1255–65.
246. Stachurski D, Miron PM, Al-Homsi S, et al. Anaplastic lymphoma kinase-positive diffuse large B-cell lymphoma with a complex karyotype and cryptic 3′ ALK gene insertion to chromosome 4 q22-24. Hum Pathol. 2007;38:940–5.
247. Panagopoulos I, Nilsson T, Domanski HA, et al. Fusion of the SEC31L1 and ALK genes in an inflammatory myofibroblastic tumor. Int J Cancer. 2006;118:1181–6.
248. Soda M, Choi YL, Enomoto M, et al. Identification of the transforming EML4-ALK fusion gene in non-small-cell lung cancer. Nature. 2007;448:561–6.

Approaches for First-Line Therapy of Peripheral T-Cell Lymphoma

12

David Sibon, Christian Gisselbrecht, and Francine Foss

Introduction

T-cell non-Hodgkin's lymphomas (NHLs) constitute about 10–15% of aggressive lymphomas. The prognostic significance of the immunophenotype has been explored in several studies and results have been reported concerning the outcome of peripheral T-cell lymphoma (PTCL) compared to that of B-cell lymphomas (BCLs). PTCL patients were found to have generally poorer prognoses than patients with BCL. However, PTCL represents a heterogeneous group of lymphomas and a wide variety of different histological subtypes have been recognized.

Patients with PTCL were treated until rituximab era with the same approach used for aggressive BCLs. In GELA prospective studies, LNH 87, LNH 93, and LNH 98, over 900 T-cell lymphoma patients were treated with conventional treatment as well as dose intensive treatments including autologous bone marrow transplantation for patients with adverse prognostic factors. When the outcomes for the T-cell lymphoma patients treated in the LNH 87 protocol with CHOP-like regimens were reviewed, the prognostic value of T-cell phenotype was studied, 5-year overall (OS) and event free survival (EFS) were 41% and 33% respectively [1]. Age, LDH, performance status, BM involvement, and non-anaplastic T-cell NHL were highly independent significant factors affecting OS, and there was no difference in outcome in the different arms of the study. In the subsequent five arm randomized LNH 93 protocol the results were similar. In these studies, the intensive regimen ACVBP was the standard control arm, and for patients less than 60 years; no difference could be seen between ACVBP and m-BACOD or CHOP for low-risk patients [2–4] or stem cell transplantation for high-risk patients or an alternating regimen with ifosfamide and etoposide for patients between 60 and 70 years [5]. Due to the limitation of such subset retrospective analysis it was not possible to determine superiority of any arm, but all regimens included anthracyclines. The retrospective T-cell Lymphoma Project demonstrated similarly that there were no significant differences in the outcomes for patients who received anthracycline-containing regimens as opposed to non-anthracycline-based regimens in the first line [6]. CHOP, therefore, has remained the standard first-line regimen.

D. Sibon
Hématologie Adulte, Hôpital Necker, AP-HP, Université Paris Descartes, Sorbonne Paris Cité, Paris, France

C. Gisselbrecht
Department of Hemato oncology, Saint Louis, Paris, France

F. Foss (✉)
Department of Medical Oncology/Hematology, Yale University School of Medicine, 333 Cedar Street, FMP 130, PO Box 208032, New Haven, CT 06520, USA
e-mail: Francine.foss@yale.edu

F. Foss (ed.), *T-Cell Lymphomas*, Contemporary Hematology,
DOI 10.1007/978-1-62703-170-7_12, © Springer Science+Business Media New York 2013

Historical Data for CHOP-Based Chemotherapy Regimens in the Different Histological Subtypes

Peripheral T-Cell Lymphoma, NOS

PTCL, not other specified (PTCLnos) represents the largest PTCL subtype in North America (60–70% of T-cell lymphomas) [6]. In the WHO classification it encompasses all of the PTCLs not classifiable as a specific disease entity in contrast to the rare, but "specified" subtypes [7]. Given the biological heterogeneity encountered in the PTCLnos, it is widely believed that it is made up of more than one disease type. PTCLnos occurs primarily in adults with a median age of 60 years. Despite being classified in as a nodal PTCL in the WHO classification, the majority of patients have extranodal site involvement including the gastrointestinal tract, liver, bone marrow, and skin. The majority of patients present with advanced stage (III–IV) and often with elevated LDH and B symptoms. The 5-year survival of patients with PTCLnos historically has approximately 30% using standard chemotherapy (CHOP and CHOP-like therapy) [6]. In one recent review, outcome has been associated with prognostic score, with patients with low IPI (0–1) having a 5-year OS of 50% vs. 11% for those with 4–5 risk factors [8].

While PTCLnos is a heterogeneous subtype, a number of prognostic markers have been identified. The overexpression of Epstein–Barr virus in 110 nodal NOS T-cell lymphomas was found in 53 patients and was associated with an even poorer prognosis [9]. Additionally for patients with the PTCL-NOS subtype, CD30 expression as well as the expression markers of proliferation such as Ki-67 has been analyzed for their prognostic ability [10]. Two chemokine receptors, CXCR3 and CCR4, were found to be expressed in 63% and 34% of PTCL-NOS cases, respectively [11, 12]. The dominant chemokine expression found in this study was CXCR3-positive/CCR4-negative; this phenotype was shown by multivariate analysis to be an independent adverse prognostic factor.

Angioimmunoblastic T-Cell Lymphoma

Angioimmunoblastic T-cell lymphoma (AITL) represents a distinct clinicopathological entity, among nodal PTCLs. It generally occurs in elderly patients presenting with generalized lymphadenopathy, hepatosplenomegaly, anemia, and hypergammaglobulinemia. Recent data concerning the identity of the normal cellular counterpart of AITL are emerging. It is now believed that AITL derives from a follicular helper T-cell subset [13, 14]. The tumor cells usually express CD4, CD10, Bcl6, and CXCL13, a phenotype that is unique among T-cell lymphomas.

To evaluate the prognostic significance of clinicobiologic and pathological features in AITL, 157 AITL patients were retrieved from the GELA LNH87-LNH93 randomized clinical trials [15]. One hundred forty-seven patients received a cyclophosphamide, doxorubicin, vincristine, and prednisone (CHOP)-like regimen with intensified courses in half of them. Median age was 62 years, with 81% advanced stage, 72% B symptoms, 65% anemia, 50% hypergammaglobulinemia, and 66% elevated LDH. Overall 7-year survival was 30%. In multivariate analysis, only male sex ($P=0.004$), mediastinal lymphadenopathy ($P=0.041$), and anemia ($P=0.042$) adversely affected overall survival. It was not possible to isolate a group of better prognosis and both IPI and PIT were of limited value. AITL portends a poor prognosis even when treated intensively. However, 30% of patients are long-term survivors, suggesting that there may be a more favorable subset [15].

Anaplastic Large Lymphoma

Primary systemic anaplastic large cell lymphoma (ALCL) accounts for 2–8% of all lymphomas and 10–15% of all childhood NHLs. Two distinct clinical forms of primary ALCL are now recognized: limited to the skin, not discussed here, and systemic. Clear clinicopathologic differences have been found between AKL-positive (ALK+) and ALK-negative (ALK−) subtypes in most studies. An increased incidence of extranodal involvement was seen in the AKL-negative group. Skin, bone, and soft tissues were commonly affected extranodal sites. ALK+ ALCL is associated with lower IPI scores than the ALK− group and is the most common ALCL occurring in children. ALK status is the most important prognostic factor in outcome for ALCL, with ALK+ patients having a 5-year overall survival of 70% and progression-free survival of 60% vs. 5-year OS of 49% and FFS of 36% for the ALK− group [16].

In children in most European studies, ALCL is considered to be a separate entity and is treated with either a short and intensive chemotherapy regimen, as for BCL or with more prolonged chemotherapy derived from T-cell lymphoma protocols. The European Intergroup Study of ALCL compared the results and prognoses of 225 children enrolled in trials designed to treat childhood ALCL with short and intensive chemotherapy [17]. Multivariate analysis revealed three significant prognostic factors: (1) mediastinal involvement, (2) visceral involvement, (3) skin lesions. For the good-prognosis group with 0 factors, the 5-years PFS was 89%; for the poor-risk group with at least one factor, the 5-years PFS was 61%.

While no large comparative studies have been published in adults with ALCL, responses to CHOP and CHOP-like regimens range from 60 to 90%. The overall survival of patients with stage I or II disease with low IPI exceeds 90%. According to the GELA study which included 146 adults with T/null- and B-cell ALCL, the 5-year overall-survival rate for patients without adverse IPI was 82%, as compared to 78% for patients with an IPI of 1, 50% for the high-intermediate-IPI group, and 25% for the high-IPI group [18]. Dose-intensive treatments have been used in this study, according to initial stratification based on prognostic factors. However, in that investigation, stratification according to ALK positivity had not been done, and results may also reflect the different percentage of ALK+ lymphomas in adults. In the good-prognosis group of ALK+ lymphomas the 5-year overall-survival rate was 94% for patients with 0–1 risk factor vs. 41% for those with two or more factors [19]. Although ALK positivity is considered a marker of better prognosis, patients with two or more IPI factors still have a poor prognosis, and new approaches are needed.

Considering the response rate and the survival of patients with ALK+ lymphoma, consolidation with ASCT is not recommended if patient achieve a complete remission. The NCCN guidelines does not recommend autologous stem cell transplant in first remission for this group of patients. For ALK− patients the debate is still open for patients with at least two IPI adverse prognostic factors, and the NCCN guidelines would suggest that such patients be consolidated with a stem cell transplant.

Extranodal Natural Killer/T-Cell Lymphoma, Nasal Type

Extranodal NK/T-cell lymphoma, nasal type, is a rare and severe disease, more frequent in Asia and South America than in Europe and North America. It shows a striking association with Epstein–Barr virus. Usually extranodal NK/T-cell lymphomas primarily involve the nasal cavity or other parts of the upper aerodigestive tract but sometimes occur in extranasal sites without involving the nasal cavity or nasopharynx (gastrointestinal tract, skin, testis, liver, spleen, bone marrow). There is no consensus treatment except that the addition of radiotherapy for early stage nasal cases results in survival benefit and can be used upfront as producing a 83% complete remission rate [20, 21]. Patients with extranodal NK/T cell lymphoma have a cumulative 5-year survival probability of 40% [21, 22]. The median overall survival is better in nasal compared to the extranasal cases in early (2.96 year vs. 0.36 year) and late stage disease (0.8 year vs. 0.28 year) [23].

For patients with refractory or relapsed extranodal NK/T-cell lymphoma, L-asparaginase-based regimens have been shown to be associated with ORR of 79% with 63% CR [24, 25]. A novel regimen that incorporates L-asparaginase along with ifosfamide, etoposide, dexamethasone, and methotrexate (SMILE) has been developed and shown to be associated in a Phase I study with a response rate of 67% in refractory patients [26]. A prospective phase II trial has been reported with SMILE regimen in patients with newly diagnosed stage IV or relapsed refractory NK/T-cell lymphomas [27]. Of 39 enrolled patients, 29 (74%) completed the planned treatment. The responses were complete remission (CR) in 15, partial remission in 14, and early death due to infection in 4. Overall response rate and CR were 74% (95% CI, 58–87) and 38%, respectively. The most common grade 3 nonhematologic toxicity was infection (41%).

Enteropathy-Type T-Cell Lymphoma

EATL is a rare type of T-cell lymphoma, often associated with a history of celiac disease, that usually arises in the jejunum but can involve other gastrointestinal tract sites (e.g., stomach and colon). There are two histological groups of EATL that correlate with clinical and immunophenotypic features. Pleomorphic-anaplastic ETL is usually associated with a history of celiac disease and histologic evidence of enteropathy and is most often CD56–. Monomorphic ETL often occurs without a history of celiac disease, has variable histological evidence of enteropathy, and is usually CD56. The most commonly used regimen for patients with enteropathy-type intestinal T-cell lymphoma is CHOP. However, the use of combination chemotherapy is difficult, and less than 50% of patients can complete their planned courses of chemotherapy, often because of poor nutritional status. Observed complications of treatment are gastrointestinal bleeding, small-bowel perforation, and the development of enterocolic fistulae. Relapses occurred in 79% of patients who respond to initial therapy. Response data are available mainly from study of Gale et al. [28]. Of 24 patients treated with combination chemotherapy, ten (41%) achieved a complete remission and four (16%) a partial response. The regimens included an intensive weekly combination of vincristine, doxorubicin, prednisolone, and high-dose methotrexate ($n=5$); cyclophosphamide, doxorubicin, vincristine, and prednisolone (CHOP) at 21-day intervals ($n=12$); alternating 21-day cycles of CHOP with procarbazine, etoposide, and prednisolone orally on days 3–7, and doxorubicin intravenously on day 1 ($n=1$); cyclophosphamide, vincristine, doxorubicin, and prednisolone ($n=1$); and alternating weekly cycles of prednisolone, doxorubicin, cyclophosphamide, and etoposide with prednisolone, bleomycin, vincristine, and methotrexate (PEACE-BOM; $n=3$). Less than 50% of patients completed their planned chemotherapy courses, largely because of complications of treatment. Poor nutritional status was common, requiring parenteral nutrition during chemotherapy in ten patients and enteral feeding in another two. Gastrointestinal bleeding occurred in one patient 5 days after starting treatment. Four patients suffered small-bowel perforation. In three, this occurred after the first cycle of treatment (at 1, 2, and 4 days) and proved a fatal event. The actuarial 1-year and 5-year overall-survival rates were 39% and 20% respectively.

Hepatosplenic T-Cell Lymphoma

Hepatosplenic T-cell Lymphoma (HSTCL) is a rare aggressive type of extranodal lymphoma characterized by hepatosplenomegaly, bone marrow involvement, and peripheral blood cytopenias. Most cases express the gamma-delta T-cell receptor, but cases can have an alpha/beta phenotype and are considered to be a variant of the disease. Many patients have a history of immunosuppression. The median age is ~30 years, with a male predominance. Prognosis of HSTCL is poor; response data are available mainly from two studies [29, 30]: median survival time is ~12 months, and almost all patients ultimately die despite consolidative or salvage high-dose therapy. Current treatment modalities appear to be ineffective in most patients. The question of whether aggressive treatment improves the overall survival is unresolved. Possibly transplantation after a short attempt to induce remission might be a suggestion.

Data with More Intensive Regimens

Given the overall inferiority of CHOP-line BCL regimens in the retrospective studies, more aggressive infusional regimens, including hyper-CVAD and hyper-CHOP, among others, were evaluated in patients with aggressive T-cell lymphomas. A retrospective study from MD Anderson Cancer Center explored alternative higher dose regimens and compared those against CHOP in 135 patients with PTCL. Among those patients with non-ALCL disease, there was no significant difference in outcome between those treated with CHOP and aggressive alternatives (3-year OS: 43% vs. 49%) [31]. However, these results are difficult to interpret, as the study was not randomized.

Mercadal et al. reported results from a study of patients who were treated in the first line with mega CHOP/ESHAP followed by autologous stem cell transplant for patients achieving remission [32]. Forty-one patients were enrolled and received three courses of high-dose cyclophosphamide 2,000 mg/m^2/day, adriamycin 90 mg/m^2/day, vincristine and prednisone alternating with three courses of etoposide, cisplatin, cytarabine, and prednisone (ESHAP). The histological distribution of the patients included PTCL unspecified, 20 cases (49%); angioimmunoblastic,12 cases (29%); hepatosplenic, 2 cases (5%); extranodal NK nasal type, 2 cases (5%); panniculitis like, 2 cases (5%) and others. Sixty-eight percent of patients received the planned treatment. After chemotherapy, 20 patients reached complete response (CR) and 4 had a partial response, for an overall response rate of 58%. The outcome of the 16 patients who showed primary refractoriness to mega-CHOP/ESHAP was extremely poor, with a median OS of 8 months. Grade 3 or 4 hematologic toxicity occurred in 63 and 68% of patients after CHOP and ESHAP respectively. Thirty-eight and 15% of patients in the CHOP and ESHAP courses respectively required hospitalizations for infections and one patient died of sepsis. Overall, the CR rate in this study (50%) was not better than with CHOP alone in studies done by the same group, suggesting no advantage to this more aggressive approach.

Recently the German High Grade Non-Hodgkin's Lymphoma Study group explored the use of dose intensive CHOP or the addition of etoposide to CHOP for aggressive lymphomas. They reported results for patients with aggressive T-cell lymphomas treated on seven trials with 6–8 courses of CHOP or CHOEP (Hi-CHOEP or MegaCHOEP) [33]. Of 343 T-cell patients enrolled in these studies, 70 had PTCLnos, 28 had AITL, 78 had ALK+ ALCL, and 113 had ALK− ALCL. When analyzed for prognostic factors, B-symptoms were most frequent in AITL patients and bulky disease was seen more often in ALCL, either ALK-positive or -negative, than in other subtypes. Over half of all ALCL (ALK-positive or -negative) patients, 46% of PTCLnos, and 21% of AITL patients were in the low-risk group by IPI.

As an aggregate, the younger patients demonstrated an improvement in EFS for both etoposide containing regimens (75% vs. 51%) compared to the non-etoposide regimen, but there was no overall survival difference. The positive effect of etoposide on EFS was seen even in the favorable ALK+ patients. For the elderly patients, neither shortening of the time interval from 3 to 2 weeks (CHOP-21 vs. CHOP-14), administration of eight instead of six courses of CHOP-14, or the addition of etoposide (CHOEP) significantly improved EFS or OS and increased toxicity was seen with the more intensive regimens. EFS for the different subtypes was 41% for PTCLu, 45% for ALK− ALCL, 50% for AITL, and 76% for ALK+ ALCL. Outcomes in this study were related to IPI for the non-ALK+ patients. Those with IPI 0 and 1 had a favorable 3-year EFS above 50%. Patients with IPI of 2 or greater showed a 3-year EFS below 34%. The conclusions from this study which is one of the largest randomized studies of first-line regimens is that younger patients may benefit from the addition of etoposide in terms of response rate and EFS, which would therefore potentially allow more patients to undergo a consolidation autologous stem cell transplant in first remission. The standard for the elderly based on these data remains six cycles of CHOP at standard doses. Finally, the excellent outcomes in patients with low IPI suggest that this group may do well and should be distinguished from the intermediate and high IPI patients.

Another more intensive regimen explored in the GELA group was ACVBP (doxorubicin 75 mg/m² D1, cyclophosphamide 1,200 mg/m² D1, vindesine 2 mg/m² D1 and D5, bleomycin 10 mg D1 and D5, and prednisone D1–D5, followed by a sequential consolidation consisting of HD methotrexate (two courses), etoposide + ifosfamide (four courses), and cytarabine (two courses) at 2 weeks intervals). In a randomized study reported by Tilly et al., there was a statistical advantage in patients 60–70 years old for ACVBP (47 T-cell lymphomas) vs. CHOP (49 T-cell lymphomas) [34]. A further study was done adding bortezomib to the regimen (5 mg/m² was administered at D1 and D5 of each ACVBP cycle, and then at D1, D8, and D15 every 4 weeks during consolidation phase) [35]. Fifty-seven patients were enrolled and were to receive four cycles of bortezomib-ACVBP over 10 weeks; 46 patients responded and received consolidation with high-dose methotrexate, ifosfamide, etoposide, and cytarabine. Only 28 patients completed the consolidation phase of the study and 39% of patients died from lymphoma. There was no overall difference in response rate between the ACVBP-bortezomib regimen and ACVBP alone.

The Groupe Ouest Est d'Etude des Leucemies et Autres Maladies du Sang devised an alternative therapeutic schedule including etoposide, ifosfamide, cisplatin alternating with doxorubicin, bleomycin, vinblastine, dacarbazine (VIP-reinforced-ABVD; VIP-rABVD) and compared it to CHOP/21 as front-line treatment in 88 patients with non-cutaneous PTCL [36]. Patients assigned to VIP-rABVD ($n=43$) received six alternative cycles every 4 weeks (three VIP and three rABVD). VIP cycles (1, 3, and 5) included etoposide 100 mg/m²/day IV days 1–3, ifosfamide 1,000 mg/m²/day days 1–5, and cisplatin 20 mg/m²/day as a continuous infusion on days 1–5. The three cycles of rABVD (cycles 2, 4, and 6) included on days 1 and 15, doxorubicin 50 mg/m²/day, bleomycin 10 mg/m²/day, vinblastine 10 mg/m²/day, and dacarbazine 375 mg/m²/day. Eighty-eight patients were enrolled, including 57 with PTCL-nos, 15 with AITL, and 14 with ALCL. Among the 14 ALCL patients, 10 were ALK+. Grade 3 or 4 neutropenia was higher in the VIP-rABVD arm (23% vs. 8%), but treatment mortality was similar (9% vs. 8%).

The 22-year EFS of 41% vs. 45% for the CHOP-21 arm vs. the intensive regimen was no different despite the more aggressive regimen and median overall survival was 42 months for each of the arms. Outcome in this study was better for patients with ALK+ ALCL and for those with low IPI. Patients with localized disease underwent consolidative involved field radiotherapy.

New Combination Therapies for PTCL

CHOP-Based Regimens

A number of studies have investigated chemoimmunotherapy in aggressive T-cell lymphomas. Alemtuzumab is a CD52-targeted monoclonal antibody that has demonstrated activity as a single agent and in combination with CHOP. Up to 40% of PTCL cases have been shown to express CD52 by immunohistochemistry, although expression has been shown to vary by subtype [37]. One phase II study by Kim et al. enrolled 20 patients treated with CHOP combined with intravenous alemtuzumab in 3-week cycles (cycle 1: 10 mg on day 1, 20 mg on day 2; subsequent cycles: 30 mg on day 1) as frontline therapy [38]. Immunohistochemistry for CD52 expression was not required for study entry. Trimethoprim/sulfamethoxazole, twice daily, three times a week, and acyclovir 600 mg, twice daily, were administered starting on day 8 and continued during the study and up to a minimum of 2 months following discontinuation of the alemtuzumab therapy. The overall response rate to this combination was 65% CR and 15% PR. Responses were seen in all ten pts with PTCLnos, one of three with extranodal NK/T-cell lymphoma, two of three with AITL, and one of two with ALK- ALCL and SPTCL respectively. Nearly all patients (90%) experienced grade 4 neutropenia and 5 of 20 experienced CMV-reactivation. Additionally, there were two treatment-related deaths, including one who died from pseudomonas pneumonial and lung abscess. The high complete response rate of 65.0%, 1-year event-free survival rate of 43.3%, and 1-year overall survival rate of 44.3% in this study was comparable to other studies with CHOP but toxicity was high and the regimen was significantly immunosuppressive in this population.

Gallamini et al. conducted a study of CHOP plus alemtuzumab combination in which alemtuzumab 30 mg was given subcutaneously on day 1 in cycles 1–4 in the first cohort of patients and then for all eight courses in the second cohort [39]. There were 14 patients with PTCLu, 6 with AITL, 3 with ALK− ALCL, and 1 with EATL. Of 24 evaluable patients, 71% had CR, including all 6 with AITL, all 3 with ALK− ALCL, 7 of 14 with PTCLu, and the one with EATL. The ORR was 75%. Neutropenia was seen in 34% of the treatment cycles and CMV reactivation in 9%. There was one patient who had reactivation of Jakob-Creutzfeldt virus and two who developed aspergillosis. At a median follow-up of 16 months at the time of the report (range, 5–42 months), 14 patients were alive, 9 had died from progressive disease, and 1 had died from pneumonia at day 198 while in CR. The overall median duration of response was 11 months. This study demonstrated that subcutaneous alemtuzumab was better tolerated and associated with a lower but still significant incidence of opportunistic infections.

A phase I study evaluated alemtuzumab combined with dose-adjusted EPOCH (etoposide, prednisone, vincristine, cyclophosphamide, doxorubicin) in PTCL patients [40]. In this study, alemtuzumab was administered at doses of 30, 60, or 90 mg prior to each EPOCH cycle. Significant bone marrow aplasia occurred in two of three patients at both the 60 and 90 mg dose groups; therefore, phase II study accrual is continuing at the 30 mg dose of alemtuzumab. Infections were reported in 11 of 14 patients, including bacterial, fungal, and viral pathogens. Patients underwent ongoing CMV surveillance and received prophylactic therapy with acyclovir and trimethoprim–sulfamethoxazole.

Based on these encouraging data with alemtuzumab and CHOP, the alemtuzumab-CHOP combination is being compared to CHOP-21 in the first line by the Nordic Lymphoma Group and the German High Grade Lymphoma Groups (the ACT Trial). Patients over age 60 will be randomized between the two arms and will then be followed until progression. Patients under age 60 will be randomized to either six cycles of CHOP-14 or four cycles of alemtuzumab-CHOP-14 and two cycles of CHOP-14 without alemtuzumab vs. six cycles of CHOP-14. Patients in remission will then undergo an autolous stem cell transplant.

Another targeted agent that has been combined with CHOP in first-line therapy for PTCL has been the interleukin-2 fusion toxin protein, denileukin diftitox. Denileukin diftitox combines the interleukin-2 receptor-binding domain with diphtheria toxin, and is FDA approved for patients with relapsed or refractory cutaneous T-cell lymphomas whose tumors express the CD25 subunit of the interleukin-2 receptor. In a single center phase II study at MD Anderson Cancer Center, denileukin diftitox was administered to 27 patients with relapsed aggressive T-cell lymphomas at the standard dose of 18 μg/kg/day for 5 days on a 21 day cycle [41]. The overall response rate was 48% in heavily pretreated patients with relapsed PTCL. Responses were seen in four of ten patients with PTCL-NOS, two of three with AITL, and two of two with ALCL. The progression-free survival was 6 months. In this trial, the expression of CD25 by immunohistochemistry was not predictive of response to denileukin diftitox.

Based on these encouraging data in relapsed patients, a multi-center prospective phase II trial evaluated the efficacy and safety of the combination of denileukin diftitox with CHOP in 49 untreated patients with aggressive PTCL subtypes [42]. In this study, denileukin diftitox was administered at a dose of 18 μg/kg/day on days 1 and 2 and CHOP was given on day 3; this was followed by growth factor support on day 4 every 21 days. Histologic subtypes included: ALCL 8, AILT 10, PTCLnos 19, EATL 3, panniculitis-like TCL 5, NK/T 1, hepatosplenic TCL 1. The median cycles was six with seven pts completing only one cycle of therapy; three pts died with PD after cycle one, and four patients were taken off study for toxicity. The ORR in 47 pts was 68% with 57% CR. In the efficacy-evaluable pts (≥2 cycles completed) the ORR was 86% (CR 75%). All patients with AITL, ALCL, and EATL responded, as did 3 of 5 with SPTCL and 9 of 12 with PTCLnos. Median PFS for the 47 pts was 12 months and 2-year estimated OS was 60%. The median response duration for the 33 responders was 29 months. The most frequent grade 3 or 4 adverse events were bone marrow suppression and febrile neutropenia, which occurred in 12% of patients. Denileukin diftitox-associated toxicities included infusion related rigor in seven pts, hypoalbuminemia in 17, and acute hypersensitivity in 1. There was no prolonged immunosuppression, or opportunistic infections, and a randomized study of CHOP with or without denileukin diftitox is ongoing.

In another study by the GELA, CHOP was combined with rituximab in elderly patients (age 59–79) with AITL in an attempt to target non-neoplastic B lymphocytes which may provide paracrine growth factors to the malignant T cells. Twenty-five patients aged 59–79 years with newly diagnosed AITL were enrolled and treated with a combination of eight cycles of rituximab (375 mg/m^2 at day 1 of each cycle) and CHOP chemotherapy delivered every 3 weeks (R-CHOP21). Most of the patients had advanced disease (stage IV: 92% and B symptoms: 68%). Twenty-one patients completed the eight cycles of R-CHOP. The overall response rate was 80%, with 44% achieving a complete response. With a median follow-up of 24 months, the progression free survival was 42 and the 2-year overall survival was 62%. It was concluded that R-CHOP21 did not improve the complete response rate or outcome compared to historical data with CHOP.

CHOP has also been combined with the bevacizumab, the anti-VEGF receptor growth factor monoclonal antibody. Several PTCL subtypes, especially AITL, are characterized by the overexpression of angiogenic factors, such as VEGF. At least one relapsed AITL patient has achieved a CR following treatment with bevacizumab [43]. A combination of CHOP and bevacizumab has been studied in patients with PTCL or NK-cell neoplasms by the Eastern Cooperative Oncology Group. Patients received bevacizumab at a dose of 15 mg/kg on day 1 followed by maintenance bevacizumab. However, this trial has been suspended when a preliminary analysis reported a high incidence of cardiac events related to the therapy, including four cases of congestive heart failure [44].

Gemcitabine-Based Regimens

Gemcitabine has demonstrated significant activity as a single agent in patients with cutaneous T-cell lymphomas and has been used in a number of combination regimens for PTCL [45]. Zinzani reported results from 19 patients with CTCL and 20 patients with PTCL who received gemcitabine at a dose of 1,200 mg/m^2 on days 1, 8, 15 schedule every 28 days. All patients had been heavily pretreated. The overall response rate was 51%; MF patients had a CR rate of 16% and a PR rate of 32%, while PTCL patients had a CR rate of 30% and a PR rate of 25%.

A combination of gemcitabine with cisplatin (GEM-P) was tested in a phase II study [46]. The regimen consisted of gemcitabine given at 1,000 mg/m^2 on days 1, 8, 15 with cisplatin 100 mg/m^2 on day 8 and methylprednisolone 1,000 mg/m^2 on days 1–5 of a 28-day cycle. Of 27 patients treated, the response rate was 73% overall and 80% in first-line patients. Grade 3 or 4 neutropenia occurred in 41% of treated patients.

The combination of gemcitabine with vinorelbine and filgrastim was also found to be active in a pilot study. Patients received vinorelbine 25 mg/m^2 and gemcitabine 1,000 mg/m^2 on days 1 and 8 of each 21-day cycle [47]. The overall response rate was 70% for the PTCL patients ($n=10$) treated with this regimen. Febrile neutropenia occurred in 6% of cycles.

In another study, gemcitabine was combined in a CHOP-based regimen (CHOP-EG, CHOP plus etoposide and gemcitabine) as first-line treatment [48]. The regimen consisted of classical CHOP plus etoposide 100 mg/m^2 intravenously on day 1 and gemcitabine 600 mg/m^2 on day 1 in a 3-week interval. Fourteen of 26 enrolled patients had PTCLnos and 8 had NK/T-cell lymphomas, 2 had AITL and 2 had ALK− ALCL. Responses were seen in 10 of 14 PTCL, 7 of 8 NK/T, one of two AILT and both ALCL patients. The overall response rate was 76.9%. Median survival has not yet been reached, while median EFS was 7 months at a median follow-up duration of 383 days. Estimated overall survival at 1 year was 69.6%. The most severe adverse event was grade 4 neutropenia in 14 patients (53.8%) and febrile neutropenia in four patients (15.4%). While active, this regimen did not appear to be superior to studies with CHOP-etoposide and incidence of myelosuppression was higher.

The Southwest Oncology Group has recently completed a study of gemcitabine, cisplatin, etoposide, and Solu-Medrol (PEGS) for patients with untreated or relapsed PTCL. The majority of the patients (79%) were untreated at the time of study entry. The 1-year event-free survival was reported to be 38%.

Another regimen incorporating gemcitabine was the GIVOX regimen (gemcitabine, ifosfamide, and oxaliplatin). In a group of high-risk PTCL patients, the response rate was 86% with 67% CR and the 5-year EFS was 49%. Toxicities were primarily hematologic with grade 4 thrombocytopenia and anemia occurring in 38% and 24% of patients respectively.

Transplantation as a Consolidation Therapy

The role of autologous or allogeneic stem cell transplanation in first remission has been explored in a number of prospective nonrandomized trials. The largest studies are from the Nordic and the German groups, who report overall EFS ranging from 30 to 50% and transplant rates of 40–70% based on intent to treat analysis. The Nordic group reported results from 160 patients treated with CHOEP-14 followed by BEAM conditioning [49]. At a median follow-up of 4 years, the OS was 50% and the PFS was 48%. Outcome results were similar for the nodal subtypes of PTCL. In the German study reported by Reimer et al., 83 patients were treated with CHOP ×4, followed by Dexa BEAM or ESHAP [50]. The conditioning regimen for the transplant was high-dose cyclophosphamide and total body irradiation. In this study, the CR rate to CHOP was 39%, and only 66% of patients were able to be transplanted. At a mean follow-up of 33 months, the OS was 48% and the EFS was 53%.

Based on the poor outcomes for most patients with PTCL, the NCCN guidelines recommends that autologous stem cell transplantation be considered in first remission all but the ALK+ ALCL group. A randomized study comparing outcomes with and without transplantation is underway as is a study comparing outcomes with autologous or allogeneic stem cell transplantation. However, more data is needed to identify prognostic factors which predict which patients will benefit from these approaches.

Summary of First-Line Treatment Approaches for PTCL

Because of the inferior outcomes with CHOP-based regimens and the paucity of data exploring other regimens in a randomized setting, treatment strategies for patients with aggressive T-cell lymphomas are not clearly defined. In the United States, the NCCN has established evidence-based treatment approaches for T-cell lymphoma and stratifies patients based on stage (Table 12.1). For early stage patients with localized disease, chemotherapy should be followed by involved field radiotherapy. It is recommended that all patients except for those with low IPI be consolidated with autologous stem cell transplant. ALK+ ALCL is identified as the one subtype which has an excellent outcome and should not be transplanted in first remission. Recent data suggest that ALK+ patients with high IPI could be an exception to this rule. In prospective trials where up to 40% of patients do not undergo a complete remission and therefore cannot be consolidated with transplant, new approaches are necessary.

Selection of first-line therapy based on histopathologic features has not yet been widely employed but should be considered. For nodal T-cell lymphomas (PTCL-NOS, AITL, ALCL)

Table 12.1 Approach to patients with T-cell lymphoma

Patient population	Induction therapy	Consolidation therapy
ALK-positive ALCL	CHOP+RT	Not needed if in remission
All other subtypes: stage I–II (low/low-intermediate risk)	Clinical trial preferred Multiagent chemotherapy (4–6 cycles) with adjuvant locoregional RT	Consider consolidation with high-dose therapy and stem cell rescue for all patients except low-risk (aaIPI)
All other subtypes: stage I–II (high/high-intermediate risk), stage III–IV	Clinical trial preferred Multiagent chemotherapy (6–8 cycles) ± RT	

Table 12.2 First-line therapies for T-cell lymphoma

First-line therapy	Clinical trial preferred CHOP (cyclophosphamide, doxorubicin, vincristine, and prednisone) for ALCL, ALK+ CHOEP (cyclophosphamide, doxorubicin, vincristine, etoposide, and prednisone) CHOP q 2–3 weeks CHOP followed by ICE (ifosfamide, carboplatin, and etoposide) or IVE (ifosfamide, etoposide, and epirubicin) HyperCVAD (cyclophosphamide, vincristine, doxorubicin, and dexamethasone) alternating with high-dose methotrexate and cytarabine
First-line consolidation	All patients except low-risk (aaIPI) should be consolidated for high-dose therapy and autologous stem cell transplantation ALK-1+ ALCL subtype has a good prognosis and does not need consolidative transplant if in remission

the standard regimen used is a CHOP-based therapy (Table 12.2). For extranodal subtypes, regimens may be individualized. NK/T-cell lymphoma patients have also had inferior outcomes with CHOP-based regimens, and consideration of alternative regimens such as SMILE and asparaginase combinations should be strongly considered for these patients.

References

1. Gisselbrecht C, Gaulard P, Lepage E, et al. Prognostic significance of T-cell phenotype in aggressive non-Hodgkin's lymphomas. Groupe d'Etudes des Lymphomes de l'Adulte (GELA). Blood. 1998;92: 76–82.
2. Tilly H, Mounier N, Lederlin P, et al. Randomized comparison of ACVBP and m-BACOD in the treatment of patients with low-risk aggressive lymphoma: the LNH87-1 study. Groupe d'Etudes des Lymphomes de l'Adulte. J Clin Oncol. 2000;18:1309–15.
3. Bonnet C, Fillet G, Mounier N, et al. CHOP alone compared with CHOP plus radiotherapy for localized aggressive lymphoma in elderly patients: a study by the Groupe d'Etude des Lymphomes de l'Adulte. J Clin Oncol. 2007;25:787–92.
4. Reyes F, Lepage E, Ganem G, et al. ACVBP versus CHOP plus radiotherapy for localized aggressive lymphoma. N Engl J Med. 2005;352:1197–205.
5. Bosly A, Lepage E, Coiffier B, et al. Outcome is not improved by the use of alternating chemotherapy in elderly patients with aggressive lymphoma. Hematol J. 2001;2:279–85.
6. Vose J, Armitage J, Weisenburger D. International peripheral T-cell and natural killer/T-cell lymphoma study: pathology findings and clinical outcomes. J Clin Oncol. 2008;26:4124–30.
7. Kluin PM, Feller A, Gaulard P, et al. Peripheral T/NK-cell lymphoma: a report of the IXth Workshop of the European Association for Haematopathology. Histopathology. 2001;38:250–70.
8. Savage KJ, Chhanabhai M, Gascoyne RD, Connors JM. Characterization of peripheral T-cell lymphomas in a single North American institution by the WHO classification. Ann Oncol. 2004;15:1467–75.
9. Dupuis J, Emile JF, Mounier N, et al. Prognostic significance of Epstein-Barr virus in nodal peripheral T-cell lymphoma, unspecified: a Groupe d'Etude des Lymphomes de l'Adulte (GELA) study. Blood. 2006;108:4163–9.
10. Went P, Agostinelli C, Gallamini A, et al. Marker expression in peripheral T-cell lymphoma: a proposed

clinical-pathologic prognostic score. J Clin Oncol. 2006;24:2472–9.
11. Ishida T, Utsunomiya A, Iida S, et al. Clinical significance of CCR4 expression in adult T-cell leukemia/lymphoma: its close association with skin involvement and unfavorable outcome. Clin Cancer Res. 2003;9:3625–34.
12. Ishida T, Inagaki H, Utsunomiya A, et al. CXC chemokine receptor 3 and CC chemokine receptor 4 expression in T-cell and NK-cell lymphomas with special reference to clinicopathological significance for peripheral T-cell lymphoma, unspecified. Clin Cancer Res. 2004;10:5494–500.
13. de Leval L, Gisselbrecht C, Gaulard P. Advances in the understanding and management of angioimmunoblastic T-cell lymphoma. Br J Haematol. 2010; 148:673–89.
14. de Leval L, Rickman DS, Thielen C, et al. The gene expression profile of nodal peripheral T-cell lymphoma demonstrates a molecular link between angioimmunoblastic T-cell lymphoma (AITL) and follicular helper T (TFH) cells. Blood. 2007;109:4952–63.
15. Mourad N, Mounier N, Briere J, et al. Clinical, biologic, and pathologic features in 157 patients with angioimmunoblastic T-cell lymphoma treated within the Groupe d'Etude des Lymphomes de l'Adulte (GELA) trials. Blood. 2008;111:4463–70.
16. Savage KJ, Harris NL, Vose JM, et al. ALK- anaplastic large-cell lymphoma is clinically and immunophenotypically different from both ALK+ ALCL and peripheral T-cell lymphoma, not otherwise specified: report from the International Peripheral T-Cell Lymphoma Project. Blood. 2008;111:5496–504.
17. Le Deley MC, Reiter A, Williams D, et al. Prognostic factors in childhood anaplastic large cell lymphoma: results of a large European intergroup study. Blood. 2008;111:1560–6.
18. Tilly H, Gaulard P, Lepage E, et al. Primary anaplastic large-cell lymphoma in adults: clinical presentation, immunophenotype, and outcome. Blood. 1997;90: 3727–34.
19. Falini B, Pileri S, Zinzani PL, et al. ALK+ lymphoma: clinico-pathological findings and outcome. Blood. 1999;93:2697–706.
20. Au WY, Ma SY, Chim CS, et al. Clinicopathologic features and treatment outcome of mature T-cell and natural killer-cell lymphomas diagnosed according to the World Health Organization classification scheme: a single center experience of 10 years. Ann Oncol. 2005;16:206–14.
21. Oshimi K. Progress in understanding and managing natural killer-cell malignancies. Br J Haematol. 2007;139:532–44.
22. Bossard C, Belhadj K, Reyes F, et al. Expression of the granzyme B inhibitor PI9 predicts outcome in nasal NK/T-cell lymphoma: results of a Western series of 48 patients treated with first-line polychemotherapy within the Groupe d'Etude des Lymphomes de l'Adulte (GELA) trials. Blood. 2007;109:2183–9.
23. Au WY, Weisenburger DD, Intragumtornchai T, et al. Clinical differences between nasal and extranasal NK/T-cell lymphoma: a study of 136 cases from the International Peripheral T-cell Lymphoma Project. Blood. 2009;113(17):3931–7.
24. Jaccard A, Gachard N, Marin B, et al. Efficacy of L-asparaginase with methotrexate and dexamethasone (AspaMetDex regimen) in patients with refractory or relapsing extranodal NK/T-cell lymphoma, a phase II study. Blood. 2011;117(6):1834–9.
25. Yong W, Zheng W, Zhang Y, et al. L-asparaginase-based regimen in the treatment of refractory midline nasal/nasal-type T/NK-cell lymphoma. Int J Hematol. 2003;78:163–7.
26. Yamaguchi M, Suzuki R, Kwong YL, et al. Phase I study of dexamethasone, methotrexate, ifosfamide, L-asparaginase, and etoposide (SMILE) chemotherapy for advanced-stage, relapsed or refractory extranodal natural killer (NK)/T-cell lymphoma and leukemia. Cancer Sci. 2008;99:1016–20.
27. Yamaguchi M, Kwong Y, Maeda Y, et al. Phase II study of SMILE chemotherapy for newly-diagnosed stage IV, relapsed or refractory extranodal NK/T-cell lymphoma, nasal type: NKTSG study. ASCO Meeting Abstracts. 2010;28:8044.
28. Gale J, Simmonds PD, Mead GM, Sweetenham JW, Wright DH. Enteropathy-type intestinal T-cell lymphoma: clinical features and treatment of 31 patients in a single center. J Clin Oncol. 2000;18:795–803.
29. Weidmann E. Hepatosplenic T cell lymphoma. A review on 45 cases since the first report describing the disease as a distinct lymphoma entity in 1990. Leukemia. 2000;14:991–7.
30. Belhadj K, Reyes F, Farcet JP, et al. Hepatosplenic gammadelta T-cell lymphoma is a rare clinicopathologic entity with poor outcome: report on a series of 21 patients. Blood. 2003;102:4261–9.
31. Escalon MP, Liu NS, Yang Y, et al. Prognostic factors and treatment of patients with T-cell non-Hodgkin lymphoma: the M. D. Anderson Cancer Center experience. Cancer. 2005;103:2091–8.
32. Mercadal S, Briones J, Xicoy B, et al. Intensive chemotherapy (high-dose CHOP/ESHAP regimen) followed by autologous stem-cell transplantation in previously untreated patients with peripheral T-cell lymphoma. Ann Oncol. 2008;19:958–63.
33. Schmitz N, Trumper L, Ziepert M, et al. Treatment and prognosis of mature T-cell and NK-cell lymphoma: an analysis of patients with T-cell lymphoma treated in studies of the German High-Grade Non-Hodgkin Lymphoma Study Group. Blood. 2010;116:3418–25.
34. Tilly H, Lepage E, Coiffier B, et al. Intensive conventional chemotherapy (ACVBP regimen) compared with standard CHOP for poor-prognosis aggressive non-Hodgkin lymphoma. Blood. 2003;102:4284–9.
35. Delmer A, Fitoussi O, Gaulard P, et al. A phase II study of bortezomib in combination with intensified CHOP-like regimen (ACVBP) in patients with previously untreated T-cell lymphoma: Results of the

GELA LNH05-1T trial. ASCO Meeting Abstracts. 2009;27:8554.
36. Simon A, Peoch M, Casassus P, et al. Upfront VIP-reinforced-ABVD (VIP-rABVD) is not superior to CHOP/21 in newly diagnosed peripheral T cell lymphoma. Results of the randomized phase III trial GOELAMS-LTP95. Br J Haematol. 2010;151:159–66.
37. Piccaluga PP, Agostinelli C, Righi S, Zinzani PL, Pileri SA. Expression of CD52 in peripheral T-cell lymphoma. Haematologica. 2007;92:566–7.
38. Kim JG, Sohn SK, Chae YS, et al. Alemtuzumab plus CHOP as front-line chemotherapy for patients with peripheral T-cell lymphomas: a phase II study. Cancer Chemother Pharmacol. 2007;60:129–34.
39. Gallamini A, Zaja F, Patti C, et al. Alemtuzumab (Campath-1H) and CHOP chemotherapy as first-line treatment of peripheral T-cell lymphoma: results of a GITIL (Gruppo Italiano Terapie Innovative nei Linfomi) prospective multicenter trial. Blood. 2007; 110:2316–23.
40. Janik JEPS, et al. A pilot study of Campath-1 with dose-adjusted EPOCH in CD52 expressing aggressive T-cell malignancies. Blood. 2005;106:33348.
41. Dang NH, Pro B, Hagemeister FB, et al. Phase II trial of denileukin diftitox for relapsed/refractory T-cell non-Hodgkin lymphoma. Br J Haematol. 2007;136:439–47.
42. Foss FM, Sjak-Shie NN, Goy A, Advani R, Jacobsen ED. Phase II study of denileukin diftitox with CHOP chemotherapy in newly-diagnosed PTCL: CONCEPT trial. ASCO Meeting Abstracts 2010;28:8045.
43. Bruns I, Fox F, Reinecke P, et al. Complete remission in a patient with relapsed angioimmunoblastic T-cell lymphoma following treatment with bevacizumab. Leukemia. 2005;19:1993–5.
44. Advani RH, Hong F, Ganjoo KN, et al. Cardiac toxicity associated with the Anti-VEGF monoclonal antibody bevacizumab (Avastin) in combination with CHOP (A-CHOP) chemotherapy for peripheral T cell lymphoma (PTCL): The ECOG 2404 Trial. Blood (ASH Annual Meeting Abstracts). 2009;114:1671.
45. Zinzani PL, Venturini F, Stefoni V, et al. Gemcitabine as single agent in pretreated T-cell lymphoma patients: evaluation of the long-term outcome. Ann Oncol. 2010;21:860–3.
46. Arkenau HT, Chong G, Cunningham D, et al. Gemcitabine, cisplatin and methylprednisolone for the treatment of patients with peripheral T-cell lymphoma: the Royal Marsden Hospital experience. Haematologica. 2007;92:271–2.
47. Spencer A, Reed K, Arthur C. Pilot study of an outpatient-based approach for advanced lymphoma using vinorelbine, gemcitabine and filgrastim. Intern Med J. 2007;37:760–6.
48. Kim JG, Sohn SK, Chae YS, et al. CHOP plus etoposide and gemcitabine (CHOP-EG) as front-line chemotherapy for patients with peripheral T cell lymphomas. Cancer Chemother Pharmacol. 2006;58:35–9.
49. d'Amore F, Jantunen E, Relander T. Hemopoietic stem cell transplantation in T-cell malignancies: who, when, and how? Curr Hematol Malig Rep. 2009;4:236–44.
50. Reimer P, Rudiger T, Geissinger E, et al. Autologous stem-cell transplantation as first-line therapy in peripheral T-cell lymphomas: results of a prospective multicenter study. J Clin Oncol. 2009;27:106–13.

Autologous and Allogeneic Stem Cell Transplantation for T-Cell Lymphomas

13

José Rodríguez and Paolo Corradini

Introduction

Peripheral T-cell lymphoma (PTCL) is a heterogeneous group of diseases with variable histologies, immunophenotype features, geographic and ethnic frequencies, and clinical natural history [1]. At present, the standard treatment for PTCL is chemotherapy based on the CHOP regimen designed for the largest group of aggressive B-cell lymphomas. However, with the exception of ALK$^+$ ALCL the outcome is poor with low number of complete responses and early progression. These facts translate into a poor outcome with 5 year overall survival values of 25–35% and a subsequent pattern of early and continuous relapses [2].

Until very recently no specific drugs for T-cell lymphomas have been incorporated to the therapeutic armamentarium, and retrospective studies suggest that anthracyclines do not add benefit for these patients, so CHOP is still the most commonly used regimen. Intensification of treatment with high-dose therapy and autologous stem cell transplantation or a graft-versus-PTCL effect with allogeneic hematopoietic stem cell transplantation have been shown to be associated with prolonged disease-free survival in selected PTCL patients.

J. Rodríguez (✉)
Department of Internal Medicine, Hospital Universitario Severo Ochoa, Avenida Orellana, S/N, 28911, Leganés, Spain
e-mail: joseguez89@hotmail.com

P. Corradini
Division of Hematology, Fondazione IRCCS Istituto Nazionale dei Tumori Milano, Milan, Italy

Retrospective Studies of ASCT for PTCL

Autologous SCT is the standard procedure after salvage chemotherapy in relapsing and refractory aggressive B-cell lymphomas, provided that the tumor has proven chemosensitivity to the salvage regimen [3]. When this strategy is applied to PTCL, results are similar in these types of lymphomas to the corresponding larger group of aggressive B-cell lymphomas.

As shown in Table 13.1, the results for autologous stem cell transplantation in the salvage setting across a number of studies demonstrate an OS of 30–45% and a corresponding PFS of 25–35% at 3–5 years.

The transplant-related mortality (TRM) is generally low at 3–10% despite the fact that many of the patients are heavily pretreated. Benefit from autologous transplantation is most evident in patients who demonstrate chemosensitivity to the salvage regimen. In the largest series reported by the Spanish GELTAMO group, the results in 123 patients (25% of the patients with diagnosis of ALCL) demonstrate at 5 years a 45 and 34% of OS and PFS respectively. Only chemosensitive patients had benefit in terms of PFS [4].

Multivariate analysis revealed two prognostic adverse factors (adjusted-international prognostic

F. Foss (ed.), *T-Cell Lymphomas*, Contemporary Hematology,
DOI 10.1007/978-1-62703-170-7_13,

Table 13.1 Main retrospective series on the use of ASCT in PTCL (Reprinted from Gutierrez et al. [45], with permission from Nature Publishing Group)

Study	Cases	% ALCL	Clinical setting	Survival	TRM (%)	Comment
Rodriguez [47]	29	NA	Salvage	3 year-OS: 36% 3 year-PFS: 28%	10	Results similar to DLCL
Blystad [48]	40	35	Frontline 1st CR Salvage	3 year-OS: 58% 3 year-PFS: 48%	7.5	Good results if chemosensitive
Song et al. [33]	36	55	Salvage	3 year-OS: 48% 3 year-PFS: 37%	17	Results similar to DLCL
Jantunen et al. [7]	19	38	Frontline 1st CR Salvage	5 year-OS: 45% 5 year-PFS: 28%	11	Better results in ALCL
Kewalramani [49]	24	0	Salvage	5 year-OS: 33% 5 year-PFS: 24%	NA	Results similar to DLCL
Smith [50]	32	65	Salvage	5 year-OS: 34% 5 year-DFS: 18%	3	Results worst than in DLCL
Feyler et al. [6]	33	31	Salvage	2 year-OS: 49% 2 year-PFS: 49%	3	Good results if chemosensitive
Rodriguez et al. [4, 5, 11]	74	31	Frontline 1st CR	5 year-OS: 68% 5 year-PFS: 63%	4	Very good results in 1st CR Worst if PIT>2
Rodriguez et al. [4, 5, 11]	123	25	Salvage	5 year-OS: 45% 5 year-PFS: 34%	5	Results similar to DLCL Worst if a-IPI>1 and B2M

ALCL anaplastic large cell lymphoma; *TRM* transplant-related mortality; *NA* nonavailable; *OS* overall survival; *PFS* progression-free survival; *DLCL* diffuse large-cell lymphoma; *CR* complete response; *PIT* prognostic index for peripheral T-cell lymphoma, : Elevated beta-2-microglobulin

index 2–3 and elevated beta-2 microglobulin) associated with favorable outcome in terms of PFS and OS. Using these and other covariates, a new prognostic index was defined for patients treated with ASCT in the salvage setting. As shown in Fig. 13.1, the value of this index relies on the identification of a subset of patients with the two adverse prognostic factors that, together with truly chemoresistant cases, do not benefit from ASCT consolidation and for whom other innovative therapies, including Allo-HSCT, should be tested.

The question as to the benefit of consolidation in first CR with transplant has benefit has been addressed in a number of prospective and retrospective studies. The largest prospective series by the GELTAMO group [5] describes the results of 74 patients who underwent ASCT consolidation after achieving a CR to induction chemotherapy regimen with CHOP or CHOP-like regimens.

With a prolonged follow-up of more than 60 months, the OS and PFS were 68 and 63%. In this study the only independent prognostic index able to identify a subset of patients who do not benefit from the ASCT as frontline consolidation at first CR was the presence of more than two adverse factors of the PIT (prognostic index for PTCL) index described by Gallamini and colleagues.

In another prospective study of 82 patients, 64 of them underwent ASCT with 50% of them in first CR. The OS and PFS at 2 years of these patients consolidated with ASCT in first CR were 62 and 59%, respectively supporting data of other series that show a substantial benefit of consolidation with ASCT in patients in first CR [6]. Similarly, another series from Finland reported 5-year OS and PFS of 63 and 64%, respectively. These results may be confounded by inclusion of ALK$^+$ patients, who have a more favorable outcome [7].

However, other studies are not so encouraging. The GELA performed a subset analysis of patients with PTCL included in the LNH93-3 aggressive lymphoma study [8]. Seventy-six patients with T-cell phenotype were analyzed in a randomized study of poor risk IPI patients comparing the GELA standard regimen ACVBP (doxorubicin, cyclophosphamide, epirubicin, vincristine, and prednisone) for

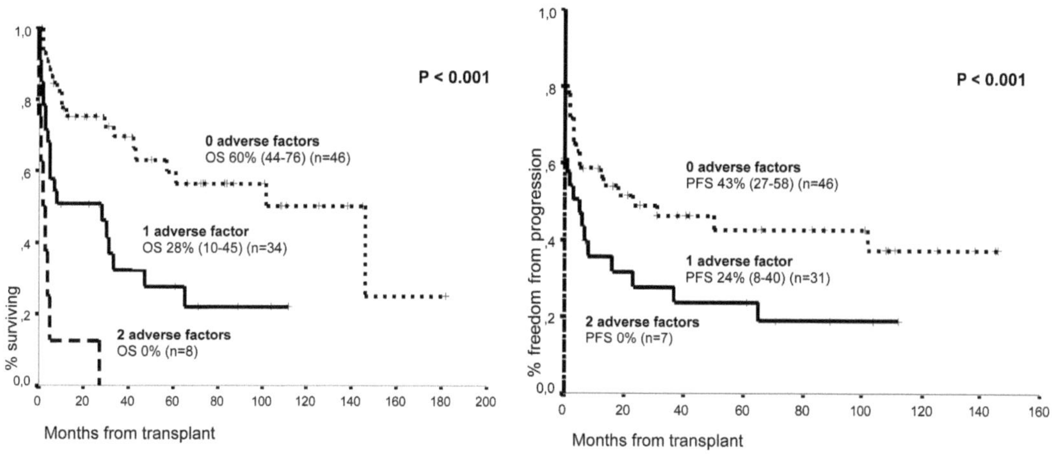

Fig. 13.1 Pretransplant value of a-IPI and beta-2-microglobulin for PTCL in the salvage setting; *OS* overall survival; *PFS* progression-free survival (Based on data from Rodríguez et al. [46])

four cycles and the experimental arm of CEOP/ECVBP (cyclophosphamide, epirubicin, vincristine, prednisone/epirubicin, cyclophosphamide, vindesine, bleomycin, and prednisone) followed by consolidation with BEAM and ASCT. Results of this and pooled analysis of the prior LNH-87 study lead to the GELA investigators to state that consolidation with transplant did not add benefit to standard therapy even in CR patients.

In summary, review of these retrospective studies demonstrates several points. First ASCT is relatively safe with a low mortality. Second, most studies are based on BEAM or BEAM-like conditioning regimens with only a few studies using total body irradiation (TBI) in the conditioning regimen. Third, only chemosensitive patients are likely to benefit from the transplant.

Prospective Studies

At present, five prospective studies testing the hypothesis that consolidation with transplant in patients in remission after induction therapy have been reported (Table 13.2). The first study reported by Reimer et al. [9] describes the outcome of 83 patients with nodal aggressive histological subtypes: PTCL-NOS, AIL, and ALCL (ALK$^-$). The treatment plan consisted of four initial courses of CHOP with two additional cycles allowed if no CR was obtained. Only chemosensitive patients advanced to ASCT. The conditioning regimen was based on myeloablative radiochemotherapy (fractionated TBI and high-dose cyclophosphamide).

Of the initial 83 patients, 55 (66%) were able to undergo the transplant. At the time of transplant, 73% of the patients were in CR and 27% were in PR. After the transplant 87% of the patients achieved a CR. The results in an intent to treat analysis showed that 58% of the population obtained a CR and 8% a PR. With a median observation time of 33 months, the estimated 3-year OS, DFS, and PFS were 48, 53, and 36%, respectively. Of note that the 3-year OS of the patients who were transplanted was 71%.

Corradini et al. [10] reported the outcome of 62 patients transplanted at a median follow-up of 76 months. The 5-year OS and PFS were 54 and 40% respectively. As suggested by the authors, only patients with ALCL (ALK$^+$), patients with an age-adjusted international prognostic index of 0–1, or patients in first CR obtained benefit from the procedure.

The GELTAMO group [11] reported their prospective trial of 26 patients who were treated with three cycles of MegaCHOP (2 g/m^2 CY, 90 mg/m^2 Doxorubicin 1.4 mg/m^2, Vincristine 60 mg/m^2, Prednisone and mesna). After these three cycles, patients were evaluated with computerized tomography and gallium scan. At that point, the patients that were in CR received one or two more cycles of MegaCHOP and were transplanted. However those patients in less than CR received

Table 13.2 Prospective series on the use of frontline ASCT in high-risk PTCL (Reprinted from Gutierrez et al. [45], with permission from Nature Publishing Group)

	Corradini et al.	Reimer et al.	D'Amore et al.	Rodríguez et al.	Mercadal et al.
n	62 (19 ALK+)	83 No ALK+	121 No ALK+	26 No ALK+	41 No ALK+
Median age (years)	43	46	55	44	47
Regimen	(1) 2×APO>2× DHAP>HD MTX/Mel (2) MACOP-B>HD AraC/Mito/Mel	4-6×CHOP+ DexaBEAM> HD Cy+TBI	6×CHOEP-14>BEAM	MegaCHOP/IFE>BEAM	3×MegaCHOP+3×E-SHAP BEAM or BEAC
ASCT (%)	74	66	73	77	41
CR/PR pretransplant (%/%)	56/16	47/26	50/35	61/16	49/10
TRM (%)	4.8	3	4	0	3
OS (%)	34 (12 years)	48 (3 years)	67 (3 years)	75 (3 years)	39 (4 years)
PFS (%)	30 (12 years)	36	NA	53	30(4 years)
Follow-up (months)	76	33	24	24 postransplant	47
Risk status of patients	PTCL AA stage II–IV	PTCL AA stage II–IV Excluding ALK+	PTCL AA stage II–IV Excluding ALK+	PTCL a-IPI 2 or 3 a-IPI 1 & B2M Excluding ALK+	PTCL AA stage II–IV Excluding ALK+

ALK anaplastic lymphoma kinase; *APO* vincristine, doxorubicin, and prednisone; *DHAP* cisplatin, cytarabine, dexamethasone; *HD* MTX/Mel high-dose methotrexate and melphalan; *MACOP-B* methotrexate, leucovorin, doxorubicin, cyclophosphamide, vincristine, bleomycin, prednisone; *HD AraC/Mito/Mel* high-dose cytarabine, mitoxantrone, melphalan; *DexaBEAM* dexamethasone, BCNU, etoposide, cytarabine, melphalan; *HD Cy + TBI* high-dose cyclophosphamide plus total body irradiation; *CHOEP-14* cyclophosphamide, vincristine, doxorubicin, etoposide, and prednisone; *BEAM BCNU*, etoposide, cytarabine, melphalan; *MegaCHOP* cyclophosphamide, vincristine, doxorubicin, etoposide, and dexamethasone; *IFE* iphosphamide, etoposide; *E-SHAP* etoposide, cisplatin, cytarabine, prednisone; *BEAC BCNU* etoposide, cytarabine, cyclophosphamide; *CR* complete response; *PR* partial response; *TRM* transplant-related mortality; *OS* overall survival; *PFS* progression-free survival; *AA* Ann Arbor; *a-IPI* adjusted-international prognostic index; □ elevated; B2M beta-2-microglobulin

3 cycles of the salvage regimen Ifosfamide and Etoposide and if in at least PR went to the transplant. With this strategy the OS and PFS at 3 years were 72 and 53% respectively. Interestingly still 23% of the patients did not receive the transplant, mainly due to early progression. In addition, there was no difference in outcome in early responders compared to the group that received the salvage regimen after not being in CR with the initial induction regimen.

The largest prospective study was reported by the Nordic Lymphoma Group [12]. With a median of 3 years of follow-up, they reported approximately 60% of transplanted patients were still alive. In this study the induction regimen was a dose-dense regimen of CHOEP-14.

Another study reported by Mercadal et al. [13] from the GELCAB Spanish group included 41 patients who were treated with chemotherapy and then transplant if in remission. Only 17 out of 41 patients (41%) underwent the planned transplant due to progression and toxicity. Interestingly, only 23% of the patients transplanted in chemosensitive remission relapsed vs. 57% of those patients who were chemosensitive but non-transplanted for various reasons. Similarly the 4-year PFS was 59% for the patients transplanted vs. 29% for the chemosensitive non-transplanted group. This study confirms the earlier retrospective data that only patients in chemosensitive are likely to benefit from consolidation with the autologous stem cell transplantation.

Although these results are encouraging, approximately 20–30% of the patients do not get to transplant for early progression or toxicity and another 20–30% of those in CR after the transplant relapse of their disease. Thus better induction regimens with new drugs and therapeutic maneuvers to maintain the remission posttransplant should be the focus of the next clinical research efforts.

In summary the existing data suggests that patients who do not benefit from the ASCT in the salvage setting are those who are chemorefractory pretransplant and/or those with an age adjusted IPI ≥2 and an elevated beta-2 microglobulin. These patients need new approaches including allogeneic stem cell transplantation procedures or innovative experimental treatments.

In addition, retrospective data suggest that only patients in low-risk groups of the PIT system and in remission after induction therapy seem to obtain benefit from the ASCT consolidation. Randomized studies are needed to confirm that consolidation with ASCT improves the outcome of these patients.

Stem Cell Transplant in Angioimmunoblastic T-Cell Lymphoma

Angioimmunoblastic T-cell lymphomas are a subset of aggressive T-cell lymphomas in which the data suggests that there may be a benefit for autologous transplantation in first remission. A retrospective multicenter study of 146 AITL patients has been reported by the European Bone Marrow Transplant group (EBMT) [14]. At a median follow-up of 31 months, they reported a 59% overall survival and a relapse rate of 51%. Interestingly the non-relapse mortality was 7% at 24 months. Disease status at transplantation was identified as the major factor associated with the outcome. Patients transplanted in CR had a PFS of 56% at 48 months vs. 30 and 23% respectively for those chemosensitive and chemorefractory disease patients.

These data highlight once again, the fact, that basically patients in CR prior to the transplant are the ones who benefit the most. However, 25% of refractory patients also had benefit. Autologous transplantation could be considered in selected refractory patients, and early transplantation might represent the best option for patients in CR.

Other smaller series by the GELTAMO (Grupo español de linfomas y trasplante autologo de médula ósea) reported similar outcomes.

In this study [11], 19 patients underwent a transplant in first remission (15 cases) and in the salvage setting (4 cases). After the transplant, 79% achieved a CR and at 3 years the PFS and OS were 55 and 60%, respectively. In this study, patients who were transplanted in a refractory disease status did not benefit from this procedure.

Thus, with the small experience available and without the robustness of a randomized study, it seems that consolidation with transplant in AITL patients chemosensitive prior to the transplant demonstrated benefit in both PFS and OS. However, longer follow-up and especially data from the ongoing randomized studies are needed to warrant this therapeutic modality as the new standard frontline therapy of these lymphomas.

Autologous Stem Cell Transplantation in Cutaneous Lymphomas

Patients with cutaneous T-cell lymphomas who have advanced disease with extensive nodal involvement, cutaneous tumors, or large cell transformation have a poor prognosis with an estimated median survival of 1–4 years. Current therapy based on systemic standard regimens for aggressive lymphomas yields usually responses that generally are short lived with a recurrent pattern of relapses. Therefore, intensification of treatment has been a logical step to take in these malignancies. However, there is a paucity of data concerning ASCT in these lymphomas. In fact, only case reports or small series with no more than ten patients have been reported. CTCL, subcutaneous panniculitis-like T-cell lymphoma, primary cutaneous gamma–delta T-cell lymphomas, and CD30-cutaneous large T-cell lymphoma report responses to high-dose therapy that are short lived with short progression-free survival rates [15–17]. In this setting, the experience with allogeneic HSCT is much more promising [18]. Consolidation with autologous stem cell transplantation is not considered a standard of care in these patients.

Autologous Transplantation in Extranodal NK/T-Cell Lymphoma

Treatment outcomes for NK/T-cell lymphoma vary according to disease stage and location. Overall, long-term survival is reported as 30–40% for patients with upper aerodigestive nasal locations and significantly lower for patients with widespread disease [19]. Due to these unfavorable results with standard chemo-radiotherapy regimens, ASCT has been tested in both: as consolidation of first remission or in the salvage setting.

Although the experience with consolidation with ASCT is small, there may be a trend toward improved survival when compared with historical controls. In a multinational, multicenter, controlled trial, Lee et al. [20] reported a significantly higher disease-specific survival in the ASCT group in patients who were in complete remission at the time of the procedure, 87% for the ASCT group vs. 68% for the standard treatment group ($P=0.02$). In contrast, the patients transplanted not in CR did not benefit from the procedure. Au et al. reported a similar finding in a series of 18 patients [21].

Thus, with the small experience available at present and without randomized studies to convince us the superiority of consolidation with ASCT, it seems that patients in first CR benefit from the procedure. For patients in refractory disease or in second remission in the salvage setting, the available results are generally poor; therefore, other options including allogeneic transplant procedures if feasible should be offered as would be discussed later in this chapter.

Prognostic Factors in the Transplant Setting

Several systems have been proposed for PTCL and NK/T-cell lymphoma. However the impact of these systems for patients treated with ASCT is not known. In one series, the PIT (prognostic index for PTCL) [22] as described by Gallamini et al., which system take into account, age, PS (ECOG, LDH, and bone marrow involvement as discrete covariates), predicted outcome in patients consolidated in first CR with ASCT better than the IPI [5]. In the salvage setting, the GELTAMO group proposed a new system based on two discrete variables: the IPI and the beta-2 microglobulin. In their series, patients who presented with both age-adjusted IPI higher than one and an elevated B2m had an inferior outcome with ASCT in the salvage setting. Clearly these patients need other therapeutic options including if feasible, allogeneic transplant [4].

Allogeneic Transplantation for PTCL and Cutaneous T-cell Lymphomas (CTCL)

Allogeneic stem cell transplantation (alloSCT) is an effective salvage treatment for some histotypes of relapsed non-Hodgkin lymphomas (NHL). Its peculiar efficacy is partly ascribed to the so-called *graft*-versus-*lymphoma* (GVL) *effect*, an immune mediated reaction operated by the transplanted immune system against the lymphoma cells. The existence of a GVL effect is mainly supported by three evidence: (1) tumor responses were observed after immune suppression withdrawal, (2) donor lymphocyte infusions (DLI) alone can cause tumor regression, (3) concomitant to the onset of acute graft-versus-host disease (GVHD) [23, 24] a lymphoma regression has been sometimes observed. Low grade NHLs have shown the most striking results, since alloSCT can provide a tumor-free graft and the indolent course of the disease allows the full exploitation of the GVL effect [25–27]. On the other hand, less data are available for aggressive histologies, and in particular for rare entities such as T-cell lymphomas [28–30].

In this chapter, the clinical results obtained in the most common subtypes of T-NHL, such as PTCL and primary CTCL, have been reported. In the largest prospective study published so far, 288 PTCL patients treated with different antracycline-containing regimens showed a 5-year overall survival (OS) and event-free survival (EFS) significantly worse compared with diffuse large B-cell lymphomas (DLBCL), with the exception of Alk-positive anaplastic T-cell lymphomas [31]. High-dose chemotherapy and autologous stem cell transplantation (autoSCT) in relapsed or newly diagnosed PTCL significantly changed the course of the disease in selected subsets of patients. Disease-free survival (DFS) and OS ranged between 35 and 45% respectively in most of the studies for relapsed patients [32, 33]. In a prospective study of high-dose chemotherapy as up-front therapy for PTCL, the outcome was improved only for patients with an age-adjusted international prognostic index (aaIPI) of 0–1, or in complete remission (CR) before transplantation or in case of Alk-positivity [10]. In general the main cause of treatment failure in autoSCT studies was disease progression before transplantation, suggesting that more intensive therapies and new drugs are needed to improve disease control [5, 10].

Similarly, in relapsed and advanced stage CTCL (Sezary syndrome (SS) and mycosis fungoides (MF)], there is no effective standard care and chemotherapy regimens usually induce transient responses that are not able to change the prognosis of these patients. The experience with autoSCT is very limited and not encouraging since most of the patients relapsed. The reinfusion of malignant cells with the graft and the failure of T-cell depletion procedures contributed to the poor results published so far [18]. The concept emerging from this brief introduction is that different mechanisms of tumor-killing are required to improve the outcome of Alk-negative PTCL and advanced CTCL.

Peripheral T-Cell Lymphomas

A retrospective analysis by Kim et al. on 233 relapsed lymphoma patients receiving a myeloablative alloSCT from a related or an unrelated donor showed a 2-year cumulative incidence of relapse of 21%, whereas the cumulative incidence of TRM was 40%. While they included a large number of aggressive lymphomas ($n=111$) in this study, there were 51 patients with PTCL. The 2-year OS for aggressive lymphomas was 42%, and patients with PTCL had a better survival than those affected by DLBCL, suggesting that T-cells can be a good target for donor-derived immune cells [34]. In this series, chemorefractory disease and a failed autoSCT were identified as adverse prognostic factors for both OS and TRM.

Le Gouill et al. have recently reported a retrospective review of allogeneic stem cell transplantation in 77 patients with PTCL (anaplastic large cell lymphoma (ALCL) ($n=27$), PTCL-unspecified ($n=27$), angioimmunoblastic T-cell lymphoma (AIL) ($n=11$), and rare subtypes ($n=12$)]. The majority of the patients (74%) received myeloablative conditioning and were allografted from HLA identical siblings (78%). This study included mainly patients with chemosensitive disease (70%). The results of this study were rather encouraging

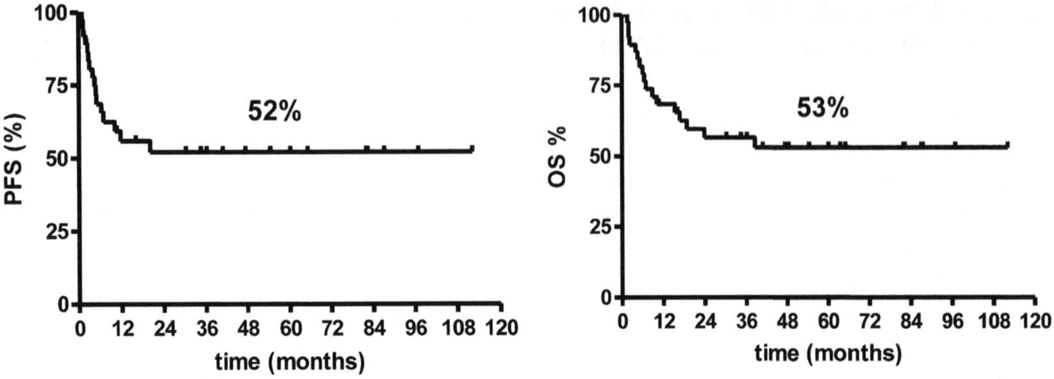

Fig. 13.2 Survival curves of relapsed patients affected by PTCL receiving RIC allogeneic stem cell transplantation; *PFS* progression-free survival; *OS* overall survival

with a 57 and 53% 5-year OS and EFS, respectively. In addition, they reported several interesting observations: (1) the OS was better in the nodal subtypes (55–80%) as compared to other histopathological subtypes (33%), (2) better OS and EFS were observed in patients receiving fewer prior therapies before alloSCT and/or with chemosensitive disease, (3) the authors observed an unexpected 5-year OS of 30 in patients with chemorefractory disease [35]. While survival was encouraging, but toxicity is still too high.

In order to decrease the toxicity and TRM of myeloablative alloSCT, reduced-intensity or nonmyeloablative conditioning (RIC) regimens have been developed from the beginning of 1990s. Unlike myeloablative conditioning which relies mainly upon high-dose chemotherapy and/or radiotherapy to eradicate the malignant cells, RIC regimens based their activity more on the GVL effect. Most of the studies performed to date have shown that RIC regimens are associated with a reduced TRM; therefore, this strategy can be offered to the elderly or heavily pretreated patients or patients affected by comorbidities [36].

A small pilot study first showed that RIC alloSCT is feasible and effective in relapsed PTCLs [37]. After a thiotepa–fludarabine–cyclophosphamide based regimen 17 patients received HLA-identical allogeneic stem cells. The 2-year TRM was 6%, supporting the feasibility of this strategy. Fourteen of seventeen enrolled patients were alive (12 in complete remission) after a median follow-up of 28 months with an estimated 3-year OS and progression-free survival (PFS) of 81 and 64%, respectively. Notably 15 of 17 patients were chemosensitive at transplant, and this can also explain the good clinical results (Fig. 13.2).

A recent update of that pilot study including 38 patients confirmed the original observations. Patients were transplanted at relapse, after a median of two lines of therapy (range, 1–4) and 54% of them had failed a previous autoSCT. Thirty-five percent of the patients were in CR at transplant, whereas 40% were in partial remission (PR). The lymphoma subtypes were distributed as follows: unspecified PTCL $n=15$, ALCL $n=9$ (Alk-negative=6, Alk-positive=3), angioimmunoblastic $n=6$, intestinal $n=3$, others $n=5$. At a median follow-up of 50 months, 21 of 38 patients were alive ($n=19$ in CR, $n=2$ with disease), 12 died of disease, and 5 died of TRM (Fig. 13.1). The median time to relapse was 140 days (range, 38–603). In 34 of 38 evaluable patients the incidence of acute and chronic GVHD was 47 and 42%, respectively. The PFS was influenced by histotype and disease status before transplant. In fact, 3-year PFS was 75% for both angioimmunoblastic and unspecified PTCL and 40% for ALCL and the other subtypes. Patients in CR, PR, or chemorefractory at transplant experienced a 3-year PFS of 66, 52, and 25%, respectively. Eight patients received DLI with or without chemotherapy for relapsed or persistent disease: three patients achieved a long-lasting CR (median follow-up of 65 months (range, 84–64)), one patient achieved PR, and the others showed progressive disease [38].

A recent phase II prospective trial on 194 patients undergoing an RIC alloSCT has further supported our previous observation that alloSCT may overcome the unfavorable prognostic impact of T-cell phenotype. In fact, at a median follow-up of 5 years, PFS and OS were not significantly different between patients with relapsed aggressive lymphoma of B- or T-cell origin (PFS: 63 vs. 57% at 5 years, $p=0.45$; OS: 67 vs. 55% at 5 years, $p=0.51$) [39].

A recent retrospective analysis of the European Blood and Marrow Transplantation group has been conducted in 45 patients affected by AIL: 25 transplants were myeloablative and 20 were based on reduced-intensity conditioning. In this cohort of patients, mainly with chemosensitive disease, the cumulative incidence of relapse was limited (20% at 3 years). The 3-year OS and PFS were 64 and 54%, respectively, with a plateau in the survival curve after the first year from the transplant [40]. The intensity of conditioning regimen did not have a significant impact on NRM, relapse risk, and overall survival (Table 13.3).

Although these results are encouraging, the disease progression before transplantation remains an unresolved issue affecting approximately 30% of the patients at diagnosis. In the attempt to identify an active salvage regimen, alemtuzumab has been associated with chemotherapy. After eight courses of CHOP-Campath, 17 out of 24 patients achieved CR (71%), and 13 of them had a median duration of 11 months [41]. Wulf et al. demonstrated that alemtuzumab, associated or not to chemotherapy, was able to induce lymphoma remission before alloSCT in six of ten patients with advanced PTCL [42]. Although the follow-up was very short (only 7 months), six of these patients remained in remission after allografting.

Cutaneous T-Cell Lymphomas

The first experience of alloSCT in patients affected by CTCL was restricted to ten young patients receiving myeloablative conditioning regimens [18]. Four of ten patients relapsed after alloSCT, but responded to the withdrawal of immunosuppressive medication and/or donor lymphocytes infusions suggesting the existence of "graft-versus-CTCL effect."

CTCL typically affects the elderly (median age at diagnosis 60 years); therefore RIC regimens have been explored also in this setting. Molina et al. conducted a retrospective study, including eight patients heavily pretreated ($n=5$ SS, $n=3$ MF). Half of them received an RIC regimen consisting of fludarabine and melphalan, and four of eight were allografted from unrelated donors [43]. All the patients achieved a clinical remission, but two of them died of TRM. Interestingly, before alloSCT, six patients showed clonal T-cell receptor γ-chain gene rearrangements (TCRγ R) in peripheral blood or bone marrow, that resulted negative in the posttransplant PCR studies. Patients affected by MF with cytogenetic abnormalities usually have a very poor outcome. In this study, all the patients with such abnormalities achieved a cytogenetic remission.

Onida et al. reported the outcome of 15 patients with advanced CTCL ($n=9$ MF, $n=6$ SS), refractory to a median of three previous lines of treatment. At median follow-up of 41 months, the results were encouraging with an estimated 5-year PFS of 60% [44] (Table 13.4).

The optimal conditioning regimen and the better timing for alloSCT are currently unknown, but these preliminary results are interesting and should stimulate novel collaborative efforts for prospective trials.

In summary, RIC alloSCT (a) was able to decrease significantly TRM, thus elderly and/or heavily pretreated patients can become eligible for alloSCT; (b) can produce clinical results supporting the existence of a "graft-versus-T-cell lymphoma" effect; (c) an up-front strategy with RIC alloSCT can be considered in patients below 65 years of age in the context of controlled prospective trials.

The challenge still remains for the 30% of patients who progress despite any treatment at diagnosis, and for them we need novel agents to induce a remission state before any transplant procedure. For those responding and then relapsing, thus showing a story of chemosensitive disease, alloSCT might be a reasonable option up to 65 years of age.

In conclusion, with the available information concerning these two stem cell transplantation procedures, we propose a working treatment algorithm for PTCL excluding anaplastic large T-cell lymphomas ALK^{+} cases that is depicted in Fig. 13.3.

Table 13.3 Allogeneic stem cell transplantation in relapsed PTCL

Author	No. Pts	Chemosensitive disease (%) before alloSCT	Type of conditioning regimen	NRM (%)	PFS (%)	OS (%)
Kim et al. [34]	58	–	Myeloablative (100%)	42[b] (2 years)	–	70 (2 years) PTCL-unspec.
	PTCL-unspec. ($n = 22$)					30 (2 years) NK/T-cell
	Others ($n = 36$)					
Corradini et al. [37]	17	10 (60%)	RIC (100%)	6 (1 year)	64 (3 years)	81 (3 years)
	PTCL-unspec. ($n = 8$)					
	Others ($n = 9$)					
Corradini et al. [39][a]	28	22 (79%)	RIC (100%)	15[b] (1 year)	57 (5 years)	55 (5 years)
Le Gouill et al. [35]	77	54 (70%)	Myeloablative (74%)	34 (5 years)	53 (5 years)[c]	57 (5 years)
	PTCL-unspec. ($n = 27$)		RIC (26%)			
	ALCL ($n = 27$)					
	AITL ($n = 11$)					
	Others ($n = 12$)					
Kyriakou et al. [40]	45	27 (60%)	Myeloablative (56%)	25 (1 year)	54 (3 years)	64 (3 years)
	All AITL		RIC (44%)			

Pts patients; *alloSCT* allogeneic stem cell transplantation; *NRM* non-relapse mortality; *PFS* progression-free survival; *OS* overall survival; *PTCL-unspec.* peripheral T-cell lymphomas unspecified; *ALCL* anaplastic large cell lymphoma; *AITL* angioimmunoblastic T-cell lymphomas; *RIC* reduced-intensity conditioning

[a]Abstract report

[b]The value was the NRM for all lymphomas not only PTCL

[c]The value reported is the event-free survival

Table 13.4 Allogeneic stem cell transplantation in relapsed CTCL

Authors	No. Pts	Chemosensitive disease before allo-SCT	Type of conditioning regimen	NRM (%)	PFS (%)	OS (%)
Molina et al. [43]	8 4 SS 4 MF	All refractory	Myeloablative (50%) RIC (50%)	25[b] (4 years)	–	75[b] (4 years)
Onida et al. [44]	15 6 SS 9 MF	All refractory	RIC (100 %)	20[b] (3 years)	60 (3 years)	–

Pts patients; *alloSCT* allogeneic stem cell transplantation; *NRM* non-relapse mortality; *PFS* progression-free survival; *OS* overall survival, SS Sezary Syndrome, MF Mycosis Fungoides, RIC reduced-intensity conditioning
[a]Abstract report
[b]The value was given as frequency

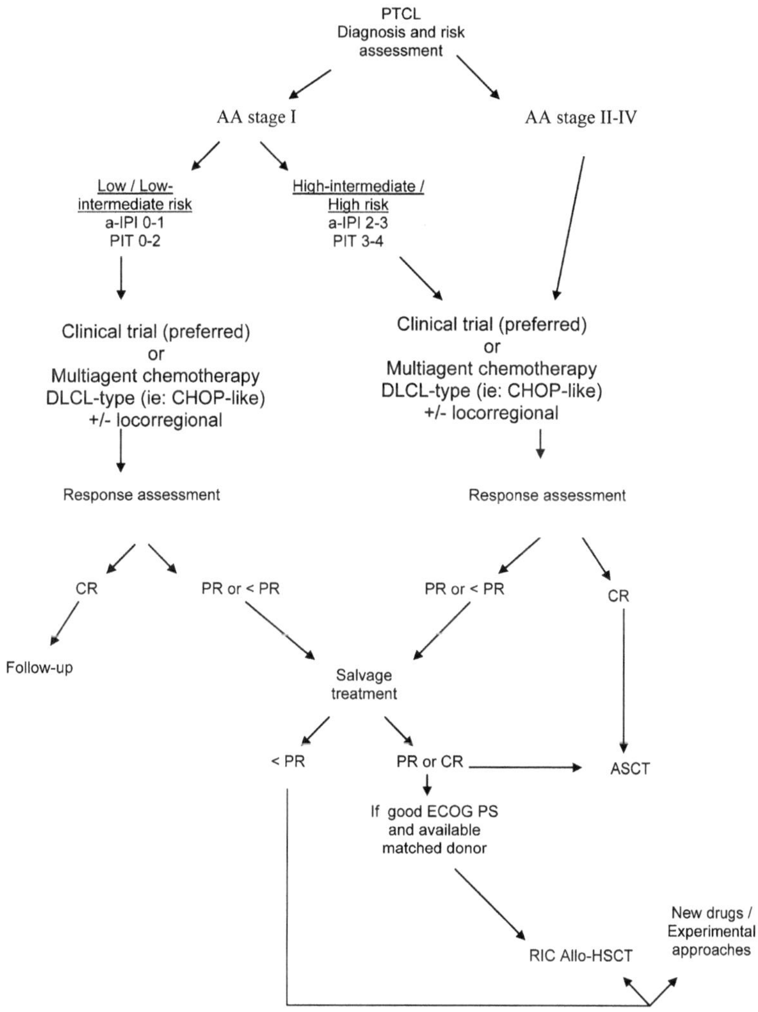

Fig. 13.3 Proposed treatment algorithm for PTCL (excluding ALK+cases). *PTCL* peripheral T-cell lymphoma; *AA* Ann Arbor; *a-IPI* adjusted International Prognostic Index; *PIT* prognostic index for peripheral T-cell lymphoma;, *DLCL* diffuse large-cell lymphoma; *CR* complete response; PR partial response; *ASCT* autologous stem cell transplantation; *ECOG* PS Eastern Cooperative Oncology Group Performance Status; *RIC* reduced-intensity conditioning; *Alo-HSCT* allogeneic hematopoietic stem cell transplantation

Since, these groups of lymphomas are currently a very active area of research, new upcoming information might modify this therapeutic proposal.

References

1. Swerdlow SH, Campo E, Harris NL, Jaffe ES, Pileri S, Stein H, et al. WHO classification of tumours of haematopoietic and lymphoid tissues. Lyon, France: IARC press; 2008.
2. Armitage JO, Vose JM, Weisenburger DD. Towards understanding the peripheral T-cell lymphomas. Ann Oncol. 2004;15(10):1447–9.
3. Philip T, Armitage JO, Spitzer G, Chauvin F, Jagannath S, Cahn JY, et al. High-dose therapy and autologous bone marrow transplantation after failure of conventional chemotherapy in adults with intermediate-grade or high-grade non-Hodgkin's lymphoma. N Engl J Med. 1987;316(24):1493–8.
4. Rodriguez J, Conde E, Gutierrez A, Lahuerta JJ, Arranz R, Sureda A, et al. The adjusted International Prognostic Index and beta-2-microglobulin predict the outcome after autologous stem cell transplantation in relapsing/refractory peripheral T-cell lymphoma. Haematologica. 2007;92(8):1067–74.
5. Rodriguez J, Conde E, Gutierrez A, Arranz R, Leon A, Marin J, et al. The results of consolidation with autologous stem-cell transplantation in patients with peripheral T-cell lymphoma (PTCL) in first complete remission: the Spanish Lymphoma and Autologous Transplantation Group experience. Ann Oncol. 2007;18(4):652–7.
6. Feyler S, Prince HM, Pearce R, Towlson K, Nivison-Smith I, Schey S, et al. The role of high-dose therapy and stem cell rescue in the management of T-cell malignant lymphomas: a BSBMT and ABMTRR study. Bone Marrow Transplant. 2007;40(5):443–50.
7. Jantunen E, Wiklund T, Juvonen E, Putkonen M, Lehtinen T, Kuittinen O, et al. Autologous stem cell transplantation in adult patients with peripheral T-cell lymphoma: a nation-wide survey. Bone Marrow Transplant. 2004;33(4):405–10.
8. Gisselbrecht C, Lepage E, Molina T, Quesnel B, Fillet G, Lederlin P, et al. Shortened first-line high-dose chemotherapy for patients with poor-prognosis aggressive lymphoma. J Clin Oncol. 2002;20(10):2472–9.
9. Reimer P, Rudiger T, Geissinger E, Weissinger F, Nerl C, Schmitz N, et al. Autologous stem-cell transplantation as first-line therapy in peripheral T-cell lymphomas: results of a prospective multicenter study. J Clin Oncol. 2009;27(1):106–13.
10. Corradini P, Tarella C, Zallio F, Dodero A, Zanni M, Valagussa P, et al. Long-term follow-up of patients with peripheral T-cell lymphomas treated up-front with high-dose chemotherapy followed by autologous stem cell transplantation. Leukemia. 2006;20(9):1533–8.
11. Rodriguez J, Conde E, Gutierrez A, Arranz R, Leon A, Marin J, et al. Frontline autologous stem cell transplantation in high-risk peripheral T-cell lymphoma: a prospective study from The Gel-Tamo Study Group. Eur J Haematol. 2007;79:32–8.
12. d'Amore F, Relander T, Lauritzsen G, Jantunen E, Hagberg H, Anderson H, et al. Dose-dense induction followed by autologous stem cell transplant (ASCT) as 1st Line treatment in peripheral T-cell lymphomas (PTCL)—a phase II study of the Nordic lymphoma group (NLG). Blood. 2006;108:401a.
13. Mercadal S, Briones J, Xicoy B, Pedro C, Escoda L, Estany C, et al. Intensive chemotherapy (high-dose CHOP/ESHAP regimen) followed by autologous stem-cell transplantation in previously untreated patients with peripheral T-cell lymphoma. Ann Oncol. 2008;19:958–63.
14. Kyriakou C, Canals C, Goldstone A, Caballero D, Metzner B, Kobbe G, et al. High-dose therapy and autologous stem-cell transplantation in angioimmunoblastic lymphoma: complete remission at transplantation is the major determinant of Outcome-Lymphoma Working Party of the European Group for Blood and Marrow Transplantation. J Clin Oncol. 2008;26(2):218–24.
15. Hashimoto H, Sawada K, Koizumi K, Nishio M, Endo T, Takashima T, et al. Effective CD34+ selected autologous peripheral blood stem cell transplantation in a patient with subcutaneous panniculitic T cell lymphoma (SPTCL) transformed into leukemia. Bone Marrow Transplant. 1999;24(12):1369–71.
16. Nishio M, Koizumi K, Endo T, Takashima H, Haseyama Y, Fujimoto K, et al. Effective high-dose chemotherapy combined with CD34+-selected autologous peripheral blood stem cell transplantation in a patient with cutaneous CD30-negative large T cell lymphoma. Bone Marrow Transplant. 2000;25(12):1315–7.
17. Koizumi K, Sawada K, Nishio M, Katagiri E, Fukae J, Fukada Y, et al. Effective high-dose chemotherapy followed by autologous peripheral blood stem cell transplantation in a patient with the aggressive form of cytophagic histiocytic panniculitis. Bone Marrow Transplant. 1997;20(2):171–3.
18. Duarte RF, Schmitz N, Servitje O, Sureda A. Haematopoietic stem cell transplantation for patients with primary cutaneous T-cell lymphoma. Bone Marrow Transplant. 2008;41(7):597–604.
19. Chim CS, Ma SY, Au WY, Choy C, Lie AK, Liang R, et al. Primary nasal natural killer cell lymphoma: long-term treatment outcome and relationship with the International Prognostic Index. Blood. 2004;103(1):216–21.
20. Lee J, Au WY, Park MJ, Suzumiya J, Nakamura S, Kameoka J, et al. Autologous hematopoietic stem cell transplantation in extranodal natural killer/T cell lymphoma: a multinational, multicenter, matched controlled study. Biol Blood Marrow Transplant. 2008;14(12):1356–64.
21. Au WY, Lie AK, Liang R, Kwong YL, Yau CC, Cheung MM, et al. Autologous stem cell transplantation for

nasal NK/T-cell lymphoma: a progress report on its value. Ann Oncol. 2003;14(11):1673–6.
22. Gallamini A, Stelitano C, Calvi R, Bellei M, Mattei D, Vitolo U, et al. Peripheral T-cell lymphoma unspecified (PTCL-U): a new prognostic model from a retrospective multicentric clinical study. Blood. 2004;103(7):2474–9.
23. van Besien KW, de Lima M, Giralt SA, Moore Jr DF, Khouri IF, Rondon G, et al. Management of lymphoma recurrence after allogeneic transplantation: the relevance of graft-versus-lymphoma effect. Bone Marrow Transplant. 1997;19(10):977–82.
24. Mandigers CM, Verdonck LF, Meijerink JP, Dekker AW, Schattenberg AV, Raemaekers JM. Graft-versus-lymphoma effect of donor lymphocyte infusion in indolent lymphomas relapsed after allogeneic stem cell transplantation. Bone Marrow Transplant. 2003;32(12):1159–63.
25. Hosing C, Saliba RM, McLaughlin P, Andersson B, Rodriguez MA, Fayad L, et al. Long-term results favor allogeneic over autologous hematopoietic stem cell transplantation in patients with refractory or recurrent indolent non-Hodgkin's lymphoma. Ann Oncol. 2003;14(5):737–44.
26. Khouri IF, Saliba RM, Giralt SA, Lee MS, Okoroji GJ, Hagemeister FB, et al. Nonablative allogeneic hematopoietic transplantation as adoptive immunotherapy for indolent lymphoma: low incidence of toxicity, acute graft-versus-host disease, and treatment-related mortality. Blood. 2001;98(13):3595–9.
27. Corradini P, Dodero A, Farina L, Fanin R, Patriarca F, Miceli R, et al. Allogeneic stem cell transplantation following reduced-intensity conditioning can induce durable clinical and molecular remissions in relapsed lymphomas: pre-transplant disease status and histotype heavily influence outcome. Leukemia. 2007; 21(11):2316–23.
28. Mollee P, Lazarus HM, Lipton J. Why aren't we performing more allografts for aggressive non-Hodgkin's lymphoma? Bone Marrow Transplant. 2003; 31(11):953–60.
29. Dhedin N, Giraudier S, Gaulard P, Esperou H, Ifrah N, Michallet M, et al. Allogeneic bone marrow transplantation in aggressive non-Hodgkin's lymphoma (excluding Burkitt and lymphoblastic lymphoma): a series of 73 patients from the SFGM database. Societ Francaise de Greffe de Moelle. Br J Haematol. 1999;107(1):154–61.
30. Doocey RT, Toze CL, Connors JM, Nevill TJ, Gascoyne RD, Barnett MJ, et al. Allogeneic haematopoietic stem-cell transplantation for relapsed and refractory aggressive histology non-Hodgkin lymphoma. Br J Haematol. 2005;131(2):223–30.
31. Gisselbrecht C, Gaulard P, Lepage E, Coiffier B, Briere J, Haioun C, et al. Prognostic significance of T-cell phenotype in aggressive non-Hodgkin's lymphomas. Groupe d'Etudes des Lymphomes de l'Adulte (GELA). Blood. 1998;92(1):76–82.
32. Rodriguez J, Caballero MD, Gutierrez A, Marin J, Lahuerta JJ, Sureda A, et al. High-dose chemotherapy and autologous stem cell transplantation in peripheral T-cell lymphoma: the GEL-TAMO experience. Ann Oncol. 2003;14(12):1768–75.
33. Song KW, Mollee P, Keating A, Crump M. Autologous stem cell transplant for relapsed and refractory peripheral T-cell lymphoma: variable outcome according to pathological subtype. Br J Haematol. 2003; 120(6):978–85.
34. Kim SW, Tanimoto TE, Hirabayashi N, Goto S, Kami M, Yoshioka S, et al. Myeloablative allogeneic hematopoietic stem cell transplantation for non-Hodgkin lymphoma: a nationwide survey in Japan. Blood. 2006;108(1):382–9.
35. Le Gouill S, Milpied N, Buzyn A, De Latour RP, Vernant JP, Mohty M, et al. Graft-versus-lymphoma effect for aggressive T-cell lymphomas in adults: a study by the Societe Francaise de Greffe de Moelle et de Therapie Cellulaire. J Clin Oncol. 2008; 26(14):2264–71.
36. Barrett AJ, Savani BN. Stem cell transplantation with reduced-intensity conditioning regimens: a review of ten years experience with new transplant concepts and new therapeutic agents. Leukemia. 2006;20(10):1661–72.
37. Corradini P, Dodero A, Zallio F, Caracciolo D, Casini M, Bregni M, et al. Graft-versus-lymphoma effect in relapsed peripheral T-cell non-Hodgkin's lymphomas after reduced-intensity conditioning followed by allogeneic transplantation of hematopoietic cells. J Clin Oncol. 2004;22(11):2172–6.
38. Corradini P, Dodero A, Lambertenghi-Deliliers G, Onida F. Allogeneic transplantation for peripheral and cutaneous T-cell lymphomas. Hematol Meet Rep. 2009;3:139–40.
39. Corradini P, Dodero A, Farina L, Fanin R, Patriarca F, Miceli R, et al. Allogeneic stem cell transplantation following a reduced-intensity conditioning in relapsed lymphomas: 5-year follow-up of a phase II study of the Gruppo Italiano Trapianto di Midollo Osseo (GITMO). Bone Marrow Transplant. 2009;43:S64.
40. Kyriakou C, Canals C, Finke J, Kobbe G, Harousseau JL, Kolb HJ, et al. Allogeneic stem cell transplantation is able to induce long-term remissions in angioimmunoblastic T-cell lymphoma: a retrospective study from the lymphoma working party of the European group for blood and marrow transplantation. J Clin Oncol. 2009;27(24):3951–8.
41. Gallamini A, Zaja F, Patti C, Billio A, Specchia MR, Tucci A, et al. Alemtuzumab (Campath-1H) and CHOP chemotherapy as first-line treatment of peripheral T-cell lymphoma: results of a GITIL (Gruppo Italiano Terapie Innovative nei Linfomi) prospective multicenter trial. Blood. 2007;110(7):2316–23.
42. Wulf GG, Hasenkamp J, Jung W, Chapuy B, Truemper L, Glass B. Reduced intensity conditioning and allogeneic stem cell transplantation after salvage therapy integrating alemtuzumab for patients with relapsed peripheral T-cell non-Hodgkin's lymphoma. Bone Marrow Transplant. 2005;36(3):271–3.
43. Molina A, Zain J, Arber DA, Angelopolou M, O'Donnell M, Murata-Collins J, et al. Durable clinical,

cytogenetic, and molecular remissions after allogeneic hematopoietic cell transplantation for refractory Sezary syndrome and mycosis fungoides. J Clin Oncol. 2005;23(25):6163–71.
44. Onida F, Saporiti G, Berti E, DellaVolpe A, Annaloro C, Usardi P, et al. Reduced-intensity conditioning allogeneic haematopoietic stem cell transplantation in advanced mycosis fungoides and Sezary syndrome. Bone Marrow Transplant. 2007;39:S40.
45. Gutierrez A, Caballero MD, Perez-Manga G, et al. Hematopoietic SCT for peripheral T-cell lymphoma. Bone Marrow Transplant. 2008;42(12):773–81.
46. Rodríguez J, Conde E, Gutiérrez A, et al. The adjusted International Prognostic Index and β-2-microglobulin predict the outcome after autologous stem cell transplantation in relapsing/refractory peripheral T-cell lymphoma. Hematologica. 2007; 92(8):1067–74.
47. Rodriguez J, Munsell M, Yazji S, Hagemeister FB, Younes A, Andersson B, Giralt S, Gajewski J, de Lima M, Couriel D, Romaguera J, Cabanillas FF, Champlin RE, Khouri IF. Impact of high dose chemotherapy in Peripherals T cell lymphoma. J Clin Oncol. 2001;19(17):3766–70.
48. Blystad AK, Enblad G, Kvaløy S, Berglund A, Delabie J, Holte H, Carlson K, Kvalheim G, Bengtsson M, Hagberg H. High-dose therapy with autologous stem cell transplantation in patients with peripheral T cell lymphomas. Bone Marrow Transplant 2001;27(7): 711–6.
49. Kewalramani T, Zelenetz AD, Teruya-Feldstein J, Hamlin P, Yahalom J, Horwitz S, Nimer SD, Moskowitz CH. Autologous transplantation for relapsed or primary refractory peripheral T cell lymphoma. Br J Haematol. 2006;134(2):202–7. Epub 2006 Jun 6.
50. Smith SD, Bolwell BJ, Rybicki LA, Brown S, Dean R, Kalaycio M, Sobecks R, Andresen S, Hsi ED, Pohlman B, Sweetenham JW. Autologous hematopoietic stem cell transplantation in peripheral T-cell lymphoma using a uniform high-dose regimen. Bone Marrow transplant 2007; 40(3):239–43.

Monoclonal Antibodies (mAb) in the Therapy of T-Cell Lymphomas

14

Lapo Alinari, Pierluigi Porcu, and Bertrand Coiffier

Introduction

Although the use of antibodies as tumor-targeting agents dates back to 1953 when Pressman and Korngold [1] showed that radiolabeled rabbit antisera could specifically target mouse osteogenic sarcoma cells, not until 1975, with the development of the hybridoma technology [2], adequate quantities of murine monoclonal antibodies (mAbs) became available for clinical use. These early trials demonstrated that murine mAbs had some measure of antitumor activity in hematological malignancies but also highlighted the limiting effect of the human-anti-mouse humoral immune responses on multiple mAb administrations. Despite the simplicity of the concept (antibody–antigen interaction), researchers had to confront a number of technical difficulties, including the selection of a proper and stable target, efficient delivery, and immunogenicity due to the murine components of the mAbs [3].

L. Alinari (✉)
Department of Internal Medicine, The Ohio State University, 395 West 12th Avenue, 3rd floor, Columbus, OH 43210, USA
e-mail: lapo.alinari@osumc.edu

P. Porcu
Department of Hematology, The Ohio State University, Columbus, OH, USA

B. Coiffier
Department of Hematology, Hospices Civils de Lyon and Université Claude Bernard, Lyon, France

In 1997 the anti-CD20 antibody rituximab became the first recombinant chimeric mAb approved by the US Food and Drug Administration (FDA) for use in the treatment of cancer, demonstrating very limited immunogenicity and leading to the explosion of the field on mAb-based therapeutics. The methodology for the manufacturing of mAbs for clinical use has evolved substantially over the past 15 years, allowing the creation of "designer" antibody biopharmaceuticals that have fully human sequence and combine the desired antigen-binding specificity with unique biodistribution and pharmacodynamic properties. The nomenclature of mAb reflects this diversity. While the suffix *mab* defines the product as a monoclonal antibody, the letter or syllable in front of the *mab* reveals the antibody's source as murine (*-omab*), chimeric (*-ximab*), humanized (*-zumab*), or fully human (*-umab*) [4]. Thus edrocolomab is a murine anti-EpCAM antibody, galiximab is a chimeric anti-CD80 antibody, alemtuzumab is a humanized anti-CD52 antibody, and ofatumumab is a fully human anti-CD20 antibody.

One of the key goals in the clinical development of mAbs for clinical use is the identification of specific surface antigens—defined according to standardized nomenclature as clusters of differentiation (CD)—whose expression is ideally restricted to the malignant cells. Unfortunately, such degree of specificity is rarely achieved and many clinically relevant antigens represent essential components of vital activation, survival, and trafficking pathways for both malignant and

F. Foss (ed.), *T-Cell Lymphomas*, Contemporary Hematology, DOI 10.1007/978-1-62703-170-7_14, © Springer Science+Business Media New York 2013

normal cells. Therefore, the fact that cell surface antigens expressed on lymphoma cells are virtually always present on their normal counterparts continues to represent a significant limit for the clinical application of these agents. mAbs induce tumor cell death by blocking survival pathways (direct apoptosis) along with other immunologic mechanisms such as antibody-dependent cellular cytotoxicity (ADCC) and complement-dependent cytotoxicity (CDC). mAbs have been used as single agent therapy or, in the attempt to enhance their ability to destroy tumor cells, in combination with chemotherapy, other antibodies or conjugated either to radioisotopes or to immunotoxins. Based on the activity in hematologic malignancies and their safety profile, mAbs are now among the most frequently used biopharmaceutical agents.

The development of mAbs for the treatment of T-cell lymphomas (TCLs) is rooted in the early functional characterization of the T-cell receptor and other surface antigens in human T-cells [3–6], and in subsequent studies aimed at the discovery of novel immune suppressive drug for use in human transplantation. The first mAb approved for clinical use was the anti-CD3 murine antibody OKT3 (muromonab), approved in 1986 for the prevention of kidney transplant rejection. Clinical experience with OKT3 showed that the drug was potently immune suppressive, achieving the desired effect against organ rejection, but also revealed a significantly higher risk of development of post-transplant lymphoproliferative disorder (PTLD), compared to conventional antirejection drugs such as antimetabolites and calcineurin inhibitors. The progressive discovery and characterization of surface markers such as CD2, CD4, CD5, CD6, CD25, CD30, and CD52 that are expressed on various functional subsets of T-cells, led to the development of corresponding murine or chimeric mAbs for clinical use. Although early investigations of these mAbs were focused on prevention of graft versus host disease (GVHD) and solid organ allograft rejection, as well as the treatment of severe autoimmune diseases, pilot studies in select subtypes of TCL we also conducted, with encouraging results. Both early and later studies of mAb-based therapy in TCL, however, have so far failed to achieve the efficacy, flexibility of use in combination, and safety profile of rituximab. Most of the anti-T-cell mAbs in clinical development or approved for TCL interfere with T-cell activation and trafficking and result in severe and prolonged T-cell depletion. Many have been associated with reactivation of latent herperviruses, such as Epstein-Barr virus (EBV) and cytomegalovirus (CMV), and a broad spectrum of bacterial and fungal opportunistic infections. Thus, in the absence of truly tumor-specific markers, the difficulty of balancing an efficient kill of malignant T-cells with an adequate preservation of normal cell-mediated immunity remains the most challenging obstacle to the development of active and safe mAbs for the treatment of TCL. Presently a number of mAbs targeting T-cell surface antigens are being evaluated in clinical trials (Table 14.1) and the purpose of this chapter is to summarize the present and potentials roles for mAbs in the treatment of TCL.

CD2 Antigen

CD2 is an approximately 50 KD transmembrane glycoprotein expressed on dendritic cells, natural killer (NK) cells, thymocytes, and mature T-cells [6–9] with much higher expression on activated T-cells than on resting T-cells [10]. Although the specificity for T-cell activation resides in the TCR/CD3 complex, the interaction of additional accessory molecules such as CD2, CD28, and lymphocyte functional antigen-1 (LFA-1) with ligands on the antigen presenting cells (APCs), is required for complete T-cell activation to occur [11]. CD2 acts as an adhesion molecule [12] through its extracellular region which has two Ig superfamily domains, the first one binds CD58 (LFA-3) [13] and the second one binds CD59 [14], helping to localize the T-cells in proximity of APCs [11, 15–17]. CD2 acts also as a signaling molecule through its large intra-cytoplasmatic domain: as a result of CD2–CD58 interaction, the CD2 intra-cytoplasmatic domain physically associates with the Wiskott-Aldrich syndrome protein [18] and the tyrosine kinase

Table 14.1 mAbs therapy for T-cell leukemia and lymphoma

Target	Description	Targeting agent	References
CD2	LFA-3 (CD58) receptor	Alefacept (Amevive) Siplizumab (MEDI-507)	[24–30, 171, 172]
CD3	Signaling chain (CD3ζ) of the T-cell receptor (TCR)	Muromonab-CD3 (Orthoclone, OKT3)	[34–39, 173]
CD4	TCR co-receptor Anti-Leu3a M-T412	Zanolimumab (HuMax-CD4)	[43, 47–49]
CD5	Scavenger receptor family member	Anti-Leu1 T101 Anti-CD5-ricin A (CD5-Plus)	[4, 174]
CD25	IL-2 receptor α-subunit	Murine anti-Tac Daclizumab (Zenapax) Denileukin diftitox (Ontak)	[57, 63, 69, 72–76, 175]
CD122	IL-2 and IL-15 receptor β-subunit	Murine and humanized Mik-β1	[81]
CD30	TNF receptor family member	Ber-H2 Hefi-1 M67 MDX-060 SGN-30 SGN-35	[103–105, 119–122]
CD52	GPI-anchored glycoprotein	Alemtuzumab (Campath)	[124]

$p56^{lck}$ [19, 20] resulting in the initiation of the phospholipase C pathway [21, 22], in actin polymerization with further strengthening of intercellular adhesion, in the production of IL-2 and, ultimately, into T-cell activation and proliferation [23].

CD2-Targeted Therapy

The limited expression of CD2 restricted to mature T-cells, the expression of CD2 on malignant T-cells, combined with preliminary data showing that engagement of CD2 by mAbs can directly trigger apoptosis [24], provided the scientific rationale for their use in immunotherapy for TCL. A number of mAbs directed against CD2 have demonstrated the ability to inhibit T-cell activation. In particular, the rat mAb BTI-322 (MedImmune, Inc.) has been used in the prevention of allograft rejection [25] and in the therapy of GVHD [26]. Given the immunosuppressive properties of BTI-322, a humanized genetically engineered version of this molecule was developed for clinical application (Siplizumab, BioTransplant, Inc.). Siplizumab (MEDI-507) is a humanized IgG1κ monoclonal antibody initially studied in murine models of adult T-cell leukemia (ATL) [27]: severe combined immune deficiency (SCID) mice engrafted with human HTLV-1 positive T-cell leukemia cells treated with MEDI-507 survived significantly longer when compared either with mice treated with a humanized mAb direct toward CD25 or with phosphate-buffered saline (PBS) (control group). Based on this preclinical data and on the data obtained with its use in the prevention in the therapy of transplant rejection and autoimmune disease [28], phase I trials were conducted in patients with $CD2^+$ lymphomas/leukemias [29, 30]. In the 2006 report, 16 patients diagnosed with peripheral T-cell lymphoma (PTCL) ($n=9$), cutaneous T-cell lymphoma (CTCL) ($n=6$), and natural killer (NK)-large granular lymphocytic (NK-LGL) leukemia ($n=1$) were treated with biweekly infusion of escalating doses of intravenous (IV) siplizumab (range 0.7–4.8 mg/kg). Two responses were observed, one partial response (PR) in the NK-LGL patient and one complete response (CR) in a PTCL patient, both treated at 3.4 mg/kg. Dose-limiting toxicities (DLT) included one case of erythematous confluent dermatitis and one case of pulmonary edema, no maximum tolerated dose (MTD) was established. In the 2009 report, 29 patients with T-cell malignancies received escalating doses of IV siplizumab (range 0.2–4.8 mg/kg), either with a weekly schedule or biweekly schedule. Although the initial responses were encouraging, 4 patients (13.7%) (3 of 7 patients treated with the weekly schedule and 1 of 22 treated with biweekly schedule) developed an EBV-lymphoproliferative disease (LPD) and the trial was stopped. The weekly administration of siplizumab decreased the CD2 expressing cells to a greater extent than the biweekly schedule highlighting the importance of NK/T cells depletion in conjunction with no effect on the B cell compartment in the pathogenesis of EBV-LPD.

CD3 Antigen

The TCR heterodimer is associated with the polypeptide dimers of the CD3 complex which comprises five invariant polypeptide chains: γ, δ, ε, ζ, and η [31]. The CD3 complex stabilizes the TCR and participates in signal transduction through its extracellular (γ, δ, ε), transmembrane and intra-cytoplasmatic domain [32, 33]. Engagement of the TCR by antigen or mAbs anti-CD3 induces phosphorylation of CD3 γ, δ, ε, and ζ chains and internalization of the TCR. The outcome of these interactions, including activation and apoptosis, is influenced by the dynamic interactions between TCR and peptide-MHC complexes and, specifically, depends on slight differences in terms of affinity and dissociation rates of the antigen/TCR complex.

CD3-Targeted Therapy

The clinical utility of the first generation of mAbs specific for CD3 (such as muromonab-CD3, also called Orthoclone OKT3, Ortho Biotech, Inc.) has been limited by several drawbacks related to their composition. The first was the induction of neutralizing anti-mouse Ab response which reduces the re-treatment efficacy [34–36]. The second is a syndrome of adverse events which includes flu-like symptoms, respiratory distress, hypotension, and hypoglycemia [36]. This first generation of mAbs can induce T-cell activation through cross-linking of the CD3/TCR complex (via the $F(ab')_2$ arms) and Fcγ receptor (FcγR) on the surface of accessory cells (via the Fc region), with consequent release of cytokine such as tumor necrosis factor α (TNFα), interleukin-2 (IL-2), and interferon γ (IFN-γ) [37, 38]. Recently, a humanized, non-FcγR-binding, anti-CD3 mAb (visilizumab, PDL BioPharma Inc.) directed against the ε invariant chain of the CD3/TCR complex, has been evaluated for the treatment of steroid refractory acute GVHD [39]. This mAb retains the specificity for CD3 but has an engineered and modified Fc portion that fails to trigger T-cell activation and therefore is associated with significantly less cytokine release. Despite this significant structural improvement, to date, there are no published reports of the use of mAbs specific for CD3 in TCL. A phase I, multiple dose escalation trial of IV humanized anti-CD3 mAb (HuM291) in patients with $CD3^+$ TCL has been recently completed at Stanford University (clinical trial number NCT00006009); however, the results are not yet available.

CD4 Antigen

CD4 is a 55 kD single chain glycoprotein containing four immunoglobulin-like domains that project from the T-cell surface, a hydrophobic transmembrane domain and a long cytoplasmic tail [40]. In association with the TCR, CD4 acts as a co-receptor for the major histocompatibility complex (MHC) class II molecules [41]. The main physiological importance of this surface glycoprotein is signaling which takes place through its cytoplasmic tail. The intracytoplasmic region of CD4 is constitutively and non-covalently associated with a src-like tyrosine kinase ($p56^{lck}$) that initiates the transduction cascade following antigen binding [42]. CD4 is normally expressed on helper/regulatory T-cells, and, at a lower level, on monocytes, macrophages, and dendritic cells [40]. CD4 is also expressed on the malignant cells of PTCL and CTCL patients [43]. The fact that CD4 is expressed only on a subset of normal T-cells, it is brightly expressed on malignant cells from CTCL patients, it is present in all stages of disease with no down-modulation during disease progression and it is involved in cell signaling, has provided the rationale for targeting CD4 with mAbs.

CD4-Targeted Therapy

The therapeutic activity of mAbs specific for CD4, in their murine and humanized variant, has been evaluated in human inflammatory diseases such as rheumatoid arthritis and psoriasis [44–46] as well as in CTCL [43, 47, 48]. In an early study [47], seven previously treated mycosis fungoides (MF) patients were treated with a chimeric murine antibody composed of the IgG1κ human constant regions and the mouse variable regions directed against CD4 (SK3/anti-Leu3a; Becton-Dickinson, Inc.). Patients received IV doses of 10, 20, 40, or 80 mg twice a week for 3 consecutive weeks. At the 80 mg dose, the antibody was detected in skin lesions and also coating circulating $CD4^+$ T-cells in the peripheral blood, however, no significant depletion of $CD4^+$ cells was observed. In a second phase I study [48], 8 previously treated MF patients received a single IV dose (50, 100 or 200 mg) of a different chimeric murine anti-CD4 mAb directed to a distinct epitope on CD4 (cM-T412; Centocor, Inc.). Following the antibody infusion there was a depletion of peripheral blood $CD4^+$ cells in 7 of the 8 patients. The overall response rate (ORR) was 88% with 5 patients achieving a PR and 2 patients achieving a minor response (MR). The time to progression (TTP) ranged from 6 to 52 weeks, with an average of 25 weeks. More recently, HuMax-CD4 (zanolimumab, Genmab, Inc.), a fully human anti-CD4 mAb, isolated from transgenic mice as a hybridoma clone and subsequently expressed in Chinese hamster ovary cells, was able to induce significant T-cell depletion in repeated dosing and was found to be safe and well tolerated in human inflammatory diseases [45, 46]. Based on its safe profile and the preliminary encouraging results obtained with murine anti-CD4 mAbs, the therapeutic activity of zanolimumab was also evaluated in two separate but otherwise identical phase 2 clinical trials in refractory CTCL [43]. In the first of the two studies, 27 patients with early-stage MF received weekly IV infusion of zanolimumab at either 280 mg (13 patients) or 560 mg (14 patients) for a total of 16 weeks. In the second study, 11 patients with advanced-stage treatment refractory MF and 9 patients with Sezary syndrome (SS) were treated with weekly IV infusion of zanolimumab at either 280 mg (7 and 4 patients, respectively) or 960 mg (4 and 5 patients, respectively). Overall, 13 of 38 patients (34.2%) with MF and 2 of 9 patients (22.2%) with SS obtained an objective response to zanolimumab (MF: 1 CR, 3 CCRs, and 9 PRs; SS: 2 PRs). 56% of the MF patients (7 of 14 at 560 mg and 3 of 4 at 980 mg) treated at the high-dose levels achieved objective response compared with only 15% at the 280 mg dose (3 of 20). In patients with SS, the response rate was 1 in 4 at the 280 mg dose and 1 in 5 at the 980 mg dose. In patients with MF, high-dose treatment resulted in an earlier time to response with 9 of 10 responses achieved within 8 weeks (median time to response 8 weeks, range 2–12 weeks) and more durable responses (median duration of response 81 weeks, range 8–91 weeks) compared with low dose treatment (three responses obtained at 4, 8, and 12 weeks; duration of response 12, 13, and 24 weeks). In patients with SS, the two responses lasted 8 weeks (280 mg) and 61 weeks (980 mg). Overall, treatment was well tolerated with infections and eczematous dermatitis being the most frequent adverse events observed. This antibody was designed to prevent the interaction between the CD4 receptor and the MHC class II molecule, thereby interfering with T-cell activation, and, recently, the mechanism through which zanolimumab may inactivate or delete T-cells has been described [49]. Ligation of CD4 by zanolimumab inhibits the necessary $p56^{lck}$-mediated co-stimulation by uncoupling this kinase from the TCR and allowing this enzyme to transmit an inhibitory signal via Dok-1 and SHIP-1 inhibitory molecules that may also reduce AKT activity. Secondly, zanolimumab induces potent ADCC with no role played by CDC and, lastly, it may act by down-modulating CD4 itself. Despite its promising profile in terms of therapeutic activity and safety, future developments for zanolimumab and its clinical applications are on hold due to pharmaceutical company's decision.

CD25 Antigen

Interleukin-2 (IL-2) is a potent immunomodulatory cytokine whose function is the activation of T- and B-lymphocytes, NK cells, and macrophages [50]. Three polypeptide chains (α, β, and γ) are non-covalently associated to form the high affinity interleukin-2 receptor (IL-2R) [51–53]. The α (CD25 or p55) and β (CD122 or p75) chains are involved in binding IL-2, while signal transduction which involves Janus kinase-1 (Jak-1), Jak-3, and STAT-5 pathways, is carried out by the γ (CD132 or p64) chain, along with the β subunit [54–56]. CD25 is a 55 kD, heavily glycosylated, integral membrane protein which, by itself, functions as a low affinity IL-2R. CD25, initially defined using the murine mAb anti-Tac [57], is a polypeptide composed of 272 aminoacids with an extracellular, transmembrane, and a very short intracellular domain. CD25 is dimly expressed on normal, resting peripheral blood T-cells, however is rapidly upregulated following antigen or cytokines stimulation [55]. Among T-cell malignancies, CD25 is strongly expressed by ATL and ALCL [55], highly variable expressed on CTCL [58]. It has been shown that CD25 expression varies depending on tissue site from CTCL patients: CD25 has been found to be highly expressed in epidermis, down-regulated in dermis, and extensively down-regulated in lymph nodes, suggesting that the microenvironment may play a role in affecting CD25 expression [58]. It has also been shown that CD25 expression correlates with advanced stage (T status) and histological grade (large cell transformation) of CTCL, suggesting a role as prognostic marker for this antigen [59]. Recently, soluble IL2-R has been identified as a reliable marker of disease activity in patients with ATL [60].

CD25-Targeted Therapy

Several studies have established the importance of CD25 as a valuable target for immunotherapy [61–63]. A number of mAbs specific for CD25 have been evaluated in several T-cell mediated disorders including prevention of rejection of transplanted organs [64], noninfectious uveitis [65], multiple sclerosis [66], and HTLV-1-associated disorders [67]. In 1997, daclizumab, a therapeutical humanized mAb specific for CD25 (zenapax, Hoffmann-La Roche) has been approved by the FDA for use in the prevention of renal allograft rejection [68]. Also among T-cell malignancies, various forms of CD25-specific mAbs have been tested in a preclinical and clinical setting. These include the murine mAb anti-Tac [57], daclizumab [69, 70], and 7G7/B6 mAb that targets CD25 at an epitope other than the IL-2 and anti-Tac binding sites [71]. These mAbs significantly prolonged the survival of MET-1 mice (murine model of ATL), however cure was not achieved [72]. For this reason, daclizumab has been combined with flavopiridol in the MET-1 murine model in which a marked synergy between these two drugs has been observed [73]. The clinical use of the murine mAbs has been limited due to their immunogenicity associated with rapid generation of neutralizing anti-mouse Ab, short in vivo survival and modest ADCC-mediated cell death due to the reduced binding to human Fc receptors [74]. However also daclizumab, as many other unmodified mAbs, has shown only modest activity as single cytotoxic agent in ATL patients. To overcome these limitations, daclizumab has been employed as a carrier of cytotoxic agents such as radionuclides or toxins. In a phase I/II trial, 18 patients with ATL were treated with 55 doses of ^{90}Y-labeled anti-Tac mAb involving 5–15 Ci per patient [75]. Ten of the evaluable patients responded to treatment, with 8 patients achieving a PR and 2a CR. Hematologic toxicity was the limiting side effect. In an alternative approach, the antitumor activity of the anti-Tac mAb conjugated with a truncated Pseudomonas exotoxin (anti-Tac (Fv)-PE38 (LMB-2)) was evaluated in a phase I/II trial [76] in which 35 patients with a CD25$^+$ lymphoma/

leukemia were enrolled. Among these patients, 1 had CTCL/SS, 3 had PTCL unspecified and 2 ATL. Patients received escalating dose of LMB-2 on alternate days for 3 doses (1 cycle), with a starting dose of 2 μg/kg administered IV, every 3 weeks. Of the 6 patients with T-cell malignancies, 3 achieved a PR (1 with CTCL/SS, 1 with PTCL, 1 with ATL). Responding patients experienced rapid reductions of circulating malignant cells, improvement in skin lesions, and regression of lymphomatous masses and splenomegaly; however, all responses were of short duration.

CD122 Antigen

CD122 or p75 represents the β subunit shared by the heterotrimeric IL-2 and IL-15 receptors [77]. IL-15 is produced by macrophages, dendritic cells, and other non-lymphoid cells, it mainly works inducing T-cells and NK-cells maturation, enhancing the survival of $CD8^+$ cytotoxic lymphocytes and stimulating the production of TNFα, IL-1β, and other cytokines [78]. Dysregulation of IL-15 and its receptor have been reported in CTCL, acute lymphoblastic leukemia (ALL), ATL, and T-LGL leukemia [79–81].

CD122-Targeted Therapy

In a phase I trial, 12 patients with T-LGL leukemia received escalating dose of Mik-β1 murine mAb, every 3 days, with a starting dose of 0.5 mg/kg, administered IV [81]. Greater than 95% saturation of CD122 was achieved in all patients; however, no responses in terms of decreases in T-LGL cell count were observed. A phase I safety and pharmacokinetic study of the humanized form of Mik-β1 in T-LGL leukemia is now underway.

CD26 Antigen

CD26 is a 110 kD surface glycoprotein expressed by a variety of cells including epithelial cells, T-lymphocytes, and NK cells [82]. CD26 possesses an intrinsic dipeptidyl peptidase IV (DPPIV) activity in its extracellular domain [83] and plays an important role in T-cell activation [82]. CD26 expression is tightly regulated on T-cells and it is significantly enhanced after activation [84]. CD26 is capable of providing a potent costimulatory signal which can induce several activation pathways leading to proliferation and cytokines production [82]. However the mechanism of costimulation remains unclear since the cytoplasmic domain consists of only six amino-acids and lacks a phosphorylation site, leading to the conclusion that CD26 must interact with other molecules to exert this function. CD26, through its peptidase activity, can also cleave certain chemokines involved in T-cell function and monocytes function, including RANTES and LD78β [85, 86]; it has also been shown that CD26 regulates adenosine deaminase surface expression with this complex perhaps playing a role in regulating immune function [87].

CD26-Targeted Therapy

Among TCL, CD26 is absent or dimly expressed in MF/SS [88], variably expressed in T-LGL [89], and expressed at high levels in γδ hepatosplenic and ALCL [90]. An mAb specific for CD26 (1F7) has shown to have in vitro and in vivo antitumor effect in human $CD30^+$ ALCL cell lines by inducing G1–S cell cycle arrest and enhancement of $p21^{Cip1}$ expression [91]. It has also been shown that CD26 is a marker of aggressive clinical behavior and poor prognosis for T-LGL [89] and T-cell lymphoblastic leukemia/lymphoma [92]. A phase I trial, involving a humanized anti-CD26 Mab, will be conducted in relapsed/refractory patients with CD26 positive tumors, including TCL, in the near future (Dr. NH Dang, Nevada Cancer Institute).

CD30 Antigen

CD30 is a 105–120 kD type I transmembrane glycoprotein and a member of the tumor necrosis factor (TNF) receptor superfamily [93]. The mature CD30 comprises 577 amino acids, with a

365 amino acids extracytoplasmatic domain physiologically bound by CD30 ligand (CD153), a 24 amino acids transmembrane domain and a 188 amino acids intracytoplasmatic domain which regulates signaling transduction following receptor binding through its serine/threonine phosphorylation sites [94]. In normal tissues, CD30 expression is restricted to activated B- and T-lymphocytes [95]. In the immune system, CD30 functions as a costimulatory molecule in the presence of TCR stimulation, it activates T-cells production of cytokines such as IL-2, TNF, and IFNγ and it appears to be involved in the negative selection of autoreactive lymphocytes [96]. In tumor cells, CD30 was originally identified on the surface of Reed-Sternberg cells [97]; however, it has been shown to be highly expressed also on ALCL tumor cells [98] and can be expressed at variable levels on CTCL cells [99]. A cleaved form of CD30 (sCD30) can be found in the plasma of $CD30^{+}$ lymphoma patients as a result of cleavage by TNFα-converting enzyme, a zinc metalloproteinase, with serum levels of sCD30 correlating with neoplastic activity, tumor burden, response to treatment, and time to treatment failure in ALCL [100].

CD30-Targeted Therapy

Although its function has not been completely clarified, CD30-mediated signaling has been implicated in both lymphocytes death and proliferation, therefore a number of different mAbs targeting different epitopes of CD30 have been developed [101–107]. It is even more interesting that the same antibody (M67) has showed opposite effect in ALCL cell lines and Hodgkin's disease (HD) cell lines [108]. Specifically, M67 was able to induce enhanced apoptosis in ALCL cell lines; however, it had no effects on HD cell lines. CD30 binding has been associated with NF-κB activation [109] and the difference in outcome between ALCL and HD cells following anti-CD30 treatment was attributed to the inability of ALCL cells to activate NF-κB [110], in contrast with HD cells which constitutively express NF-κB [111]. Chimeric anti-CD30 mAbs have also been tested in murine xenograft model of ALCL in which treatment with these mAbs was able to significantly prolong survival of mice bearing chemotherapy resistant human ALCL [112, 113]. In the attempt to improve its in vitro and in vivo antitumor activity, Ber-H2, an mAb specific for CD30, has been conjugated with the plant ribosome-inactivating protein saporin and showed promising initial results [114]. Based on these preclinical data, mAbs targeting CD30 have been evaluated in phase I/II clinical trials. In a phase I/II trial, MDX-060 (Medarex, Inc.), a fully human anti-CD30 mAb, was administered at doses up to 15 mg/kg to 21 patients (16 with HD, 3 with ALCL, and 2 with $CD30^{+}$ TCL unspecified) [115]. Adverse events were common but primarily mild or moderate in intensity and an MTD was not defined. In phase II, an additional 51 patients were treated, 4 of which with ALCL. Of the 7 patients with ALCL, 2 (28%), with a predominantly skin disease, achieved a CR. Both CR lasted more than 1 year with both patients receiving additional cycles of therapy. In another phase I trial, SGN-30 (Seattle Genetics, Inc.), a chimeric anti-CD30 mAb, was administered at four dose levels (2, 4, 8, or 12 mg/kg) on a weekly schedule for 6 consecutive weeks, to 24 patients with refractory lymphoma (21 with HD and 3 with $CD30^{+}$ NHL) [116]. Antibody treatment was well tolerated and, although antitumor activity was not an objective of this trial, of the 3 patients with $CD30^{+}$ NHL, 1 patient (33%) with a history of cutaneous ALCL achieved a CR and 2 patients achieved stable disease (SD). Forero-Torres et al. [117] recently reported on 79 patients, 38 with refractory/relapsed HD and 41 with systemic ALCL (35 with ALK^{-} ALCL), treated in a multicenter phase II trial with SGN-30 at a dose of 6 mg/kg for 6 weeks. After the first 24 patients were enrolled, the dose was escalated to 12 mg/kg per week. Overall the treatment was well tolerated, adverse events were common but primary mild or moderate. In the ALCL group, 2 patients achieved a CR and 6 patients a PR for an ORR of 21% and with a response duration ranging from 27 to 1,460+ days. Duvic et al. [118] recently reported the results from another multicenter phase II trial in which SGN-30 was administered to patients with CD30$^+$ lymphomas. Specifically, 5 patients with primary cutaneous ALCL (pc-ALCL) and 1 patient with multiple clinical diagnosis (mixed CD30$^+$ lesions), received 1 dose of IV SGN-30 at 4 mg/kg every 3 weeks for up to six doses. Six patients with pc-ALCL, 3 with lymphomatoid papulosis (LyP), 3 with transformed MF, and 5 with multiple clinical diagnosis (mixed CD30$^+$ lesions), received 1 dose of IV SGN-30 at 12 mg/kg every 3 weeks for up to six doses. Eligible patients could receive two additional courses. Overall the treatment was well tolerated but adverse events were common, 15 patients (65%) experienced at least 1 adverse event with fatigue being the most common. 10 patients (43%) achieved a CR (6 with pc-ALCL, 1 with LyP, and 3 with mixed CD30$^+$ lesions) and 6 patients (26%) achieved a PR (3 with pc-ALCL, 1 with LyP, 1 with MF, and 1 with mixed CD30$^+$ lesions) for an ORR of 87%. However the responses were of short duration (the overall median duration of objective response, CR+PR, was 84 days, range 1–238). Overall, anti-CD30 mAbs have shown an acceptable safety profile, however, in the majority of studies, anti-CD30 mAbs as single agents showed only modest antitumor activity in most CD30$^+$ TCL, suggesting combination strategies as an attractive alternative option. Phase I/II trials with SGN-30 either in combination with chemotherapy or conjugated with drugs/toxins are now ongoing in pretreated patients with CD30$^+$ hematologic malignancies.

Better efficacy with CD30-targcting agents has been observed with brentuximab vedotin (SGN-35, Adcetris, Seattle Genetics, Inc), an antibody-drug conjugate which consists of the anti-CD30 monoclonal antibody cAC10 (SGN-30) conjugated with the cytotoxic agent monomethylauristatin E (MMAE) via a protease-cleavable linker [119, 120]. Brentuximab vedotin was recently approved by the US FDA in August 2011 for the treatment of relapsed or refractory Hodgkin's lymphoma (HL) and ALCL. In the initial phase I dose-escalation study [121], brentuximab vedotin was administered intravenously on days 1, 8, and 15, of each 28-day cycle at doses ranging from 0.4 to 1.4 mg/kg. Forty-four patients were enrolled: 38 with Hodgkin's lymphoma, 5 with systemic ALCL, and 1 with PTCL. Doses were escalated in increments of 0.2 mg/kg until DLT was observed. Antitumor assessments were carried out every two cycles. The MTD was 1.2 mg/kg. The most common adverse events were peripheral sensory neuropathy, fatigue, nausea, diarrhea, arthralgia, and fever. The majority of events were mild to moderate in severity. Tumor regression occurred in 85% of patients and the overall objective response rate was 59% ($n=24$), with 34% ($n=14$) complete remissions. The median duration of response was not reached at a median follow-up of 45 weeks on study. FDA approval was based on data from two pivotal, open-label clinical trials independent review of response rate. Brentuximab vedotin was administered intravenously at a dose of 1.8 mg/kg over the course of 30 min once every 3 weeks. Results from the Hodgkin study ($n=102$) showed an ORR of 73% (95% confidence interval [CI], 65–83%), including 32% with complete remission (95% CI, 23–42%). Response duration averaged 6.7 months (range, 1.3–21.9+ months). Data from the ALCL study ($n=58$) revealed an 86% response rate (95% CI, 77–95%), with 57% complete remission rate (95% CI, 44–70%). Median response duration was 12.6 months (range, 0.1–15.9+ months) [122]. Based on these data, brentuximab vedotin represents a welcome addition to the therapeutic tool box for CD30$^+$ lymphomas, including ALCL and HL, with high response rates and manageable toxicity. While the drug appears to be safe on early follow up, more recently the FDA issued a warning to health care professionals due to three cases of progressive multifocal leukoencephalopathy (PML), and a new boxed warning highlighting this risk has been added to the drug label [123]. In addition, a contraindication was added, warning against the use of brentuximab with the cancer drug bleomycin because of the increased risk for pulmonary toxicity.

CD52 Antigen

CD52 is a 21–28 kD, glycosylphosphatidylinositol (GPI)-anchored, heavily glycosilated, protein, encoded by a gene on human chromosome 1 [124]. The peptide component of CD52 is represented by a 12 aminoacids scaffold, which undergoes significant posttranslational modification [125]. Attempts to identify a ligand have not been successful and the physiologic function of CD52 remains to be clarified: it may mediate a variety of biological effects such as signal transduction including promotion of cell–cell adhesion and protection of the cell from environmental insult, however, CD52 knock-outs or congenitally CD52-deficient animals have not been described. Relatively recently, it has also been suggested that CD52 may contribute to the activation of $CD4^+$ regulatory T-cells [126]. CD52 is highly expressed on membrane lipids raft of all B and T lymphocytes at most stages of differentiation (except plasma cells), as well as on monocytes, macrophages, eosinophils, NK cells, and dendritic cells [124, 127–130]. The antigen is also found in the male reproductive tract, where it is strongly expressed on epithelial cells lining the epididymis, vas deferens, and seminal vesicle [131]. Notably, CD52 is not expressed on hematopoietic stem cells, erythrocytes, and platelets [132]; however, it has been found on a subpopulation of $CD34^+CD38^+$ cells which are believed to represent lymphocyte-committed progenitors [133]. CD52 is also variably expressed on subsets of tumor cells, at a particular high density on T-prolymphocytic leukemia (T-PLL) cells followed by B-CLL, hairy cell leukemia (HCL), ALL, and NHL, including TCL [128, 134, 135]. However, in contrast with B-cell malignancies, there is a great variability in terms of CD52 expression in TCL. Currently the expression of CD52 is best assessed by flow cytometry [136], in fact, a reliable assay for the detection of CD52 on paraffin-embedded, formalin-fixed tissue is not available and data on CD52 expression in various subtypes of TCL are conflicting, due to inconsistent reproducibility [134, 135, 137, 138]. Alemtuzumab has shown encouraging activity in T-cell malignancies [139], however, the variable expression of CD52 among TCL and the profound lymphopenia associated with the use of this mAb, have partially limited its use in TCL.

CD52-Targeted Therapy

Campath-1H (alemtuzumab [U.S.], mabCampath [E.U.], Genzyme, and Bayer HealthCare Pharmaceuticals Inc.) is a humanized IgG1κ mAb directed against the human CD52 antigen that is FDA approved for the management of patients with pretreated [140] and untreated B-CLL [141]. The CD52 epitope recognized by alemtuzumab corresponds to the last three aminoacids of the peptide scaffold and part of the GPI anchor [139]. The mechanisms underlying the therapeutic effect of alemtuzumab in lymphoid malignancies have not been well characterized. The spectrum of biologic effects on tumor cells is heterogeneous and the dominant mechanism of antitumor activity may differ from disease to disease. In vitro and in vivo evidence show that alemtuzumab induces CDC, ADCC, and direct apoptosis in B- and T-cell malignancies [125, 142–147]. The pharmacokinetics (PK) of alemtuzumab has been studied in B-CLL, using the approved schedule consisting of a 2 h IV infusion at a starting dose of 3 mg on day 1, 10 mg on day 2 up to the target dose of 30 mg, three times per week for up to 12 weeks [148]. Considering the fact that remarkable "first-dose" reactions consisting in fever, vomiting, rigors, skin rash, dyspnea, and hypotension have been noted in the majority of patients treated with the IV route [149], Hale et al. [148] compared blood concentrations of alemtuzumab in B-CLL patients after IV and subcutaneous (SC) dosing. SC administration was not associated with "first-dose" reactions and similar peak drug concentrations were achieved; however, a higher cumulative dose of SC alemtuzumab was required to reach concentrations similar to the IV administration. PK data with alemtuzumab (IV or SC) in T-cell malignancies are not available. Multiple studies have shown single-agent alemtuzumab to be active in T-cell malignancies (*T-PLL*: [150]; *CTCL*: [151–155]; *PTCL*: [156]); however, clinical experience with alemtuzumab treatment in T-cell malignancies has been limited to small series and approval for this indication has not been granted yet. The first suggestion of activity in T-PLL came from a phase II trial [150] in which 39 patients with previously treated T-PLL received IV alemtuzumab (30 mg, three times a week until maximum response). The ORR was 76% (60% complete response, CR, and 16% partial response, PR). The TTP was 10 months (range 3–45) and median OS was 13 months (24 months for patients in CR). The response rate and survival were significantly longer than those reported for conventional therapies [157]. In a retrospective study of 76 patients with heavily pretreated T-PLL, alemtuzumab was administered at the standard schedule for up to 12 weeks. The ORR was 50% with 28 patients (37.5%) achieving a CR. The TTF was 4.5 months, the median OS was 7.5 months (14.8 months for patients in CR) [158]. In an early, preliminary, European experience, 50 B- and T-cell NHL patients received single-agent alemtuzumab [151]. Eight of these patients had advanced refractory MF: an ORR of 50% with 2 CRs and 2 PRs was seen. These promising results led to a multicenter phase II trial with the largest reported CTCL series [152] in which 22 patients with heavily pretreated, CD52-positive, advanced stage MF/SS, were treated with single-agent alemtuzumab. Alemtuzumab was administered IV at the standard dose of 30 mg, three times per week, for up to 12 weeks. The ORR rate was 55% (32% CR, 23% PR), with better efficacy in patients with erythroderma (69% ORR) than those with plaques/skin tumors (40% ORR). Median TTF for all responders was 12 months (range 5–32). Infectious complications were observed, including asymptomatic CMV reactivation (4 patients), generalized HSV (1 patient), 1 case of fatal aspergillosis, and 1 case of fatal *Mycobacterium pneumonia*. In another phase II trial [153], 8 MF/SS patients (7 of whom with refractory disease), received IV alemtuzumab according to the standard schedule; however, the ORR was only 38%, with no CR observed and a shorter TTF (4 months). In the attempt to reduce the incidence of hematologic toxicities and the risk of infectious complications associated with the standard schedule, Zinzani et al. [154] assessed the impact of a reduced-dose schedule of IV alemtuzumab (10 mg, three times per week, for 4 weeks) in 10 pretreated patients (6 PTCL and 6 MF). Despite the dose reduction, an ORR of 75% (with no CRs) among the MF patients and an ORR of 50% (with 2 CRs) among the PTCL patients were observed. More importantly, no grade 3–4 hematologic toxicities were noticed and CMV reactivation occurred in only 1 patient. More recently Bernengo et al. [155] investigated the association of a reduced-dose schedule of alemtuzumab with the SC administration route in the attempt to also eliminate the systemic reactions associated with the IV route. Eleven relapsed/refractory MF patients and 3 untreated SS patients were enrolled, 4 of them received alemtuzumab 3 mg on day 1, 10 mg on day 3, then 15 mg on alternating days, for a total of four doses. A reduced dosage (3 mg on day 1, then 10 mg on alternating days) was administered to the remaining patients. The ORR was 85.7%, with 3 CRs (21.4%). After a median follow-up of 16 months, the median TTF was 12 months. Infectious complications occurred in 4 patients. Lenihan et al. [159] described the activity of alemtuzumab, at the standard IV 12-week dosing schedule, in 5 patients with SS. Activity was modest with only 3 PR achieved, and a variety of cardiovascular adverse events were observed, including chronic heart failure, hypotension, pulmonary thromboembolism, and atrial fibrillation, even in the absence of known cardiac risk factors. However evidence of cardiac toxicity with alemtuzumab treatment has not been confirmed [160]. A few additional small studies reporting on the activity of alemtuzumab in SS have been published [161–163]. Data on PTCL patients and single-agent alemtuzumab are even scarcer than those available for T-PLL and CTCL. In the only prospective trial in PTCL patients treated with single-agent alemtuzumab published so far [156], 14 patients with advanced relapsed/refractory disease received IV alemtuzumab following the standard schedule. The ORR was 36% with 3 patients achieving a CR and 2 patients achieving a PR. The duration of response was 2, 6, and 12 months for each of the CR patients. However, in these heavily pretreated patients, alemtuzumab therapy was associated with significant toxicity, including CMV reactivation in 6 patients, pulmonary aspergillosis in 2 patients, EBV-related hemophagocytosis in 2 patients.

In the attempt to enhance the response rate and prolong the TTF, alemtuzumab has also been administered in association with chemotherapy in the treatment of TCL patients.

In the first phase II trial, 20 patients with previously untreated PTCL (10 patients with PTCL-unspecified, 3 with angioimmunoblastic lymphoma, 3 with extranodal NK/TCL, nasal type, 2 with ALK$^-$ ALCL, and 2 with subcutaneous panniculitis-like TCL) received CHOP (cyclophosphamide, doxorubicin, vincristine, prednisone) plus alemtuzumab (10 mg IV on day 1, 20 mg on day 2 of the first cycle, then 30 mg IV on day 1 in the subsequent cycles), based on 3 week interval [164]. An ORR of 80% with a 65% CR rate was observed however the trial was prematurely closed due to two treatment-related deaths and high incidence of infectious complications as well as hematologic adverse events. An Italian prospective multicenter phase II trial evaluated the activity of alemtuzumab in combination with CHOP in 24 patients with previously untreated PTCL (8 patients with PTCL-unspecified, 7 with angioimmunoblastic lymphoma, 3 with ALK$^-$ ALCL, and 1 with enteropathy-associated TCL) [165]. SC alemtuzumab was administered at 30 mg at day 1 to 8 courses of CHOP-28. An ORR of 75% with a 71% CR rate was observed. Thirteen patients were disease free with an overall median duration of response of 11 months. Neutropenia and CMV reactivation were the most common hematologic and non-hematologic complications, occurring in 59 of 176 (34%) and 15 of 176 (9%) of CHOP chemotherapy courses, respectively. Two cases of invasive aspergillosis and 1 case of PML were also noticed. Alemtuzumab was also combined with CHOP and ESHAP (ethopside, cytarabin, cisplatin, and methylpredinsolone) in 13 patients with untreated PTCL (3 patients with PTCL-unspecified, 5 with extranodal NK/TCL, nasal type, 4 with subcutaneous panniculitis-like TCL, and 1 with enteropathy-associated TCL) [166]. SC alemtuzumab was administered at 30 mg at day 1–3 of cycle 1–5 plus CHOP (day 1 of cycle 1, 3, 5) and ESHAP (day 1 of cycle 2, 4, 6) at 28-day intervals. In the 10 evaluable patients, an ORR of 90% with a 80% CR rate was observed. Infection was the major adverse event with CMV reactivation occurring in 54% of the patients.

Recently, two phase III trials (ACT1 and ACT2) combining CHOP with alemtuzumab as primary treatment for patients with PTCL, have been opened by the European Intergroup.

In a German phase II trial, alemtuzumab was combined with fludarabine, cyclophosphamide, and doxorubicin (alemtuzumab 3, 10, 30, 30 mg, days 1–4, fludarabine 25 mg/m^2 days 2–4, cyclophosphamide 600 mg/m^2 day 3, and doxorubicin 50 mg/m^2 day 4, every 28 days) [167] to treat 19 newly diagnosed and 11 relapsed/refractory PTCL patients (13 patients with PTCL-unspecified, 9 with angioimmunoblastic lymphoma, 2 with ALK$^-$ ALCL, 2 with enteropathy-associated TCL, 2 with nasal-type NK-/TCL, 1 with an NK-cell lymphoma and 1 with a T-PLL). An ORR of 63% with a 58% CR rate and with ten ongoing remissions at the time of publication, were observed in the previously untreated patients' group. An ORR of 45% with a 28% CR rate was observed in the relapsed/refractory group. The toxicity was significant with 65% of the patients experiencing a sustained grade III/IV neutropenia, 40% of the patients had a CMV reactivation which was symptomatic in 2.

As emerged from many clinical trials, most of the TCL patients experience variable grades of cytopenia during treatment with alemtuzumab, especially if heavily pretreated and with advanced stage of disease. Thrombocytopenia is generally most common during the first 2 weeks and neutropenia is most common during weeks 5 and 6 [152]. Importantly, grade 4 neutropenia could be an indication to postpone alemtuzumab therapy but prematurely terminating treatment should be avoided especially in SS patients because, although resolution of peripheral blood lymphocytosis occurs early, bone marrow is unlikely to be clear of disease after 4 weeks of therapy [152, 155]. Monocytes, NK cells and peripheral blood but not tissue antigen-presenting dendritic cells are also profoundly depleted but this reduction is not as pronounced as for lymphocytes. Profound and sustained T and B lymphopenia is the most significant and consistent side-effect of alemtuzumab, according to the high expression of CD52 antigen on these cells' surface [152]. Granulocytes population usually returns to baseline levels early during the unmaintained follow-up while monocytes remain at around 50% of their baseline value for a prolonged period of time. B lymphocytes normalize relatively quickly, $CD8^+$ T lymphocytes recover slower, and $CD4^+$ T lymphocytes may remain subnormal for over a year [152]. The stage of the disease, the disease itself, the number of prior treatments and the myelo/immunosuppression alemtuzumab-induced, increase the susceptibility to opportunistic and other severe infections, primarily bacterial [152, 168]. The most frequent opportunistic infection is caused by CMV. The overall incidence of CMV reactivation ranges between 5 and 43% in patients treated with alemtuzumab [150–153, 155, 156] and it is usually observed shortly after the nadir in T-cell counts, between 4 and 6 weeks of therapy. Antiviral prophylaxis (acyclovir, famciclovir, valaciclovir) is a mandatory procedure in these patients but these antiviral agents do not prevent CMV reactivation, although most patients respond rapidly to IV ganciclovir. At the present, no data are available to recommend routine prophylaxis for CMV but routine weekly monitoring with CMV antigenemia is indicated. Antibacterial and anti-Pneumocystis Jiroveci prophylaxis is recommended as well. CMV monitoring and prophylaxis should be continued for 2–4 months after alemtuzumab discontinuation [168]. Recently, cases of EBV-associated B and TCL after treatment with alemtuzumab in combination with chemotherapy for TCL have been reported [169, 170]. Alemtuzumab administered with proper antimicrobial prophylaxis has shown to be active in TCL; however, hematologic toxicities and infection complications are a major concern. The infusion related events are drastically reduced by the SC administration without affecting the efficacy. Alemtuzumab as single agent does not appear to be curative, therefore combination strategies with chemotherapeutic, biological agents and emerging class of new compounds such as histone deacetylase inhibitors should be further explored.

Conclusions

TCL represent a heterogeneous group of lymphoid neoplasms, and, with the exception of ALK^+ ALCL, early stage MF and T-LGL leukemia, TCL have a suboptimal response to conventional chemotherapy and a poor prognosis. Few patients achieve CR, relapse is common and usually associated with chemo-resistance. Malignant T-cells express a number of potential targets for immunotherapy. mAbs such as alemtuzumab have shown significant clinical activity in a variety of T-cell malignancies and represent a significant improvement over previous therapy considering that durable remissions have been seen in heavily pretreated patients with TCL. However, mAbs as single agents do not appear to be curative in TCL. Therefore, although active as single agents, mAbs may have a greater role in alternative strategies such as combinations with other biological or chemotherapeutic agents, either simultaneously or sequentially, with the hope to translate durable remissions into improved survival. Maintenance therapy or retreatment based on the monitoring of malignant T-cells should also be considered although antigen mutation or modulation may limit repeated administration activity. Another insight derives from studies involving mAbs covalently bound to radioisotope or toxins to enhance their ability to destroy tumor cells. This multimodality strategy together with a personalized, tailored, stage-specific approach may represent the future management of TCL patients. Based on the number of investigational mAbs now available and the activity shown by some mAbs alone or as a part of a multimodality strategy, there is no doubt that mAbs therapy of TCL will continue to be an area of active interest and expanding clinical trials.

References

1. Pressman D, Korngold L. The in vivo localization of anti-Wagner-osteogenic-sarcoma antibodies. Cancer. 1953;6(3):619–23.

2. Köhler G, Milstein C. Continuous cultures of fused cells secreting antibody of predefined specificity. Nature. 1975;256(5517):495–7.
3. Mascelli MA, Zhou H, Sweet R, et al. Molecular, biologic, and pharmacokinetic properties of monoclonal antibodies: impact of these parameters on early clinical development. J Clin Pharmacol. 2007;47(5):553–65.
4. Dillman RO. Monoclonal antibody therapy. In: Oldham RK, Dillman RO, editors. Principles of cancer biotherapy. 5th ed. New York: Springer; 2009. p. 303–407.
5. Meuer SC, Acuto O, Hercend T, et al. The human T-cell receptor. Annu Rev Immunol. 1984;2:23–50.
6. Kamoun M, Martin PJ, Hansen JA, et al. Identification of a human T lymphocyte surface protein associated with the E-rosette receptor. J Exp Med. 1981;153(1):207–12.
7. Bernard A, Gelin C, Raynal B, et al. Phenomenon of human T cells rosetting with sheep erythrocytes analyzed with monoclonal antibodies. "Modulation" of a partially hidden epitope determining the conditions of interaction between T cells and erythrocytes. J Exp Med. 1982;155(5):1317–33.
8. Alberola-Ila J, Places L, de la Calle O, et al. Stimulation through the TCR/CD3 complex up-regulates the CD2 surface expression on human T lymphocytes. J Immunol. 1991;146(4):1085–92.
9. Crawford K, Stark A, Kitchens B, et al. CD2 engagement induces dendritic cell activation: implications for immune surveillance and T-cell activation. Blood. 2003;102(5):1745–52.
10. Ohno H, Ushiyama C, Taniguchi M, et al. CD2 can mediate TCR/CD3-independent T cell activation. J Immunol. 1991;146(11):3742–6.
11. Moingeon P, Chang HC, Wallner BP. et al CD2-mediated adhesion facilitates T lymphocyte antigen recognition function. Nature. 1989;339(6222):312–4.
12. Peterson A, Seed B. Monoclonal antibody and ligand binding sites of the T cell erythrocyte receptor (CD2). Nature. 1987;329(6142):842–6.
13. Dustin ML, Sanders ME, Shaw S, et al. Purified lymphocyte function-associated antigen 3 binds to CD2 and mediates T lymphocyte adhesion. J Exp Med. 1987;165(3):677–92.
14. Hahn WC, Menu E, Bothwell AL, et al. Overlapping but nonidentical binding sites on CD2 for CD58 and a second ligand CD59. Science. 1992;256(5065):1805–7.
15. Selvaraj P, Plunkett ML, Dustin M, et al. The T lymphocyte glycoprotein CD2 binds the cell surface ligand LFA-3. Nature. 1987;326(6111):400–3.
16. Arulanandam AR, Kister A, McGregor MJ, et al. Interaction between human CD2 and CD58 involves the major beta sheet surface of each of their respective adhesion domains. J Exp Med. 1994;180(5):1861–71.
17. Zhu DM, Dustin ML, Cairo CW, et al. Mechanisms of cellular avidity regulation in CD2-CD58-mediated T cell adhesion. ACS Chem Biol. 2006;1(10):649–58.
18. Badour K, Zhang J, Shi F, et al. The Wiskott-Aldrich syndrome protein acts downstream of CD2 and the CD2AP and PSTPIP1 adaptors to promote formation of the immunological synapse. Immunity. 2003;18(1):141–54.
19. Carmo AM, Mason DW, Beyers AD. Physical association of the cytoplasmic domain of CD2 with the tyrosine kinases p56lck and p59fyn. Eur J Immunol. 1993;23(9):2196–201.
20. Bell GM, Fargnoli J, Bolen JB, et al. The SH3 domain of p56lck binds to proline-rich sequences in the cytoplasmic domain of CD2. J Exp Med. 1996;183(1):169–78.
21. Pantaleo G, Olive D, Poggi A, et al. Transmembrane signalling via the T11-dependent pathway of human T cell activation. Evidence for the involvement of 1,2-diacylglycerol and inositol phosphates. Eur J Immunol. 1987;17(1):55–60.
22. Hubert P, Debré P, Boumsell L, et al. Tyrosine phosphorylation and association with phospholipase C gamma-1 of the GAP-associated 62-kD protein after CD2 stimulation of Jurkat T cell. J Exp Med. 1993;178(5):1587–96.
23. Meuer SC, Hussey RE, Fabbi M, et al. An alternative pathway of T-cell activation: a functional role for the 50 kd T11 sheep erythrocyte receptor protein. Cell. 1984;36(4):897–906.
24. Dumont C, Déas O, Mollereau B, et al. Potent apoptotic signaling and subsequent unresponsiveness induced by a single CD2 mAb (BTI-322) in activated human peripheral T cells. J Immunol. 1998;160(8):3797–804.
25. Schad V, Greenstein JL, Giovino-Barry V, et al. An anti-CD2 monoclonal antibody that elicits alloantigen-specific hyporesponsiveness. Transplant Proc. 1996;28(4):2051–3.
26. Przepiorka D, Phillips GL, Ratanatharathorn V, et al. A phase II study of BTI-322, a monoclonal anti-CD2 antibody, for treatment of steroid-resistant acute graft-versus-host disease. Blood. 1998;92(11):4066–71.
27. Zhang Z, Zhang M, Ravetch JV, et al. Effective therapy for a murine model of adult T-cell leukemia with the humanized anti-CD2 monoclonal antibody, MEDI-507. Blood. 2003;102(1):284–8.
28. Sorbera LA, Leeson PA, Revel L, et al. Siplizumab. Drugs Fut. 2002;27(6):558.
29. Casale DA, Bartlett NL, Hurd DD, et al. A phase I open label dose escalation study to evaluate MEDI-507 in patients with CD2-positive T-cell lymphoma/leukemia [ASH annual meeting abstracts]. Blood. 2006;108:2727.
30. O'Mahony D, Morris JC, Stetler-Stevenson M, et al. EBV-related lymphoproliferative disease complicating therapy with the anti-CD2 monoclonal antibody, siplizumab, in patients with T-cell malignancies. Clin Cancer Res. 2009;15(7):2514–22.
31. Manolios N, Letourneur F, Bonifacino JS, et al. Pairwise, cooperative and inhibitory interactions

describe the assembly and probable structure of the T-cell antigen receptor. EMBO J. 1991;10(7):1643–51.
32. Chetty R, Gatter K. CD3: structure, function, and role of immunostaining in clinical practice. J Pathol. 1994;173(4):303–7.
33. San José E, Sahuquillo AG, Bragado R, et al. Assembly of the TCR/CD3 complex: CD3 epsilon/delta and CD3 epsilon/gamma dimers associate indistinctly with both TCR alpha and TCR beta chains. Evidence for a double TCR heterodimer model. Eur J Immunol. 1998;28(1):12–21.
34. Jaffers GJ, Fuller TC, Cosimi AB, et al. Monoclonal antibody therapy. Anti-idiotypic and non-anti-idiotypic antibodies to OKT3 arising despite intense immunosuppression. Transplantation. 1986;41(5):572–8.
35. Legendre C, Kreis H, Bach JF, et al. Prediction of successful allograft rejection retreatment with OKT3. Transplantation. 1992;53(1):87–90.
36. Sgro C. Side-effects of a monoclonal antibody, muromonab CD3/orthoclone OKT3: bibliographic review. Toxicology. 1995;105(1):23–9.
37. Abramowicz D, Schandene L, Goldman M, et al. Release of tumor necrosis factor, interleukin-2, and gamma-interferon in serum after injection of OKT3 monoclonal antibody in kidney transplant recipients. Transplantation. 1989;47(4):606–8.
38. Alegre ML, Vandenabeele P, Depierreux M, et al. Cytokine release syndrome induced by the 145-2C11 anti-CD3 monoclonal antibody in mice: prevention by high doses of methylprednisolone. J Immunol. 1991;146(4):1184–91.
39. Carpenter PA, Appelbaum FR, Corey L, et al. A humanized non-FcR-binding anti-CD3 antibody, visilizumab, for treatment of steroid-refractory acute graft-versus-host disease. Blood. 2002;99(8):2712–9.
40. Springer TA. Adhesion receptors of the immune system. Nature. 1990;346(6283):425–34.
41. Leahy DJ. A structural view of CD4 and CD8. FASEB J. 1995;9(1):17–25.
42. Veillette A, Bookman MA, Horak EM, et al. The CD4 and CD8 T cell surface antigens are associated with the internal membrane tyrosine-protein kinase p56lck. Cell. 1988;55(2):301–8.
43. Kim YH, Duvic M, Obitz E, et al. Clinical efficacy of zanolimumab (HuMax-CD4): two phase 2 studies in refractory cutaneous T-cell lymphoma. Blood. 2007;109(11):4655–62.
44. Herzog C, Walker C, Müller W, et al. Anti-CD4 antibody treatment of patients with rheumatoid arthritis: I. Effect on clinical course and circulating T cells. J Autoimmun. 1989;2(5):627–42.
45. Choy EH, Connolly DJ, Rapson N, et al. Pharmacokinetic, pharmacodynamic and clinical effects of a humanized IgG1 anti-CD4 monoclonal antibody in the peripheral blood and synovial fluid of rheumatoid arthritis patients. Rheumatology (Oxford). 2000;39(10):1139–46.
46. Skov L, Kragballe K, Zachariae C, et al. HuMax-CD4: a fully human monoclonal anti-CD4 antibody for the treatment of psoriasis vulgaris. Arch Dermatol. 2003;139(11):1433–9.
47. Knox SJ, Levy R, Hodgkinson S, et al. Observations on the effect of chimeric anti-CD4 monoclonal antibody in patients with mycosis fungoides. Blood. 1991;77(1):20–30.
48. Knox S, Hoppe RT, Maloney D, et al. Treatment of cutaneous T-cell lymphoma with chimeric anti-CD4 monoclonal antibody. Blood. 1996;87(3):893–9.
49. Rider DA, Havenith CE, de Ridder R, et al. A human CD4 monoclonal antibody for the treatment of T-cell lymphoma combines inhibition of T-cell signaling by a dual mechanism with potent Fc-dependent effector activity. Cancer Res. 2007;67(20):9945–53.
50. Ma A, Koka R, Burkett P. Diverse functions of IL-2, IL-15, and IL-7 in lymphoid homeostasis. Annu Rev Immunol. 2006;24:657–79.
51. Leonard WJ, Depper JM, Uchiyama T, et al. A monoclonal antibody that appears to recognize the receptor for human T-cell growth factor; partial characterization of the receptor. Nature. 1982;300(5889):267–9.
52. Leonard WJ, Depper JM, Crabtree GR, et al. Molecular cloning and expression of cDNAs for the human interleukin-2 receptor. Nature. 1984;311(5987):626–31.
53. Sharon M, Klausner RD, Cullen BR, et al. Novel interleukin-2 receptor subunit detected by cross-linking under high-affinity conditions. Science. 1986;234(4778):859–63.
54. Leonard WJ, Depper JM, Kanehisa M, et al. Structure of the human interleukin-2 receptor gene. Science. 1985;230(4726):633–9.
55. Waldmann TA. The structure, function, and expression of interleukin-2 receptors on normal and malignant lymphocytes. Science. 1986;232(4751):727–32.
56. Sugamura K, Asao H, Kondo M, et al. The interleukin-2 receptor gamma chain: its role in the multiple cytokine receptor complexes and T cell development in XSCID. Annu Rev Immunol. 1996;14:179–205.
57. Uchiyama T, Nelson DL, Fleisher TA, et al. A monoclonal antibody (anti-Tac) reactive with activated and functionally mature human T cells. II. Expression of Tac antigen on activated cytotoxic killer T cells, suppressor cells, and on one of two types of helper T cells. J Immunol. 1981;126(4):1398–403.
58. Jones D, Ibrahim S, Patel K, et al. Degree of CD25 expression in T-cell lymphoma is dependent on tissue site: implications for targeted therapy. Clin Cancer Res. 2004;10(16):5587–94.
59. Talpur R, Jones DM, Alencar AJ, et al. CD25 expression is correlated with histological grade and response to denileukin diftitox in cutaneous T-cell lymphoma. J Invest Dermatol. 2006;126(3):575–83.
60. Janik JE, Morris JC, Pittaluga S, et al. Elevated serum-soluble interleukin-2 receptor levels in patients with anaplastic large cell lymphoma. Blood. 2004;104(10):3355–7.

61. Waldmann TA. The multi-subunit interleukin-2 receptor. Annu Rev Biochem. 1989;58:875–911.
62. Waldmann TA. The IL-2/IL-2 receptor system: a target for rational immune intervention. Immunol Today. 1993;14(6):264–70.
63. Foss FM, Waldmann TA. Interleukin-2 receptor-directed therapies for cutaneous lymphomas. Hematol Oncol Clin North Am. 2003;17(6):1449–58.
64. Kirkman RL, Shapiro ME, Carpenter CB, et al. A randomized prospective trial of anti-Tac monoclonal antibody in human renal transplantation. Transplant Proc. 1991;23(1 Pt 2):1066–7.
65. Nussenblatt RB, Fortin E, Schiffman R, et al. Treatment of noninfectious intermediate and posterior uveitis with the humanized anti-Tac mAb: a phase I/II clinical trial. Proc Natl Acad Sci U S A. 1999;96(13):7462–6.
66. Bielekova B, Richert N, Howard T, et al. Humanized anti-CD25 (daclizumab) inhibits disease activity in multiple sclerosis patients failing to respond to interferon beta. Proc Natl Acad Sci U S A. 2004;101(23):8705–8.
67. Lehky TJ, Levin MC, Kubota R, et al. Reduction in HTLV-I proviral load and spontaneous lymphoproliferation in HTLV-I-associated myelopathy/tropical spastic paraparesis patients treated with humanized anti-Tac. Ann Neurol. 1998;44(6):942–7.
68. Wiseman LR, Faulds D. Daclizumab: a review of its use in the prevention of acute rejection in renal transplant recipients. Drugs. 1999;58(6):1029–42.
69. Queen C, Schneider WP, Selick HE, et al. A humanized antibody that binds to the interleukin 2 receptor. Proc Natl Acad Sci U S A. 1989;86(24):10029–33.
70. Junghans RP, Waldmann TA, Landolfi NF, et al. Anti-Tac-H, a humanized antibody to the interleukin 2 receptor with new features for immunotherapy in malignant and immune disorders. Cancer Res. 1990;50(5):1495–502.
71. Rubin LA, Kurman CC, Biddison WE, et al. A monoclonal antibody 7G7/B6, binds to an epitope on the human interleukin-2 (IL-2) receptor that is distinct from that recognized by IL-2 or anti-Tac. Hybridoma. 1985;4(2):91–102.
72. Phillips KE, Herring B, Wilson LA, et al. IL-2Ralpha-directed monoclonal antibodies provide effective therapy in a murine model of adult T-cell leukemia by a mechanism other than blockade of IL-2/IL-2Ralpha interaction. Cancer Res. 2000;60(24):6977–84.
73. Zhang M, Zhang Z, Goldman CK, et al. Combination therapy for adult T-cell leukemia-xenografted mice: flavopiridol and anti-CD25 monoclonal antibody. Blood. 2005;105(3):1231–6.
74. Waldmann TA, White JD, Goldman CK, et al. The interleukin-2 receptor: a target for monoclonal antibody treatment of human T-cell lymphotrophic virus I-induced adult T-cell leukemia. Blood. 1993;82(6):1701–12.
75. Waldmann TA, White JD, Carrasquillo JA, et al. Radioimmunotherapy of interleukin-2R alpha-expressing adult T-cell leukemia with Yttrium-90-labeled anti-Tac. Blood. 1995;86(11):4063–75.
76. Kreitman RJ, Wilson WH, White JD, et al. Phase I trial of recombinant immunotoxin anti-Tac(Fv)-PE38 (LMB-2) in patients with hematologic malignancies. J Clin Oncol. 2000;18(8):1622–36.
77. Anderson DM, Kumaki S, Ahdieh M, et al. Functional characterization of the human interleukin-15 receptor alpha chain and close linkage of IL15RA and IL2RA genes. J Biol Chem. 1995; 270(50):29862–9.
78. Shanmugham LN, Petrarca C, Frydas S, et al. IL-15 an immunoregulatory and anti-cancer cytokine. Recent advances. J Exp Clin Cancer Res. 2006;25(4):529–36.
79. Döbbeling U, Dummer R, Laine E, et al. Interleukin-15 is an autocrine/paracrine viability factor for cutaneous T-cell lymphoma cells. Blood. 1998;92(1):252–8.
80. Cario G, Izraeli S, Teichert A, et al. High interleukin-15 expression characterizes childhood acute lymphoblastic leukemia with involvement of the CNS. J Clin Oncol. 2007;25(30):4813–20.
81. Morris JC, Janik JE, White JD, et al. Preclinical and phase I clinical trial of blockade of IL-15 using Mikbeta1 monoclonal antibody in T cell large granular lymphocyte leukemia. Proc Natl Acad Sci U S A. 2006;103(2):401–6.
82. Morimoto C, Schlossman SF. The structure and function of CD26 in the T-cell immune response. Immunol Rev. 1998;161:55–70.
83. von Bonin A, Hühn J, Fleischer B. Dipeptidyl-peptidase IV/CD26 on T cells: analysis of an alternative T-cell activation pathway. Immunol Rev. 1998;161:43–53.
84. Ishii T, Ohnuma K, Murakami A, et al. CD26-mediated signaling for T cell activation occurs in lipid rafts through its association with CD45RO. Proc Natl Acad Sci U S A. 2001;98(21):12138–43.
85. Oravecz T, Pall M, Roderiquez G, et al. Regulation of the receptor specificity and function of the chemokine RANTES (regulated on activation, normal T cell expressed and secreted) by dipeptidyl peptidase IV (CD26)-mediated cleavage. J Exp Med. 1997;186(11):1865–72.
86. Proost P, Menten P, Struyf S, et al. Cleavage by CD26/dipeptidyl peptidase IV converts the chemokine LD78beta into a most efficient monocyte attractant and CCR1 agonist. Blood. 2000;96(5): 1674–80.
87. Kameoka J, Tanaka T, Nojima Y, et al. Direct association of adenosine deaminase with a T cell activation antigen, CD26. Science. 1993;261(5120):466–9.
88. Jones D, Dang NH, Duvic M, et al. Absence of CD26 expression is a useful marker for diagnosis of T-cell lymphoma in peripheral blood. Am J Clin Pathol. 2001;115(6):885–92.
89. Dang NH, Aytac U, Sato K, et al. T-large granular lymphocyte lymphoproliferative disorder: expression of CD26 as a marker of clinically aggressive disease and characterization of marrow inhibition. Br J Haematol. 2003;121(6):857–65.

90. Ruiz P, Mailhot S, Delgado P, et al. CD26 expression and dipeptidyl peptidase IV activity in an aggressive hepatosplenic T-cell lymphoma. Cytometry. 1998;34(1):30–5.
91. Ho L, Aytac U, Stephens LC, et al. In vitro and in vivo antitumor effect of the anti-CD26 monoclonal antibody 1F7 on human CD30+ anaplastic large cell T-cell lymphoma Karpas 299. Clin Cancer Res. 2001;7(7):2031–40.
92. Carbone A, Gloghini A, Zagonel V, et al. The expression of CD26 and CD40 ligand is mutually exclusive in human T-cell non-Hodgkin's lymphomas/leukemias. Blood. 1995;86(12):4617–26.
93. Falini B, Pileri S, Pizzolo G, et al. CD30 (Ki-1) molecule: a new cytokine receptor of the tumor necrosis factor receptor superfamily as a tool for diagnosis and immunotherapy. Blood. 1995;85(1):1–14.
94. Gruss HJ, Duyster J, Herrmann F. Structural and biological features of the TNF receptor and TNF ligand superfamilies: interactive signals in the pathobiology of Hodgkin's disease. Ann Oncol. 1996;7 Suppl 4:19–26.
95. Chiarle R, Podda A, Prolla G, et al. CD30 in normal and neoplastic cells. Clin Immunol. 1999; 90(2):157–64.
96. Gilfillan MC, Noel PJ, Podack ER, et al. Expression of the costimulatory receptor CD30 is regulated by both CD28 and cytokines. J Immunol. 1998;160(5): 2180–7.
97. Schwab U, Stein H, Gerdes J, et al. Production of a monoclonal antibody specific for Hodgkin and Sternberg-Reed cells of Hodgkin's disease and a subset of normal lymphoid cells. Nature. 1982;299(5878):65–7.
98. Stein H, Mason DY, Gerdes J, et al. The expression of the Hodgkin's disease associated antigen Ki-1 in reactive and neoplastic lymphoid tissue: evidence that Reed-Sternberg cells and histiocytic malignancies are derived from activated lymphoid cells. Blood. 1985;66(4):848–58.
99. Beljaards RC, Meijer CJ, Scheffer E, et al. Prognostic significance of CD30 (Ki-1/Ber-H2) expression in primary cutaneous large-cell lymphomas of T-cell origin. A clinicopathologic and immunohistochemical study in 20 patients. Am J Pathol. 1989;135(6): 1169–78.
100. Zinzani PL, Pileri S, Bendandi M, et al. Clinical implications of serum levels of soluble CD30 in 70 adult anaplastic large-cell lymphoma patients. J Clin Oncol. 1998;16(4):1532–7.
101. Hecht TT, Longo DL, Cossman J, et al. Production and characterization of a monoclonal antibody that binds Reed-Sternberg cells. J Immunol. 1985; 134(6):4231–6.
102. Norton AJ, Isaacson PG. Detailed phenotypic analysis of B-cell lymphoma using a panel of antibodies reactive in routinely fixed wax-embedded tissue. Am J Pathol. 1987;128(2):225–40.
103. Bowen MA, Olsen KJ, Cheng L, et al. Functional effects of CD30 on a large granular lymphoma cell line, YT. Inhibition of cytotoxicity, regulation of CD28 and IL-2R, and induction of homotypic aggregation. J Immunol. 1993;151(11):5896–906.
104. Gruss HJ, Boiani N, Williams DE, et al. Pleiotropic effects of the CD30 ligand on CD30-expressing cells and lymphoma cell lines. Blood. 1994;83(8): 2045–56.
105. Borchmann P, Treml JF, Hansen H, et al. The human anti-CD30 antibody 5F11 shows in vitro and in vivo activity against malignant lymphoma. Blood. 2003;102(10):3737–42.
106. Wahl AF, Klussman K, Thompson JD, et al. The anti-CD30 monoclonal antibody SGN-30 promotes growth arrest and DNA fragmentation in vitro and affects antitumor activity in models of Hodgkin's disease. Cancer Res. 2002;62(13):3736–42.
107. Hu XF, Xing PX. MDX-060. Medarex. Curr Opin Investig Drugs. 2005;6(12):1266–71.
108. Mir SS, Richter BW, Duckett CS. Differential effects of CD30 activation in anaplastic large cell lymphoma and Hodgkin disease cells. Blood. 2000;96(13): 4307–12.
109. Duckett CS, Gedrich RW, Gilfillan MC, et al. Induction of nuclear factor kappaB by the CD30 receptor is mediated by TRAF1 and TRAF2. Mol Cell Biol. 1997;17(3):1535–42.
110. Hirsch B, Hummel M, Bentink S, et al. CD30-induced signaling is absent in Hodgkin's cells but present in anaplastic large cell lymphoma cells. Am J Pathol. 2008;172(2):510–20.
111. Bargou RC, Leng C, Krappmann D, et al. High-level nuclear NF-kappa B and Oct-2 is a common feature of cultured Hodgkin/Reed-Sternberg cells. Blood. 1996;87(10):4340–7.
112. Tian ZG, Longo DL, Funakoshi S, et al. In vivo antitumor effects of unconjugated CD30 monoclonal antibodies on human anaplastic large-cell lymphoma xenografts. Cancer Res. 1995;55(22):5335–41.
113. Pfeifer W, Levi E, Petrogiannis-Haliotis T, et al. A murine xenograft model for human CD30+ anaplastic large cell lymphoma. Successful growth inhibition with an anti-CD30 antibody (HeFi-1). Am J Pathol. 1999;155(4):1353–9.
114. Pasqualucci L, Wasik M, Teicher BA, et al. Antitumor activity of anti-CD30 immunotoxin (Ber H2/saporin) in vitro and in severe combined immunodeficiency disease mice xenografted with human CD30+ anaplastic large-cell lymphoma. Blood. 1995;85(8):2139–46.
115. Ansell SM, Horwitz SM, Engert A, et al. Phase I/II study of an anti-CD30 monoclonal antibody (MDX-060) in Hodgkin's lymphoma and anaplastic large-cell lymphoma. J Clin Oncol. 2007;25(19):2764–9.
116. Bartlett NL, Younes A, Carabasi MH, et al. A phase 1 multidose study of SGN-30 immunotherapy in patients with refractory or recurrent CD30+ hematologic malignancies. Blood. 2008;111(4):1848–54.
117. Forero-Torres A, Leonard JP, Younes A, et al. A phase II study of SGN-30 (anti-CD30 mAb) in Hodgkin lymphoma or systemic anaplastic large cell lymphoma. Br J Haematol. 2009;146(2):171–9.

118. Duvic M, Reddy SA, Pinter-Brown L, et al. A phase II study of SGN-30 in cutaneous anaplastic large cell lymphoma and related lymphoproliferative disorders. Clin Cancer Res. 2009;15(19):6217–24.
119. Younes A, Yasothan U, Kirkpatrick P. Brentuximab vedotin. Nat Rev Drug Discov. 2012;11(1):19–20.
120. Foyil KV, Bartlett NL. Brentuximab vedotin for the treatment of CD30+ lymphomas. Immunotherapy. 2011;3(4):475–85.
121. Fanale MA, Forero-Torres A, Rosenblatt JD, et al. A phase I weekly dosing study of brentuximab vedotin in patients with relapsed/refractory CD30-positive hematologic malignancies. Clin Cancer Res. 2012;18(1):248–55.
122. Younes A, Bartlett NL, Leonard JP, et al. Brentuximab vedotin (SGN-35) for relapsed CD30-positive lymphomas. N Engl J Med. 2010;363(19):1812–21.
123. Wagner-Johnston ND, Bartlett NL, Cashen A, et al. Progressive multifocal leukoencephalopathy (PML) in a patient with Hodgkin's lymphoma treated with brentuximab vedotin. Leuk Lymphoma. 2012 [Epub ahead of print].
124. Hale G, Xia MQ, Tighe HP, et al. The CAMPATH-1 antigen (CDw52). Tissue Antigens. 1990;35(3): 118–27.
125. Xia MQ, Hale G, Lifely MR, et al. Structure of the CAMPATH-1 antigen, a glycosylphosphatidylinositol-anchored glycoprotein which is an exceptionally good target for complement lysis. Biochem J. 1993;293(Pt 3):633–40.
126. Watanabe T, Masuyama J, Sohma Y, et al. CD52 is a novel costimulatory molecule for induction of CD4+ regulatory T cells. Clin Immunol. 2006;120(3):247–59.
127. Elsner J, Hochstetter R, Spiekermann K, et al. Surface and mRNA expression of the CD52 antigen by human eosinophils but not by neutrophils. Blood. 1996;88(12):4684–93.
128. Ginaldi L, De Martinis M, Matutes E, et al. Levels of expression of CD52 in normal and leukemic B and T cells: correlation with in vivo therapeutic responses to Campath-1H. Leuk Res. 1998;22(2):185–91.
129. Hale G. The CD52 antigen and development of the CAMPATH antibodies. Cytotherapy. 2001;3(3):137–43.
130. Buggins AG, Mufti GJ, Salisbury J, et al. Peripheral blood but not tissue dendritic cells express CD52 and are depleted by treatment with alemtuzumab. Blood. 2002;100(5):1715–20.
131. Hale G, Rye PD, Warford A, et al. The glycosylphosphatidylinositol-anchored lymphocyte antigen CDw52 is associated with the epididymal maturation of human spermatozoa. J Reprod Immunol. 1993;23(2):189–205.
132. Gilleece MH, Dexter TM. Effect of Campath-1H antibody on human hematopoietic progenitors in vitro. Blood. 1993;82(3):807–12.
133. Olweus J, Lund-Johansen F, Terstappen LW. Expression of cell surface markers during differentiation of CD34+, CD38-/lo fetal and adult bone marrow cells. Immunomethods. 1994;5(3):179–88.
134. Rodig SJ, Abramson JS, Pinkus GS, et al. Heterogeneous CD52 expression among hematologic neoplasms: implications for the use of alemtuzumab (CAMPATH-1H). Clin Cancer Res. 2006; 12(23):7174–9.
135. Piccaluga PP, Agostinelli C, Righi S, et al. Expression of CD52 in peripheral T-cell lymphoma. Haematologica. 2007;92(4):566–7.
136. Lapalombella R, Zhao X, Triantafillou G, et al. A novel Raji-Burkitt's lymphoma model for preclinical and mechanistic evaluation of CD52-targeted immunotherapeutic agents. Clin Cancer Res. 2008; 14(2):569–78.
137. Salisbury JR, Rapson NT, Codd JD, et al. Immunohistochemical analysis of CDw52 antigen expression in non-Hodgkin's lymphomas. J Clin Pathol. 1994;47(4):313–7.
138. Jiang L, Yuan CM, Hubacheck J, et al. Variable CD52 expression in mature T cell and NK cell malignancies: implications for alemtuzumab therapy. Br J Haematol. 2009;145(2):173–9.
139. Dearden CE, Matutes E. Alemtuzumab in T-cell lymphoproliferative disorders. Best Pract Res Clin Haematol. 2006;19(4):795–810.
140. Keating MJ, Flinn I, Jain V, et al. Therapeutic role of alemtuzumab (Campath-1H) in patients who have failed fludarabine: results of a large international study. Blood. 2002;99(10):3554–61.
141. Hillmen P, Skotnicki AB, Robak T, et al. Alemtuzumab compared with chlorambucil as first-line therapy for chronic lymphocytic leukemia. J Clin Oncol. 2007;25(35):5616–23.
142. Xia MQ, Hale G, Waldmann H. Efficient complement-mediated lysis of cells containing the CAMPATH-1 (CDw52) antigen. Mol Immunol. 1993;30(12):1089–96.
143. Zhang Z, Zhang M, Goldman CK, et al. Effective therapy for a murine model of adult T-cell leukemia with the humanized anti-CD52 monoclonal antibody, Campath-1H. Cancer Res. 2003;63(19): 6453–7.
144. Golay J, Manganini M, Rambaldi A, et al. Effect of alemtuzumab on neoplastic B cells. Haematologica. 2004;89(12):1476–83.
145. Zent CS, Chen JB, Kurten RC, et al. Alemtuzumab (CAMPATH 1H) does not kill chronic lymphocytic leukemia cells in serum free medium. Leuk Res. 2004;28(5):495–507.
146. Nuckel H, Frey UH, Roth A, et al. Alemtuzumab induces enhanced apoptosis in vitro in B-cells from patients with chronic lymphocytic leukemia by antibody-dependent cellular cytotoxicity. Eur J Pharmacol. 2005;514(2–3):217–24.
147. Lowenstein H, Shah A, Chant A, et al. Different mechanisms of Campath-1H-mediated depletion for CD4 and CD8 T cells in peripheral blood. Transpl Int. 2006;19(11):927–36.
148. Hale G, Rebello P, Brettman LR, et al. Blood concentrations of alemtuzumab and antiglobulin

responses in patients with chronic lymphocytic leukemia following intravenous or subcutaneous routes of administration. Blood. 2004;104(4):948–55.

149. Wing MG, Moreau T, Greenwood J, et al. Mechanism of first-dose cytokine-release syndrome by CAMPATH 1-H: involvement of CD16 (FcgammaRIII) and CD11a/CD18 (LFA-1) on NK cells. J Clin Invest. 1996;98(12):2819–26.
150. Dearden CE, Matutes E, Cazin B, et al. High remission rate in T-cell prolymphocytic leukemia with CAMPATH-1H. Blood. 2001;98(6):1721–6.
151. Lundin J, Osterborg A, Brittinger G, et al. CAMPATH-1H monoclonal antibody in therapy for previously treated low-grade non-Hodgkin's lymphomas: a phase II multicenter study. European Study Group of CAMPATH-1H treatment in low-grade non-Hodgkin's lymphoma. J Clin Oncol. 1998;16(10):3257–63.
152. Lundin J, Hagberg H, Repp R, et al. Phase 2 study of alemtuzumab (anti-CD52 monoclonal antibody) in patients with advanced mycosis fungoides/Sezary syndrome. Blood. 2003;101(11):4267–72.
153. Kennedy GA, Seymour JF, Wolf M, et al. Treatment of patients with advanced mycosis fungoides and Sézary syndrome with alemtuzumab. Eur J Haematol. 2003;71(4):250–6.
154. Zinzani PL, Alinari L, Tani M, et al. Preliminary observations of a phase II study of reduced-dose alemtuzumab treatment in patients with pretreated T-cell lymphoma. Haematologica. 2005;90(5):702–3.
155. Bernengo MG, Quaglino P, Comessatti A, et al. Low-dose intermittent alemtuzumab in the treatment of Sézary syndrome: clinical and immunologic findings in 14 patients. Haematologica. 2007;92(6):784–94.
156. Enblad G, Hagberg H, Erlanson M, et al. A pilot study of alemtuzumab (anti-CD52 monoclonal antibody) therapy for patients with relapsed or chemotherapy-refractory peripheral T-cell lymphomas. Blood. 2004;103(8):2920–4.
157. Absi A, Hsi E, Kalaycio M. Prolymphocytic leukemia. Curr Treat Options Oncol. 2005;6(3):197–208.
158. Keating MJ, Cazin B, Coutré S, et al. Campath-1H treatment of T-cell prolymphocytic leukemia in patients for whom at least one prior chemotherapy regimen has failed. J Clin Oncol. 2002;20(1):205–13.
159. Lenihan DJ, Alencar AJ, Yang D, et al. Cardiac toxicity of alemtuzumab in patients with mycosis fungoides/Sézary syndrome. Blood. 2004;104(3):655–8.
160. Lundin J, Kennedy B, Dearden C, et al. No cardiac toxicity associated with alemtuzumab therapy for mycosis fungoides/Sézary syndrome. Blood. 2005;105(10):4148–9.
161. Gibbs SD, Herbert KE, McCormack C, et al. Alemtuzumab: effective monotherapy for simultaneous B-cell chronic lymphocytic leukaemia and Sézary syndrome. Eur J Haematol. 2004;73(6):447–9.
162. Gautschi O, Blumenthal N, Streit M, et al. Successful treatment of chemotherapy-refractory Sézary syndrome with alemtuzumab (Campath-1H). Eur J Haematol. 2004;72(1):61–3.
163. Capalbo S, Delia M, Dargenio M, et al. Mycosis fungoides/Sézary syndrome: a report of three cases treated with Campath-1H as salvage treatment. Med Oncol. 2003;20(4):389–96.
164. Kim JG, Sohn SK, Chae YS, et al. Alemtuzumab plus CHOP as front-line chemotherapy for patients with peripheral T-cell lymphomas: a phase II study. Cancer Chemother Pharmacol. 2007;60(1):129–34.
165. Gallamini A, Zaja F, Patti C, et al. Alemtuzumab (Campath-1H) and CHOP chemotherapy as first-line treatment of peripheral T-cell lymphoma: results of a GITIL (Gruppo Italiano Terapie Innovative nei Linfomi) prospective multicenter trial. Blood. 2007;110(7):2316–23.
166. Intragumtornchai T, Bunworasate U, Nakorn TN, et al. Alemtuzumab in combination with CHOP and ESHAP as first-line treatment in peripheral T-cell lymphoma [ASH annual meeting abstracts]. Blood. 2006;108:4740.
167. Weidmann E, Hess G, Chow KU, et al. A phase II study of alemtuzumab, fludarabine, cyclophosphamide, and doxorubicin (Campath-FCD) in peripheral T-cell lymphomas. Leuk Lymphoma. 2010;51(3):447–55.
168. Osterborg A, Karlsson C, Lundin J, et al. Strategies in the management of alemtuzumab-related side effects. Semin Oncol. 2006;33(2 Suppl 5):S29–35.
169. Weisel KC, Weidmann E, Anagnostopoulos I, et al. Epstein-Barr virus-associated B-cell lymphoma secondary to FCD-C therapy in patients with peripheral T-cell lymphoma. Int J Hematol. 2008;88(4):434–40.
170. Kluin-Nelemans HC, Coenen JL, Boers JE, et al. EBV-positive immunodeficiency lymphoma after alemtuzumab-CHOP therapy for peripheral T-cell lymphoma. Blood. 2008;112(4):1039–41.
171. Majeau GR, Meier W, Jimmo B, et al. Mechanism of lymphocyte function-associated molecule 3-Ig fusion proteins inhibition of T cell responses. Structure/function analysis in vitro and in human CD2 transgenic mice. J Immunol. 1994;152(6):2753–67.
172. Branco L, Barren P, Mao SY, et al. Selective deletion of antigen-specific, activated T cells by a humanized MAB to CD2 (MEDI-507) is mediated by NK cells. Transplantation. 1999;68(10):1588–96.
173. Kung P, Goldstein G, Reinherz EL, et al. Monoclonal antibodies defining distinctive human T cell surface antigens. Science. 1979;206(4416):347–9.
174. Ravel S, Colombatti M, Casellas P. Internalization and intracellular fate of anti-CD5 monoclonal antibody and anti-CD5 ricin A-chain immunotoxin in human leukemic T cells. Blood. 1992;79(6):1511–7.
175. Foss FM. DAB(389)IL-2 (ONTAK): a novel fusion toxin therapy for lymphoma. Clin Lymphoma. 2000;1(2):110–6.

Nucleoside Analogs in the Therapy of T-Cell Malignancies

15

Varsha Gandhi and Pier Luigi Zinzani

Introduction

The nucleoside analogs (NA) are one of the most active classes of drugs in patients with T-cell lymphoma. The analogs have developed based on the discovery metabolic syndromes associated with deficiency of purine catabolizing enzymes. The lack of adenosine deaminase (ADA) enzyme was associated with a variant of severe combined immunodeficiency syndrome where patient suffered with both B- and T-lymphocytopenia [1]. Deficiency of purine nucleoside phosphorylase on the other hand leads to T-lymphocytopenia in pediatric patients [2]. ADA and PNP enzymes are involved in metabolic clearance of dAdo and dGuo, respectively. As a result in these patients there is an accumulation of these nucleosides in the plasma and triphosphate (i.e., dATP and dGTP) in the cells. Inherently, T-cells have high levels of ADA, a key enzyme in the dAdo degradation pathway. Potent inhibitors of ADA and PNP were developed and two of these, deoxycoformycin and forodesine, made to the clinic and have been tested effectively in T-cell lymphoma. Among the pyrimidine nucleoside analogs, gemcitabine has shown efficacy in T-cell malignancies. For purine nucleoside agents, cladribine and fludarabine have shown activity in mature T-cell leukemias, with overall response rates between 35 and 41% [3, 4]. Nelarabine has shown selectivity and specificity for T-cell diseases that include leukemias and lymphomas. This chapter reviews and summarizes the activity of these agents in T-cell neoplasms.

V. Gandhi
Departments of Experimental Therapeutics and Leukemia, MD Anderson Cancer Center, Houston, TX, USA

P.L. Zinzani (✉)
Institute of Hematology "Seràgnoli," University of Bologna, Via Massarenti 9, Bologna 40138, Italy
e-mail: pierluigi.zinzani@unibo.it

Pentostatin

Structure and Synthesis

Pentostatin (2′-deoxycoformycin), a natural product, is a potent transition state inhibitor of adenosine [5, 6]. Structurally it resembles the ADA substrate dAdo but binds tightly with the enzyme resulting in its inhibition (Fig. 15.1; [7]).

Metabolism and Mechanisms of Action

There is very limited phosphorylation of deoxycoformycin itself [8]. The drug directly inhibits ADA enzyme. As this enzyme mediates the normal metabolic clearance of deoxyadenosine, inhibition of this enzyme cause deoxyadenosine levels to increase in plasma [9, 10] as do the dATP in erythrocytes and leukemia cells [11–14] mimicking ADA deficiency syndrome [15].

F. Foss (ed.), *T-Cell Lymphomas*, Contemporary Hematology,
DOI 10.1007/978-1-62703-170-7_15, © Springer Science+Business Media New York 2013

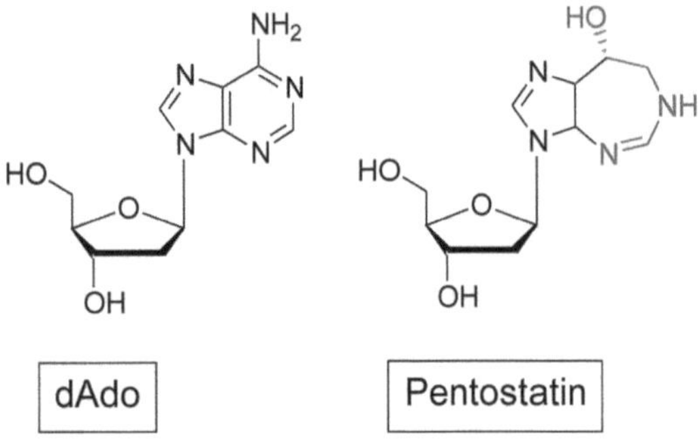

Fig. 15.1 Structures of deoxyadenosine and inhibitor of adenosine deaminase, pentostatin

Because deoxyadenosine uses deoxycytidine kinase for its phosphorylation, this enzyme is important for this drug also.

It is thought that the imbalance of deoxynucleotide pools caused by this greatly increased dATP concentration activates cell death mechanisms. More importantly, dATP is a global inactivator of the activity of ribonucleotide reductase and inhibits its conversion of all four ribodiphosphates to their deoxy-forms [16]. Hence, this perturbation of dNTP pool results in inhibition of DNA synthesis and initiation of cell death. Additionally, dATP has been demonstrated to be part of apoptosomes; these are formed by cytochrome C, Apaf-1, procaspase 9, and dATP [17]. Binding of dATP triggers the reaction leading to cleavage of procaspase 9 to caspase 9 and downstream effect on the activation of caspase 3; the route which is known as intrinsic cell death pathway. Hence accumulation of increased dATP could further activate cell death pathway [18].

Pentostatin as a Single Agent in the Clinic

Pentostatin has been the most extensively studied in T-cell lymphoma and has shown variable response rates. However, many of the reports are limited to small single-center studies. Larger prospective randomized trials will be necessary to examine this therapy and to further explore combination regimens, which may result in increased responses. In the earliest clinical trials pentostatin was used in high doses to treat patients with T acute lymphoblastic leukemia (T-ALL) [19]. This was associated with treatment limiting toxicities. Since that time pentostatin in lower, well tolerated, doses has shown remarkable activity in patients with hairy-cell leukemia, chronic lymphocytic leukemia, low-grade B-cell malignancies as well as in T-cell lymphoma [20]. The commonly used schedule now is intravenous administration of pentostatin at 4 mg/m^2 given every 1–2 weeks. Other higher dose schedules have also been used in reported studies. Dose adjustments are required if renal function is impaired.

The majority of data evaluating pentostatin in T-cell lymphomas is based on trials in cutaneous T-cell lymphoma (CTCL). There are also reports that support the activity of these agents in other mature T-cell malignancies (Table 15.1). In the early 1980s, there were small reports describing the effectiveness of pentostatin in patients with T-cell leukemias, including patients refractory to other therapy [19, 20, 27–30]. The European Organization for Research and Treatment for Cancer Leukemia Cooperative Study Group (EORTC) conducted a Phase II trial that included 76 patients with advanced T-cell malignancies, including 25 patients with what was then termed “T chronic lymphocytic leukemia” (T-CLL) [21] (Table 15.1). The response rate with pentostatin was 8% with a median disease-free survival of 22 weeks. T-CLL has been reclassified by WHO as T prolymphocytic leukemia (T-PLL), which has been shown in other studies to be responsive to pentostatin. The first case study was published in 1986, showing that two patients achieved remission following pentostatin [31]. In the early 1990s, Matutes et al. [22] published a report of 78 patients with T-PLL describing the clinical and laboratory features of the disease. Of the 78 patients, 31 were treated with pentostatin. There were 15 responses (48%) including 3 complete responses (CR) and 12 partial responses (PR). Another phase II study conducted by the EORTC treated 20 patients with T- or B-prolymphocytic leukemia with weekly pentostatin [23]. Of the 20 patients, 6 patients had T-PLL. There were nine overall responders in the entire study population

Table 15.1 Summary of ADA inhibitor, pentostatin, studies in peripheral T-cell lymphomas and other mature T-cell malignancies

Study	Dose	Total # patients	Patients subset	CR (%)	PR (%)	ORR (%)	Median overall survival
Ho et al. [21]	4 mg/m² Q week × 3 then Q 2 week × 6 then Q month × 6	N = 76 (T-cell NHL)	T-CLL = 25	0	8	8	DFS = 22 weeks
Matutes et al. [22]	4 mg/m² Q week	N = 78 (T-PLL)	Pentostatin treated = 31	9	39	48 (58)	16 months (responders) 10 months (nonresponders) 7 months (patients not treated with pentostatin)
Dohner et al. [23]	4 mg/m² Q week × 3 then Q 2 week × 3 if PR, Q month × 6	N = 20 (B & T-PLL)	T-PLL = 6	0	33	33	N/A
Dearden et al. [24]	4 mg/m² Q week × 4 then Q 2 week till optimal response	N = 68 (T-cell NHL)	T-PLL = 31 ATLL = 20 LGL = 4	9 10 25	39 5 0	48 (58) 15 (18) 25 (50)	T-PLL (10–16 months) ATLL (N/A) LGL (N/A)
Mercieca et al. [25]	4 mg/m² Q week × 4 then Q 2 week till optimal response	N = 145 (T-cell NHL)	T-PLL = 55 LGL = 5 ATLL = 25	9 40 8	40 0 4	45 40 12	N/A
Tsimberidou et al. [26]	5 mg/m²/day × 3 days q 3 weeks	N = 42	PTCL = 4 ATLL = 3 ALCL = 1	50 0 0	50 33 0	100 33 0	Median 4 months (1–61)

(45%) including two (33%) of the patients with T-PLL. All of the responses were PR and the median duration of response was 9 months (range 2–30 months). The majority of patients (85%) enrolled in this study had received prior chemotherapy. By far the largest published experience with pentostatin in mature T-cell malignancies has been at the Royal Marsden Hospital in London [24, 25, 32] (Table 15.1). A total of 165 patients who had a range of relapsed/refractory post-thymic T-cell malignancies received pentostatin at a dose of 4 mg/m^2 weekly for 4 weeks and then every 2 weeks until maximal response. Responses were seen in 34% of patients with a median response duration of 6 months (range 3 months to 15 years). Some patients had durable remissions, with disease subtypes the main predictor of response; T-PLL and Sézary syndrome (SS) had the best response rates of 45% and 62%, respectively. Only a minority (<10%) of these responses were complete. Although some of the remissions have been prolonged (up to 15 years in an SS patient) most patients relapsed within 1 year [25]. Activity in ATLL was disappointing and this has been confirmed by a number of studies in Japan. Tsimberidou et al. [26] published the most recent report of pentostatin in peripheral T-cell lymphoma (PTCL), using a different dose schedule (5 $mg/m^2 \times 3$ days).

Table 15.2 summarizes the role of pentostatin in CTCL. Forty-two patients including 32 (76%) with mycosis fungoides (MF)/SS and 10 patients (24%) with other T-cell leukemias or lymphomas were enrolled. The overall response rate was 54.8% (CR = 14.3% and PR = 40.5%). Durable responses were observed mainly in patients with SS or PTCL. The median duration of response was 4.3 months (range 1–61 months). Several other smaller studies of pentostatin as a single agent in previously treated CTCL showed an overall response rate of approximately 50% (range 26–100%) [33–36]. The first report was by Grever et al. [33] in four patients with advanced refractory MF, with two achieving CR and two PR. Subsequent trials did not confirm these high response rates for MF with responses (mostly PR) seen in 0–57%. The distinction was not always clear between MF and SS in these studies but, where stated, the best responses were seen in erythrodermic CTCL/SS. Again, response rates appear to be dose-related. There have been numerous case reports of successful treatment of other, rarer, T-cell malignancies, including T-large granular lymphocyte (LGL) leukemia [38–40], hepatosplenic T-cell lymphoma [41–43], and granulomatous slack skin disease [44].

Pentostatin Combination Therapy

A study combining pentostatin with interferon-α for the treatment of refractory CTCL showed an increased response rate compared with historic data using pentostatin alone, with a response duration of 13 months [37]. Monoclonal antibody therapy is also emerging as a promising approach to treating PTCL. The anti-CD52 antibody alemtuzumab is an effective therapy in PTCL [45] and has produced durable responses in two-thirds of heavily pretreated patients with T-PLL [46]. There is some limited experience of the combination of pentostatin and alemtuzumab [47] and this deserves further exploration. However, the increased risk of infection must be considered.

There are other agents which have also shown single agent activity in small numbers of patients with PTCL, including anti-CD4 and anti-CD25 monoclonal antibodies, denileukin diftitox (ONTAK), bexarotene, and histone deacetylase (HDAC) inhibitors. Further study will be necessary to delineate the role of any of these agents in combination with purine analogs.

Forodesine

Structure and Synthesis

Several inhibitors of PNP that block dGuo degradation have been synthesized, developed, and tested in in vitro cultures and some were brought to animal in vivo systems (reviewed in [48]). None were potent enough to be effectively used in the clinic [49, 50]. A new strategy has subsequently been used to develop powerful inhibitor by identification of the transition-state structure

Table 15.2 Summary of trials of ADA inhibitor, pentostatin, in CTCL

Study	Pentostatin dose	Total # patients	CR (%)	PR (%)	ORR(%)	Duration of response
Ho et al. [21]	4 mg/m^2 Q week × 3	21 SS	5	28	33	
	then Q 2 week × 6 then Q month × 5	22 MF	0	23	23	
Dearden et al. [24]	4 mg/m^2 week × 4	7 SS	14	86	100	(not reported)
	then QOW	6 MF	0	0	0	
Mercieca et al. [25]	4 mg/m^2 Q week × 4	16 SS	19	44	63	9 month for SS
	then Q 2 week till optional response	4 SL	0	50	50	
		13 MF	0	0	0	
Grever et al. [33]	4 mg/m^2 × 3 days then monthly	18	11	22	33	CR (7–10 month) PR (1–3 month)
Cummings et al. [34]	5 mg/m^2 x 3 days, Q 3 week	6	0	67	67	
Greiner et al. [35]	4 mg/m^2 QOW	18	11	28	39	CR (4 month–6 year) PR (1.5–6 month)
Kurzrock et al. [36]	3.75–5 mg/m^2 day × 3 days q 3 weeks	24	29	43	71	3.2 month for SS 2 month for MF
Foss et al. [37]	Alternating w/IFN	41	5	37	42	15.8 month

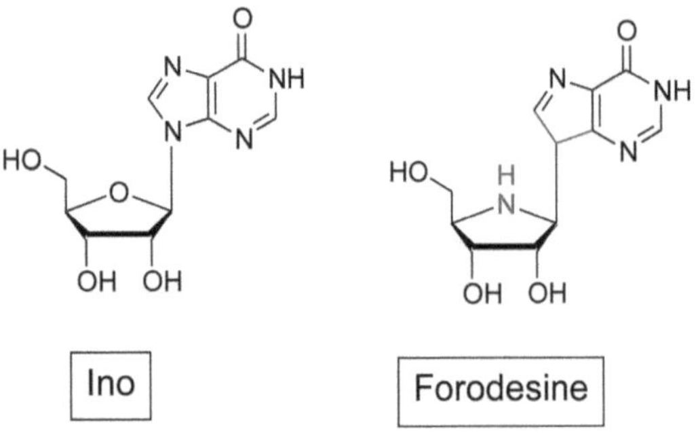

Fig. 15.2 Structures of inosine and inhibitor of purine nucleoside phosphorylase, forodesine

stabilized by the target enzyme. Using inosine as a substrate for transition-state analysis, a series of 9-deazanucleoside analogs, termed immucillins, was designed to mimic the transition-state (Fig. 15.2; [49]). The immucillins have a carbon–carbon linkage between a cyclic amine moiety that replaces ribose, and either 9-deaza-hypoxanthine (immucillin H, now forodesine, Fig. 15.2) and or 9-deaza-guanine (immucillin G), respectively. Chemically forodesine is [(1S)-1-(9-deazahypoxanthin-9-yl)-1,4-dideoxy-1,4-imino-D-ribitol]. These analogs inhibited PNP with high potency; the Ki values were in 20–80 pM range for human and bovine enzyme [51].

Metabolism and Mechanisms of Action

Forodesine itself is a poor substrate for phosphorylation and no metabolites were detected in cells when incubated with this compound [51]. Hence forodesine's actions are through PNP inhibition. Consistent with this statement, cells incubated with forodesine alone (without deoxyguanosine) did not have any cytotoxic effects. Because in the body PNP is responsible for metabolic clearance of deoxyguanosine; the levels of dGuo increases in the plasma when animals are infused with forodesine [52].

In vitro cytotoxicity to T-lineage leukemia cells requires deoxycytidine kinase and the presence of dGuo. This was associated with elevation of dGTP (154-fold), which was significantly higher than dGTP accumulation in normal lymphocytes (15-fold) [51, 53]. The proposed mechanism of action of forodesine is that the high accumulation of dGTP inhibits the ribonucleotide reductase. However, decrease in pyrimidine deoxynucleotides was not observed in leukemia blasts during therapy. Although the exact mechanism is not known, the nuclear consequence of the deregulated levels of deoxynucleotide pools inhibits DNA synthesis that eventually leads to cellular death [54].

Pharmacology studies demonstrated that cytotoxicity was associated with elevated plasma deoxyguanosine [54] and the pronounced intracellular accumulation of dGTP [54]. Models of this metabolic disease demonstrated that immature T lymphocytes and T-lymphoblastoid cells were selectively sensitive to treatment with deoxyguanosine, whereas lymphocytes of B cell lineage did not accumulate high levels of dGTP and were much less sensitive to deoxyguanosine [55–58]. Hence, for forodesine dGuo acts as a drug. Primary leukemia cells when incubated with forodesine and deoxyguanosine showed cytotoxicity which was directly correlated to levels of dGTP increase in leukemia cells [59] and resulted in increase in proapoptotic Bim protein [60].

Forodesine as a Single Agent in the Clinic

A phase I clinical trial, performed by Gandhi et al. [54], was designed to determine the maximum tolerated dose for forodesine and to correlate the drug pharmacodynamics to the administered dose. The patients with relapsed or refractory T-cell disorders were treated with forodesine at a dose of 40 mg/m^2 over 30 min of IV infusion on the first day, then the treatment was continued for days 2–5 at the same dose administered twice daily and repeated every 21–28 days. Recently, Furman et al. [61] have presented spectacular results of phase IIa, multicenter, open-label, single-arm, repeated dose, ongoing clinical trial in patients with advanced precursor T-ALL or T-PLL. Forodesine was administered intravenously, at the dose 40 mg/m^2 for 5 days weekly for a total of six cycles. In total

Table 15.3 Results of clinical trials with PNP inhibitor, forodesine

Drug	Phase	Disease	N	CR (%)	PR (%)	ORR (%)	Author
Forodesine	I	T-ALL T-PLL	5	0	0	0	Gandhi et al. [54]
	II	T-ALL T-PLL	34	21	11	32	Furman et al. [61]
	II	T-ALL	3	100	–	100	Stelljes et al. [62]
	I/II	CTCL	28	7	46	53	Duvic et al. [64]

34 pretreated patients, OR rate was 32.4% and CR was achieved in 20.6%. Time to progression for CR patients was 77–398 days and OS were 77–459 days. In the analyzed group only two patients died. In another report by Stelljes et al. [62], forodesine was given at 40 mg/m^2 for 5 days up to six cycles in three patients with refractory/relapsed T-ALL (two patients were prior to and one post-allogeneic hematopoietic stem cells transplantation; HSCT). Up to the publication of the study all three were alive and in CR with survival of 215+, 398+, and 180+ days, respectively. In authors' opinion, forodesine used in monotherapy can be effective before and after allogeneic HSCT with minimal toxicity and without affecting potential graft versus leukemia effect. Recently, Gore et al. [63] have shown that forodesine contributed to a primary antileukemic cytotoxic effect as well as a secondary immunologic effect by allowing the development of an ongoing graft-versus leukemia effect in T-ALL patients who relapsed following allogeneic HSCT and were treated with this drug.

Forodesine is clinically active also in CTCL. In a multicenter phase I/II, dose-escalation study, forodesine was administered IV at doses between 40 and 135 mg/m^2 [64]. In this study one CR (8%) and two PR (15%) were obtained. Recently, the same authors submitted results of phase I/II open-label a dose-escalation study, evaluating efficacy of oral forodesine administration at the doses from 40 to 320 mg/m^2 in 28 refractory CTCL patients. The OR rate was 53.6% (7.1% with CR and 46.4% with PR). Only lymphopenia of grade 3 or 4 was observed in two patients (5%) [65]. Results of clinical trials with forodesine used as monotherapy are presented in Table 15.3.

Gemcitabine

Structure and Synthesis

Gemcitabine was synthesized at Eli Lilly by Larry Hertel [66] based on the fact that the atomic radius of hydrogen is similar to that of fluorine which suggested that metabolic enzymes may utilize a fluorine substituted nucleoside analog with high efficiency. This postulate was correct as gemcitabine is the best substrate known for deoxycytidine kinase with Km value of 1–10 μM [67, 68]. The positioning of geminal fluorine at the 2′-position inspired the generic name of the drug (Fig. 15.3).

Metabolism and Mechanisms of Action

Similar to cytarabine, gemcitabine is cleared rapidly by deamination [69], although because it is a much better substrate for phosphorylation by deoxycytidine kinase, high levels of gemcitabine triphosphate accumulate in different cell types during in vitro incubations [70, 71] and during therapy [72–74].

Gemcitabine has multiple mechanisms of actions and most of these actions are DNA-directed. The diphosphate of gemcitabine has been studied extensively regarding its biochemical actions on both subunits of ribonucleotide reductase to illustrate a mechanism-based irreversible inactivation of the enzyme [75, 76]. X-ray crystallographic studies with ribonucleotide reductase bound to gemcitabine diphosphate illustrates that the binding is different than the natural substrate CDP [77]. Unlike other known

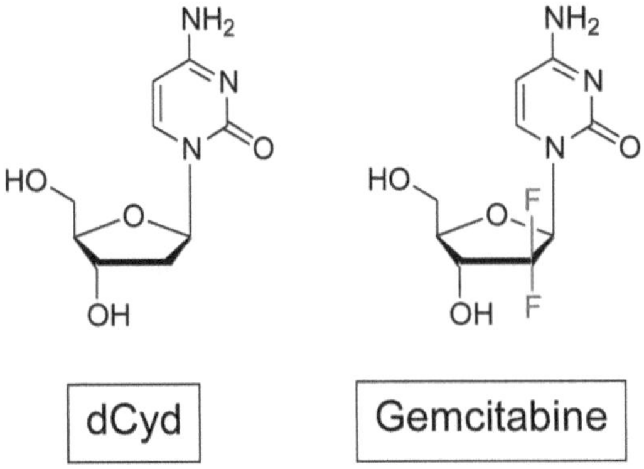

Fig. 15.3 Structures of deoxycytidine and its analog gemcitabine

ribonucleotide reductase inhibits, such as hydroxyurea, fludarabine, cladribine, and clofarabine triphosphate and dATP (accumulates with pentostatin), gemcitabine diphosphate is irreversible inhibitor. Hence the activity of the enzyme is restored only after new synthesis of the enzyme once the inhibitor is removed. Studies have demonstrated role of this action on cytotoxicity especially combination chemotherapy [78]. In addition, inhibition of ribonucleotide reductase results in a decrease in cellular dCTP pool which activates deoxycytidine kinase activity [67] and may facilitate incorporation of gemcitabine triphosphate into DNA [79, 80].

The activities of gemcitabine are DNA-directed in that the nucleoside and its nucleotides interact with numerous metabolic enzymes in the deoxycytidine salvage pathway acting as inhibitory alternative substrates for some. [70]. Gemcitabine is novel among nucleoside analogs as it is active against numerous solid tumors.

Incorporation of the analog in DNA is considered as the primary cytotoxic lesion leading to cell death [81]. Incorporation into DNA is followed by a DNA damage response and recent data suggest that the MRN complex (Mre11-Rad50-Nbs1 complex), which is involved in recognition and repair of double strand breaks is activated in response to gemcitabine-mediated stalled replication forks [82, 83]. Also role of ATM and DNA-PK as molecular sensors for replication halt has been identified [81, 82].

Gemcitabine as a Single Agent in the Clinic

In hematopoietic malignancies, gemcitabine has shown a high level of activity as a single agent in relapsed or refractory Hodgkin's disease and some degree of efficacy in aggressive and indolent non-Hodgkin's lymphoma. Among the several second-line and experimental drugs for PTCL and CTCL, gemcitabine should be considered among the most suitable options to date for pretreated PTCLU and MF patients. Gemcitabine has been demonstrated to be an effective monotherapy with a 60–70% overall response rate in patients with advanced, heavily pretreated patients [84–87]. In a phase II trial, Zinzani et al. [86] treated 44 consecutive, previously treated patients with MF (30 cases) and PTCLU (14 cases) with exclusive skin involvement. Gemcitabine was given to all patients on days 1,8, and 15 of a 28-day schedule at a dose of 1,200 mg/m for a total of three cycles. Of the 44 patients, 5 (11.5%) achieved CR, 26 (59%) PR, and the remaining 13 showed no benefit from the treatment. Two of the CRs were histologically confirmed. The complete and partial response rates were the same for patients with MF and those with PTCLU, respectively. No difference in terms of overall response rate was observed between relapsed and refractory patients. The median durations of CR and PR were 15 months and 10 months, respectively. Two other studies have shown good activity when using gemcitabine for the treatment of patients with refractory T-cell lymphoma. Sallah et al. [85] reported their experience in ten patients with refractory and relapsed T-cell malignancies treated with gemcitabine. Two patients had CTCL, two T-PLL, two nodal PTCL, two small lymphocytic lymphoma, one anaplastic, and one angiocentric lymphoma. The drug dose was the conventional 1,200 mg/m^2 on days 1, 8, and 15 of each 28-day cycle. Of the ten patients, two achieved a complete response (one T-PLL and one anaplastic) and four a partial response (two CTCL, one angiocentric, one PTCL) for an overall response rate of 60%. The median and mean duration of response was 13 months and 16 months, respectively. The second trial was conducted at the M.D. Anderson

Cancer Center [84]. Thirty-three pretreated CTCL patients received gemcitabine at a lower dose of 1,000 mg/m^2 for six or more cycles. Thirty-one patients had MF; the overall response rate was 68% including three CR. These findings show that gemcitabine has substantial activity and acceptable toxicity in previously treated patients with MF and PTCL.

In addition, there are also interesting data in untreated patients [88] and few data describing the efficacy of gemcitabine combinations in patients with T-cell lymphoma [89–93]. For these reasons we ran a phase IIb multicenter study with gemcitabine as primary chemotherapy of patients with advanced CTCL (or pretreated only with PUVA or radiotherapy). The patients were recruited from the Italian Cutaneous Lymphoma Study Group. Thirty-two patients with untreated MF, PTCLU, and SS were treated with gemcitabine in seven Italian institutions. Twenty-six of 32 patients had a diagnosis of MF, 5 were diagnosed with PTCLU, and only 1 patient had SS. The median age of the patients was 58 years (range *25–77* year); 22 patients were male and 10 were female. Of the 32 patients studied, 4 had been previously treated with local radiotherapy, 10 had received previous PUVA therapy, and 8 had been treated previously with PUVA and radiotherapy, whereas 10 patients had not received any previous treatment. Gemcitabine was given to all patients on days 1, 8, and 15 of a 28-day schedule at a dose of 1,200 mg/m2 per day for a total of six cycles. The overall response rate (CR+PR) was 75% (24 of 32 patients). The CR were 22% (7 of 32 patients) and 53% (17 of 32 patients), respectively. Patients with MF had a CR rate of 23% (6 of 26 patients) and a PR rate of 50% (13 of 26 patients). Conversely, patients with PTCLU had a CR rate of 20% (1 of 5 patients) and a PR rate of 80% (4 of 5 patients). Of the seven patients who achieved a CR, three were still in disease remission after a median follow-up of 10 months (range 4–22). The median PFS and OS were, respectively, 10 months and 19 months.

Its modest toxicity profile and the easy schedule of administration make gemcitabine an ideal agent for consideration in the development of chemotherapy regimens. In particular, it would be interesting to evaluate the use of two different nucleoside analogs (fludarabine or pentostatin plus gemcitabine) in modulating the entry route into DNA and their action in terms of direct cytotoxicity and apoptosis, respectively. Earlier investigations demonstrated the possibility of potentiating fludarabine with low doses of gemcitabine. In addition, combinations of gemcitabine with other compounds are under investigation. For example pralatrexate, a 10-deazaaminopterin derivative is a novel antifolate designed to have high affinity for the reduced folate carrier type I [94]. The combination of pralatrexate with gemcitabine is currently being explored in a phase I/II clinical trial.

Hematologic toxicities: anemia of WHO grade III was observed in 5–10% of patients, neutropenia of WHO grades III and IV in 20% and 10% of patients, respectively, WHO grade III and IV thrombocytopenia in 20% and 10% of patients, respectively. Non-hematologic toxicity: transient elevations in liver transaminases were observed in 5–10% of patients. Renal and pulmonary toxicity was very rare; WHO grade III and IV less than 1%. Flu-like symptoms with headache, fever, myalgias, and fatigue occurred in up to 10% of patients. No alopecia usually occurs during gemcitabine therapy. Neurotoxicity in connection with gemcitabine is rare. Peripheral edema occurs in 10% of patients. These toxicities were usually mild and reversible after the end of therapy.

Nelarabine

Structure and Synthesis

Nelarabine (Arranon®) resembles arabinosylguanine and acts as a prodrug of ara-G which is an analog of natural nucleoside deoxyguanosine (Fig. 15.2). Chemically it is 2-amino-9-β-D-arabinofuranosyl-6-methoxy-9H-purine and also known as compound-506U78, and GW506U. There were two reasons for an interest in ara-G prodrug. First, due to the success of cytarabine arabinosyl analogs were created with other bases

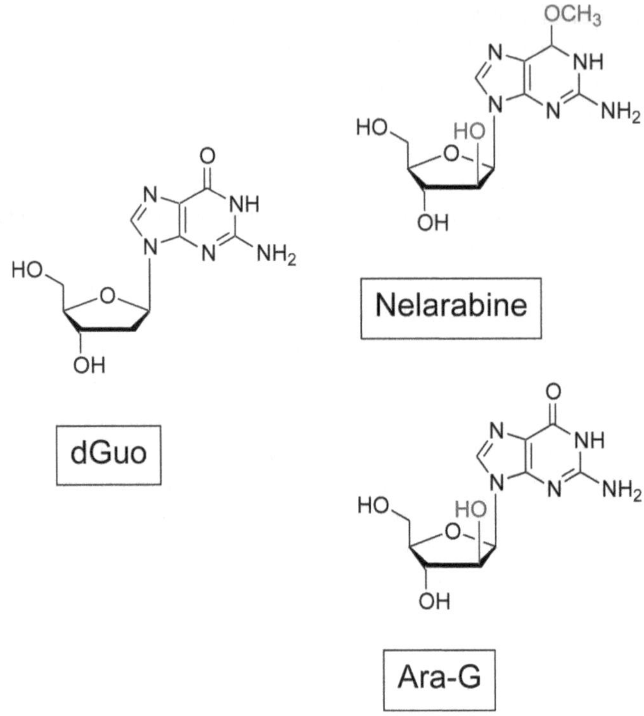

Fig. 15.4 Structures of deoxyguanosine and its analog nelarabine which acts as a prodrug for analog arabinosylguanine

such as adenine and guanine. Second, as mentioned earlier, the discovery that genetic deficiency of PNP results in a profound T-cell lymphopenia suggested that analog of dGuo which is resistant to PNP may show selectivity to T-cells.

Reist and Goodman [95] devised procedures for the chemical synthesis of 9-β-D-arabinosylguanine (ara-G). Despite this compelling evidence for its T-cell specificity and the pressing need for active agents in these diseases, ara-G had not been evaluated in clinical trials, probably due to the low solubility of the compound. The recent development of a more soluble 6-methoxy-prodrug (2-amino-9-B-D-arabinofuranosyl-6-methoxy-9H-purine, 506U, Compound-506U78, nelarabine; Fig. 15.4) of ara-G by Burroughs Wellcome Co. has now made such trials possible [96].

Metabolism and Mechanisms of Action

Nelarabine is a poor substrate for direct phosphorylation, which prohibits further anabolism of the parent drug [96]. When infused to patients, ara-G is liberated when ADA demethoxylates nelarabine. Although nelarabine is a poor substrate for this enzyme with a Km value of 170 μM (rel. Vmax = 2% of adenosine), the abundance of this enzyme in large body organs (including spleen and thymus) results in a rapid conversion. With respect to T-cell diseases, it is of importance to note that there are high levels of ADA in RBCs, which are probably responsible for the conversion in the circulation [97]. The generation of ara-G in the plasma of monkeys and humans infused with nelarabine was rapid [96, 97]. The t½ of nelarabine was 11 min in monkeys and between 14 and 17 min in humans with a concomitant peak of ara-G, reflecting the metabolic conversion to ara-G by ADA and a smaller element of renal clearance.

Ara-G is transported into T-lymphoblastoid cells via nucleoside transport system [98]. Despite the relatively low affinity of these systems, they have a generally high capacity that is not likely to limit cellular metabolism of ara-G but the initial phosphorylation of ara-G to its monophosphate appears to be the rate-limiting step in triphosphate formation. This step is catalyzed by two enzymes [99]; high affinity (Km dGuo, 7 μM; ara-G, 7 μM), low specific activity mitochondrial deoxyguanosine

Table 15.4 Results of clinical trials with nelarabine as monotherapy

Drug	Phase	Disease	N	CR (%)	PR (%)	ORR (%)	Author
Nelarabine	I	Pediatric T-ALL	26	27	15	42	Kurzberg et al. [116]
		Adult T-ALL	13	15	62	80	
		T-CLL/T-PLL	7	0	29	29	
		B-ALL/Pre-B-ALL	10	0	10	10	
		B-CLL/B-PLL	4	0	25	25	
		B-NHL	6	0	17	17	
		AML-CML-BC	8	13	0	13	
	II	T-ALL	106	26	8	32	Berg et al. [117]
	II	T-ALL	26	31	10	41	DeAngelo et al. [118]
		T-lymphoma	13				

kinase [100, 101] and low affinity (Km dCyd, <1 μM, ara-G, >100 μM) cytosolic deoxycytidine kinase [96, 101–103]. Subsequent phosphorylation steps are required to generate the triphosphate ara-GTP. As expected from experience with other nucleoside analogs, T-cell lines accumulated higher levels of ara-GTP [104–106], which was retained for a longer time [107]. Greater accumulation of analog triphosphate was also observed in primary leukemia cells [108, 109].

For its mechanism of actions, the triphosphate of ara-G behaves similar to other nucleoside analogs. It is the proximal active metabolite which competes with natural substrate dGTP for incorporation into DNA. Because dGTP levels are low in cells, the analog triphosphate incorporation is favored. Following analog incorporation, the modified DNA is resistant to further deoxynucleotide addition in DNA replication and repair reactions [110]. Using in vitro DNA primer extension assays, it has been demonstrated that the molecular basis for ara-GTP-induced inhibition of DNA synthesis is due in part to incorporation of the nucleoside analog [111, 112]. T-cell selective cytotoxicity investigations illustrated that in addition to higher accumulation of ara-GTP, induction of Fas-mediated cell death pathway further enhanced the cell killing in T-cell types [113].

Nelarabine as a Single Agent in the Clinic

Nelarabine is a potent agent for the treatment of hematologic malignancies with major efficacy in T-cell disorders [114–116]. Kurtzberg et al. [116] reported the clinical outcome of pediatric and adult patients with refractory hematological malignancies treated with nelarabine. The OR rate was 31%, however this rate was 54% in the subgroups of patients with T-ALL who achieved a complete or PR after one or two cycles of nelarabine (Table 15.4). The efficacy of intravenous nelarabine in patients with refractory or relapsed T-ALL or T-lymphoblastic lymphoma (T-LBL) was evaluated in phase II, noncomparative, open-label, multicentre trials in children and young adults aged <21 years when first diagnosed [117], and adolescents and adults aged ≥16 years [118], and in the GMALL (German Multicentre Study Group for Adult ALL) trial in adults aged ≥19 years [119]. The pediatrics [114] and adult [118] trials recruited 153 and 40 patients; of these, 39 [117] and 28 [118] had not responded to, or had relapsed following treatment with, at least two prior chemotherapy regimens. In the initial group of pediatric patients, nelarabine 1.2 g/m²/day was infused over 1 h for 5 consecutive days every 3 weeks, but was reduced to 650 mg/m²/day for 5 days in subsequent patients. In adult patients, the treatment regimen for the first three patients was nelarabine 2,200 mg/m²/day infused over 2 h on days 1, 3, and 5, but for subsequent patients, the dose was reduced to 1,500 mg/m². In the GMALL trial, of 49 evaluable patients, 34 were in first relapse (of these, 32 were refractory to at least one salvage chemotherapy regimen), 7 were in second relapse, 7 were in second relapse after stem cell transplantation and 2 patients never reached a CR. Patients received nelarabine 1,500 mg/m²/day on days 1, 3, and 5 (number of cycles not stated) [119].

Nelarabine treatment induced CR or CR-incomplete (CRi; it was defined as CR without full hematological recovery) in approximately one-fifth of pediatric and adult patients who had not responded to, or had relapsed following treatment with two or more prior chemotherapy regimens. The CR rate in pediatric patients was 13% and a further 10% had a CRi, for a total of CR/CRi response rate of 23%. In the adult trial, 18% had a CR and a further 3% had a CRi, for a total CR/CRi response rate of 21% (Table 15.4). For responders as a group, the duration of CR ranged from 4.7 to 36.4 weeks in pediatric patients and from 15.1 through >195.4 weeks in adult patients. In the GMALL trial, 25 patients (51%) achieved a CR and 19 patients went on to receive stem cell transplantation. Neurological adverse events are the most likely adverse events to limit treatment with nelarabine.

The drug is approved for the treatment of pediatric and adult patients with T-ALL and T-LBL whose disease has not responded to, or has relapsed after treatment with at least two prior chemotherapy regimens. The recommended dose of the drug in adults is 1,500 mg/m²/day infused undiluted over 2 h on day 1, 3, and 5, and repeated every 21 days. In pediatric patients the recommended dose is 650 mg/m²/day infused intravenously undiluted over 1 h for 5 consecutive days, repeated every 21 days. The efficacy of nelarabine in combination chemotherapy for newly diagnosed T-ALL is currently being investigated in a large, multinational, phase III trial in patients aged 1–30 years.

Acknowledgements Authors are thankful to Dr. Lisa Chen for critically reading the manuscript, assisting with reference list, and drawing chemical structures.

References

1. Giblett ER, Anderson JE, Cohen F, Pollara B, Meuwissen HJ. Adenosine-deaminase deficiency in two patients with severely impaired cellular immunity. Lancet. 1972;2:1067–9.
2. Giblett ER, Ammann AJ, Wara DW, Sandman R, Diamond LK. Nucleoside-phosphorylase deficiency in a child with severely defective T-cell immunity and normal B-cell immunity. Lancet. 1975;1:1010–3.
3. Kantarjian HM, Childs C, O'Brien S, Huh Y, Beran M, Schachner J, et al. Efficacy of fludarabine, a new adenine nucleoside analogue, in patients with prolymphocytic leukemia and the prolymphocytoid variant of chronic lymphocytic leukemia. Am J Med. 1991;90:223–8.
4. O'Brien S, Kurzrock R, Duvic M, Kantarjian H, Stass S, Robertson LE, et al. 2-Chlorodeoxyadenosine therapy in patients with T-cell lymphoproliferative disorders. Blood. 1994;84:733–8.
5. Agarwal RP. Inhibitors of adenosine deaminase. Pharmacol Ther. 1982;17:399–429.
6. Woo PWK, Dion HW, Lange SM, Dahl LF, Durham LJ. Novel adenosine and ara-A deaminase inhibitor, (R)-3-(2-deoxy-beta -D-erythro-pentofuranosyl)-3,6,7,8-tetrahydroimidazo[4,5-d][1,3]diazepin-8-ol. J Heterocycl Chem. 1974;11:641–3.
7. O'Dwyer PJ, Wagner B, Leyland-Jones B, Wittes RE, Cheson BD, Hoth DF. 2'-Deoxycoformycin (pentostatin) for lymphoid malignancies. Rational development of an active new drug. Ann Intern Med. 1988;108:733–43.
8. Siaw MF, Coleman MS. In vitro metabolism of deoxycoformycin in human T lymphoblastoid cells. Phosphorylation of deoxycoformycin and incorporation into cellular DNA. J Biol Chem. 1984;259: 9426–33.
9. Gray DP, Grever MR, Siaw MF, Coleman MS, Balcerzak SP. 2'-deoxycoformycin (DCF) and 9-beta-D-arabinofuranosyladenine (Ara-A) in the treatment of refractory acute myelocytic leukemia. Cancer Treat Rep. 1982;66:253–7.
10. Major PP, Agarwal RP, Kufe DW. Clinical pharmacology of arabinofuranosyladenine in combination with deoxycoformycin. Cancer Chemother Pharmacol. 1983;10:125–8.
11. Koller CA, Mitchell BS, Grever MR, Mejias E, Malspeis L, Metz EN. Treatment of acute lymphoblastic leukemia with 2'-deoxycoformycin: clinical and biochemical consequences of adenosine deaminase inhibition. Cancer Treat Rep. 1979;63: 1949–52.
12. Russell NH, Prentice HG, Lee N, Piga A, Ganeshaguru K, Smyth JF, et al. Studies on the biochemical sequelae of therapy in Thy-acute lymphoblastic leukaemia with the adenosine deaminase inhibitor 2' deoxycoformycin. Br J Haematol. 1981;49:1–9.
13. Siaw MF, Mitchell BS, Koller CA, Coleman MS, Hutton JJ. ATP depletion as a consequence of adenosine deaminase inhibition in man. Proc Natl Acad Sci USA. 1980;77:6157–61.
14. Venner PM, Glazer RI, Blatt J, Sallan S, Rivera G, Holcenberg JS, et al. Levels of 2'-deoxycoformycin,

adenosine, and deoxyadenosine in patients with acute lymphoblastic leukemia. Cancer Res. 1981;41: 4508–11.
15. Agarwal RP, Blatt J, Miser J, Sallan S, Lipton JM, Reaman GH, et al. Clinical pharmacology of 9-beta-D-arabinofuranosyladenine in combination with 2'-deoxycoformycin. Cancer Res. 1982;42:3884–6.
16. Reichard P. Regulation of deoxyribotide synthesis. Biochemistry. 1987;26:3245–8.
17. Liu X, Kim CN, Yang J, Jemmerson R, Wang X. Induction of apoptotic program in cell-free extracts: requirement for dATP and cytochrome c. Cell. 1996;86:147–57.
18. Chandra D, Bratton SB, Person MD, Tian Y, Martin AG, Ayres M, et al. Intracellular nucleotides act as critical prosurvival factors by binding to cytochrome C and inhibiting apoptosome. Cell. 2006;125: 1333–46.
19. Yu AL, Mendelsohn J, Matsumoto SS. Induction of complete remission in T-cell acute lymphoblastic leukemia with deoxycoformycin (dcf) and 9-beta-D-arabinofuranosyladenine (ara-A). Adv Exp Med Biol. 1986;195(Pt A):491–6.
20. Spiers AS, Ruckdeschel JC, Horton J. Effectiveness of pentostatin (2'-deoxycoformycin) in refractory lymphoid neoplasms. Scand J Haematol. 1984;32: 130–4.
21. Ho AD, Suciu S, Stryckmans P, De Cataldo F, Willemze R, Thaler J, et al. Pentostatin in T-cell malignancies—a phase II trial of the EORTC. Leukemia Cooperative Group. Ann Oncol. 1999;10: 1493–8.
22. Matutes E, Brito-Babapulle V, Swansbury J, Ellis J, Morilla R, Dearden C, et al. Clinical and laboratory features of 78 cases of T-prolymphocytic leukemia. Blood. 1991;78:3269–74.
23. Dohner H, Ho AD, Thaler J, Stryckmans P, Sonneveld P, de Witte T, et al. Pentostatin in prolymphocytic leukemia: phase II trial of the European Organization for Research and Treatment of Cancer Leukemia Cooperative Study Group. J Natl Cancer Inst. 1993;85:658–62.
24. Dearden C, Matutes E, Catovsky D. Pentostatin treatment of cutaneous T cell lymphoma. Oncology. 2000;14:37–40.
25. Mercieca J, Matutes E, Dearden C, MacLennan K, Catovsky D. The role of pentostatin in the treatment of T-cell malignancies: analysis of response rate in 145 patients according to disease subtype. J Clin Oncol. 1994;12:2588–93.
26. Tsimberidou AM, Giles F, Duvic M, Fayad L, Kurzrock R. Phase II study of pentostatin in advanced T-cell lymphoid malignancies: update of an M.D. Anderson Cancer Center series. Cancer. 2004; 100:342–9.
27. Daenen S, Rojer RA, Smit JW, Halie MR, Nieweg HO. Successful chemotherapy with deoxycoformycin in adult T-cell lymphoma-leukaemia. Br J Haematol. 1984;58:723–7.
28. Spiers AS, Davis MP, Levine M, Li CY, Mangan KF, Mazza JJ, et al. T-cell chronic lymphocytic leukaemia: anomalous cell markers, variable morphology, and marked responsiveness to pentostatin (2'-deoxycoformycin). Scand J Haematol. 1985;34:57–67.
29. Yamaguchi K, Yul LS, Oda T, Maeda Y, Ishii M, Fujita K, et al. Clinical consequences of 2'-deoxycoformycin treatment in patients with refractory adult T-cell leukaemia. Leuk Res. 1986;10:989–93.
30. Lofters W, Campbell M, Gibbs WN, Cheson BD. 2'-Deoxycoformycin therapy in adult T-cell leukemia/lymphoma. Cancer. 1987;60:2605–8.
31. el'Agnaf MR, Ennis KE, Morris TC, Robertson JH, Markey G, Alexander HD. Successful remission induction with deoxycoformycin in elderly patients with T-helper prolymphocytic leukaemia. Br J Haematol. 1986;63:93–104.
32. Dearden C, Matutes E, Catovsky D. Deoxycoformycin in the treatment of mature T-cell leukaemias. Br J Cancer. 1991;64:903–6.
33. Grever MR, Leiby JM, Kraut EH, Wilson HE, Neidhart JA, Wall RL, et al. Low-dose deoxycoformycin in lymphoid malignancy. J Clin Oncol. 1985;3:1196–201.
34. Cummings FJ, Kim K, Neiman RS, Comis RL, Oken MM, Weitzman SA, et al. Phase II trial of pentostatin in refractory lymphomas and cutaneous T-cell disease. J Clin Oncol. 1991;9:565–71.
35. Greiner D, Olsen EA, Petroni G. Pentostatin (2'-deoxycoformycin) in the treatment of cutaneous T-cell lymphoma. J Am Acad Dermatol. 1997; 36:950–5.
36. Kurzrock R, Pilat S, Duvic M. Pentostatin therapy of T-cell lymphomas with cutaneous manifestations. J Clin Oncol. 1999;17:3117–21.
37. Foss FM, Ihde DC, Breneman DL, Phelps RM, Fischmann AB, Schechter GP, et al. Phase II study of pentostatin and intermittent high-dose recombinant interferon alfa-2a in advanced mycosis fungoides/ Sezary syndrome. J Clin Oncol. 1992;10:1907–13.
38. Aribi A, Huh Y, Keating M, O'Brien S, Ferrajoli A, Faderl S, et al. T-cell large granular lymphocytic (T-LGL) leukemia: experience in a single institution over 8 years. Leuk Res. 2007;31:939–45.
39. Dincol G, Diz-Kucukkaya R, Bicakci E. T-cell large granular lymphocytic leukaemia: successful response to 2-deoxycoformycin. Neth J Med. 2008; 66:85–7.
40. Tsirigotis P, Venetis E, Kapsimali V, Rontogianni D, Varvitsioti E, Pappa V, et al. 2-deoxycoformycin in the treatment of T-large granular lymphocyte leukemia. Leuk Res. 2003;27:865–7.
41. Aldinucci D, Poletto D, Zagonel V, Rupolo M, Degan M, Nanni P, et al. In vitro and in vivo effects of 2'-deoxycoformycin (Pentostatin) on tumour cells from human gammadelta+ T-cell malignancies. Br J Haematol. 2000;110:188–96.
42. Corazzelli G, Capobianco G, Russo F, Frigeri F, Aldinucci D, Pinto A. Pentostatin (2'-deoxycoformycin) for the treatment of hepatosplenic gammadelta T-cell lymphomas. Haematologica. 2005; 90:ECR14.

43. Grigg AP. 2'-Deoxycoformycin for hepatosplenic gammadelta T-cell lymphoma. Leuk Lymphoma. 2001;42:797–9.
44. Osuji N, Fearfield L, Matutes E, Wotherspoon AC, Bunker C, Catovsky D. Granulomatous slack skin disease—disease features and response to pentostatin. Br J Haematol. 2003;123:297–304.
45. Gallamini A, Zaja F, Patti C, Billio A, Specchia MR, Tucci A, et al. Alemtuzumab (Campath-1H) and CHOP chemotherapy as first-line treatment of peripheral T-cell lymphoma: results of a GITIL (Gruppo Italiano Terapie Innovative nei Linfomi) prospective multicenter trial. Blood. 2007; 110:2316–23.
46. Dearden CE, Matutes E, Cazin B, Tjonnfjord GE, Parreira A, Nomdedeu B, et al. High remission rate in T-cell prolymphocytic leukemia with CAMPATH-1 H. Blood. 2001;98:1721–6.
47. Ravandi F, Kantarjian HM, Faderl S, Verstovsek S, Koller CA, Odinga S, et al. Combination therapy with alemtuzumab and pentostatin is effective and has acceptable toxicity in patients with T-lymphoid neoplasms. Blood. 2006;108:4971 (abstr).
48. Gandhi V, Balakrishnan K. Pharmacology and mechanism of action of forodesine, a T-cell targeted agent. Semin Oncol. 2007;34:S8–12.
49. Schramm VL. Development of transition state analogues of purine nucleoside phosphorylase as anti-T-cell agents. Biochim Biophys Acta. 2002;1587: 107–17.
50. Viegas TX, Omura GA, Stoltz RR, Kisicki J. Pharmacokinetics and pharmacodynamics of peldesine (BCX-34), a purine nucleoside phosphorylase inhibitor, following single and multiple oral doses in healthy volunteers. J Clin Pharmacol. 2000;40:410–20.
51. Kicska GA, Long L, Horig H, Fairchild C, Tyler PC, Furneaux RH, et al. Immucillin H, a powerful transition-state analog inhibitor of purine nucleoside phosphorylase, selectively inhibits human T lymphocytes. Proc Natl Acad Sci USA. 2001;98: 4593–8.
52. Kilpatrick JM, Morris PE, Serota Jr DG, Phillips D, Moore DR, Bennett JC, et al. Intravenous and oral pharmacokinetic study of BCX-1777, a novel purine nucleoside phosphorylase transition-state inhibitor. In vivo effects on blood 2'-deoxyguanosine in primates. Int Immunopharmacol. 2003;3:541–8.
53. Bantia S, Ananth SL, Parker CD, Horn LL, Upshaw R. Mechanism of inhibition of T-acute lymphoblastic leukemia cells by PNP inhibitor—BCX-1777. Int Immunopharmacol. 2003;3:879–87.
54. Gandhi V, Kilpatrick JM, Plunkett W, Ayres M, Harman L, Du M, et al. A proof-of-principle pharmacokinetic, pharmacodynamic, and clinical study with purine nucleoside phosphorylase inhibitor immucillin-H (BCX-1777, forodesine). Blood. 2005;106:4253–60.
55. Cohen A, Lee JW, Dosch HM, Gelfand EW. The expression of deoxyguanosine toxicity in T lymphocytes at different stages of maturation. J Immunol. 1980;125:1578–82.
56. Gelfand EW, Lee JJ, Dosch HM. Selective toxicity of purine deoxynucleosides for human lymphocyte growth and function. Proc Natl Acad Sci USA. 1979;76:1998–2002.
57. Gudas LJ, Ullman B, Cohen A, Martin Jr DW. Deoxyguanosine toxicity in a mouse T lymphoma: relationship to purine nucleoside phosphorylase-associated immune dysfunction. Cell. 1978;14:531–8.
58. Mitchell BS, Mejias E, Daddona PE, Kelley WN. Purinogenic immunodeficiency diseases: selective toxicity of deoxyribonucleosides for T cells. Proc Natl Acad Sci USA. 1978;75:5011–4.
59. Balakrishnan K, Nimmanapalli R, Ravandi F, Keating MJ, Gandhi V. Forodesine, an inhibitor of purine nucleoside phosphorylase, induces apoptosis in chronic lymphocytic leukemia cells. Blood. 2006;108:2392–8.
60. Alonso R, Lopez-Guerra M, Upshaw R, Bantia S, Smal C, Bontemps F, et al. Forodesine has high antitumor activity in chronic lymphocytic leukemia and activates p53-independent mitochondrial apoptosis by induction of p73 and BIM. Blood. 2009;114: 1563–75.
61. Furman RR, Iosava G, Isola L, et al. Forodesine (FodosineTM), a PNP inhibitor active in relapsed or refractory T-cell leukemia patients (Phase II study). Blood. 2005;106:881 (abstr).
62. Stelljes M, Kienast J, Berning B, et al. Forodesine in patients with refractory/relapsed T-ALL can induce prolonged stable remission with minimal toxicity before and after allogeneic hematopoietic stem cell transplantation. Blood. 2005;106:1832 (abstr).
63. Gore L, Stelljes M, Quinones R. Forodesine treatment and post-transplant graft-versus-host disease in two patients with acute leukemia: facilitation of graft-versus-leukemia effect? Semin Oncol. 2007;34: S35–9.
64. Duvic M, Foss FM, Olsen EA, Forero-Torres A, Bennett JC, Bantia S, et al. Intravenous Forodesine (BCX-1777), a novel purine nucleoside phosphorylase (PNP) inhibitor, demonstrates clinical activity in patients with refractory cutaneous T-cell lymphoma. Blood. 2004;104:2491 (abstr).
65. Duvic M, Forero-Torres A, Foss FM, Olsen EA, Kim Y. Oral forodesine (BCX-1777) is clinically active in refractory cutaneous T-cell lymphoma: results of a phase I/II study. Blood. 2006;108:698a. (abstr) 899.
66. Hertel LW, Boder GB, Kroin JS, Rinzel SM, Poore GA, Todd GC, et al. Evaluation of the antitumor activity of gemcitabine (2',2'-difluoro-2'-deoxycytidine). Cancer Res. 1990;50:4417–22.
67. Gandhi V, Plunkett W. Modulatory activity of 2',2'-difluorodeoxycytidine on the phosphorylation and cytotoxicity of arabinosyl nucleosides. Cancer Res. 1990;50:3675–80.
68. Shewach DS, Reynolds KK, Hertel L. Nucleotide specificity of human deoxycytidine kinase. Mol Pharmacol. 1992;42:518–24.

69. Abbruzzese JL, Grunewald R, Weeks EA, Gravel D, Adams T, Nowak B, et al. A phase I clinical, plasma, and cellular pharmacology study of gemcitabine. J Clin Oncol. 1991;9:491–8.
70. Plunkett W, Huang P, Xu YZ, Heinemann V, Grunewald R, Gandhi V. Gemcitabine: metabolism, mechanisms of action, and self-potentiation. Semin Oncol. 1995;22:3–10.
71. van Moorsel CJ, Veerman G, Ruiz van Haperen VW, Bergman AM, Jensen PB, Sehested M, et al. Differential effects of gemcitabine on nucleotide pools of 19 solid tumor cell lines. Adv Exp Med Biol. 1998;431:661–5.
72. Gandhi V, Plunkett W, Du M, Ayres M, Estey EH. Prolonged infusion of gemcitabine: clinical and pharmacodynamic studies during a phase I trial in relapsed acute myelogenous leukemia. J Clin Oncol. 2002;20:665–73.
73. Grunewald R, Abbruzzese JL, Tarassoff P, Plunkett W. Saturation of 2',2'-difluorodeoxycytidine 5'-triphosphate accumulation by mononuclear cells during a phase I trial of gemcitabine. Cancer Chemother Pharmacol. 1991;27:258–62.
74. Patel SR, Gandhi V, Jenkins J, Papadopolous N, Burgess MA, Plager C, et al. Phase II clinical investigation of gemcitabine in advanced soft tissue sarcomas and window evaluation of dose rate on gemcitabine triphosphate accumulation. J Clin Oncol. 2001;19:3483–9.
75. van der Donk WA, Yu G, Perez L, Sanchez RJ, Stubbe J, Samano V, et al. Detection of a new substrate-derived radical during inactivation of ribonucleotide reductase from Escherichia coli by gemcitabine 5'-diphosphate. Biochemistry. 1998;37:6419–26.
76. Wang J, Lohman GJ, Stubbe J. Enhanced subunit interactions with gemcitabine-5'-diphosphate inhibit ribonucleotide reductases. Proc Natl Acad Sci USA. 2007;104:14324–9.
77. Xu H, Faber C, Uchiki T, Racca J, Dealwis C. Structures of eukaryotic ribonucleotide reductase I define gemcit abine diphosphate binding and subunit assembly. Proc Natl Acad Sci USA. 2006;103:4028–33.
78. Shewach DS, Lawrence TS. Antimetabolite radiosensitizers. J Clin Oncol. 2007;25:4043–50.
79. Huang P, Chubb S, Hertel LW, Grindey GB, Plunkett W. Action of 2',2'-difluorodeoxycytidine on DNA synthesis. Cancer Res. 1991;51:6110–7.
80. Huang P, Plunkett W. Fludarabine- and gemcitabine-induced apoptosis: incorporation of analogs into DNA is a critical event. Cancer Chemother Pharmacol. 1995;36:181–8.
81. Achanta G, Pelicano H, Feng L, Plunkett W, Huang P. Interaction of p53 and DNA-PK in response to nucleoside analogues: potential role as a sensor complex for DNA damage. Cancer Res. 2001;61:8723–9.
82. Ewald B, Sampath D, Plunkett W. Nucleoside analogs: molecular mechanisms signaling cell death. Oncogene. 2008;27:6522–37.
83. Ewald B, Sampath D, Plunkett W. ATM and the Mre11-Rad50-Nbs1 complex respond to nucleoside analogue-induced stalled replication forks and contribute to drug resistance. Cancer Res. 2008;68:7947–55.
84. Duvic M, Talpur R, Wen S, Kurzrock R, David CL, Apisarnthanarax N. Phase II evaluation of gemcitabine monotherapy for cutaneous T-cell lymphoma. Clin Lymphoma Myeloma. 2006;7:51–8.
85. Sallah S, Wehbie R, Lepera P, Sallah W, Bobzien W. The role of 2-chlorodeoxyadenosine in the treatment of patients with refractory angioimmunoblastic lymphadenopathy with dysproteinemia. Br J Haematol. 1999;104:163–5.
86. Zinzani PL, Baliva G, Magagnoli M, Bendandi M, Modugno G, Gherlinzoni F, et al. Gemcitabine treatment in pretreated cutaneous T-cell lymphoma: experience in 44 patients. J Clin Oncol. 2000;18:2603–6.
87. Zinzani PL, Magagnoli M, Bendandi M, Orcioni GF, Gherlinzoni F, Albertini P, et al. Therapy with gemcitabine in pretreated peripheral T-cell lymphoma patients. Ann Oncol. 1998;9:1351–3.
88. Marchi E, Alinari L, Tani M, Stefoni V, Pimpinelli N, Berti E, et al. Gemcitabine as frontline treatment for cutaneous T-cell lymphoma: phase II study of 32 patients. Cancer. 2005;104:2437–41.
89. Arkenau HT, Chong G, Cunningham D, Watkins D, Sirohi B, Chau I, et al. Gemcitabine, cisplatin and methylprednisolone for the treatment of patients with peripheral T-cell lymphoma: the Royal Marsden Hospital experience. Haematologica. 2007;92:271–2.
90. Crump M, Shepherd L, Lin B. A randomized phase III study of gemcitabine, dexamethasone, and cisplatin versus dexamethasone, cytarabine, and cisplatin as salvage chemotherapy followed by posttransplantation rituximab maintenance therapy versus observation for treatment of aggressive B-Cell and T-Cell non-Hodgkin's lymphoma. Clin Lymphoma. 2005;6:56–60.
91. Emmanouilides C, Colovos C, Pinter-Brown L, Hernandez L, Schiller G, Territo M, et al. Pilot study of fixed-infusion rate gemcitabine with cisplatin and dexamethasone in patients with relapsed or refractory lymphoma. Clin Lymphoma. 2004;5:45–9.
92. Evens AM, Gordon LI, Patton D, Rosen ST, Winter JN, Kline J, et al. Phase I results of combination gemcitabine and bortezomib (Velcade) for relapsed/refractory nodal T-cell non-Hodgkin lymphoma (T-NHL) and aggressive B-cell NHL (B-NHL). Blood. 2008;112:2005. (abstr).
93. Ng M, Waters J, Cunningham D, Chau I, Horwich A, Hill M, et al. Gemcitabine, cisplatin and methylprednisolone (GEM-P) is an effective salvage regimen in patients with relapsed and refractory lymphoma. Br J Cancer. 2005;92:1352–7.
94. Toner LE, Vrhovac R, Smith EA, Gardner J, Heaney M, Gonen M, et al. The schedule-dependent effects of the novel antifolate pralatrexate and gemcitabine

are superior to methotrexate and cytarabine in models of human non-Hodgkin's lymphoma. Clin Cancer Res. 2006;12:924–32.
95. Reist EJ, Goodman L. Synthesis of 9-Beta-D-Arabinofuranosylguanine. Biochemistry. 1964;3: 15–8.
96. Lambe CU, Averett DR, Paff MT, Reardon JE, Wilson JG, Krenitsky TA. 2-Amino-6-methoxypurine arabinoside: an agent for T-cell malignancies. Cancer Res. 1995;55:3352–6.
97. Kisor DF, Plunkett W, Kurtzberg J, Mitchell B, Hodge JP, Ernst T, et al. Pharmacokinetics of nelarabine and 9-beta-D-arabinofuranosyl guanine in pediatric and adult patients during a phase I study of nelarabine for the treatment of refractory hematologic malignancies. J Clin Oncol. 2000;18:995–1003.
98. Prus KL, Averett DR, Zimmerman TP. Transport and metabolism of 9-beta-D-arabinofuranosylguanine in a human T-lymphoblastoid cell line: nitrobenzylthio-inosine-sensitive and -insensitive influx. Cancer Res. 1990;50:1817–21.
99. Rodriguez Jr CO, Mitchell BS, Ayres M, Eriksson S, Gandhi V. Arabinosylguanine is phosphorylated by both cytoplasmic deoxycytidine kinase and mitochondrial deoxyguanosine kinase. Cancer Res. 2002;62:3100–5.
100. Lewis RA, Link L. Phosphorylation of arabinosyl guanine by a mitochondrial enzyme of bovine liver. Biochem Pharmacol. 1989;38:2001–6.
101. Wang L, Karlsson A, Arner ES, Eriksson S. Substrate specificity of mitochondrial 2'-deoxyguanosine kinase. Efficient phosphorylation of 2-chlorodeoxyadenosine. J Biol Chem. 1993;268:22847–52.
102. Carson DA, Kaye J, Seegmiller JE. Lymphospecific toxicity in adenosine deaminase deficiency and purine nucleoside phosphorylase deficiency: possible role of nucleoside kinase(s). Proc Natl Acad Sci USA. 1977;74:5677–81.
103. Krenitsky TA, Tuttle JV, Koszalka GW, Chen IS, Beacham 3rd LM, Rideout JL, et al. Deoxycytidine kinase from calf thymus. Substrate and inhibitor specificity. J Biol Chem. 1976;251:4055–61.
104. Cohen A, Lee JW, Gelfand EW. Selective toxicity of deoxyguanosine and arabinosyl guanine for T-leukemic cells. Blood. 1983;61:660–6.
105. Shewach DS, Daddona PE, Ashcraft E, Mitchell BS. Metabolism and selective cytotoxicity of 9-beta-D-arabinofuranosylguanine in human lymphoblasts. Cancer Res. 1985;45:1008–14.
106. Ullman B, Martin Jr DW. Specific cytotoxicity of arabinosylguanine toward cultured T lymphoblasts. J Clin Invest. 1984;74:951–5.
107. Verhoef V, Fridland A. Metabolic basis of arabinonucleoside selectivity for human leukemic T- and B-lymphoblasts. Cancer Res. 1985;45:3646–50.
108. Rodriguez Jr CO, Legha JK, Estey E, Keating MJ, Gandhi V. Pharmacological and biochemical strategies to increase the accumulation of arabinofuranosylguanine triphosphatein primary human leukemia cells. Clin Cancer Res. 1997;3:2107–13.
109. Shewach DS, Mitchell BS. Differential metabolism of 9-beta-D-arabinofuranosylguanine in human leukemic cells. Cancer Res. 1989;49: 6498–502.
110. Rodriguez Jr CO, Gandhi V. Arabinosylguanine-induced apoptosis of T-lymphoblastic cells: incorporation into DNA is a necessary step. Cancer Res. 1999;59:4937–43.
111. Gandhi V, Mineishi S, Huang P, Chapman AJ, Yang Y, Chen F, et al. Cytotoxicity, metabolism, and mechanisms of action of 2',2'-difluorodeoxyguanosine in Chinese hamster ovary cells. Cancer Res. 1995; 55:1517–24.
112. Gandhi V, Mineishi S, Huang P, Yang Y, Chubb S, Chapman AJ, et al. Difluorodeoxyguanosine: cytotoxicity, metabolism, and actions on DNA synthesis in human leukemia cells. Semin Oncol. 1995; 22:61–7.
113. Rodriguez Jr CO, Stellrecht CM, Gandhi V. Mechanisms for T-cell selective cytotoxicity of arabinosylguanine. Blood. 2003;102:1842–8.
114. Czuczman MS, Porcu P, Johnson J, Niedzwiecki D, Kelly M, Hsi ED, et al. Results of a phase II study of 506U78 in cutaneous T-cell lymphoma and peripheral T-cell lymphoma: CALGB 59901. Leuk Lymphoma. 2007;48:97–103.
115. Gandhi V, Plunkett W, Rodriguez Jr CO, Nowak BJ, Du M, Ayres M, et al. Compound GW506U78 in refractory hematologic malignancies: relationship between cellular pharmacokinetics and clinical response. J Clin Oncol. 1998;16:3607–15.
116. Kurtzberg J, Ernst TJ, Keating MJ, Gandhi V, Hodge JP, Kisor DF, et al. Phase I study of 506U78 administered on a consecutive 5-day schedule in children and adults with refractory hematologic malignancies. J Clin Oncol. 2005;23:3396–403.
117. Berg SL, Blaney SM, Devidas M, Lampkin TA, Murgo A, Bernstein M, et al. Phase II study of nelarabine (compound 506U78) in children and young adults with refractory T-cell malignancies: a report from the Children's Oncology Group. J Clin Oncol. 2005;23:3376–82.
118. DeAngelo DJ, Yu D, Johnson JL, Coutre SE, Stone RM, Stopeck AT, et al. Nelarabine induces complete remissions in adults with relapsed or refractory T-lineage acute lymphoblastic leukemia or lymphoblastic lymphoma: Cancer and Leukemia Group B study 19801. Blood. 2007;109:5136–42.
119. Gokbuget N, Arnold R, Atta J, et al. High single dose activity of compound GW506U78 in relapsed T-lymphoblastic leukaemia (T-ALL) and T-lymphoblastic lymphoma (T-LBL) offers option for cure with stem cell transplantation. Haematologica. 2006;90:157 (abstr).

16 Current Epigenetic Therapy for T-Cell Lymphoma

Michael Dickinson, Chan Cheah, and H. Miles Prince

Introduction

Cutaneous T-cell lymphoma (CTCL) is challenging to treat. Patients with advanced disease typically only enjoy brief responses to conventional chemotherapeutics, and are at particularly high risk of infectious complications during the treatment with chemotherapy. Combination and intensification of conventional chemotherapeutics fails to cure the vast majority of patients of patients with CTCL or other forms of peripheral T-cell lymphoma (PTCL). In this context, biological agents, and in particular the histone deacetylase inhibitors (HDACis), present an attractive alternative because they lack many of the side effects of conventional chemotherapy and appear to overcome chemotherapy resistance.

M. Dickinson, M.B.B.S. (Hons), F.R.A.C.P., F.R.C.P.A. (✉)
Division of Cancer Medicine,
Peter MacCallum Cancer Centre, Locked Bag1, Melbourne 8006, VIC, Australia

Sir Peter MacCallum Department of Oncology, The University of Melbourne, Parkville, Melbourne 3010, VIC, Australia
e-mail: Michael.Dickinson@petermac.org

C. Cheah, M.B.B.S. (Hons)
Division of Cancer Medicine,
Peter MacCallum Cancer Centre, Locked Bag1, Melbourne 8006, VIC, Australia

H.M. Prince, M.B.B.S. (Hons), M.D., M.R.A.C.M.A., F.R.A.C.P., F.R.C.P.A.
Sir Peter MacCallum Department of Oncology, Division of Cancer Medicine, Peter MacCallum Cancer Centre, Parkville, Melbourne, VIC, Australia

The HDACis target not only the epigenome but also numerous nucleic and cytoplasmic non-histone proteins and are powerful and selective inducers of cancer cell apoptosis and modifiers of the tumour microenvironment. To date, the best data for their use comes from trials in the lymphoid malignancies and CTCL is the only condition for which HDACis are currently registered. The FDA has approved romidepsin and vorinostat for use in relapsed/refractory CTCL and these agents provide patients with a new opportunity for durable clinical response. Similarly, romidepsin has potent activity in nodal PTCLs, with emerging data supporting a future role in clinical practice, either alone or in combination with conventional therapies.

Here we discuss the concept of epigenetic modifying agents, briefly review the putative targets for the HDACis and discuss key clinical trials supporting their use in T-cell lymphoma.

Epigenetics and Epigenetic Therapies

The term "epigenetics" refers to changes in gene expression that are not coded in the DNA sequence itself, which are heritable in the progeny of cells after mitosis [1]. Epigenetic therapies, therefore, target the dysregulated gene expression of neoplasia by altering the structure of chromatin or DNA promoter regions, rather than by addressing defects in the primary DNA code of conventional oncogenes or tumour suppressor genes.

F. Foss (ed.), *T-Cell Lymphomas*, Contemporary Hematology,
DOI 10.1007/978-1-62703-170-7_16, © Springer Science+Business Media New York 2013

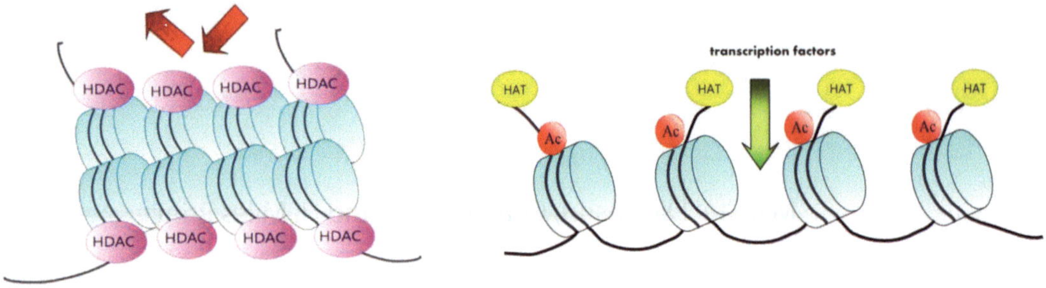

Figure 16.1 HDACs remove acetyl groups from the lysine tails of histones. Conversely HATs result in histone hyperacetylation, open chromatin formation and increased accessibility of target genes to transcription factors.

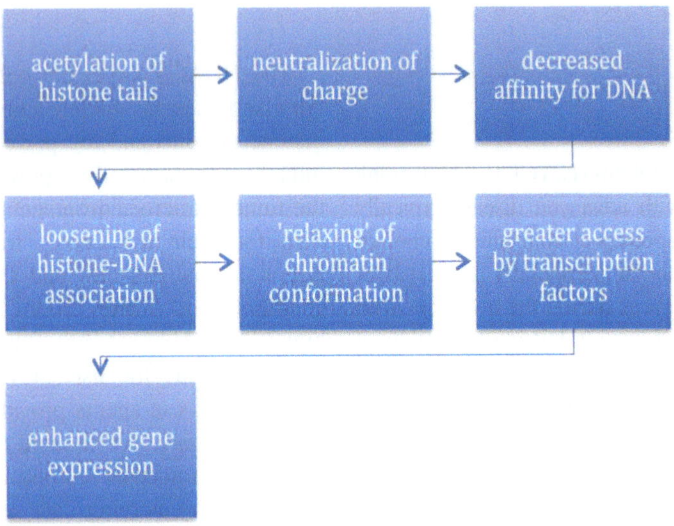

Figure 16.2 Relaxation of chromatin leads to increased gene expression

Drugs in clinical use today target two epigenetic mechanisms. Methylation of the CpG dinucleotides in the promoter regions of genes is heritable and suppresses gene expression. This mechanism is targeted by the DNA-methyltransferase inhibitors azacitidine and decitabine. The DNA demethylating agents are predominantly used in myeloid malignancies although trials continue in the lymphoid malignancies, particularly in combination with other agents. The HDACis are a broad and novel class of agents that target one aspect of the "histone code," lysine-acetylation. Histones are octomeric proteins largely responsible for the structure of chromatin and the packaging of DNA within the cell. Condensed chromatin results in tightly packaged DNA, limiting access to transcription factors. A variety of modifications to the histone tail, including acetylation, methylation, ubiquitination, phosphorylation and sumoylation, alter histone charge and subsequently chromatin structure and gene expression [2]. The archetypal and most successfully druggable example applying to all of the agents in this chapter is histone acetylation. The key enzymes involved are histone acetyltransferases (HATs) and histone deacetylases (HDACs), which have contradictory effects on the acetylation status of histones and on chromatin structure [1]. Histone acetylation by HATs results in neutralisation of charge, decreased affinity for DNA, loosening of the histone–DNA interaction and open chromatin structure—making it more accessible to transcription factors and enhanced gene expression. (figure 16.1, and 16.2) [3] Conversely, histone deacetylation by HDACs leads to a more compact chromatin structure and gene repression. Following this logic, the HDACi could be considered de-repressors of gene expression, although in truth they have a far more complex set of effects and are probably best considered *modulators* of gene expression.

Targets of HDACi

Histone Targets

HDACs can be grouped according to their structure and homology to yeast enzymes. Classes I, II and IV are the zinc-dependent. Class III HDACs are the NAD-dependent deacetylases, sirtuins, which are not targets of the HDACis in current clinical use. Class I enzymes (HDAC 1,2,3,8) are found primarily in the nucleus, as is the single member of class IV, HDAC 11. Class II can be divided into two subgroups, IIa (HDAC 4,5,7,9) which can shuttle between the nucleus and cytoplasm, and IIb (HDAC 6,10) which is predominantly cytoplasmic [4]. Knowledge of the specific function of each HDAC isoenzyme (and therefore the effect of inhibition) continues to accumulate, but distinguishing the individual properties can be a difficult undertaking given the complexity of the cellular pathways involved. (Figure 16.3) One useful property of HDAC inhibition is that transformed cells are more sensitive to their pro-apoptotic effect than normal cells [4]. This is probably due to the dependence of malignant cells on HDACs for tumour cell growth, differentiation and apoptosis that provide a differential survival advantage [5].

HDACis share a common mechanism of action in binding a zinc ion critical to HDAC function. At present, the simplest method of grouping HDACi is based on specificity. HDACis which inhibit most or all zinc-dependent HDACs (pan-HDAC inhibitors) include the hydroxamic acid derivatives (trichostatin A, vorinostat [SAHA],

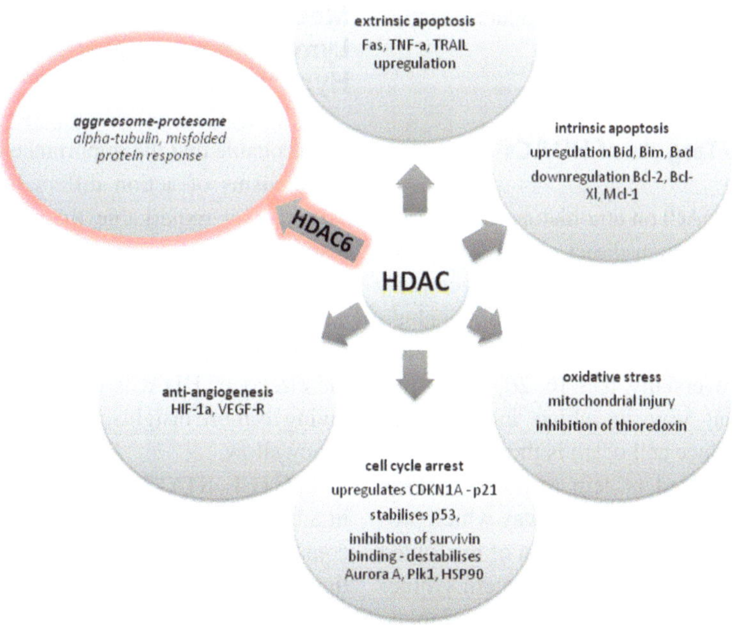

Figure 16.3 Exposure to HDACi leads a wide spectrum of biological effects including induction of apoptosis, inhibition of angiogenesis, induction of cellular senescence and disruption of the aggresome/Proteasome and endoplasmic reticulum.

panobinostat [LBH589]). Class I-specific HDACis include benzamide derivatives (entinostat, mocetinostat) and cyclic tetrapeptides (romidepsin [previously called depsipeptide]) [6]. These are summarised in Table 16.1. Cytoplasmic HDAC6 has effects on cell motility and proteasome and aggresome pathways which, along with inhibition of HDACs 1 and 2, is considered to be responsible for much of the anti-cancer effects of these drugs [6]. A key difference between the pan-HDACs and the class 1-specific HDACis is thought to be the inhibition of cytoplasmic HDAC6.

In cancer cells, HDACis induce caspase-dependent cell death, apparently through increased expression and activation of pro-apoptotic members of the intrinsic pathway (bax, bim, bak, etc.) and down-regulation of BCL-2 pro-survival proteins [7–12]. HDACi may induce sensitivity of cells to death-receptor pathway-induced apoptosis; this appears to occur either through increased expression of death receptors [13, 14] or thorough mechanisms independent of death receptor expression [15–17].

In addition to apoptosis, HDACis induce cell cycle arrest at G1/S or G2/M through a number of mechanisms including, in particular, the induction of p21. [18–21] They also induce reactive oxygen species. [22–24]

Non-Histone Targets of HDACs

The effects of HDACi on non-histone targets may be more important than direct changes in chromatin modification for anti-tumour effect [25]. Putative non-histone targets of HDACs include the STAT proteins, alpha-tubulin, HSP90, NF-KB and more controversially, p53. [6, 26]

An important way in which inhibition of HDAC6 may induce cell death is through disruption of the misfolded protein response (MPR). The MPR is a three pronged pathway which protects the cell from the accumulation of misfolded proteins that arise from defective protein synthesis [27]. Protein folding occurs in the endoplasmic reticulum, and requires the chaperone function of HSP90. [28, 29] Misfolded proteins accumulate into aggresomes by means of an HDAC6-dependent microtubule, and are then earmarked for destruction by the autophagosome. [30] This system thereby serves as a homeostatic mechanism which protects the cell from proteosomal dysfunction [6] and suggests the appeal of synergistic anti-cancer activity between proteasome inhibitors and HDACis. [31] HDACis induce both acetylation and dysfunction of HSP90, and disruption of the aggresome through acetylation of the tubulin. This is part of the rationale for the use of HDACi in myeloma; however, despite the evidence for HDACi causing dysfunction of the aggresome–proteasome pathway [32] clinical studies of HDACi have shown the class I-selective HDACi romidepsin can rescue patients with bortezomib-refractory myeloma. [33] Moreover, there is no suggestion that this potential mechanistic difference between the pan-HDACi and the isotype-selective HDACi effects the response rates in other cancers: as we shall show, response rates to the pan-DAC inhibitor vorinostat in CTCL are similar to those of romidepsin. [34] Key pharmacokinetic properties of the approved agents are listed in table 16.2.

Mechanism of Action in T-Cell Lymphoma—Biomarkers and Hypotheses

It is probable that the importance of these various mechanisms of action differs by disease being treated, and remarkable that the diseases most responsive to HDACis bare profound immunological and cytokine-signalling perturbation. The accessibility of the skin for biopsy means that CTCL provides an opportunity for the study of the effects of HDACis on tumour cells, in vivo, giving us more insights than other types of malignancy allow.

In CTCL, STAT3 phosphorylation is increased in a cytokine-independent manner, possibly as a consequence of defective T-cell receptor signalling [35–40]. Duvic and colleagues explored the mechanisms of action of HDACi using immunohistochemistry on primary patient samples in the phase II study of vorinostat [11, 41]. They showed that phospho-STAT3 was increased in the

Table 16.1 Classes of DAC inhibitors, their HDAC targets and HDAC cellular distribution. HDACs 6 and 10 are typically found in the cytoplasm [68]; however, both have also been found in the nucleus and are likely to affect transcription. [69, 70]

		HDAC specificity			
	HDAC Cellular distribution	Nuclear	Nuclear, cytoplasmic	Cytoplasmic [1]	Nuclear
	HDAC Class	I	IIa	IIb	IV
HDACi class	HDAC	1 2 3 8	4 5 7 9	6 10	11
Short chain fatty acids	Butyrate				
	Valproate				
Hydroxamic acid derivative	Trichostatin A				
	Vorinostat (suberoylanilide hydroxamic acid, SAHA)				
	Panobinostat (LBH589)*				
	Belinostat (PXD101)				
	Tubacin				
Benzamide	Entinostat (MS-275)				
	Mocetinostat (MGCD0103)				
Cyclic tetrapeptide	Romidepsin (depsipeptide)				

[Reprinted from Dickinson M, Johnstone RW, Prince HM. Histone deacetylase inhibitors: potential targets responsible for their anti-cancer effect. Invest New Drugs 2010;28 Suppl 1:S3–20. With permission from Springer Science+Business Media.]

Table 16.2 Pharmacokinetic properties of registered HDACis

	Vorinostat PO [71–73]	Romidepsin IV [74, 75]
t1/2	1.5–2 h	3 h
Protein binding (%)	71	>90
Metabolism	Hepatic (glucoronidation)	CYP3A4, 5 (minor)
Excretion	<1% intact drug excreted renally	66% excreted in bile in pre-clinical models
Bioavailability	43%	N/A

cytoplasm and the nucleus of lymphocytes and keratinocytes at baseline in all patients in whom biopsies were performed. Repeat immunohistochemistry after 4 weeks of treatment showed reduced levels of phospho-STAT3 in the nucleus in 9 of 11 patients with clinical improvement and in only 3 of 16 who did not show a clinical improvement. Interestingly, overall pSTAT-3 was *increased* in the cytoplasmic compartment, suggesting that vorinostat does not alter expression of pSTAT3, but rather it impedes its ability to translocate to the nucleus and function as a transcription factor. Fantin [11] went on to examine more baseline samples and suggested that patients with higher baseline nuclear p-STAT3, and baseline nuclear p-STAT1 were likely to be resistant to vorinostat. Researchers investigating the mechanism of panobinostat using in vitro and in vivo models, have suggested that vorinostat resistance in particular CTCL cell lines could be overcome by panobinostat, via reduction in the overall quantity of activated p-STAT3 in cells [42, 43]. These findings have not been replicated by other investigators and the differences in methodology make it difficult to make definitive statements about the precise effect of HDACi on STAT3 signalling; however, it is reasonable to conclude that reduced STAT3 signalling represents both a potential mechanism of action and resistance for HDACi in CTCL and further investigation is required.

In addition to the observations on STAT3, the immunohistochemical work of Duvic et al. showed that thrombospondin 1, an inhibitor of angiogenesis, is upregulated after exposure to vorinostat, supporting the hypothesis anti-angiogenic effects are important to HDACi activity in CTCL. [41] Work from *Ellis* et al. [44] has provided further support for the anti-angiogenesis hypothesis. They performed serial gene-expression profiling on samples from ten patients with CTCL treated with panobinostat and showed consistent changes in expression in a set of 23 genes, including down-regulation of expression the angiogenic genes GUCY1A3 and ANGPT1.

Following a genome-wide loss of function screen on cell lines which suggested that cells with higher expression of RAD23B/HR23B [45], Khan and colleagues went on to show that patients whose tumours had higher levels of expression HR23B by immunohistochemistry at baseline were more likely to have responsive disease. HR23B has a ubiquitin-like domain and shuttles proteins to the proteasome for degradation. The finding supported the concept that disruption of the proteasome is important in CTCL, and the authors suggested that it could be a useful biomarker. Further studies elucidating the precise mechanism and whether romidepsin exerts a similar effect are required.

Clinical Studies

Cutaneous T-Cell Lymphoma

The selection of CTCL and PTCL as a candidate diseases for the HDACi came through results from conventionally designed, broadly inclusive clinical phase I trials as opposed to a clear preclinical rationale. [46] HDACi therapy induces objective responses in a significant minority of patients, in the order of 25–30% across studies. The responses take a median of 8 weeks and up to 2 years to occur, and appear to last somewhere between 6 months and a year in responding patients; however, median treatment duration was in only about 3 months across the studies.

A proportion of patients benefit from protracted clinical responses as well as significant improvements in more subjective symptomatic end-points such as erythema and pruritis. This comes at the cost of other symptoms such as asthenia and gastrointestinal side effects, as well as reversible thrombocytopenia, which appear to vary between the various HDACis and doses administered.

Response Criteria

Consensus response criteria for CTCL have only recently been published, but warrant discussion here because variations in response criteria affect interpretation of studies of CTCL [47]. The new consensus criteria incorporate a composite assessment of responses in the skin, blood, nodes and viscera. Cutaneous response criteria utilise changes in the mSWAT tool (Table 16.3) [48] in which overall body surface area involvement and disease type is incorporate in the overall score. Unfortunately all CTCL response criteria are somewhat subject to inter-observer variability. An important aspect of the consensus criteria is that responses, including progression, require confirmation at least 4 weeks after the initial observation. This stipulation prevents patients coming off-study due to a temporary disease flare or the typical minor clinical fluctuations characteristic of CTCL.

The studies presented here all precede the release of the consensus criteria and so the trials of HDACi in CTCL are difficult both to interpret, and to compare with each other. (Table 16.4) Interestingly, some do not incorporate visceral responses, and others do not include the mSWAT. For example, criteria for progression in the panobinostat study mandated patients come off study after minor progression (25% increase in mSWAT) which after a deep response might still represent a significant improvement over the patient's baseline condition. The authors of the conventional response criteria do not provide a single agreed measure of the pruritis that accompanies Sézary syndrome. Choice of that endpoint varies across the studies presented here but most commonly a 30 mm or 30% reduction in a 100 mm visual/analogue scale was considered as consistent with a significant clinical symptomatic response.

Table 16.3 *The mSWAT (modified severity weight assessment tool).* Patch = any size lesion without induration or significant elevation above the surrounding uninvolved skin; plaque = any size lesion that is elevated or indurated; crusting, ulceration or poikiloderma may be present tumour = any solid or nodular lesion ≥ 1 cm in diameter with evidence of deep; Tumour = infiltration in the skin and/or vertical growth. [47, 48]

Body region (%BSA)	Patch*	Plaque*	Tumour*
Head (7)			
Neck (2)			
Anterior trunk (13)			
Arms (8)			
Forearms (6)			
Hands (5)			
Posterior trunk (13)			
Buttocks (5)			
Thighs (19)			
Legs (14)			
Feet (7)			
Groin (1)			
Subtotal of lesion BSA			
Weighting factor	X 1	X 2	X 4
Subtotal lesion BSA x weighting factor			
mSWAT score = summation of each column line above			

Table 16.4 Response assessment methods varied considerably in studies of all patients in studies of CTCL

Drug	First author	Notes on response assessments
Vorinostat	Olsen [50]	Skin: mSWAT [48]
		PR: 50% reduction in mSWAT
		CR:100% clearing of skin disease
		PD: 25% worsening of mSWAT from baseline or ≥50% increase in SPD of nodal disease
		Date of relapse: mSWAT score from nadir to a more than 50% difference between the baseline and the nadir
		Confirmation of CR/PR: ≥4 weeks
		Confirmation of SD: not defined
		Pruritis: VAS with 30 mm reduction for at least 4 weeks considered significant, with no increase in use of anti-pruritis medications
		Separate reporting of nodal response, not reported in overall response results—≥50% reduction in nodal disease or ≥25% reduction in blood tumour burden
	Duvic [41]	Physician's Global Assessment of Clinical Condition (PGA) [76]
		PR: ≥50% improvement in either BSA or skin score with reduction of lymph nodes or blood when involved
		PD: ≥25% increase in the number or area of clinically abnormal nodes, or % of BSA or new visceral disease or increase in circulating Sézary cells
		Pruritis: 30% reduction of VAS for 4 weeks
		Confirmation of CR/PR: 4 weeks
		Confirmation of SD: 8 weeks
		Confirmation of PD: 4 weeks
Romidepsin	Whitakker [52]	LN: RECIST [77]
		Skin: Composite of SWAT [48] score and erythroderma scores. [78]
		PR: 50% improvement in the *sum of* Cheson, SWAT and erythroderma scores but with ≥30% improvement in skin, and no worsening at any site
		PD: new cutaneous or non-cutaneous tumour or >25% improvement in the sum of the three assessments or ≥15% worsening of skin
		CR: response at all sites
		Pruritis: VAS with 30 mm reduction for at least two cycles considered significant.
	Piekarz [51]	Skin or Viscera: RECIST [77]
		LN: IWG/Cheson [56]
		Erythroderma: present or absent
		Flow presence: present or absent
		PR: either a response in the skin or lymph nodes
		CR: a response in all sites of disease
Panobinostat	Duvic [53]	Skin: mSWAT, PGA
		Lymph nodes: Confirmatory CTs were performed to excluded disease progression in the nodes at the time of response in the skin
		PD: ≥25% increase in mSWAT compared to nadir
		Confirmation of progression not required

Abbreviations: PGA Physician's global assessment of clinical condition, mSWAT-modified severity weighted assessment tool

Efficacy

Vorinostat

Vorinostat (suberoylanilide hydroxamic acid, SAHA) was the first HDACi approved by the FDA, in 2006, for patients with CTCL who had failed two prior systemic therapies. [49] Clinical response data came from two phase II studies: a pivotal, single-arm study of 74 patients [50] and a smaller 3-arm, sequential, non-randomised study that recruited 33 patients to treatment on one of the three treatment schedules of vorinostat. [41]

In the pivotal study by Olsen et al., subjects received 400 mg/day, now the FDA-recommended dose. 61 of the 74 patients (82%) had clinically advanced disease, 30 (40.5%) had Sézary syndrome and all had been exposed to two (median 3) prior systemic therapies: 96% to oral bexarotene; 64% to interferon and 60.8% to systemic chemotherapeutics. Reported response rates were limited to cutaneous responses, and based on reductions in the mSWAT. Although baseline computed tomography scans were performed, and visceral disease monitored during the study, formal response criteria and response data did not include visceral disease. (Table 16.4) The overall response rate was 29.7% (95% CI 19.7–41.5) and a response was seen in a third of patients with Sézary syndrome; however, only 1 patient experienced a complete remission. (Figure 16.4) An additional 48% had a measurable disease improvement (See diagram). Pruritis improvement (rather then resolution) was experienced by a third of the 65 patients who recorded a score of 3 or above at baseline. Responses occurred after a median of 8 weeks and lasted a median of 6.1 months.

Duvic et al. simultaneously conducted a second study, exploring 3 dose levels of vorinostat. Patient characteristics were similar to the pivotal study by Olsen. Patients were sequentially enrolled into the open dose level: 400 mg daily ($n=13$), 300 mg bd 3,4 or 5 days a week ($n=11$) and 300 mg bd x 14 days, with 7 days rest, with 200 mg bd maintenance ($n=9$). Each of these doses had been established as MTDs in previous phase I studies. The overall response rate was comparable between the three dose levels, although was perhaps poorer for the intermittent dosing schedule (group 2). The overall response rate was 24%. The authors described a "clinical benefit", as determined by stable disease, pruritis relief, or both in an additional 19 (58%) of the study patients. In common with the study by

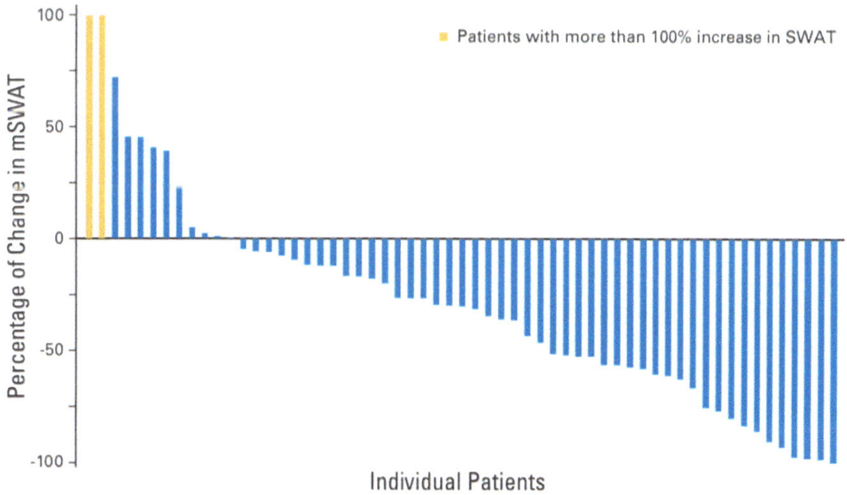

Figure 16.4 Percentage change in mSWAT in the pivotal study of vorinotsat, 47 of 61 patients had a reduced MSWAT score. [Reprinted from Olsen EA, Kim YH, Kuzel TM, et al. Phase IIb multi-centre trial of vorinostat in patients with persistent, progressive or treatment refractory cutaneous T-cell lymphoma. J Clin Oncol 2007;25:3109–15. With permission from American Socicty of Clinical Oncology.]

Olsen, was the observation that a broad range of clinical CTCL presentations, with responses seen in patients with and without Sézary syndrome and of clinical symptoms such as pruritis. Although statistical comparisons were not possible, it was argued that the intermittent dosing schedule was probably less effective due to a relative, albeit unproven, reduction in drug-induced histone hyperacetylation. The onset of response was similar in tempo to the study by Olsen, as was the time to progression. Those who achieved an objective response were able to maintain it for 9.4–19.6 months (median of 15.1). In both studies, the median duration of treatment was 8 months (range, 1–67).

Romidepsin

The cyclic peptide romidepsin (depsipeptide, FK228, FR901228) is, by contrast to vorinostat, a more specific inhibitor of class-I histone deacetylases. However this does not appear to have been detrimental to clinical effect. To its potential disadvantage, romidepsin is only available as an intravenous formulation. Data is available from two large phase II studies, an international study based at the NCI in the United States [51], the other, European [52]. The treatment schedule was identical across both studies, 14 mg/m^2 intravenously, days 1, 8 and 15 of a 28-day cycle.

The NCI study by Piekarz [51] included patients with both CTCL and PTCL and utilised the RECIST criteria which is typically reserved for studies of non-haematological solid tumours. These criteria stipulate the selection of a limited number of measurable lesions at baseline (minimum 10 mm by calliper), and a partial response requires a 30% reduction in the maximal diameter of all target lesions. The system is perhaps not well suited to the patches and plaques of CTCL, nor to the potential for multiple lesions below the measurable length required for the baseline assessment. Nodal assessment used the Cheson/IWG criteria, in which a partial response requires a 50% reduction in the sum of the product of the diameters of the target lesions. Symptomatic responses, such as improvement in pruritis, were not reported.

The study design was the Simon 2-stage, with the initial cohort of patients not having received more than two systemic therapies. The 44 patients recruited in the second stage of the study had been more heavily treated and in the overall study, patients had received a median of four prior regimens. The severity of disease was similar to the other studies of HDACi in CTCL (Table 16.5). The overall response rate of 34% included four complete remissions. Three of these occurred in the relatively treatment naïve first-stage study. Of the 20 patients that experienced a partial response, 13 had involvement of blood, nodes or viscera. The response duration was 13.7 months for the 24 patients achieving a CR or PR, and 4 months for those with stable disease. As with the vorinostat studies, responses occurred at a median of 8 weeks.

The pivotal 33-centre phase II study of romidepsin by Whittaker et al. [52]. confirmed the observations by Piekarz et al. 96 patients were treated. Response criteria were more rigorous in regard to the skin, using the mSWAT tool (Table 16.3, 16.4) but were more inclusive for lymph nodes, using the RECIST criteria. The authors had an umbrella response score that incorporated all domains of disease (skin, blood and nodes). Nevertheless, they were able to demonstrate an identical response rate of 34%; time-to-response of 8 weeks and response duration of 15 (0–19.8) months. (Fig. 16.5, Table 16.6) This study included assessment of pruritis by a visual scale, as used in the vorinostat studies, and ≥30 mm reduction was seen in 43% of the 65 patients with pruritis, including those without objective disease responses.

Panobinostat

Like vorinostat, panobinostat is also available in oral formulation. Of the studies presented here, the response criteria used in the study for panobinostat were the most comprehensive; however, the criteria used did not require a second confirmation of progression prior withdrawal of patients from the study. In an attempt to adjust for this difference the authors presented multiple post hoc

Table 16.5 Patient characteristics in clinical studies of HDAC inhibitors for cutaneous T-cell lymphoma

	Vorinostat		Romidepsin		Panobinostat
First Author	Olsen [50]	Duvic [41]	Whitakker [52]	Piekarz [51]	Duvic [53]
Total number	74	33	96	71	139
Age; Median (range)	60 (39–83)	67 (26–82)	57 (mean)	57 (28–84)	
CTCL stage (*n*, %)					
IA	0	1 (3)	0	1 (1.4)	36 (25.9)
IB	11 (14.9)	3 (9)	15 (16)	6 (8.5)	
IIA	2 (2.7)	1 (3)	13 (14)	2 (2.8)	
IIB	19 (25.7)	5 (15)	21 (22)	15 (2.1)	70 (50.4)
III	20 (27)	5 (15)	23 (24)	6 (8.5)	
IVA	18 (24.3)	10 (30)	25 (25)	28 (3.9)	0
IVB	4 (5.4)	8 (24)	0	13 (18.3)	33 (23.7)
Number of prior therapies; *n* (range)	3 (1–12)	5 (1–15)	4 (1–11)	4 (0–14)	4 (1–15)
Time from original diagnosis years (range)	2.9 (0.7–27.3)	3.3 (0.2–27.2)	3 (1–26)	–	2.8 (0.1–42)
Sézary syndrome	30 (40.5)	11 (33)	37 (39)	–	38(23.7)
Prior oral bexarotene	71 (95.9)	22 (67)	32 (33)	45 (63.4)	79 (57)
Prior chemotherapy	45 (60.8)	29 (88)	74 (77)	65 (91.5)	–

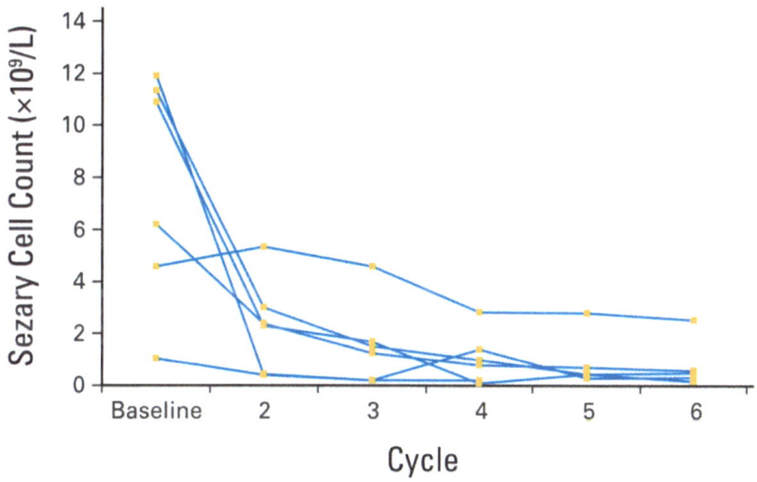

Figure 16.5 Sézary cell counts for 6 of 13 patients with higher blood tumour burden in the study of romidepsin by Whittaker et al. [52] [Reprinted from Whittaker SJ, Demierre M-F, Kim EJ, et al. Final Results From a Multicenter, International, Pivotal Study of Romidepsin in Refractory Cutaneous T-Cell Lymphoma. Journal of clinical oncology. 2010;28(29):4485–4491. With permission from American Society of Clinical Oncology.]

analyses of patient outcomes, adjusting for the variation in criteria for progression. Patients entering this study were stratified by whether they had received systemic bexarotene as it was hypothesised that the response rate would be less in those who had. That hypothesised difference was not born out in the crude number of responses; however, bexarotene naive patients appeared to enjoy a (statistically insignificant) longer response. Taken together, the lower RR in this study is difficult to place into context of the results reported with vorinostat or romidepsin and at this time it is not possible to determine whether this drug has inferior efficacy (Table 16.6).

Specifically, 139 patients were treated in the study (see Table 16.5). 79 patients (59%) had

Table 16.6 Results from key studies of HDAC inhibitors for CTCL . Abbreviations: TTP: time to progression

	Vorinostat		Romidepsin		Panobinostat
First Author	Olsen [50]	Duvic [41]	Whitakker [52]	Piekarz [51]	Duvic [53]
Total number	74	33	96	71	139
Overall response (%)	29.7	24.2	34	34	17.3
Complete responses; *n* (%)	1 (1.4)	0	6 (6)	4 (7)	2 (1.4)
Median weeks to response (range)	7.9 (4–24.4)	11.9 (3.6–21.9)	8 (3.6–19.2)	8 (4–24)	10.8 (range not available)
Median duration of response; months (range)	NR but estimated ≥6.16 (1–14.7)	15.1 (9.4–19.6)	15 (0–19.8)	13.7 (1–76)	5.6 months in bexarotene exposed and not reached in the bexarotene naïve group.
TTP (months)	4.9 (≥9.8 for stage IIb or greater)	2.82	8 (0–21.7)	15.1 for those responding 5.9 for SD 1.9 for the rest	??
Duration of treatment; median months (range)	8 (4–67)	8 (1–67)	–	4 (1–72)	3 (0.2–29.6)

previously been treated with oral bexarotene [53]. Patients had similar characteristics to those included in other HDACi studies. The overall response rate was 17.3%; 15.2% in those previously exposed to bexarotene and 20% in those who were not. Conversely, the crude response rate was higher in bexarotene-exposed patients with Sézary syndrome (6 of 21, 28.6%) than bexarotene-naïve Sézary patients (2 of 12, 16.7%). The median duration of response in bexarotene-exposed patients was 5.6 months, and was not reached at a median follow up of months (Table 16.6). By applying alternative response criteria similar to those used in the other studies, where confirmation of progression at least 4 weeks after first documentation was required, the adjusted duration of response was reported as 9.2 months in the bexarotene-exposed group. A quarter of the 97 patients with pruritis experienced relief, somewhat less impressive than the results for vorinostat and romidepsin.

The authors attributed the lower response rate of CTCL to panobinostat to two possible causes: insufficient dose and premature withdrawal of patients due to progression that was not confirmed with a period of observation. After re-analysis of the data, only 7 of the 84 patients who progressed during the study period would not have been considered to have progressed if a second conformation was required. This analysis raised the overall response to 19.4%.Whether attempts to develop panobinostat at higher doses for CTCL will proceed, remains to be seen. Selected phase II dose was based on phase I data from other indications, and experience in Hodgkin lymphoma suggests that higher doses of panobinostat are likely to be more effective. At the time of writing, panobinostat is being developed primarily for use in myeloma in combination with other agents. Overall the clinical findings from studies of HDACi with CTCL are consistent, demonstrating responses in about a third of patients lasting from 6 months to beyond 18 months in a significant minority. This class of agent also offers some symptomatic pruritis relief and appears to be safe.

Romidepsin in PTCL

Presently, no HDACis are approved for the treatment of PTCL. The majority of the clinical data come from the studies of romidepsin. The NCI-led study of romidepsin by Piekarz et al., referred to above, reported the outcomes of patients with PTCL separately from that of CTCL [54]. Response assessment for nodal disease in this and in the other major study in PTCL was by

Table 16.7 Patient characteristics in studies with PTCL. Central reviewa

First Author	Piekarz [54]	Coiffier [55]
Total patient number	47	130
Median Age (range)	59 (27–84)	61 (20–83)
Stage III/IV (%)	45 (96%)	70
Marrow involvement (%)	14 (28%)	36 (28%)
Elevated LDH	26 (55%)	
PTCL NOS	27 (57%)	27 (21%)
Angioimmunoblastic	7 (15%)	27 (21%)
ALCL ALK Positive	2 (4%)	1 (0.7%)
ALCL ALK negative	2 (4%)	21 (16%)
Cutaneous ALCL	2 (4%)	–
Other	4 (8%)	12 (9.2%)
DLBCLa	1(2%)	
Overall response	16 (38%)	38 (39%)b
Complete response	8 (18%)	18 (14)
Median response duration, months (range)	8.9 (2–74)	3 (<1–28+)
Median time to response, months	1.8	1.8
Response duration in complete responders, months (range)	29.4 (3–74)	14 (1.2–26.7+)
Response duration in partial responders, months (range)	5.2 (2–23, ongoing)	17 (0.5–34, ongoing)[a]
Response duration in patients with stable disease	6 (3–12)	Not provided
Median duration of treatment, months (range)	3 (1–57)	1.4 (mean 4.2)

standard lymphoma IWG guidelines [55, 56]. All patients with PTCL had been exposed to systemic chemotherapy and 38% to stem cell transplantation; 40% of patients had previously received radiation. The dose and administration was the same as for patients with CTCL; 14 mg days 1,8 and 15 of a 28-day cycle. Responses are listed in Table 16.7. The overall response rate was 38%, with complete responses observed in eight patients (18%). The time to response was comparable to that seen in CTCL—approximately 2 months. Those with only stable disease ($n = 5$) had a median time to progression of 6 (range 3–12) months, with those with PR (9,20%) had a median response of 5.2 months, with some experiencing protracted periods of time on treatment. Overall, the median number of cycles delivered was three (1–57), with 22 of 47 patients receiving less than or equal to two cycles. Toxicities are discussed below.

A multi-centre, international study of 131 patients from 48 centres has recently been completed and reported by Coiffier et al. [55]. The mean age of patients was 59, and a median of 2 prior systemic therapies had been given. 16% of patients had received autologous stem cell transplantation, and all but one systemic chemotherapy. 38% were refractory to the immediate prior therapy. The overall response rate was 30%, which included 21 patients (16%) with a CRu or better. 17% of patients withdrew because of adverse events. The authors noted that the response rate was similarly high in patients who had been refractory to their most recent therapy, reassuring evidence that the HDACis are targeting genuinely novel molecular pathways from those of conventional chemotherapy.

There does not appear to be a particular difference in efficacy across the PTCL subtypes; however, the frequency of specific entities other than PTCL-NOS is low in both trials. The largest subtype of PTCL studied in the romidepsin trials other than PTCL, NOS was angioimmunoblastic lymphoma. While only one of six patients (16%, 95% CI 0.04–64%) with angioimmunoblastic lymphoma responded in the NCI study, [54] 8 of 27 (29%, 95%CI 13.75–50.18%) patients responded in the study by Coiffier et al., similar to the overall response rate for PTCL, NOS. The numbers of patients

Table 16.8 Common toxicities from studies of HDAC inhibitors in CTCL. Approximate ranges are given and rates of toxicities are generally similar between the agents, with the probable exception of diarrhoea which appears to be less common for romidepsin

Most frequent toxicities (all grades)	Diarrhoea ~50% for pan-HDACi and ~10% for romidepsin
	Fatigue ~40%
	Nausea ~20–40%
	Anorexia ~20%
	Thrombocytopenia ~11–50%
	Taste disturbance ~10–50%
Grade III/IV toxicities	Fatigue/aesthenia ~5–7%
	Thrombocytopenia 5–20%
	Anaemia 2–8%
	Neutropenia ~10%
	Sepsis 1–5%

with other subtypes of PTCL are fewer, thus no clear conclusions about differential responses can be made.

Safety and toxicities

As a class of agents, the HDACis share common toxicities, which, with the exception of diarrhoea, do not seem to differ by the HDAC specificity of the agent. Key toxicities in the studies in CTCL are summarised in (Table 16.8). While they appear dose-dependent, they are on the whole across the five studies and the three agents discussed here. In practical use, the most consistent and troublesome toxicities are the mild fatigue and asthenia experienced by approximately half of patients. Similarly common are disorders of taste. Nausea is frequent but more easily treated with standard antiemetics. Thrombocytopenia occurred in up to 40% and was severe (grade III/IV) in up to 20%. The thrombocytopenia of HDACis is rapidly reversible upon withdrawal of the drug and does not appear to relate to cumulative drug exposure. [57] While megakaryocyte numbers increase in response to HDACi, platelet budding is defective, owing to drug-induced phosphorylation of the myosin light chain. [58]

Readers familiar with the treatment of advanced CTCL with systemic chemotherapy will immediately notice the low rates of grade III/IV neutropenia, sepsis or febrile neutropenia associated with the use of HDACis (see Table 16.8). This difference is one of the key advantages of the HDACi, in that they can induce systemic responses without requiring the aggressive prophylaxis against infection or hospitalisation frequently required in patients receiving myelosuppressive combination therapy (especially those with Sézary syndrome).

As consequence of rare episodes of cardiac dysrhythmia in the phase I studies, ECG assessments were systematically performed in the larger HDACi studies. ECG changes have been observed in each of the HDACi discussed here but only rarely have they been of clinical significance. Clinically insignificant QTc prolongation was recorded in 3 patients in the study of vorinostat by Olsen [50] and was not reported in the study by Duvic. [41] T wave flattening was seen in 71% of patients in on the NCI romidepsin study, and ST depression in 9%. Clinically significant QTc prolongation was reported in two patients on the European romidepsin study, which also reported an average prolongation of the QTc interval of 4.6 ms. [51, 59] More detailed study of the initial 42 patients in that trial, which included Holter monitoring in nine patients, showed that the changes in QTc were not associated with elevated cardiac troponin or to changes in left ventricular ejection fraction. [60] One patient had a QTc of >500 ms; however, this occurred in association with abnormal potassium and magnesium levels. Panobinostat and vorinostat also have reports of prolongation of the QTc, rarely as long as 60 ms in the case of panobinostat [61] or 30 ms after a single supratherapeutic dose of vorinostat [62]. QTc prolongation may well be dose and schedule dependent [63]. Despite prolongation of the QTc less than what would usually be considered as significant by regulators, regular ECG monitoring remains a component of the ongoing prospective trials. Replenishment of potassium and magnesium (which may be especially lowered in CTCL) [64] to within normal limits prior to therapy is recommended, particularly prior to administration of intravenous romidepsin. In addition, drugs which are known to cause prolongation of the QTc should be avoided.

All HDACis should be considered contraindicated in pregnancy. Romidepsin competes with oestrogen for its receptor and therefore, and as is usually the case with other anti-cancer agents, it cannot be assumed that the oral contraceptive pill provides sufficient protection against conception.

Placing HDACi in the overall therapy of T-cell lymphoma, future directions

Based on the evidence and label restrictions, we reserve HDACi for second or subsequent-line therapy of CTCL, and a future role for HDACi in other forms of PTCL seems likely [65]. The possibility of protracted responses makes HDACi an attractive option for patients with advanced and symptomatic CTCL. HDACis are also effective in earlier stages of disease. These agents are generally well tolerated; however, the later onset of response makes HDACi a poor choice if rapid control of symptoms is desired. We frequently find that palliative doses of corticosteroids are needed to ease symptoms in CTCL while a response to the HDACi is anticipated. Combinations with other agents to improve response rates present an attractive concept, with a strong rationale existing for combinations with proteasome inhibitors and other biological therapies [66]. HDACi may also be useful as a chemo- or radiotherapy-sensitising agent. [67] Combination with conventional chemotherapeutics is being tested in Groupe d'Etude des Lymphomes de l'Adulte-led dose escalation study of romidepsin in combination with CHOP chemotherapy (Ro-CHOP, NCT01280526) for PTCL. The results of these trials are eagerly awaited.

References

1. Egger G, Liang G, Aparicio A, Jones PA. Epigenetics in human disease and prospects for epigenetic therapy. Nature. 2004;429:457–63.
2. Bolden JE, Peart MJ, Johnstone RW. Anticancer activities of histone deacetylase inhibitors. Nat Rev. 2006;5:769–84.
3. Narlikar GJ, Fan HY, Kingston RE. Cooperation between complexes that regulate chromatin structure and transcription. Cell. 2002;108:475–87.
4. Lane AA, Chabner BA. Histone deacetylase inhibitors in cancer therapy. J Clin Oncol. 2009;27:5459–68.
5. Johnstone RW. Histone-deacetylase inhibitors: novel drugs for the treatment of cancer. Nat Rev. 2002;1:287–99.
6. Dickinson M, Johnstone RW, Prince HM. Histone deacetylase inhibitors: potential targets responsible for their anti-cancer effect. Invest New Drugs. 2010;28 Suppl 1:S3–20.
7. Minucci S, Pelicci PG. Histone deacetylase inhibitors and the promise of epigenetic (and more) treatments for cancer. Nat Rev Cancer. 2006;6:38–51.
8. Peart MJ, Smyth GK, van Laar RK, et al. Identification and functional significance of genes regulated by structurally different histone deacetylase inhibitors. Proc Natl Acad Sci USA. 2005;102:3697–702.
9. Zhang XD, Gillespie SK, Borrow JM, Hersey P. The histone deacetylase inhibitor suberic bishydroxamate regulates the expression of multiple apoptotic mediators and induces mitochondria-dependent apoptosis of melanoma cells. Mol Cancer Ther. 2004;3:425–35.
10. Buglio D, Georgakis GV, Hanabuchi S, et al. Vorinostat inhibits STAT6-mediated TH2 cytokine and TARC production and induces cell death in Hodgkin lymphoma cell lines. Blood. 2008;112:1424–33.
11. Fantin VR, Loboda A, Paweletz CP, et al. Constitutive activation of signal transducers and activators of transcription predicts vorinostat resistance in cutaneous T-cell lymphoma. Cancer Res. 2008;68:3785–94.
12. Ruefli AA, Ausserlechner MJ, Bernhard D, et al. The histone deacetylase inhibitor and chemotherapeutic agent suberoylanilide hydroxamic acid (SAHA) induces a cell-death pathway characterized by cleavage of Bid and production of reactive oxygen species. Proc Natl Acad Sci USA. 2001;98:10833–8.
13. Nakata S, Yoshida T, Horinaka M, Shiraishi T, Wakada M, Sakai T. Histone deacetylase inhibitors upregulate death receptor 5/TRAIL-R2 and sensitize apoptosis induced by TRAIL/APO2-L in human malignant tumor cells. Oncogene. 2004;23:6261–71.
14. Fandy TE, Shankar S, Ross DD, Sausville E, Srivastava RK. Interactive effects of HDAC inhibitors and TRAIL on apoptosis are associated with changes in mitochondrial functions and expressions of cell cycle regulatory genes in multiple myeloma. Neoplasia. 2005;7:646–57.
15. Inoue S, Harper N, Walewska R, Dyer MJS, Cohen GM. Enhanced Fas-associated death domain recruitment by histone deacetylase inhibitors is critical for the sensitization of chronic lymphocytic leukemia cells to TRAIL-induced apoptosis. Mol Cancer Ther. 2009;8:3088–97.
16. Klener P, Molinsky J, Simonova T, Necas E, Andera L, Zivny J. Acquired resistance to tumor necrosis factor-related apoptosis-inducing ligand (TRAIL): histone deacetylase inhibitors resensitize TRAIL-resistant jurkat acute lymphocytic leukemia cells. ASH Annual Meeting Abstracts. 2008;112:5032 EP.

17. Frew AJ, Lindemann RK, Martin BP, et al. Combination therapy of established cancer using a histone deacetylase inhibitor and a TRAIL receptor agonist. Proc Natl Acad Sci USA. 2008;105: 11317–22.
18. Vrana JA, Decker RH, Johnson CR, et al. Induction of apoptosis in U937 human leukemia cells by suberoylanilide hydroxamic acid (SAHA) proceeds through pathways that are regulated by Bcl-2/Bcl-XL, c-Jun, and p21CIP1, but independent of p53. Oncogene. 1999;18:7016–25.
19. Johnstone RW, Licht JD. Histone deacetylase inhibitors in cancer therapy: is transcription the primary target? Cancer Cell. 2003;4:13–8.
20. Marks PA, Richon VM, Rifkind RA. Histone deacetylase inhibitors: inducers of differentiation or apoptosis of transformed cells. J Natl Cancer Inst. 2000;92:1210–6.
21. Richon VM, Sandhoff TW, Rifkind RA, Marks PA. Histone deacetylase inhibitor selectively induces p21WAF1 expression and gene-associated histone acetylation. Proc Natl Acad Sci USA. 2000;97: 10014–9.
22. Ungerstedt JS, Sowa Y, Xu WS, et al. Role of thioredoxin in the response of normal and transformed cells to histone deacetylase inhibitors. Proc Natl Acad Sci USA. 2005;102:673–8.
23. Rosato RR, Almenara JA, Grant S. The histone deacetylase inhibitor MS-275 promotes differentiation or apoptosis in human leukemia cells through a process regulated by generation of reactive oxygen species and induction of p21CIP1/WAF1 1. Cancer Res. 2003;63:3637–45.
24. Rosato RR, Kolla SS, Hock SK, et al. Histone deacetylase inhibitors activate NF-kappaB in human leukemia cells through an ATM/NEMO-related pathway. J Biol Chem. 2010;285:10064–77.
25. Piekarz RL, Sackett DL, Bates SE. Histone deacetylase inhibitors and demethylating agents: clinical development of histone deacetylase inhibitors for cancer therapy. Cancer J. 2007;13:30–9.
26. Spange S, Wagner T, Heinzel T, Krämer OH. Acetylation of non-histone proteins modulates cellular signalling at multiple levels. Int J Biochem Cell Biol. 2009;41:185–98.
27. Rodriguez-Gonzalez A, Lin T, Ikeda AK, Simms-Waldrip T, Fu C, Sakamoto KM. Role of the aggresome pathway in cancer: targeting histone deacetylase 6-dependent protein degradation. Cancer Res. 2008; 68:2557–60.
28. Davenport EL, Morgan GJ, Davies FE. Untangling the unfolded protein response. Cell Cycle. 2008; 7:865–9.
29. Todd DJ, Lee A-H, Glimcher LH. The endoplasmic reticulum stress response in immunity and autoimmunity. Nat Rev Immunol. 2008;8:663–74.
30. Kawaguchi Y, Kovacs JJ, McLaurin A, Vance JM, Ito A, Yao TP. The deacetylase HDAC6 regulates aggresome formation and cell viability in response to misfolded protein stress. Cell. 2003;115:727–38.
31. Buglio D, Mamidipudi V, Khaskhely NM, et al. The class-I HDAC inhibitor MGCD0103 induces apoptosis in Hodgkin lymphoma cell lines and synergizes with proteasome inhibitors by an HDAC6-independent mechanism. Br J Haematol. 2010;151(4):387–96.
32. Boyault C, Sadoul K, Pabion M, Khochbin S. HDAC6, at the crossroads between cytoskeleton and cell signaling by acetylation and ubiquitination. Oncogene. 2007;26:5468–76.
33. Harrison SJ, Quach H, Link E, et al. A high rate of durable responses with romidepsin, bortezomib, and dexamethasone in relapsed or refractory multiple myeloma. Blood. 2011;118:6274–83.
34. Piekarz RL, Frye R, Turner M, et al. Phase II multi-institutional trial of the histone deacetylase inhibitor romidepsin as monotherapy for patients with cutaneous T-cell lymphoma. J Clin Oncol. 2009;27:5410–7.
35. Mitchell TJ, John S. Signal transducer and activator of transcription (STAT) signalling and T-cell lymphomas. Immunology. 2005;114:301–12.
36. Brender C, Nielsen M, Kaltoft K, et al. STAT3-mediated constitutive expression of SOCS-3 in cutaneous T-cell lymphoma. Blood. 2001;97:1056–62.
37. Eriksen KW, Kaltoft K, Mikkelsen G, et al. Constitutive STAT3-activation in Sezary syndrome: tyrphostin AG490 inhibits STAT3-activation, interleukin-2 receptor expression and growth of leukemic Sezary cells. Leukemia. 2001;15:787–93.
38. Nielsen M, Kaltoft K, Nordahl M, et al. Constitutive activation of a slowly migrating isoform of Stat3 in mycosis fungoides: tyrphostin AG490 inhibits Stat3 activation and growth of mycosis fungoides tumor cell lines. Proc Natl Acad Sci USA. 1997;94:6764–9.
39. Nielsen M, Nissen MH, Gerwien J, et al. Spontaneous interleukin-5 production in cutaneous T-cell lymphoma lines is mediated by constitutively activated Stat3. Blood. 2002;99:973–7.
40. Wozniak MB, Villuendas R, Bischoff JR, et al. Vorinostat interferes with the signaling transduction pathway of T cell receptor and synergizes with PI3K inhibitors in cutaneous T-cell lymphoma. Haematologica. 2010;95:613–21.
41. Duvic M, Talpur R, Ni X, et al. Phase 2 trial of oral vorinostat (suberoylanilide hydroxamic acid, SAHA) for refractory cutaneous T-cell lymphoma (CTCL). Blood. 2007;109:31–9.
42. Shao W, Growney JD, Feng Y, et al. Activity of deacetylase inhibitor panobinostat (LBH589) in cutaneous T-cell lymphoma models: Defining molecular mechanisms of resistance. Int J Cancer. 2010; 127:2199–208.
43. Tiffon C, Adams J, van der Fits L, et al. The histone deacetylase inhibitors vorinostat and romidepsin downmodulate IL-10 expression in cutaneous T-cell lymphoma cells. Br J Pharmacol. 2011;162:1590–602.
44. Ellis L, Pan Y, Smyth GK, et al. Histone deacetylase inhibitor panobinostat induces clinical responses with associated alterations in gene expression profiles in cutaneous T-cell lymphoma. Clin Cancer Res. 2008; 14:4500–10.

45. Fotheringham S, Epping MT, Stimson L, et al. Genome-wide loss-of-function screen reveals an important role for the proteasome in HDAC inhibitor-induced apoptosis. Cancer Cell. 2009;15:57–66.
46. Piekarz RL, Robey R, Sandor V, et al. Inhibitor of histone deacetylation, depsipeptide (FR901228), in the treatment of peripheral and cutaneous T-cell lymphoma: a case report. Blood. 2001;98:2865–8.
47. Olsen EA, Whittaker S, Kim YH, et al. Clinical end points and response criteria in mycosis fungoides and Sezary syndrome: a consensus statement of the International Society for Cutaneous Lymphomas, the United States Cutaneous Lymphoma Consortium, and the Cutaneous Lymphoma Task Force of the European Organisation for Research and Treatment of Cancer. J Clin Oncol. 2011;29:2598–607.
48. Stevens SR, Ke MS, Parry EJ, Mark J, Cooper KD. Quantifying skin disease burden in mycosis fungoides-type cutaneous T-cell lymphomas: the severity-weighted assessment tool (SWAT). Arch Dermatol. 2002;138:42–8.
49. Mann BS, Johnson JR, Cohen MH, Justice R, Pazdur R. FDA approval summary: vorinostat for treatment of advanced primary cutaneous T-cell lymphoma. Oncologist. 2007;12:1247–52.
50. Olsen EA, Kim YH, Kuzel TM, et al. Phase IIb multicenter trial of vorinostat in patients with persistent, progressive, or treatment refractory cutaneous T-cell lymphoma. J Clin Oncol. 2007;25:3109–15.
51. Piekarz R, Frye R, Turner M, et al. Phase II multi-institutional trial of the histone deacetylase inhibitor romidepsin as monotherapy for patients with cutaneous T-cell lymphoma. J Clin Oncol. 2009;27(32):5410–7.
52. Whittaker SJ, Demierre M-F, Kim EJ, et al. Final results from a multicenter, international, pivotal study of romidepsin in refractory cutaneous T-cell lymphoma. J Clin Oncol. 2010;28(29):4485–91.
53. Duvic M, Dummer R, Becker J, et al. Panobinostat activity in both bexarotene-exposed and -naïve patients with refractory cutaneous T-cell lymphoma: results of a phase II trial. Eur J Haematol. 2011 [Epub ahead of print].
54. Piekarz RL, Frye R, Prince HM, et al. Phase II trial of romidepsin in patients with peripheral T-cell lymphoma. Blood. 2011;117(22):5827–34.
55. Coiffier B, Pro B, Prince HM, et al. Final results from a pivotal, multicenter, international, open-label, phase 2 study of romidepsin in progressive or relapsed peripheral T-cell lymphoma (PTCL) following prior systemic therapy. ASH Annual Meeting Abstracts. 2010;116:114.
56. Cheson BD, Horning SJ, Coiffier B, et al. Report of an international workshop to standardize response criteria for non-Hodgkin's lymphomas. NCI Sponsored International Working Group. J Clin Oncol. 1999;17: 1244.
57. Lin R, Hu J, Paul S, et al. Characteristics of thrombocytopenia in patients treated with oral panobinostat (LBH589). ASH Annual Meeting Abstracts. 2009; 114:2740 EP.
58. Bishton MJ, Harrison SJ, Martin BP, et al. Deciphering the molecular and biological processes that mediate histone deacetylase inhibitor-induced thrombocytopenia. Blood. 2011;117(13):3658–68.
59. Cabell C, Bates S, Piekarz R, et al. Systematic assessment of potential cardiac effects of the novel histone deacetylase (HDAC) inhibitor romidepsin. ASCO Meeting Abstracts. 2009;27:e19533 EP.
60. Piekarz RL, Frye AR, Wright JJ, et al. Cardiac studies in patients treated with depsipeptide, FK228, in a phase II trial for T-cell lymphoma. Clin Cancer Res. 2006;12:3762–73.
61. Weber H, Tai F, Paul S, et al. QT interval measurements in patients with hematologic malignancies and solid tumors treated with oral panobinostat (LBH589). ASH Annual Meeting Abstracts. 2009;114:3781 EP.
62. Munster PN, Rubin EH, Van Belle S, et al. A single supratherapeutic dose of vorinostat does not prolong the QTc interval in patients with advanced cancer. Clin Cancer Res. 2009;15:7077–84.
63. Zhang L, Lebwohl D, Masson E, Laird G, Cooper MR, Prince HM. Clinically relevant QTc prolongation is not associated with current dose schedules of LBH589 (panobinostat). J Clin Oncol. 2008;26:332–3. discussion 3–4.
64. Morgan M, Maloney D, Duvic M. Hypomagnesemia and hypocalcemia in mycosis fungoides: a retrospective case series. Leuk Lymphoma. 2002;43:1297–302.
65. Prince HM, Whittaker S, Hoppe RT. How I treat mycosis fungoides and Sézary syndrome. Blood. 2009;114:4337–53.
66. Bots M, Johnstone RW. Rational combinations using HDAC inhibitors. Clin Cancer Res. 2009;15:3970–7.
67. Sharma SV, Lee DY, Li B, et al. A chromatin-mediated reversible drug-tolerant state in cancer cell subpopulations. Cell. 2010;141:69–80.
68. Hubbert C, Guardiola A, Shao R, et al. HDAC6 is a microtubule-associated deacetylase. Nature. 2002;417:455–8.
69. Guardiola AR, Yao T-P. Molecular cloning and characterization of a novel histone deacetylase HDAC10. J Biol Chem. 2002;277:3350–6.
70. Wang Z, Zang C, Cui K, et al. Genome-wide mapping of HATs and HDACs reveals distinct functions in active and inactive genes. Cell. 2009;138(5):1019–31.
71. Fujiwara Y, Yamamoto N, Yamada Y, et al. Phase I and pharmacokinetic study of vorinostat (suberoylanilide hydroxamic acid) in Japanese patients with solid tumors. Cancer Sci. 2009;100:1728–34.
72. Kelly WK, Richon VM, O'Connor O, et al. Phase I clinical trial of histone deacetylase inhibitor: suberoylanilide hydroxamic acid administered intravenously. Clin Cancer Res. 2003;9:3578–88.
73. O'Connor OA. Clinical experience with the novel histone deacetylase inhibitor vorinostat (suberoylanilide hydroxamic acid) in patients with relapsed lymphoma. Br J Cancer. 2006;95:S7–12.
74. Piekarz RL, Frye R, Prince HM, et al. Phase 2 trial of romidepsin in patients with peripheral T-cell lymphoma. Blood. 2011;117:5827–34.
75. Woo S, Gardner ER, Chen X, et al. Population pharmacokinetics of romidepsin in patients with cutaneous T-cell lymphoma and relapsed peripheral T-cell lymphoma. Clin Cancer Res. 2009;15:1496–503.

76. Duvic M, Hymes K, Heald P, et al. Bexarotene is effective and safe for treatment of refractory advanced-stage cutaneous T-cell lymphoma: multinational phase II-III trial results. J Clin Oncol. 2001;19:2456–71.
77. Therasse P, Arbuck SG, Eisenhauer EA, et al. New guidelines to evaluate the response to treatment in solid tumors. European Organization for Research and Treatment of Cancer, National Cancer Institute of the United States, National Cancer Institute of Canada. J Natl Cancer Inst. 2000;92:205–16.
78. Olsen E, Duvic M, Frankel A, et al. Pivotal phase III trial of two dose levels of denileukin diftitox for the treatment of cutaneous T-cell lymphoma. J Clin Oncol. 2001;19:376–88.

Novel Therapies for T-cell Lymphomas

17

Christiane Querfeld and Steven T. Rosen

Introduction

Advanced stages of mycosis fungoides (MF) and Sézary syndrome (SS) are often refractory to treatment and have an unfavorable prognosis. It is not clear what mechanisms are adopted by the malignant T-lymphocytes to proliferate and to escape immune surveillance. Immune dysregulation is demonstrated by the constitutive phosphorylation of STAT-3 protein in neoplastic T-cells [1, 2]. These cells may express the IL-2 alpha receptor (CD25) which is a target for biologic therapy with denileukin diftitox. Naturally occurring regulatory T-cells (Tregs) also express the CD25 molecule. They suppress the activity of other immune cells, thus maintaining immunological tolerance. Features of Tregs appear to play a role in the immunosuppression of advanced stages, but their role in CTCL is still controversial [3, 4]. Strategies for driving immune responses to lymphoma have been investigated, including the use of immunomodulatory drugs (IMiDs), which target immune cells rather than the malignant lymphocytes [5]. Mutations affecting the *p16*, *FAS*, and *JUNB* genes and alterations of death receptor signaling have been identified in patients with MF/SS [6–9]. The clonal expansion of the malignant T-cells is proposed to be at least in part due to defective regulation of apoptosis. Some of the investigational therapies used in cutaneous T-cell lymphoma (CTCL) such as enzastaurin are able to induce apoptosis via activation of the AKT and caspase-9-dependent pathway [10]. Other important novel agents include the Bcl-2-antagonists; a novel antifolate, pralatrexate, and the proteasome inhibitor bortezomib. The mechanisms of action of the novel agents are reviewed as well as available clinical data.

C. Querfeld (✉)
Section of Dermatology, University of Chicago, 5841 South Maryland Avenue, MC 5067, Chicago, IL, USA 60637
e-mail: christiane.querfeld@uchospitals.edu

S.T. Rosen
Department of Medicine, Division of Hematology/Oncology, Robert H. Lurie Comprehensive Cancer Center, Northwestern University, Chicago, IL, USA

Bortezomib

The ubiquitin–proteasome pathway plays a critical role in the degradation of proteins involved in cell cycle, survival, and apoptosis. It modulates cell cycle proteins such as the cyclins, cyclin-dependent kinases, and their inhibitors p21 and p27, but is also central to the regulation of transcription, through its control of NF-κB levels. The proteasome pathway is activated in malignant cells and inhibition of this activity is thought to induce antitumor effects. Bortezomib, first approved by the US Food and Drug Administration (FDA) for the treatment of

F. Foss (ed.), *T-Cell Lymphomas*, Contemporary Hematology,
DOI 10.1007/978-1-62703-170-7_17, © Springer Science+Business Media New York 2013

relapsed and refractory multiple myeloma (MM), was the first proteasome inhibitor to enter clinical trials for MM and is now being widely tested in clinical trials for other malignancies [11–14]. The best evidence of single-agent activity is in patients with mantle cell lymphoma (MCL) in which response rates (RR) of 30–40% were seen [12]. Responses have been infrequent in patients with other refractory B-cell non-Hodgkin lymphomas (NHLs) [14].

Recently, the mechanism by which bortezomib leads to tumor cell apoptosis in T-cell lymphoma was investigated using CTCL and adult T-cell leukemia/lymphoma cell lines [15]. Bortezomib treatment was found to induce mitochondrial membrane injury mediated by Noxa, an apoptosis-inducible BH3-only protein, which interacts with and inactivates Mcl-1, an antiapoptotic Bcl-2 family protein, and triggers mitochondrial membrane permeabilization leading to apoptosis. Clinical trials were exploring the activity of bortezomib in patients with CTCL and peripheral T-cell lymphoma (PTCL). A phase I trial of cyclophosphamide, hydroxydaunorubicin, oncovin, prednisone, and bortezomib in 13 previously untreated patients with PTCL or aggressive NK/T-cell lymphoma showed overall RR and CR of 61.5% (eight patients). Three patients relapsed at 3, 4, and 12 months [16]. NF-κB is constitutively activated in CTCL, which may be crucial for its resistance to apoptosis [17]. Bortezomib at nanomolar concentrations inhibited constitutive activation of NF-κB and induced apoptosis in CTCL cell lines and provided a rationale for its clinical use in CTCL [18]. A phase II study of bortezomib in patients with relapsed or refractory CTCL and PTCL with isolated skin involvement showed promising activity with an overall RR of 67%, with six (17%) complete (CR) and six (50%) partial remissions (PR) among the 12 patients enrolled lasting 7 to 12+ months [19]. The most significant toxicity was sensory neuropathy in 50% of patients followed by neutropenia and thrombocytopenia in 17% of patients.

Two recent laboratory studies have shown that bortezomib and the histone deacetylase inhibitor SAHA synergistically induces apoptosis in T-cell leukemia/lymphoma cells [20, 21]. Moreover, bortezomib inhibits tumor growth in a murine xenograft model [21]. Future clinical applications of combined bortezomib/SAHA regimen in T-cell lymphomas are warranted.

Pralatrexate

The reduced folate carrier-type 1 (RFC-1), an oncofetoprotein predominantly expressed in the membranes of fetal and tumor cells, mediates cellular uptake of folates and antifolate drugs. Alterations of the RFC-1 protein have been associated with resistance to methotrexate (MTX). Pralatrexate [PDX (RS)-10-propargyl-10-deaza-aminopterin] is a 10-deaza-aminopterin-analog of MTX, and is a novel targeted antifolate that has shown higher affinity to the RFC-1, increased accumulation and polyglutamylation in tumor cells compared to MTX [22–24]. In prior studies, pralatrexate exhibited enhanced efficacy over MTX in human solid tumor xenografts [25].

Pralatrexate has marked activity in patients with relapsed and/or chemotherapy-resistant T-cell lymphoma that has led to FDA approval for its use as a single agent for the treatment of patients with relapsed or refractory PTCL [26]. In an early phase study of pralatrexate with various B-and T-cell NHL, all four patients with refractory aggressive T-cell lymphoma achieved CR [27]. More recently, a phase I/II study of two different doses and schedules of pralatrexate in patients with relapsed/refractory NHL or Hodgkin disease (HD) showed an overall RR of 55% in T-cell NHL on the phase I study weekly schedule and 50% on the phase II study including 44% and 19% CR/unconfirmed complete remission (CRu), respectively, while only minimal responses in B-cell NHL (10% RR) were seen. The dose-limiting toxicity for pralatrexate in the phase I with a treatment schedule of 135–150 mg/m^2 every other week used for non-small-cell lung cancer has been stomatitis. Symptoms have been ameliorated by a reduced weekly schedule of 30 mg/m^2 for 6 of 7 weeks with folate and B12 supplementation. Risk factors contributing to pralatrexate-related mucositis are homocysteine levels greater than or equal to

10 μmol/L and methylmalonic acid levels greater than or equal to 200 nmol/L. On the basis of the activity in T-cell NHL a pivotal phase II, non-randomized, open-label, international study (PROPEL) in patients with relapsed/refractory PTCL has been completed using the same weekly schedule showed a lower overall RR of 29% with CR in 10% of patients [28]. Most patients were heavily pretreated with a median of three prior treatments and had advanced disease. The most common grades 3 and 4 toxicities were mucositis and thrombocytopenia.

A phase I trial in patients with relapsed CTCL showed impressive activity of pralatrexate with responses seen in 11 of 18 patients (two CR and nine PR) [29]. Patients with MF, SS, and C-ALCL were included. Dose-limiting toxicity was mucositis. The optimal dose and schedule that provided activity with tolerability for CTCL was determined to be pralatrexate 15 mg/m^2 weekly on 3 of 4 weeks. A phase II study is ongoing. An interesting case of pralatrexate-induced tumor cell apoptosis within epidermal Pautrier microabscesses presenting as innumerable skin erosions in a patient with advanced adult T-cell lymphoma/leukemia was recently published [30]. Histologic examination revealed that epidermal Pautrier microabscesses showed extensive cellular debris, with normal-appearing adjacent keratinocytes. The erosions healed within a few days and a complete resolution of disease was observed while continued on pralatrexate. Pralatrexate was also given at weekly doses in a patient with relapsed CD4+ CD56+ hematodermic/plasmacytoid dendritic cell tumor presenting with skin lesions only that resulted in a remarkable clinical response with regression of cutaneous tumors after two treatments [31]. Response lasted for about 4 months.

Preclinical data reported synergy for the combination with gemcitabine. A recent phase I study of pralatrexate with gemcitabine in patients with lymphoproliferative malignancies have been reported [32]. Thirty-four patients: 13 with B-cell lymphoma, 11 with T/NK-cell lymphoma, 7 with HD, and 3 with "other" lymphoma were included. Three treatment schedules were applied ranging from once weekly sequential-day dosing (pralatrexate 10–15 mg/m^2 and gemcitabine 300–400 mg/m^2), sequential-day dosing every 2 weeks, to same day dosing every 2 weeks. Preliminary results showed activity in 21% (7/34) of patients with acceptable toxicities with every 2 week dosing. Dose limiting toxicities were grade 3 to 4 hematologic toxicities.

Lenalidomide

Lenalidomide is probably the most extensively studied compound of a new class of agents which are known as IMiDs [33]. It is a 4-amino-gultaramide derivative of thalidomide and was designed to enhance the immunological and antitumor properties of thalidomide with improved safety profile. It is a lead therapeutic in multiple myeloma and myelodysplastic syndromes associated with the deletion of 5q cytogenetic abnormality (del-5q MDS). Lenalidomide has been FDA approved for previously treated multiple myeloma in combination with dexamethasone and del-5q MDS [34].

The mechanisms of action remain uncertain, but appear to involve direct cytotoxic action in some cell types, the modulation of immunity via altered cytokine production and cellular changes both on the malignant cell and reactive T- and NK-cells, and the suppression of angiogenesis by downregulation of vascular endothelial growth factor (VEGF). In multiple myeloma, lenalidomide has been demonstrated to directly induce apoptosis via caspase-8 activation, to inhibit VEGF, and to reduce adhesion of myeloma cells to bone marrow stroma. In preclinical observations, lenalidomide inhibits or modulates various cytokines including tumor necrosis factor-alpha (TNF-α), interleukin (IL)-1β, IL-6, and IL-12. Furthermore it has demonstrated its ability to increase T- and NK-cell stimulation, T-cell proliferation, and production of IL-2 and interferon-γ (IFN-γ) by T-cells, and to inhibit expression and function of Tregs [35, 36].

Lenalidomide has been shown activity against chronic lymphocytic leukemia (CLL), relapsed or refractory NHL, and various solid cancers in phase II studies. In general the activity seen in patients with recurrent and refractory lymphoma has been moderate with RR between 22 and 50%. An overall RR of 35–50% with lenalidomide was reported in patients with CLL. Results from phase I/II trials in relapsed multiple myeloma show RR of 14–29% with lenalidomide alone.

Cytopenias are the primary adverse events associated with the administration of lenalidomide, particularly in subjects with compromised bone marrow. However, these are manageable with dose interruptions and reductions. Other side effects include malaise, fatigue, diarrhea, rash, and muscle cramps. An increased risk of thromboembolism has been noted when lenalidomide is combined with steroids. A "flare" phenomenon has been observed in CLL prior to disease response [37]. The recommended starting dose is 10 mg. Patients with multiple myeloma typically receive 25 mg daily for three weeks followed by a 1-week rest period.

There have been two recent reports of lenalidomide for the treatment in T-cell lymphoma. The immunomodulatory properties of lenalidomide such as T-cell co-stimulation with induction of Th1 cytokine production and cytotoxic activity along with antiangiogenic, anti-proliferative, and pro-apoptotic properties provided the rationale to use this agent in CTCL [38]. Preliminary results of 25 patients show that lenalidomide has clinical activity in patients with advanced CTCL with a toxicity profile similar to that previously reported. The first fifteen patients received 25 mg lenalidomide daily for 21 days of a 28-day cycle that was adjusted to an initial dose of 10 mg with dose escalation up to 25 mg. Seven patients have achieved a PR. Responding patients received a median of nine cycles of therapy; median time to best response was 6 months. Four of the responding patients developed new skin lesions. Eight patients had stable disease (SD) ≥ 4 months. A regrowth of disease-related hair loss was observed in some patients. The most common side effects were anemia, fatigue/malaise, skin burning, pruritus, diarrhea, and lower leg edema.

The mechanism of the observed antitumor effects remains unclear. An initial flare reaction manifested by a temporary increase in the size, number, and discomfort of skin lesions and/or tender swelling of lymph nodes and/or increase in Sézary cell count was noted in some patients during the first cycle of treatment and/or each cycle for the remainder of therapy with subsequent improvement of symptoms and/or disease. The cause of this phenomenon has not been studied in CTCL and could be related to the co-stimulatory or cytotoxic activity of lenalidomide and represent an immune response against the disease with enhanced $CD8^+$ T-cell and NK-cell cytotoxic activity, but may, in fact, represent a combination of cytotoxic and cytokine-mediated events. One could suggest that the flare reaction could actually predict the subsequent antitumor response in CTCL patients. Correlative biologic studies will include analysis of antiangiogenic and immunomodulatory activity on skin biopsies and peripheral blood samples.

Twenty-four patients with relapsed and refractory T-cell lymphomas other than MF were treated in a phase II trial with lenalidomide 25 mg daily on days 1 to 21 of each 28-day cycle with standardized dose reductions for toxicity [39]. Twenty-three patients were eligible for response with seven patients (30%) achieving PR. Responses were seen in patients with anaplastic large cell lymphoma (ALCL), angioimmunoblastic lymphoma, and PTCL, unspecified. Two patients had SD for ≥3 cycles. Median overall survival (OS) was 8 months. The most common grade 3 and 4 toxicities were thrombocytopenia, neutropenia, neutropenic fever, and pain. Although moderate responses are seen in patients with T-cell NHL, lenalidomide holds considerable promise for both combination and maintenance treatment given its oral availability.

Enzastaurin

Enzastaurin (LY317615), an acyclic bisindolylmaleimide, is a novel orally available protein kinase C (PKC) inhibitor. Tumor-induced angiogenesis requires the activation of PKC-β, a key modulator of the VEGF signaling pathway, and enzastaurin was originally evaluated in human tumor xenograft mice models for its antiangiogenic activity upon PKC-β inhibition [40]. However, in addition to its antiangiogenic effects, enzastaurin, at concentrations reached in clinical trials, directly suppressed proliferation and induced apoptosis of tumor cells in culture and in human colon and glioblastoma xenografts through the inhibition of the PI3Kinase/AKT/glycogen synthase kinase-3 signaling pathway [41].

PKC consists of a family of at least 12 serine-threonine protein kinases, which are divided into the classical (α, βI, βII, γ), novel (δ, ε, η, θ), and atypical (ζ, λ/ι) subtypes based on their second messenger requirements [42]. PKC-μ/PKD and PKC-ν were recently added to the PKC superfamily based on homology within the catalytic domain [43].

PKC isoenzymes exhibit distinct tissue distribution and play a distinct role in various cellular events including cell survival, growth factor response, proliferation and tumorigenesis in solid tumors, and several hematologic malignancies. PKC-β is the major PKC isoform involved in B-cell receptor signaling. Specifically, PKC-β mediates growth and survival of diffuse large B-cell lymphoma (DLBCL), cell proliferation in CLL, as well as migration and cell growth in multiple myeloma and Waldenström macroglobulinemia [44–48]. Overexpression in treatment-refractory DLBCL is associated with shortened survival [45]. In contrast, enzastaurin had no effect on normal mononuclear cells or hematopoietic progenitor cells suggesting a favorable therapeutic index.

The conventional PKC (α, β , γ, ε, and ζ) isoforms are not necessary for proliferation as previously shown in cloned cell lines derived from the CTCL cell line HuT-78 [49]. Functionally, PKC-β is critical for IL-2 secretion in HuT-78 cells, and for promoting the epidermotropism of CTCL, but its role in T-cell malignancies has not been determined yet [50]. PKC-θ mediates pre-TCR signaling and contributes to Notch3-induced T-cell leukemia [51].

Enzastaurin competes with ATP for the nucleotide triphosphate-binding site of PKC, thereby blocking its activation, but the exact mechanism of action of enzastaurin malignancies is not well defined. It is not completely specific to PKC-β as it inhibits several PKC isoforms. A recent multicenter phase I study evaluated dose escalation and pharmacokinetics of oral enzastaurin in 47 adult patients with advanced cancer [52]. The 525 mg daily dose produced the targeted steady-state concentration of 1.4 μmol/L and was selected as the recommended dose for phase II studies. The most common toxicities were grade 1 chromaturia, fatigue, and gastrointestinal toxicities; no clinically significant grade 3 or 4 toxicities occurred. Three cases of significant QTc prolongation occurred.

Enzastaurin has been administered to more than 620 cancer patients as a single agent or in combination with other antitumor drugs in a variety of hematological and solid tumor malignancies. Enzastaurin has shown clinical activity in relapsed and/or refractory DLBCL, relapsed/refractory MCL and Waldenström macroglobulinemia [44, 45, 48]. Importantly, enzastaurin enhanced in vitro antitumor activity of rituximab, bortezomib, fludarabine, and dexamethasone that supports the therapeutic combination of these agents.

Recently, the significance of enzastaurin activity on two CTCL cell lines HuT-78 and HH was demonstrated [10]. Enzastaurin, at clinically relevant concentrations, caused growth inhibition of CTCL cell lines. Enzastaurin was reported to block AKT activity, affected both caspase-mediated apoptosis and cell cycle regulatory pathways, but may involve other biochemical mechanisms. The promising preclinical activity has prompted the initiation of a multicenter phase II trial in patients with advanced CTCL and enrollment is ongoing.

Apoptosis Antagonists

Defective regulation of apoptosis is a central feature of the pathology of several lymphoma types such as CTCL and ALCL. Apoptosis can be triggered by death receptors that belong to the tumor necrosis factor-receptor (TNF-R) family or by aberrations in expression of the B-cell lymphoma-2 (Bcl-2) family. Six death receptors (DR) are known including Fas (CD95, Apo-1), TRAIL-receptor 1 (DR4), TRAIL-R2 (Apo-2, DR5), TNF-R1, TRAMP (WSL-1, Apo-3, DR3), and

DR6. All contain a death domain protein that bridges the death receptors with downstream caspases. Their activation leads to apoptosis. Fas gene mutations leading to defective Fas/FasL signaling have been shown to result in autoimmune lymphoproliferative syndromes as a consequence of lymphocyte accumulation [53]. There are limited studies describing defects in proteins regulating apoptosis in CTCL, but loss of Fas and/or defects in Fas-mediated and TNF-R1-mediated apoptosis have been described in early and advanced stages of CTCL [8, 54–57].

Cellular caspase-8 (FLICE)-like inhibitory protein (cFLIP) was originally identified as an inhibitor of death-receptor signaling through competition with caspase-8 upon triggering Fas-mediated apoptosis. Resistance to Fas ligand (FasL) and TNF-related apoptosis-inducing ligand (TRAIL)-mediated apoptosis in malignant T-cells from patients with SS was associated with impaired death receptor and overexpression of cFLIP [58]. Overexpression of c-FLIP protects anaplastic lymphoma kinase (ALK)+ ALCL cells from death-receptor-induced apoptosis [59]. The overexpression of TRAIL in CTCL is not clear. TRAIL is a member of the TNF receptor/ligand family and a powerful inducer of apoptosis. It shares homology to other members of the TNF cytokine family, especially to FasL CD95L (FasL/APO-1L). TRAIL is known to effectively induce apoptosis in numerous tumor cell lines but not in the majority of normal cells. Currently, TRAIL-receptor-targeted therapies including the untagged recombinant Apo2L/TRAIL and agonistic antibodies to TRAIL-R1 and TRAIL-R2 are in clinical phase I and II studies in various tumors.

The intrinsic pathway of apoptosis is critically regulated by the Bcl-2 protein family. Few studies have analyzed the expression of the pro- and antiapoptotic Bcl-2 protein family proteins (Bax, Bak, Bcl-2, Bcl-x_L, Bcl-x, Mcl-1) in CTCL [60]. Overexpression of Bcl-2 and its family members confers resistance of lymphomas to various chemotherapies and biological agents. Investigational drugs targeting the antiapoptotic Bcl-2 protein family have preclinical activity as single agents and in combination with other antineoplastic agents. Cotreatment with the Bcl-2/Bcl-xL antagonist ABT-737 and panabinostat decreased resistance and synergistically induced apoptosis of human CTCL cell lines [61]. Clinical trials of several Bcl-2 antagonists (oblimersen sodium, AT-101, gossypol, obatoclax [GX15-070], ABT-737) in various solid and hematologic malignancies are ongoing.

Clinical phase III studies with oblimersen, a Bcl-2 antisense phosphorothioate oligonucleotide in patients with CLL have been completed. Despite modest single-agent activity in relapsed/refractory CLL, oblimersen combined with fludarabine offers responding patients (CR and PR) a significant survival benefit [62, 63]. The best-characterized target is the BH3 domain of the antiapoptotic Bcl-2, Bcl-XL, and Mcl-1 proteins, with several small molecule inhibitors being tested for their potential as enhancers of the cytotoxicty of conventional anti-lymphoma drugs. AT-101, an enantiomer of the natural compound gossypol, is a BH3-mimetic, which has shown promising results in CLL in vitro. Obatoclax (GX15-070) is a pan-BCL-2 inhibitor that has shown efficacy against various hematologic malignancies such as CLL, AML, MDS, and MM in early clinical studies [64]. It has also shown the potential to overcome Mcl-1-mediated resistance to bortezomib [65, 66]. The combination of obatoclax and bortezomib induced complete remission in some heavily pretreated chemo-refractory MCL patients [67]. One of the most common grade 3 adverse effects of these BH3-mimetics is thrombocytopenia due to the induction of apoptosis in platelets [68].

Conclusions

T-cell NHLs represent a spectrum of uncommon and heterogeneous malignancies with a wide range of genomic and cytogenetic aberrations that affect cell growth and regulation of apoptosis. It is important to identify the biology and immunology of these lymphomas to develop new and promising therapeutic targets.

Despite the lack of significant single-agent activity most of the novel therapeutics discussed hold considerable promise for combination with other agents given their low toxicity profile and/or oral availability.

References

1. Eriksen KW, Kaltoft K, Mikkelsen G, et al. Constitutive STAT3-activation in Sezary syndrome: tyrphostin AG490 inhibits STAT3-activation, interleukin-2 receptor expression and growth of leukemic Sezary cells. Leukemia. 2001;15(5):787–93.
2. Nielsen M, Kaltoft K, Nordahl M, et al. Constitutive activation of a slowly migrating isoform of Stat3 in mycosis fungoides: tyrphostin AG490 inhibits Stat3 activation and growth of mycosis fungoides tumor cell lines. Proc Natl Acad Sci USA. 1997;94(13): 6764–9.
3. Heid JB, Schmidt A, Oberle N, et al. FOXP3+CD25-tumor cells with regulatory function in Sezary syndrome. J Invest Dermatol. 2009;129(12):2875–85.
4. Tiemessen MM, Mitchell TJ, Hendry L, Whittaker SJ, Taams LS, John S. Lack of suppressive CD4+CD25+FOXP3+ T cells in advanced stages of primary cutaneous T-cell lymphoma. J Invest Dermatol. 2006;126(10):2217–23.
5. Querfeld C, Kuzel TM, Guitart J, Rosen ST. Preliminary results of a phase II study of CC-5013 (Lenalidomide, Revlimid™) in patients with cutaneous T-cell lymphoma. Blood. 2005;106(11):936a–7.
6. van Doorn R, van Kester MS, Dijkman R, et al. Oncogenomic analysis of mycosis fungoides reveals major differences with Sezary syndrome. Blood. 2009;113(1):127–36.
7. Mao X, Orchard G, Lillington DM, Russell-Jones R, Young BD, Whittaker SJ. Amplification and overexpression of JUNB is associated with primary cutaneous T-cell lymphomas. Blood. 2003;101(4):1513–9.
8. Zoi-Toli O, Vermeer MH, De Vries E, Van Beek P, Meijer CJ, Willemze R. Expression of Fas and Fas-ligand in primary cutaneous T-cell lymphoma (CTCL): association between lack of Fas expression and aggressive types of CTCL. Br J Dermatol. 2000;143(2):313–9.
9. Navas IC, Ortiz-Romero PL, Villuendas R, et al. p16(INK4a) gene alterations are frequent in lesions of mycosis fungoides. Am J Pathol. 2000;156(5): 1565–72.
10. Querfeld C, Rizvi MA, Kuzel TM, et al. The selective protein kinase C beta inhibitor enzastaurin induces apoptosis in cutaneous T-cell lymphoma cell lines through the AKT pathway. J Invest Dermatol. 2006;126(7):1641–7.
11. Richardson P. Management of the relapsed/refractory myeloma patient: strategies incorporating lenalidomide. Semin Hematol. 2005;42(4 Suppl 4):S9–15.
12. Goy A, Bernstein SH, Kahl BS, et al. Bortezomib in patients with relapsed or refractory mantle cell lymphoma: updated time-to-event analyses of the multicenter phase 2 PINNACLE study. Ann Oncol. 2009;20(3):520–5.
13. Fisher RI, Bernstein SH, Kahl BS, et al. Multicenter phase II study of bortezomib in patients with relapsed or refractory mantle cell lymphoma. J Clin Oncol. 2006;24(30):4867–74.
14. Goy A, Younes A, McLaughlin P, et al. Phase II study of proteasome inhibitor bortezomib in relapsed or refractory B-cell non-Hodgkin's lymphoma. J Clin Oncol. 2005;23(4):667–75.
15. Ri M, Iida S, Ishida T, et al. Bortezomib-induced apoptosis in mature T-cell lymphoma cells partially depends on upregulation of Noxa and functional repression of Mcl-1. Cancer Sci. 2009;100(2):341–8.
16. Lee J, Suh C, Kang HJ, et al. Phase I study of proteasome inhibitor bortezomib plus CHOP in patients with advanced, aggressive T-cell or NK/T-cell lymphoma. Ann Oncol. 2008;19(12):2079–83.
17. Izban KF, Ergin M, Qin JZ, et al. Constitutive expression of NF-kappa B is a characteristic feature of mycosis fungoides: implications for apoptosis resistance and pathogenesis. Hum Pathol. 2000;31(12):1482–90.
18. Sors A, Jean-Louis F, Pellet C, et al. Down-regulating constitutive activation of the NF-kappaB canonical pathway overcomes the resistance of cutaneous T-cell lymphoma to apoptosis. Blood. 2006;107(6):2354–63.
19. Zinzani PL, Musuraca G, Tani M, et al. Phase II trial of proteasome inhibitor bortezomib in patients with relapsed or refractory cutaneous T-cell lymphoma. J Clin Oncol. 2007;25(27):4293–7.
20. Heider U, Rademacher J, Lamottke B, et al. Synergistic interaction of the histone deacetylase inhibitor SAHA with the proteasome inhibitor bortezomib in cutaneous T cell lymphoma. Eur J Haematol. 2009;82(6):440–9.
21. Zhang QL, Wang L, Zhang YW, et al. The proteasome inhibitor bortezomib interacts synergistically with the histone deacetylase inhibitor suberoylanilide hydroxamic acid to induce T-leukemia/lymphoma cells apoptosis. Leukemia. 2009;23(8):1507–14.
22. Mould DR, Sweeney K, Duffull SB, et al. A population pharmacokinetic and pharmacodynamic evaluation of pralatrexate in patients with relapsed or refractory non-Hodgkin's or Hodgkin's lymphoma. Clin Pharmacol Ther. 2009;86(2):190–6.
23. Izbicka E, Diaz A, Streeper R, et al. Distinct mechanistic activity profile of pralatrexate in comparison to other antifolates in in vitro and in vivo models of human cancers. Cancer Chemother Pharmacol. 2009;64(5):993–9.
24. Wang ES, O'Connor O, She Y, Zelenetz AD, Sirotnak FM, Moore MA. Activity of a novel anti-folate (PDX, 10-propargyl 10-deazaaminopterin) against human lymphoma is superior to methotrexate and correlates with tumor RFC-1 gene expression. Leuk Lymphoma. 2003;44(6):1027–35.
25. Sirotnak FM, DeGraw JI, Colwell WT, Piper JR. A new analogue of 10-deazaaminopterin with markedly enhanced curative effects against human tumor xenografts in mice. Cancer Chemother Pharmacol. 1998;42(4):313–8.

26. Thompson CA. FDA approves pralatrexate for treatment of rare lymphoma. Am J Health Syst Pharm. 2009;66(21):1890.
27. O'Connor OA, Hamlin PA, Portlock C, et al. Pralatrexate, a novel class of antifol with high affinity for the reduced folate carrier-type 1, produces marked complete and durable remissions in a diversity of chemotherapy refractory cases of T-cell lymphoma. Br J Haematol. 2007;139(3):425–8.
28. OConnor O, Pro B, Pinter-Brown L, et al. PROPEL: results of the pivotal, multicenter, phase II study of pralatrexate in patients with relapsed or refractory peripheral T-cell lymphoma (PTCL). J Clin Oncol. 2009;27:15s (suppl; abstr 8561).
29. Horwitz SM, Duvic M, Kim Y, et al. Pralatrexate is active in cutaneous T-cell lymphoma (CTCL): results of a multicenter, dose-finding trial. Blood. 2009; 114(22):a379 (abstract 919).
30. Marneros AG, Grossman ME, Silvers DN, et al. Pralatrexate-induced tumor cell apoptosis in the epidermis of a patient with HTLV-1 adult T-cell lymphoma/leukemia causing skin erosions. Blood. 2009;113(25):6338–41.
31. Leitenberger JJ, Berthelot CN, Polder KD, et al. CD4+ CD56+ hematodermic/plasmacytoid dendritic cell tumor with response to pralatrexate. J Am Acad Dermatol. 2008;58(3):480–4.
32. Horwitz SM, Vose JM, Advani R, et al. Pralatrexate and gemcitabine in patients with relapsed or refractory lymphoproliferative malignancies: phase 1 results. Blood. 2009;114(22):a667–8 (abstract 1674).
33. Bartlett JB, Dredge K, Dalgleish AG. The evolution of thalidomide and its IMiD derivatives as anticancer agents. Nat Rev Cancer. 2004;4(4):314–22.
34. Galustian C, Dalgleish A. Lenalidomide: a novel anticancer drug with multiple modalities. Expert Opin Pharmacother. 2009;10(1):125–33.
35. LeBlanc R, Hideshima T, Catley LP, et al. Immunomodulatory drug costimulates T cells via the B7-CD28 pathway. Blood. 2004;103(5):1787–90.
36. Galustian C, Meyer B, Labarthe MC, et al. The anticancer agents lenalidomide and pomalidomide inhibit the proliferation and function of T regulatory cells. Cancer Immunol Immunother. 2009;58(7):1033–45.
37. Ferrajoli A, Lee BN, Schlette EJ, et al. Lenalidomide induces complete and partial remissions in patients with relapsed and refractory chronic lymphocytic leukemia. Blood. 2008;111(11):5291–7.
38. Querfeld C, Kuzel TM, Guitart J, Rosen ST. Preliminary results of a phase II study of CC-5013 (Lenalidomide, Revlimid®) in patients with cutaneous T-cell lymphoma. Blood. 2005;106:936a–7 (abstract 3351).
39. Dueck GS, Chua N, Prasad A, et al. Activity of lenalidomide in a phase II trial for T-cell lymphoma: report on the first 24 cases. J Clin Oncol. 2009;27(15S):8524.
40. Keyes KA, Mann L, Sherman M, et al. LY317615 decreases plasma VEGF levels in human tumor xenograft-bearing mice. Cancer Chemother Pharmacol. 2004;53(2):133–40.
41. Graff JR, McNulty AM, Hanna KR, et al. The protein kinase Cbeta-selective inhibitor, Enzastaurin (LY317615.HCl), suppresses signaling through the AKT pathway, induces apoptosis, and suppresses growth of human colon cancer and glioblastoma xenografts. Cancer Res. 2005;65(16):7462–9.
42. Mellor H, Parker PJ. The extended protein kinase C superfamily. Biochem J. 1998;332(Pt 2):281–92.
43. Hayashi A, Seki N, Hattori A, Kozuma S, Saito T. PKCnu, a new member of the protein kinase C family, composes a fourth subfamily with PKCmu. Biochim Biophys Acta. 1999;1450(1):99–106.
44. Robertson MJ, Kahl BS, Vose JM, et al. Phase II study of enzastaurin, a protein kinase C beta inhibitor, in patients with relapsed or refractory diffuse large B-cell lymphoma. J Clin Oncol. 2007;25(13):1741–6.
45. Hans CP, Weisenburger DD, Greiner TC, et al. Expression of PKC-beta or cyclin D2 predicts for inferior survival in diffuse large B-cell lymphoma. Mod Pathol. 2005;18(10):1377–84.
46. Holler C, Pinon JD, Denk U, et al. PKCbeta is essential for the development of chronic lymphocytic leukemia in the TCL1 transgenic mouse model: validation of PKCbeta as a therapeutic target in chronic lymphocytic leukemia. Blood. 2009;113(12):2791–4.
47. Rizvi MA, Ghias K, Davies KM, et al. Enzastaurin (LY317615), a protein kinase C beta inhibitor, inhibits the AKT pathway and induces apoptosis in multiple myeloma cell lines. Mol Cancer Ther. 2006;5(7): 1783–9.
48. Moreau AS, Jia X, Ngo HT, et al. Protein kinase C inhibitor enzastaurin induces in vitro and in vivo antitumor activity in Waldenstrom macroglobulinemia. Blood. 2007;109(11):4964–72.
49. Long A, Kelleher D. Conventional protein kinase C isoforms are not essential for cellular proliferation of a T cell lymphoma line. FEBS Lett. 1993;333(3):243–7.
50. Long A, Kelleher D, Lynch S, Volkov Y. Cutting edge: protein kinase C beta expression is critical for export of Il-2 from T cells. J Immunol. 2001;167(2):636–40.
51. Felli MP, Vacca A, Calce A, et al. PKC theta mediates pre-TCR signaling and contributes to Notch3-induced T-cell leukemia. Oncogene. 2005;24(6):992–1000.
52. Carducci MA, Musib L, Kies MS, et al. Phase I dose escalation and pharmacokinetic study of enzastaurin, an oral protein kinase C beta inhibitor, in patients with advanced cancer. J Clin Oncol. 2006;24(25):4092–9.
53. Rieux-Laucat F, Le Deist F, Hivroz C, et al. Mutations in Fas associated with human lymphoproliferative syndrome and autoimmunity. Science. 1995;268(5215):1347–9.
54. Dereure O, Portales P, Clot J, Guilhou JJ. Decreased expression of Fas (APO-1/CD95) on peripheral blood CD4+ T lymphocytes in cutaneous T-cell lymphomas. Br J Dermatol. 2000;143(6):1205–10.
55. Contassot E, French LE. Targeting apoptosis defects in cutaneous T-cell lymphoma. J Invest Dermatol. 2009;129(5):1059–61.
56. Wu J, Nihal M, Siddiqui J, Vonderheid EC, Wood GS. Low FAS/CD95 expression by CTCL correlates with

reduced sensitivity to apoptosis that can be restored by FAS upregulation. J Invest Dermatol. 2009; 129(5):1165–73.
57. Braun FK, Fecker LF, Schwarz C, et al. Blockade of death receptor-mediated pathways early in the signaling cascade coincides with distinct apoptosis resistance in cutaneous T-cell lymphoma cells. J Invest Dermatol. 2007;127(10):2425–37.
58. Contassot E, Kerl K, Roques S, et al. Resistance to FasL and tumor necrosis factor-related apoptosis-inducing ligand-mediated apoptosis in Sezary syndrome T-cells associated with impaired death receptor and FLICE-inhibitory protein expression. Blood. 2008;111(9):4780–7.
59. Oyarzo MP, Medeiros LJ, Atwell C, et al. c-FLIP confers resistance to FAS-mediated apoptosis in anaplastic large-cell lymphoma. Blood. 2006;107(6):2544–7.
60. Zhang CL, Kamarashev J, Qin JZ, Burg G, Dummer R, Dobbeling U. Expression of apoptosis regulators in cutaneous T-cell lymphoma (CTCL) cells. J Pathol. 2003;200(2):249–54.
61. Chen J, Fiskus W, Eaton K, et al. Cotreatment with BCL-2 antagonist sensitizes cutaneous T-cell lymphoma to lethal action of HDAC7-Nur77-based mechanism. Blood. 2009;113(17):4038–48.
62. O'Brien SM, Cunningham CC, Golenkov AK, Turkina AG, Novick SC, Rai KR. Phase I to II multicenter study of oblimersen sodium, a Bcl-2 antisense oligonucleotide, in patients with advanced chronic lymphocytic leukemia. J Clin Oncol. 2005;23(30): 7697–702.
63. O'Brien S, Moore JO, Boyd TE, et al. 5-year survival in patients with relapsed or refractory chronic lymphocytic leukemia in a randomized, phase III trial of fludarabine plus cyclophosphamide with or without oblimersen. J Clin Oncol. 2009;27(31):5208–12.
64. Schimmer AD, O'Brien S, Kantarjian H, et al. A phase I study of the pan bcl-2 family inhibitor obatoclax mesylate in patients with advanced hematologic malignancies. Clin Cancer Res. 2008;14(24): 8295–301.
65. Nguyen M, Marcellus RC, Roulston A, et al. Small molecule obatoclax (GX15-070) antagonizes MCL-1 and overcomes MCL-1-mediated resistance to apoptosis. Proc Natl Acad Sci USA. 2007;104(49): 19512–7.
66. Trudel S, Li ZH, Rauw J, Tiedemann RE, Wen XY, Stewart AK. Preclinical studies of the pan-Bcl inhibitor obatoclax (GX015-070) in multiple myeloma. Blood. 2007;109(12):5430–8.
67. Goy A, Ford P, Feldman T, et al. A phase 1 trial of the pan Bcl-2 family inhibitor obatoclax mesylate (GX15-070) in combination with bortezomib in patients with relapsed/refractory mantle cell lymphoma. Blood. 2007;110:757a (abstract 2569).
68. Mason KD, Carpinelli MR, Fletcher JI, et al. Programmed anuclear cell death delimits platelet life span. Cell. 2007;128(6):1173–86.

18 Immunotherapy for Cutaneous T-Cell Lymphoma

Badri Modi, Francine Foss, Richard L. Edelson, and Michael Girardi

Introduction

The immunopathophysiology of CTCL has made it a favorable target for immunotherapy treatments. Prior to the development of extracorporeal photopheresis (ECP) in 1987, the first-line treatment for CTCL was nonspecific chemotherapy and offered a very poor response rate. The elucidation of the immune dysregulation seen in the disease not only spurred the introduction of biologic therapies such as interferons (IFNs), interleukins, and toll-like receptor (TLR) agonists, but also led to the investigation of the immunomodulatory impact of the other systemic therapies, such as retinoids and histone deacetylase inhibitors (HDIs), not traditionally classified as immunotherapy.

In review of the various available immune influencing treatment modalities and biologic agents for CTCL, we have considered their capacity to stimulate the immune system and restore a normal immunologic environment. The following sections include a discussion on the immune rationale, clinical efficacy, and combination regimens available for each therapeutic modality.

B. Modi • R.L. Edelson • M. Girardi
Department of Dermatology, Yale University School of Medicine, New Haven, CT, USA

F. Foss (✉)
Department of Medical Oncology/Hematology, Yale University School of Medicine, 333 Cedar Street, FMP 130, PO Box 208032, New Haven, CT, USA 06520
e-mail: Francine.foss@yale.edu

Extracorporeal Photopheresis

Although the exact mechanism of action is not yet elucidated, ECP therapy is regarded as an immunotherapy supported by several clinical studies and laboratory models, as well as the subsequent discoveries of clinical benefit in other T-cell-mediated diseases (e.g., graft-versus-host disease, organ transplant rejection). During the ECP procedure, the patient undergoes discontinuous pheresis cycles to harvest the leukocyte-rich buffy coat. The separated leukocytes are exposed to 8-methoxypsoralen (8-MOP) and irradiated with UVA light before reinfusion back into the patient. 8-MOP is a photoactivated, DNA-intercalating agent that forms cross-links after UVA-activation and induces apoptosis, particularly within activated and proliferating T cells.

The earliest clues to support the immunomodulating effects of ECP appeared in the initial clinical trial by Edelson et al [1]. The original goal of ECP was simply to induce CTCL cells to undergo apoptosis and reduce tumor burden. However, given that only a minor portion of total circulating T cells undergo extracorporeal treatment, it was evident that there must be another process in play, perhaps involving antigen presentation of apoptotic tumor cells. ECP's effects on circulating leukocytes appear to selectively target lymphoma cells. CTCL patients treated

F. Foss (ed.), *T-Cell Lymphomas*, Contemporary Hematology,
DOI 10.1007/978-1-62703-170-7_18,

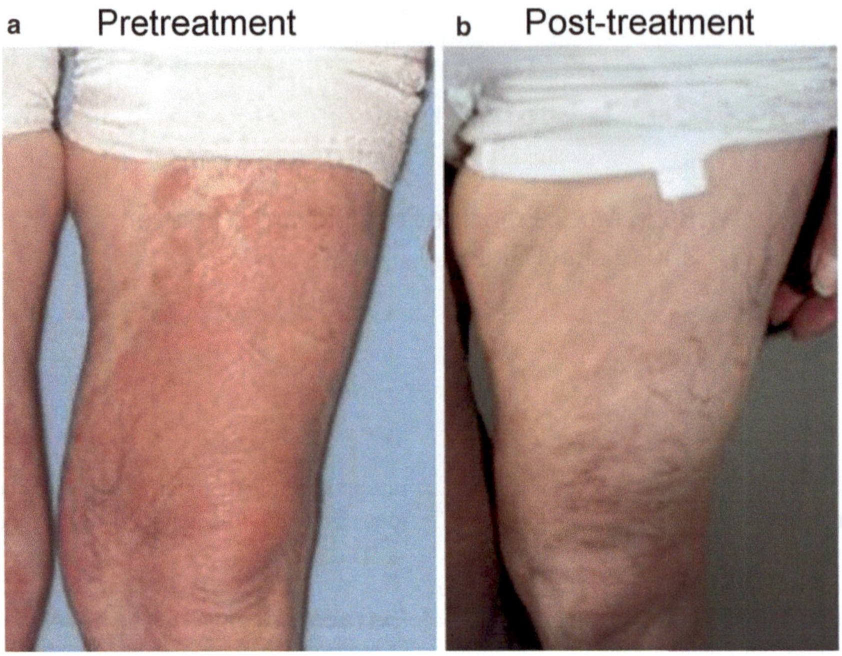

Figure 18.1 Patient with Sezary syndrome before (A) and six months after (B) extracorporeal photopheresis. Treatment was administered for two consecutive days every 4 weeks.

with ECP maintain their absolute number of normal T cells with a disproportionately greater decrease in their total body burden of malignant T cells. In addition, response rates to ECP are higher in individuals with normal or near normal natural killer and cytotoxic T-cell numbers and function [2]. ECP has also been shown to increase the production of TNF-α and shift the balance of Th1 and Th2 cytokines. Taken together, these data suggest that ECP induces an antitumor cellular immune response.

The mechanisms by which ECP cultivates an adaptive immune environment have recently been explored. As the patient's blood passes through the photopheresis apparatus, monocytes appear to be stimulated to mature into antigen presenting dendritic cells. Flow cytometric and DNA microarray analyses of passaged monocytes demonstrate an increased expression of dendritic cell markers [3]. Furthermore, these dendritic cells are functional in vitro in their capacity to stimulate allogeneic CD4+ T cells to proliferate as well as differentiate CD8+ T cells into cytotoxic cells. Thus, ECP-generated dendritic cells have the ability to ingest the apoptotic malignant T cells, ultimately leading to the potential production and reinfusion of putative CTCL tumor-loaded APC. These cells may therefore stimulate the production of specific antitumor cytotoxic T cells against the malignant lymphocytes.

The initial multicenter trial of erythrodermic patients demonstrated a 73% response rate, with a quarter of patients experiencing full remission. Their protocol consisted of two consecutive days of ECP treatment, repeated every 4 weeks. Figure 18.1 shows a representative patient with Sezary syndrome who had a complete clinical response. Since then, there have been approximately 30 trials of varying stages of CTCL that clinically confirm the benefit of ECP as monotherapy—in more than 1,000 patients treated worldwide with ECP, the response rate ranges from 43–100% with a complete response in 0–62% of patients [4]. Further investigation revealed a set of prognostic factors that predict a better response to ECP and include (1) absence of tumor-stage skin lesions, (2) shorter disease course, (3) absence of significant internal organ involvement or bulky lymphadenopathy, and (4) minimal pretreatment with chemotherapy [2, 5].

A minority of patients treated with ECP monotherapy will be refractory to the disease, and it is important to consider the addition of other broad therapeutic categories, including skin-directed therapies, biologic response modifiers, and low-dose chemotherapy. Skin-directed therapies are thought to significantly enhance response rates by reducing tumor burden. These include radiotherapy, psoralen plus ultraviolet A (PUVA), and topical chemotherapy. Wilson and colleagues investigated the combination of ECP and total skin electron beam therapy (TSEBT) and found significantly longer progression-free survival periods and decreased CTCL-related mortality, compared to TSEBT alone [6]. Furthermore, skin-directed therapies are an obvious choice in patients who develop patch or plaque lesions after ECP initiation, as improving erythroderma often unveils cutaneous disease.

Biologic response modifier agents include cytokines, retinoids, and toxin–cytokine fusion proteins, and each is approved as a monotherapy for CTCL. Several retrospective studies comparing ECP and ECP plus biologic response modifiers suggest higher clinical response rates and longer survival in the combination cohort [7]. The addition of IFNα (3–18 MU (million units), three times per week) to ECP showed significantly improved response rates compared to ECP alone [8, 9]. The retinoid etretinate combined with ECP therapy in patients with recalcitrant palmer and plantar hyperkeratosis in erythrodermic CTCL results in marked improvement in the hyperkeratosis [10]. Similar favorable results are observed with the use of bexarotene, an RXR-specific retinoid. A small number of patients showed promising results after the combination of ECP and granulocyte-macrophage colony-stimulating factor (sargramostim) treatment. Finally, the combination of ECP and two other agents (IFNs, retinoids, GM-CSF) has been investigated in 28 patients with SS, achieving an overall response rate of 89% [2].

Although chemotherapy as a single agent has not been shown to improve response rates, combination of ECP and chemotherapy is shown to be beneficial to CTCL patients. As the disease advances, chemotherapy is thought to exacerbate immunosuppression in patients with an already blunted immune system. In the setting of ECP where cell-mediated immune response thrives, the introduction of apoptosis-inducing agents like chemotherapy may enhance the development of an antitumor response. The combination of ECP and low-dose methotrexate at 15–25 mg per week has been shown to be safe and enhance efficacy [11].

In conclusion, ECP is a rigorously studied and widely accepted monotherapy for patients with erythrodermic CTCL, which derives a significant portion of its clinical efficacy by modulating the body's natural immune system. ECP has a very limited side effect profile, and the major contraindication to its use is related to the ability of the patient's cardiovascular system to sustain the hemodynamic challenges posed by ECP cycles. With several small-scale, prospective studies suggesting the benefit of ECP in combination with other therapeutic categories, there is an obvious need for further investigation to clearly demonstrate these effects. As basic science models continue to explore the immunomodulatory mechanisms, it will both improve the efficacy of ECP and suggest novel approaches for the treatment of CTCL.

Cytokine-based therapy: Interferons and Interleukins

IFNα and IFNγ

The role of IFNs in innate immunity, immunomodulation, and cancer has been of great scientific interest. IFN alter the interaction between the body's own immune system and tumor cells, and in CTCL, play an important role in boosting antitumor immunity. They are normally secreted by a variety of cells—for example, lymphocytes, fibroblasts, epithelial cells, activated T cells, and natural killer cells—all of which express TLRs on their surface membranes or on internal endosomes. TLR ligands—including viral, bacterial, fungal products—naturally induce synthesis of

IFNs that can bind to specific receptors and cause antiviral, immunoregulatory, and antitumor effects. IFNs are a large family of secreted proteins classified into three different types, each of which has its own receptor targets and causes activation of unique signaling pathways. Th1 CD4+ T-helper cells secrete IFNγ, which activates cytotoxic CD8+ T cells and NK cells. IFNα directly inhibits the secretion Th2 cytokines, including IL-4 and IL-5 [12]. Also, IFNs prime plasmacytoid DCs for antigen presentation by upregulating MHC II expression and enabling effector CD8+ T cells for antigen recognition by upregulating expression of MHC I genes [13]. These immunomodulatory effects may help offset the Th1/Th2 imbalance characteristic of CTCL and restore cell-mediated immunity, providing the rationale for its use as therapy.

IFN-α, IFN-β, and IFN-γ represent the majority of IFNs that have been used as therapy for CTCL. The two most commonly used commercially available synthetic IFNs are IFN-α2a and IFN-α2b, both of which are injected subcutaneously. There have been at least 14 trials that demonstrate the clinical efficacy of IFN-α, examining various doses and dosing schedules; however, no consensus exists regarding which treatment regimen is most effective. The earliest trial, by Bunn and coworkers in 1984, delivered high doses of 50 MU TIW and resulted in clinical responses, but also substantial toxicities [14]. A subsequent trial comparing 3–36 MU per day confirmed that response rate is dose dependent [15], and 18 MU is generally considered the highest tolerable dose. In the largest trial examining IFN monotherapy, 43 patients with all stages of disease underwent a 12-week dose-escalation phase starting at 3 MU per day, followed by a 6-month maintenance phase at the maximal tolerated dose TIW. A partial response was observed in 49% of patients, and a complete response in 26% [16]. Thus, in order to optimize clinical efficacy and reduce toxicity, it is recommended to initiate treatment at 1 MU per day and escalate to 5 MU until a response or a dose-limiting side effect is observed. Patients who achieve remission are advised to continue treatment for 3 months beyond the last signs of disease, while a second agent may be introduced to patients who fail to achieve a response at the maximal tolerated dose [17]. IFN can also be administered directly into skin lesions, as intralesional injections are reported to have maximal benefit in both the injected and non-injected lesions [18]. Unlike other therapies, clinical stage at initiation is not a significant predictor of response, although patients with tumor-stage disease typically benefit less from IFN [17, 19]. Furthermore, an antibody reaction has been observed against synthetic IFNs and may blunt the therapeutic response [20]. Although there is no consensus yet about the clinical relevance of these antibodies [21], neutralizing antibodies may represent a mechanism of resistance and explain refractory disease in the setting of IFN therapy [22].

Iatrogenic elevation of inflammatory cytokines causes both immediate and long-term effects. Acutely, IFN therapy may induce a "flu-like" syndrome of fever, chills, arthralgias, and myalgias, lasting for approximately 1 week. These symptoms can be mitigated with prophylactic acetaminophen or ibuprofen 1–2 h prior to IFN injection. Importantly, infection must be ruled out in all patients who present with fever, regardless of their medication list. Chronic use of IFNs may lead to cachexia characterized by weight loss, fatigue, and anorexia. Other concerning side effects of long-term use include hypothyroidism, depression, rhabdomyolysis, and cardiac toxicity. Thus, a thorough workup that encompasses endocrine, renal, hepatic, and cardiac systems is warranted prior to initiating IFN therapy [17, 23].

Several other IFN-based therapeutic strategies are currently being examined, including those to enhance IFN-γ and IL-12 levels. Important cytokines of the Th1 effector response, IFN-γ, and IL-12 offer many theoretical benefits to CTCL patients. The addition of IFNγ to patients on ECP has shown efficacy in early and late stage disease. While the use of IFNγ as a monotherapy is promising, it is limited due to pharmacokinetic shortcomings such as its short half-life [5]. Innovative strategies for cytokine delivery exploit genetically modified, non-pathologic viruses expressing IFNγ and have already been well tolerated in early phase trials [24, 25]. In addition, in a phase

II trial investigating recombinant IL-12 in early stage MF, a partial response was observed in 43% of patients. Although most adverse effects were mild to moderate, one patient in partial response died from severe hemolytic anemia, which may have been exacerbated by IL-12 therapy [26].

IL-2-directed therapies

Interleukin-2 is an important growth factor for most types of T cells. Antigen engagement with a CD4+ lymphocyte's T-cell receptor induces rapid production of IL-2 followed by expression of the high-affinity IL-2R, enabling selective expansion of only the antigen-activated T cells [27]. The IL-2R is composed of three subunits—CD25 (α), CD122 (β), and CD132 (γ). Any combination of subunits may be found on T cells, but receptors with all three have the highest affinity for IL-2. While less than 5% of PBMCs from a healthy volunteer express IL-2R, more than half of all CTCL patients have malignant lymphocytes that over express this T-cell growth factor receptor [28]. Thus, IL-2R offers an attractive therapeutic strategy for targeting tumor cells, and monoclonal antibodies like daclizumab have already been developed to exploit this pathway. Unfortunately, daclizumab lacked strong cytocidal activity in clinical trials, and therefore other strategies were needed to direct more cytotoxic activity to IL-2R positive cells [29].

Denileukin-diftitox (DD) addresses this need by fusing a recombinant IL-2 molecule with the cytotoxic subunit of the diphtheria toxin. Engagement with IL-2R leads to internalization via receptor-mediated endocytosis, and allows the diphtheria subunit to block protein synthesis and cause cell death [30]. Due to the theoretical requirement of IL-2R affinity, most clinical trials assessing the efficacy of DD have required that a significant percentage—usually greater than 20%—of lymphocytes are CD25 or CD122 positive. Prince et al. conducted a phase III, placebo-controlled, randomized trial on 144 patients with CD25+ CTCL who had less than three previous therapies. Patients were enrolled into one of the three arms: (1) placebo group, (2) 9 μg/kg/day DD, and (3) 18 μg/kg/day DD. While the treatment groups experienced response rates similar to reports from previous trials (9 μg/kg/day DD: PR = 26.7 and CR = 11.1; 18 μg/kg/day DD: PR = 40% and CR = 9.1; placebo group: PR = 13.6% and CR = 2.3%), this trial demonstrated that "clinical responses" can also occur in the placebo group without treatment, suggesting the potentially confounding role of the disease's waxing and waning natural history when investigating novel therapies [31].

The most common toxicity observed in the DD clinical trials was infusion-related hypersensitivity, which included fever, rash, hypotension, chest tightness, or shortness of breath and can be controlled with steroid pretreatment [32]. Physicians should be aware of vascular leak syndrome, characterized by increased vascular permeability, and resulting in extravasation of fluid and subsequent hypotension, hypoalbuminemia, and edema. Patients with liver disease are at higher risk because they are unable to compensate for albumin loss. Increased muscular intracompartmental pressure may lead to rhabdomyolysis.

Since clinical response hinges on IL-2R expression, strategies to upregulate IL-2R expression in the presence of DD therapy have been investigated. Bexarotene has clinical efficacy against CTCL as a monotherapy and is known to have anti-proliferative, pro-apoptotic, and immune-modulating effects. In preclinical trials, bexarotene upregulated the expression of CD25 and CD122 subunits on T-cell leukemia lines and enhanced their susceptibility to DD [33]. The phase I clinical trial to test the in vivo reproducibility of this finding enrolled 14 patients with progressive disease after one systemic therapy. DD 18 μg/kg/day × 3 days every 21 days was combined with daily oral bexarotene in a dose-escalation fashion (75–300 mg/day) to upregulate IL-2R. Of the 14 patients, including one patient who had previously been refractory to eight cycles of DD monotherapy, four patients (33%) each achieved a partial response and complete response. Notably, all four patients who achieved a complete response also demonstrated significant upregulation of CD25 expression after bexarotene treatment; CD25 expression increased in only one out of four patients who experienced a partial response. A potentially negative effect of this combination regimen is upregulation of CD25 expression in normal cells, enhancing their susceptibility to DD [34].

TLR Agonists

TLRs represent a class of ten pattern-recognition receptors found on various cells that signal the presence of infection and direct the innate and adaptive immune system to mount a response against the antigen [35]. TLRs detect pathogen-associated molecular patterns and stimulate immune cells via the MyD88-dependent interleukin 1 receptor (IL-1R) – TLR signaling pathway, which leads to activation of the transcription factor NF-κB [36]. The TLRs most relevant to CTCL immunotherapy appear to be TLR 4, 9, 7, and 8. TLR4 is found on myeloid DCs and recognizes the lipopolysaccharides of Gram-negative bacteria cell walls, resulting in secretion of IL-12, IL-4, and TNFα. Similarly, specific sequences of unmethylated DNA highly present in to bacterial and viral genomes known as "CpG motifs" activate TLR9 on plasmacytoid DCs and induce a cytokine response consisting predominantly of IFNα. TLR7 and TLR8 are found on both DC types and play a role in detection of viral ssRNA [37, 38]. TLRs are a critical mediator of the Th1 effector response [35], and thus are an attractive target for CTCL therapy to mediate restoration of the cytokine profile balance.

Imiquimod is a synthetic agonist for TLR7 and stimulates the production of numerous Th1 cytokines, including IFNα, IFNγ, TNFα, and IL-12 [39]; for this reason, 5% topical cream has been used off-label for stage IA disease. Approved for the treatment of basal cell carcinoma, actinic keratosis and genital warts, imiquimod shows a benefit in cancer by facilitating induction of an antitumor cellular response and apoptosis in some tumor cells. Clinical uses have been anecdotal and limited to skin-directed therapy for patches/plaques of early stage disease, but have suggested a clinical benefit even in patients refractory to other early stage treatments, including PUVA and low-dose retinoids [7, 40].

Synthetic oligodeoxynucleotides contain regions of unmethylated CpG motifs (CpG ODN) and are an excellent example of the translation of immunobiology into targeted therapy for cancer. This class of compounds is well described in its ability to potently stimulate DC activation, differentiation, and production of cytokines. Intralesional injection's ability to generate antitumor cytotoxic T-cell responses and induce a response has been demonstrated in murine melanoma models [41] and in human basal cell carcinoma and melanoma [42]. Culturing PBMCs from CTCL patients in the presence of CpG ODNs resulted in marked induction of IFN-α and significant activation of NK cells and CD8+ T cells, as measured by CD69 expression, compared to PBMCs from normal donors. These data provide the rationale for the development of clinical trials assessing the therapeutic benefits of CpG ODNs for CTCL [42].

A phase I dose-escalation study in 28 patients with treatment refractory stage IB to IVA was conducted to evaluate the safety and efficacy of PF-3512676 (0.08–0.36 mg/kg), a novel member of class-B CpG ODNs that targets TLR9. Patients tolerated the 24 weekly injections well, experiencing mostly grade 1 or 2 adverse events. Notably, no patients developed autoimmune disease, a concern with any novel immunomodulatory therapy. Although this study was not designed to rigorously assess efficacy, response rates of 32% (11% CR, 21% PR) suggest a clinical benefit of this therapy [43]. Further investigation is warranted, including the possible combination of TLR-agonists with other modalities of treatment.

Immune considerations for other systemic therapies: Retinoids and HDAC inhibitors

Retinoids

Retinoids are derivatives of vitamin A widely used as topical and oral therapy for dermatologic conditions including psoriasis, acne, and

CTCL. Their clinical effects are mediated through interactions with the transcription factors retinoid A receptors (RAR) and retinoid X receptors (RXR). They impact cell cycle progression through the modulation of cyclins, CDKs, and cell cycle inhibitors [44], and are known to induce apoptosis in vitro in cancer cell lines, including immortalized cells from CTCL patients [45].

Although retinoids are not traditionally classified as immunotherapy, clear evidence exists regarding their immunomodulatory role in CTCL, and this effect may contribute to their therapeutic value. In the epidermis, retinoids stimulate Langerhans cells to upregulate expression of MHC II and CD11c molecules, and thereby enhance the capacity to present antigen and generate a T-cell-mediated immune response [46]. As mentioned previously, some retinoids augment T-cell expression of IL-2R, and this specific effect is exploited to increase target sites for combination therapy with DD [47, 48]. Moreover, retinoids have a significant impact on the Th1/Th2 imbalance seen in CTCL by enhancing production of Th1 cytokines. In the presence of monocytes and IL-2, retinoids induce both normal and malignant T-cells to secrete IFN-γ through an IL-12-dependent mechanism [49]. Additionally, retinoids enhance the cytotoxicity of natural killer cells and CD8+ T cells, boosting the depressed cellular immunity seen in CTCL [50, 51].

Clinical use of retinoids for CTCL patients has been successful and includes both topical and systemic formulation. Bexarotene 1% gel demonstrated a 44% overall response rate (8% complete response rate) in patients with refractory early stage disease when applied every other day [52]. Oral bexarotene has been evaluated in both early and late stage patients, showing 54% and 45% response rates, respectively, at a dose of 300 mg/kg/day [53, 54]. Side effects include hyperlipidemia, central hypothyroidism, and headaches. Potential resistance remains a concern in the long-term therapeutic properties of bexarotene and may be mediated via epigenetic silencing of RXR genes [55].

HDI

HDIs have shown promise in the treatment of hematologic malignancies, including CTCL. Histone deacetylases are involved in the remodeling of chromatin, which impacts the level of access to regions of DNA available to transcriptional machinery. These epigenetic modifications have the potential of exerting cancer-promoting effects through changes in expression of critical oncogenes or tumor suppressor genes. Moreover, these inhibitors have recently been shown to deacetylate numerous nonhistone substrates, resulting in several anticancer effects ranging from cell cycle arrest to angiogenesis reduction to immunomodulation [56]. Evidence suggests that histone deacetylases are overexpressed in CTCL [57], which has led to the inclusion of HDI in the arsenal of therapy against CTCL.

The mechanistic basis of benefit seen from HDI therapy in CTCL patients has also been investigated. Induction of apoptosis is a well-described effect of HDI in both CTCL cell lines and ex vivo malignant cells, and this process is thought to be mediated through regulation of p21 expression [58]. The precise immunological impact of HDI remains to be clarified, but various immune responses have been reported. HDIs seem to promote the restoration of the effector cytokine response balance. Both primary cells and immortalized cell lines from CTCL patients show a dramatic reduction in Th2 cytokines IL-10, IL-2, and IL-4 [59]. Furthermore, in response to HDI treatment, the cell line Hut78 upregulates IL-2R expression and is subsequently more susceptible to the treatment with DD, the cytotoxic IL-2 chimeric compound that can only gain access to cells via IL-2R [58, 60]. Moreover, in vitro and ex vivo data suggests that HDI suppress the cell-mediated cytotoxic immune response, providing rationale for the use of HDI in the treatment of autoimmune conditions [61]. While other CTCL therapies typically enhance NK cell activation and dendritic cell maturation, HDIs seem to impair this process and further weaken the overall immunologic status. Preliminary data suggests that addition of a more classic immunotherapy such as TLR agonist may be able to overcome HDI-induced immunosuppression [62]. Even despite these effects on the immune system, HDI monotherapy leads to a clinical benefit in CTCL patients.

Vorinostat and romidepsin are two HDI therapies approved for the treatment of CTCL. The pivotal, multicenter trial of vorinostat enrolled 74 patients with stage IB or higher CTCL who were refractory or resistant to other therapies; treatment with 400 mg of oral vorinostat daily produced an overall response rate of 30%, consistent even in patients with advanced disease including Sezary syndrome and T3 (tumor) stage [63]. The efficacy of romidepsin was assessed in two clinical trials of patients with all stages of diseases, including a significant majority of patients with poor prognoses who were refractory to at least one other therapy and often two. Even with the inclusion of patients with advanced disease, a 34% overall response rate was reported in both trials [64, 65]. Although safe and effective, significant cardiovascular and hematological adverse effects were reported in the HDI clinical trials, but the precise risk associated with these drugs is not clear [66, 67].

References

1. Edelson R, Berger C, Gasparro F, et al. Treatment of cutaneous T-cell lymphoma by extracorporeal photochemotherapy. Preliminary results. N Engl J Med. 1987;316:297–303.
2. Knobler R, Barr ML, Couriel DR, et al. Extracorporeal photopheresis: past, present, and future. J Am Acad Dermatol. 2009;61:652–65.
3. Berger C, Hoffmann K, Vasquez JG, et al. Rapid generation of maturationally synchronized human dendritic cells: contribution to the clinical efficacy of extracorporeal photochemotherapy. Blood. 2010;116:4838–47.
4. Scarisbrick JJ, Taylor P, Holtick U, et al. U.K. consensus statement on the use of extracorporeal photopheresis for treatment of cutaneous T-cell lymphoma and chronic graft-versus-host disease. Br J Dermatol. 2008;158:659–78.
5. Lansigan F, Foss FM. Current and emerging treatment strategies for cutaneous T-cell lymphoma. Drugs. 2010;70:273–86.
6. Wilson LD, Jones GW, Kim D, et al. Experience with total skin electron beam therapy in combination with extracorporeal photopheresis in the management of patients with erythrodermic (T4) mycosis fungoides. J Am Acad Dermatol. 2000;43:54–60.
7. Suchin KR, Cucchiara AJ, Gottleib SL, et al. Treatment of cutaneous T-cell lymphoma with combined immunomodulatory therapy: a 14-year experience at a single institution. Arch Dermatol. 2002;138:1054–60.
8. Dippel E, Schrag H, Goerdt S, Orfanos CE. Extracorporeal photopheresis and interferon-alpha in advanced cutaneous T-cell lymphoma. Lancet. 1997; 350:32–3.
9. Wollina U, Looks A, Meyer J, et al. Treatment of stage II cutaneous T-cell lymphoma with interferon alfa-2a and extracorporeal photochemotherapy: a prospective controlled trial. J Am Acad Dermatol. 2001; 44:253–60.
10. Lim HW, Harris HR. Etretinate as an effective adjunctive therapy for recalcitrant palmar/plantar hyperkeratosis in patients with erythrodermic cutaneous T cell lymphoma undergoing photopheresis. Dermatol Surg. 1995;21:597–9.
11. Zackheim HS, Epstein Jr EH. Low-dose methotrexate for the Sezary syndrome. J Am Acad Dermatol. 1989;21:757–62.
12. Suchin KR, Cassin M, Gottleib SL, et al. Increased interleukin 5 production in eosinophilic Sezary syndrome: regulation by interferon alfa and interleukin 12. J Am Acad Dermatol. 2001;44:28–32.
13. Borden EC, Sen GC, Uze G, et al. Interferons at age 50: past, current and future impact on biomedicine. Nat Rev Drug Discov. 2007;6:975–90.
14. Bunn Jr PA, Foon KA, Ihde DC, et al. Recombinant leukocyte A interferon: an active agent in advanced cutaneous T-cell lymphomas. Ann Intern Med. 1984;101:484–7.
15. Olsen EA, Rosen ST, Vollmer RT, et al. Interferon alfa-2a in the treatment of cutaneous T cell lymphoma. J Am Acad Dermatol. 1989;20:395–407.
16. Papa G, Tura S, Mandelli F, et al. Is interferon alpha in cutaneous T-cell lymphoma a treatment of choice? Br J Haematol. 1991;79 Suppl 1:48–51.
17. Olsen EA. Interferon in the treatment of cutaneous T-cell lymphoma. Dermatol Ther. 2003;16:311–21.
18. Wolff JM, Zitelli JA, Rabin BS, Smiles KA, Abell E. Intralesional interferon in the treatment of early mycosis fungoides. J Am Acad Dermatol. 1985;13:604–12.
19. Springer EA, Kuzel TM, Variakojis D, Kaul K, Rosen ST, Roenigk Jr HH. Correlation of clinical responses with immunologic and morphologic characteristics in patients with cutaneous T-cell lymphoma treated with interferon alfa-2a. J Am Acad Dermatol. 1993; 29:42–6.
20. Steis RG, Smith 2nd JW, Urba WJ, et al. Resistance to recombinant interferon alfa-2a in hairy-cell leukemia associated with neutralizing anti-interferon antibodies. N Engl J Med. 1988;318:1409–13.
21. Itri LM, Sherman MI, Palleroni AV, et al. Incidence and clinical significance of neutralizing antibodies in patients receiving recombinant interferon-alpha 2a. J Interferon Res. 1989;9 Suppl 1:S9–15.

22. Olsen EA, Bunn PA. Interferon in the treatment of cutaneous T-cell lymphoma. Hematol Oncol Clin North Am. 1995;9:1089–107.
23. Rook AH, Kuzel TM, Olsen EA. Cytokine therapy of cutaneous T-cell lymphoma: interferons, interleukin-12, and interleukin-2. Hematol Oncol Clin North Am. 2003;17:1435–48. ix.
24. Dummer R, Hassel JC, Fellenberg F, et al. Adenovirus-mediated intralesional interferon-gamma gene transfer induces tumor regressions in cutaneous lymphomas. Blood. 2004;104:1631–8.
25. Heinzerling L, Kunzi V, Oberholzer PA, Kundig T, Naim H, Dummer R. Oncolytic measles virus in cutaneous T-cell lymphomas mounts antitumor immune responses in vivo and targets interferon-resistant tumor cells. Blood. 2005;106:2287–94.
26. Duvic M, Sherman ML, Wood GS, et al. A phase II open-label study of recombinant human interleukin-12 in patients with stage IA, IB, or IIA mycosis fungoides. J Am Acad Dermatol. 2006;55:807–13.
27. Gaffen SL, Liu KD. Overview of interleukin-2 function, production and clinical applications. Cytokine. 2004;28:109–23.
28. Foss FM, Borkowski TA, Gilliom M, et al. Chimeric fusion protein toxin DAB486IL-2 in advanced mycosis fungoides and the Sezary syndrome: correlation of activity and interleukin-2 receptor expression in a phase II study. Blood. 1994;84:1765–74.
29. Lansigan F, Stearns DM, Foss F. Role of denileukin diftitox in the treatment of persistent or recurrent cutaneous T-cell lymphoma. Cancer Manag Res. 2010;2:53–9.
30. Kadin ME, Vonderheid EC. Targeted therapies: Denileukin diftitox–a step towards a 'magic bullet' for CTCL. Nat Rev Clin Oncol. 2010;7:430–2.
31. Prince HM, Duvic M, Martin A, et al. Phase III placebo-controlled trial of denileukin diftitox for patients with cutaneous T-cell lymphoma. J Clin Oncol. 2010;28:1870–7.
32. Olsen E, Duvic M, Frankel A, et al. Pivotal phase III trial of two dose levels of denileukin diftitox for the treatment of cutaneous T-cell lymphoma. J Clin Oncol. 2001;19:376–88.
33. Gorgun G, Foss F. Immunomodulatory effects of RXR rexinoids: modulation of high-affinity IL-2R expression enhances susceptibility to denileukin diftitox. Blood. 2002;100:1399–403.
34. Foss F, Demierre MF, DiVenuti G. A phase-1 trial of bexarotene and denileukin diftitox in patients with relapsed or refractory cutaneous T-cell lymphoma. Blood. 2005;106:454–7.
35. Medzhitov R. Toll-like receptors and innate immunity. Nat Rev Immunol. 2001;1:135–45.
36. Jurk M, Heil F, Vollmer J, et al. Human TLR7 or TLR8 independently confer responsiveness to the antiviral compound R-848. Nat Immunol. 2002; 3:499.
37. Krieg AM. CpG motifs: the active ingredient in bacterial extracts? Nat Med. 2003;9:831–5.
38. Heil F, Hemmi H, Hochrein H, et al. Species-specific recognition of single-stranded RNA via toll-like receptor 7 and 8. Science. 2004;303:1526–9.
39. Martinez-Gonzalez MC, Verea-Hernando MM, Yebra-Pimentel MT, Del Pozo J, Mazaira M, Fonseca E. Imiquimod in mycosis fungoides. Eur J Dermatol. 2008;18:148–52.
40. Dummer R, Urosevic M, Kempf W, Kazakov D, Burg G. Imiquimod induces complete clearance of a PUVA-resistant plaque in mycosis fungoides. Dermatology. 2003;207:116–8.
41. Lonsdorf AS, Kuekrek H, Stern BV, Boehm BO, Lehmann PV, Tary-Lehmann M. Intratumor CpG-oligodeoxynucleotide injection induces protective antitumor T cell immunity. J Immunol. 2003; 171:3941–6.
42. Wysocka M, Benoit BM, Newton S, Azzoni L, Montaner LJ, Rook AH. Enhancement of the host immune responses in cutaneous T-cell lymphoma by CpG oligodeoxynucleotides and IL-15. Blood. 2004;104:4142–9.
43. Kim YH, Girardi M, Duvic M, et al. Phase I trial of a Toll-like receptor 9 agonist, PF-3512676 (CPG 7909), in patients with treatment-refractory, cutaneous T-cell lymphoma. J Am Acad Dermatol. 2010;63:975–83.
44. Tang XH, Gudas LJ. Retinoids, retinoic acid receptors, and cancer. Annu Rev Pathol. 2011;6:345–64.
45. Fontana JA, Rishi AK. Classical and novel retinoids: their targets in cancer therapy. Leukemia. 2002; 16:463–72.
46. Meunier L, Bohjanen K, Voorhees JJ, Cooper KD. Retinoic acid upregulates human Langerhans cell antigen presentation and surface expression of HLA-DR and CD11c, a beta 2 integrin critically involved in T-cell activation. J Invest Dermatol. 1994;103:775–9.
47. Kempf W, Kettelhack N, Duvic M, Burg G. Topical and systemic retinoid therapy for cutaneous T-cell lymphoma. Hematol Oncol Clin North Am. 2003; 17:1405–19.
48. Foss FM, Waldmann TA. Interleukin-2 receptor-directed therapies for cutaneous lymphomas. Hematol Oncol Clin North Am. 2003;17:1449–58.
49. Fox FE, Kubin M, Cassin M, et al. Retinoids synergize with interleukin-2 to augment IFN-gamma and interleukin-12 production by human peripheral blood mononuclear cells. J Interferon Cytokine Res. 1999;19:407–15.
50. Pigatto PD, Bersani L, Colotta F, Morelli M, Altomare GF, Polenghi MM. Effect of retinoids on natural killer cell activity. Arch Dermatol Res. 1986;278:507–9.
51. Gordy C, Dzhagalov I, He YW. Regulation of CD8(+) T cell functions by RARgamma. Semin Immunol. 2009;21:2–7.
52. Heald P, Mehlmauer M, Martin AG, Crowley CA, Yocum RC, Reich SD. Topical bexarotene therapy for patients with refractory or persistent early-stage cutaneous T-cell lymphoma: results of the phase III clinical trial. J Am Acad Dermatol. 2003;49:801–15.

53. Duvic M, Hymes K, Heald P, et al. Bexarotene is effective and safe for treatment of refractory advanced-stage cutaneous T-cell lymphoma: multinational phase II–III trial results. J Clin Oncol. 2001;19:2456–71.
54. Duvic M, Martin AG, Kim Y, et al. Phase 2 and 3 clinical trial of oral bexarotene (Targretin capsules) for the treatment of refractory or persistent early-stage cutaneous T-cell lymphoma. Arch Dermatol. 2001; 137:581–93.
55. Lin JH, Kim EJ, Bansal A, et al. Clinical and in vitro resistance to bexarotene in adult T-cell leukemia: loss of RXR-alpha receptor. Blood. 2008;112:2484–8.
56. Choudhary C, Kumar C, Gnad F, et al. Lysine acetylation targets protein complexes and co-regulates major cellular functions. Science. 2009;325:834–40.
57. Mercurio C, Minucci S, Pelicci PG. Histone deacetylases and epigenetic therapies of hematological malignancies. Pharmacol Res. 2010;62:18–34.
58. Piekarz RL, Robey RW, Zhan Z, et al. T-cell lymphoma as a model for the use of histone deacetylase inhibitors in cancer therapy: impact of depsipeptide on molecular markers, therapeutic targets, and mechanisms of resistance. Blood. 2004;103:4636–43.
59. Tiffon C, Adams J, van der Fits L, et al. The histone deacetylase inhibitors vorinostat and romidepsin downmodulate IL-10 expression in cutaneous T-cell lymphoma cells. Br J Pharmacol. 2011;162:1590–602.
60. Shao RH, Tian X, Gorgun G, Urbano AG, Foss FM. Arginine butyrate increases the cytotoxicity of DAB(389)IL-2 in leukemia and lymphoma cells by upregulation of IL-2Rbeta gene. Leuk Res. 2002; 26:1077–83.
61. Wang L, de Zoeten EF, Greene MI, Hancock WW. Immunomodulatory effects of deacetylase inhibitors: therapeutic targeting of FOXP3+ regulatory T cells. Nat Rev Drug Discov. 2009;8:969–81.
62. Kelly-Sell M BB, Kim Y, Harrison C, Sutherland K, Showe L, Maria W, Rook A. The histone deacetylase inhibitor, romidepsin, suppresses in vivo immune functions of cutaneous T-cell lymphoma patients. J Invest Dermatol. 2011;131:Suppl; abstr 520.
63. Olsen EA, Kim YH, Kuzel TM, et al. Phase IIb multicenter trial of vorinostat in patients with persistent, progressive, or treatment refractory cutaneous T-cell lymphoma. J Clin Oncol. 2007;25:3109–15.
64. Piekarz RL, Frye R, Turner M, et al. Phase II multi-institutional trial of the histone deacetylase inhibitor romidepsin as monotherapy for patients with cutaneous T-cell lymphoma. J Clin Oncol. 2009;27:5410–7.
65. Whittaker SJ, Demierre MF, Kim EJ, et al. Final results from a multicenter, international, pivotal study of romidepsin in refractory cutaneous T-cell lymphoma. J Clin Oncol. 2010;28:4485–91.
66. Bates SE, Rosing DR, Fojo T, Piekarz RL. Challenges of evaluating the cardiac effects of anticancer agents. Clin Cancer Res. 2006;12:3871–4.
67. Piekarz RL, Frye AR, Wright JJ, et al. Cardiac studies in patients treated with depsipeptide, FK228, in a phase II trial for T-cell lymphoma. Clin Cancer Res. 2006;12:3762–73.

Syndromes and Clinical Management Issues Associated with T-Cell Lymphomas

19

Merry Jennifer Markham and Nam H. Dang

Introduction

T-cell lymphomas have been associated with specific clinical syndromes and characteristics, often requiring special attention by the clinician. In addition, some of the drugs used to treat T-cell malignancies have specific side effects or distinctive risks associated with their use. In this chapter, we will review some of the unique clinical syndromes that may occur in patients with T-cell lymphomas, either as a result of the disease or as a result of the treatments for the malignancy.

Clinical Syndromes

Poor Prognosis

Lymphomas derived from T-lymphocytes have been associated with the presence of more adverse features and a worse prognosis than lymphomas of B-cell origin [1–4]. Retrospective evaluation of patients enrolled in two GELA (Groupe d'Etude des Lymphomes Aggressives) studies has yielded data on the implication of the T-cell phenotype on prognosis [1, 2]. While adverse features are more likely to be present in patients with T-cell lymphomas, it appears that the T-cell histology itself is an independent poor prognostic factor [2, 3].

Of 361 patients with lymphoma treated on the LNH-84 regimen for aggressive lymphoma, 108 had peripheral T-cell lymphoma and 253 had B-cell lymphomas [1]. When compared to patients with B-cell lymphomas, those with peripheral T-cell lymphomas were more likely to have stage IV disease (53% vs. 45%) and B-symptoms (58% vs. 42%). In addition, those with T-cell histology had a higher rate of relapse (43% vs. 29%) and a shorter freedom-from-relapse survival (34 months vs. not reached). Overall survival was shorter in the patients with T-cell lymphomas (42 months vs. 50 months); however, this difference was not statistically significant.

The multicenter LNH-87 trial enrolled patients with intermediate or high-grade non-Hodgkin's lymphoma, and Gisselbrecht et al. reported on the prognostic significance of the T-cell phenotype in patients treated on that protocol [2]. Of 1,883 evaluable patients, 288 (15%) had peripheral T-cell lymphomas and 1,595 (85%) had B-cell lymphomas. While B-cell lymphoma patients had more bulky disease (41% vs. 26%), T-cell lymphoma patients had more bone marrow involvement (31% vs. 17%) and advanced stage disease (78% vs. 58%). Peripheral T-cell lymphoma patients were also more likely to have B-symptoms (57% vs. 40%) and increased B2-microglobulin (50% vs. 34%) than those with

M.J. Markham • N.H. Dang (✉)
Department of Medicine, Division of Hematology and Oncology, University of Florida, 1600 SW Archer Road, Box 100278, Room M410A, Gainesville, FL 32610, USA
e-mail: nam.dang@medicine.ufl.edu

F. Foss (ed.), *T-Cell Lymphomas*, Contemporary Hematology,
DOI 10.1007/978-1-62703-170-7_19,

B-cell lymphomas. Complete remission rates (54% vs. 63%), 5-year overall survival rates (41% vs. 53%), and event-free survival rates (33% vs. 42%) were worse for patients with T-cell lymphomas compared to B-cell lymphomas.

Investigators at the M. D. Anderson Cancer Center reviewed six front-line chemotherapy clinical trials in aggressive non-Hodgkin's lymphoma that were performed at the institution from 1984 to 1995 [3]. Of 560 evaluable patients, 492 (88%) were of B-cell phenotype and 68 (12%) were peripheral T-cell lymphomas. The 5-year overall survival rate for those patients with peripheral T-cell lymphomas was 38% compared to 55% for those with B-cell lymphomas. T-cell lymphoma patients with an International Prognostic Index (IPI) score of more than two (poor prognosis) had a 5-year overall survival of 10% compared to 40% ($p=0.011$) in those patients with B-cell lymphomas. T-cell lymphoma patients with an M. D. Anderson prognostic tumor score (MDATS) of more than two (poor prognosis) had a 5-year overall survival of 24% compared to 41% ($p=0.02$) in those with B-cell lymphomas. Multivariate analysis confirmed that the most significant independent predictors of overall survival were the MDATS, the IPI score, and the T-cell phenotype.

Hemophagocytic Syndrome

The hemophagocytic syndrome (HPS) is characterized by fever, pancytopenia, hepatosplenomegaly, and liver dysfunction. The clinical syndrome results from activated macrophages, and evidence of hemophagocytosis can be found in the bone marrow and other tissues. HPS has been associated with T-cell lymphomas [5–7]. While the syndrome has been associated with the Epstein–Barr virus, malignancy-associated HPS such as that found in patients with T-cell lymphomas is not necessarily due to viral infection [6, 8]. Diagnostic criteria have been established for HPS, mostly arising from literature on the familial form of the disease [9]. Five out of the following eight criteria are required to make a diagnosis of HPS: (1) fever; (2) splenomegaly; (3) cytopenias in at least two cell lines; (4) hypertriglyceridemia and/or hypofibrinogenemia; (5) ferritin more than 500 mg/L; (6) decreased or absent NK-cell activity; (7) sCD25 more than 2,400 U/mL; (8) hemophagocytosis documented in the bone marrow, cerebrospinal fluid, or lymph nodes [9].

Lymphoma-associated HPS was evaluated in a retrospective series of 29 patients treated between 1994 and 2006 [10]. The authors found that of the 29 patients with HPS, 11 patients (37.9%) had aggressive NK/T-cell leukemia; 8 (27.6%) had peripheral T-cell lymphoma, not otherwise specified (NOS); 3 (10.3%) had extranodal NK/T-cell lymphoma, nasal type; and 2 patients (6.9%) had anaplastic large cell lymphoma (ALCL). Just 17% (five patients) had diffuse large B-cell lymphoma. In comparison to those patients with B-cell lymphoma-associated HPS, those patients with T- or NK-cell malignancies were more likely to be younger than 60, have evidence of disseminated intravascular coagulation (DIC), and have bone marrow involvement. For all patients, the most frequent symptom was fever (100%) followed by hepatosplenomegaly (93.1%). Of the 23 patients who received combination chemotherapy for their malignancy, four achieved a complete remission and three achieved partial remission. The median survival of all patients was 36 days (range 2 to 1,991+ days). Univariate analysis revealed that poor prognostic factors included poor performance status, the presence of jaundice, the presence of DIC, poor response to therapy, and T- or NK-cell lymphoma.

More evidence supporting the poor prognosis of T-cell lymphoma-associated HPS comes from a review of 113 patients with aggressive T-cell lymphoma of whom 28 had HPS [11]. Fever was identified in 100% of the 28 patients with HPS and in 48% of those without HPS. Hepatosplenomegaly was identified in 100% of the patients with HPS compared to 39% of those without HPS. Cytopenias in more than one cell line (100% vs. 20%) and bone marrow involvement (57% vs. 32%) were also more likely to be present in the T-cell lymphoma patients with HPS. Patients were treated with combination chemotherapy. Eleven of the 28 patients with T-cell lymphoma associated HPS died of multiorgan failure prior to receiving chemotherapy. The median survival of the HPS group was 40 days compared to a median survival of 8 months in those without HPS.

Tong et al. recently reviewed data from 173 patients diagnosed with peripheral T-cell lymphoma to assess the role of bone marrow involvement in the prognosis and outcome of the disease [12]. In their evaluation, 70 of the 173 patients (40%) with peripheral T-cell lymphoma had bone marrow involvement. Of those patients with bone marrow involvement, the HPS was identified in 36% compared with only 8% of those patients without bone marrow involvement. The highest frequency of bone marrow involvement was found in angioimmunoblastic T-cell lymphoma with 64% having bone marrow involvement. Marrow involvement was also identified in 46% of the peripheral T-cell lymphoma, NOS, patients; in 29% of the anaplastic large T-cell lymphoma patients; in 23% of extranodal NK/T-cell lymphoma patients; and in 13% of patients with enteropathy-type T-cell lymphoma. The diagnosis of HPS was associated with a worse 1-year overall survival in those with bone marrow involvement (5%) than without bone marrow involvement (49%) [12].

Skin Infections

Patients with cutaneous T-cell lymphoma (CTCL) are at risk for morbidity and mortality from infection caused by bacterial and viral pathogens. In a retrospective cohort study of 356 patients with mycosis fungoides or Sézary syndrome, infection was noted to be an important cause of morbidity [13]. The most common infections were cutaneous bacterial infections which accounted for 17 infections per 100 patient years. Following cutaneous bacterial infections were cutaneous herpes simplex and herpes zoster virus infection (3.8 infections per 100 patient-years), bacteremia (2.1 infections per 100 patient-years), bacterial pneumonia (1.7 infections per 100 patient-years), and urinary tract infections (1.4 infections per 100 patient-years). Twenty-seven patients (36%) in the cohort died from infection, and pneumonia or bacteremia was present in 88% of those who died of infection. Using regression models, the most important risk factor for recurrent bacterial skin infection, disseminated herpes virus infection, bacteremia, and death from infection was the presence of advanced stage (stages III and IV) of the lymphoma.

Tokura et al. have demonstrated that circulating Sézary cells have a response to bacterial superantigens, such as the toxins produced by *Staphylococcus aureus*—exfoliating toxin (ExT), staphylococcal enterotoxins (SE), and toxic shock syndrome toxin-1 (TSST-1) [14]. In two patients with CTCL whose skin was colonized with *S. aureus*, treatment with antibacterial agents lessened the severity of CTCL-associated skin manifestations and eliminated the *S. aureus* [15]. Peripheral blood mononuclear cells (PBMC)—which contained a high proportion of circulating Sézary cells—taken from one of the patients demonstrated marked proliferation when exposed to staphylococcal exotoxin. Superinfections of the skin with *S. aureus* may play a role in the exacerbation of the disease course of CTCL.

Two recent studies have provided data on the rates of *S. aureus* colonization in patients with CTCL [16, 17]. In the first study, researchers at Northwestern University prospectively evaluated 50 patients with CTCL, 25 patients with psoriasis to serve as controls, and 25 healthy control patients [16]. *S. aureus* colonization was identified in 44% of the CTCL patients, 48% of those patients with psoriasis, and in 28% of healthy controls. Because of small sample size, no significant difference was identified in the rates among groups. Higher rates of methicillin-sensitive *Staphylococcus aureus* (MSSA) colonization were identified in CTCL patients (42%) compared to healthy controls (20%); however, this difference only trended toward statistical significance.

In the second and larger study, Talpur et al. performed skin and nares cultures in a prospective manner in 106 patients with newly or recently diagnosed mycosis fungoides or Sézary syndrome [17]. Patients with positive nasal cultures were treated with topical nasal mupirocin to suppress colonization, and those with positive skin cultures received oral antibiotics. Sixty-seven patients (63%) had skin colonization with *S. aureus*, and 57 patients (54%) had nasal colonization with the bacteria. The highest rates of colonization were seen in patients with erythrodermic Sézary syndrome (48%), and the lowest rates were seen in CTCL without erythroderma (26%). Historical data used for comparison revealed that the *S. aureus* colonization rate seen in atopic dermatitis is 64%. The colonization rate in psoriasis is 21%, and the rate in the general population is 10% [17]. Eradication of the bacterial colonization with oral or topical antibiotics reduced the *S. aureus* colonization by 85–91%, and over half of those treated experienced clinical improvement in their disease symptoms [17].

Fatigue and Edema in Cutaneous T-Cell Lymphoma

Patients with CTCL may have increased rates of peripheral edema and fatigue. Negro-Vilar et al. presented preliminary data from the phase III, double-blind, placebo-controlled trial of denileukin diftitox in patients with CTCL and demonstrated that denileukin diftitox was superior to placebo [18]. Eighty-six percent (124 of 144 patients randomized) had received one or more prior treatment regimens, including single agent chemotherapy, systemic retinoids, phototherapy, or external beam radiotherapy. While there was a higher rate of adverse events in the experimental arms, there was also noted to be a relatively high percentage of patients experiencing fatigue and peripheral edema in the placebo arm. Peripheral edema was experienced by patients in the denileukin diftitox 9-μg/kg arm (20%) and in the 18-μg/kg arm (25.5%); in the placebo arm, the rate was 22.7%. Fatigue was noted both in the 9 μg/kg arm (46.7%) and in the 18 μg/kg arm (43.6%); the fatigue rate in the placebo arm was 31.8%.

Tumor Lysis Syndrome

Tumor lysis syndrome (TLS) is a well-known oncologic emergency that may occur in patients with aggressive hematologic malignancies upon the initiation of cytotoxic chemotherapy. Cairo and Bishop defined two types of TLS—laboratory TLS and clinical TLS—in their 2004 publication on the subject [19]. Laboratory TLS was defined as having at least two serum lab values with the following abnormalities: potassium ≥6.0 mmol/L; uric acid ≥8 mg/dL, phosphate ≥4.5 mg/dL in adults or ≥6.5 mg/dL in children, calcium ≤7 mg/dL. Having laboratory TLS plus one clinical manifestation (increased serum creatinine concentration ≥1.5 times upper limit of normal, cardiac arrhythmia/sudden death, or seizure) characterized clinical TLS. These defining features of TLS must be present within 3 days before or 7 days after the initiation of chemotherapy.

There is a paucity of literature available on the incidence of TLS in T-cell malignancies. TLS has been reported in peripheral T-cell lymphoma and in ALCL [20–23]. There have been at least three case reports of TLS occurring after initiation of corticosteroid monotherapy in T-cell lymphoblastic lymphoma [24–26]. The first case reported was a patient with untreated T-cell lymphoblastic lymphoma who received two doses of hydrocortisone prior to a platelet transfusion who subsequently developed laboratory TLS [25]. A 20-year-old man with T-cell lymphoblastic lymphoma developed acute renal failure requiring hemodialysis after receiving prednisolone [26]. A recently reported case involved a 60-year-old woman who received dexamethasone for her diagnosis of precursor T-lymphoblastic lymphoma/leukemia and subsequently developed laboratory evidence of TLS, also requiring hemodialysis [24].

TLS has recently been reported in human T-lymphotropic virus (HTLV)-1 adult T-cell leukemia/lymphoma (ATLL). A 49-year-old woman with an 8-year history of systemic lupus erythematosus (SLE) was diagnosed with HTLV-1-associated ATLL after presenting with fevers, malaise, and lymphadenopathy [27]. She developed TLS with hyperkalemia, hyperphosphatemia, and hypocalcemia; and she died 3 days after chemotherapy with cyclophosphamide, doxorubicin, and prednisone was initiated. Bouaziz et al. reported their experience with a

50-year-old man with ATLL with skin involvement who later experienced leukemic conversion of the ATLL [28]. When the patient was treated with combination chemotherapy for his disease, he developed skin erosions in the areas of prior cutaneous leukemic infiltration. Histopathological examination of the skin erosions showed atypical T-lymphocytes (CD3+, CD4+, and CD25+) with apoptosis. Because of this skin finding, the authors suggest a new term to describe the entity—"cutaneous tumor lysis" [28].

TLS has been reported in one patient with CTCL. A 65-year-old man with mycosis fungoides had failed therapy with bexarotene and photophoresis when he was admitted for fever and dyspnea [29]. Since a chest X-ray showed bilateral infiltrates, therapy with antibiotics and intravenous corticosteroids was initiated for presumed *Pneumocystis carinii* infection. Over the next 4 days, he developed laboratory evidence of TLS requiring therapy with rasburicase (recombinant urate oxidase).

Central Nervous System Involvement

T-cell lymphomas may manifest as primary central nervous system (CNS) lymphomas, or CNS involvement may occur as a secondary phenomenon resulting from spread of the initial disease site(s). Lymphomas of T-cell histology comprise a minority of the cases of primary and secondary CNS lymphoma; the majority of cases are of B-cell origin [30, 31].

The incidence of primary CNS lymphoma in the United States was 5.1 per one million person-years in 1998 [32]. There are case reports of primary CNS lymphoma of T-cell origin, including individual case reports of primary CNS manifestations of ALCL, adult T-cell lymphoma/leukemia, and extranodal NK/T-cell lymphoma [33–36]. To characterize primary CNS T-cell lymphoma, Shenkier et al. performed a retrospective review of 45 patients from 12 cancer centers in seven countries [37]. The median age of the patients was 60 years (range, 3–84 years), and none of the patients had systemic lymphoma at presentation. Median disease-specific survival was 25 months, and the 5-year disease specific survival was 51%. Good Eastern Cooperative Oncology Group (ECOG) performance status (PS of 0 or 1) and the use of methotrexate were associated with improved outcome.

In addition to presenting with brain involvement, primary CNS lymphoma may also present with leptomeningeal involvement as the primary site of disease [37–39]. Levin et al. reviewed their cases of primary CNS lymphoma treated over the past 10 years [38]. Out of 100 cases, five patients (5%) had lymphomas of T-cell histology. Each of those five patients presented with leptomeningeal involvement rather than brain involvement, and four of the patients had neuronal lymphomatosis at presentation. Each of the five patients had evidence of cranial or peripheral nerve dysfunction. Four of the five died within 10–19 months and one patient was alive at 36 months from the date of report publication.

Primary CNS lymphoma of T-cell origin can be difficult to diagnose and may, in fact, be under recognized [40]. Performing T-cell receptor gene rearrangements on the tumor biopsy samples may increase the accuracy of diagnosis and may distinguish between reactive lymphoid infiltrates [40]. Clinicians might also consider meningeal or nerve biopsy in the setting of symptoms of neuronal lymphomatosis, especially in the setting where cerebrospinal fluid cytology findings are not conclusive [38].

Salzburg et al. evaluated the patterns of secondary CNS involvement in childhood and adolescent non-Hodgkin's lymphoma and found that CNS involvement was associated with advanced stage of lymphoma [31]. CNS involvement was found in 5.9% of 2,381 patients. Among the T-cell lymphoma subtypes, CNS involvement was identified in 3.3% of ALCL cases and in 3.2% of T-cell lymphoblastic lymphoma cases. Other T-cell lymphoma subtypes may spread to the CNS, including NK/T-cell lymphoma and mycosis fungoides. Mycosis fungoides, with or without large cell transformation, has been associated with secondary CNS involvement [41–43]. Nasal-type extranodal NK/T-cell lymphoma may rarely present with primary CNS involvement [36]. More likely is relapse within the CNS or direct extension from the nasal area into the CNS [44–47]. Hon et al. report a 78-year-old woman who presented with stage IE nasal-type natural killer cell lymphoma with the primary cite of disease located in a left elbow ulceration [45]. Three months later, the patient presented with blurry vision and was found to have bilateral hypopyon. An aqueous tap and lumbar puncture confirmed that NK cells were present, and a computed tomography scan revealed hemorrhagic lymphomatous infiltration. Luther et al. described a 37-year-old man with direct extension of nasal NK/T-cell lymphoma to the brain from the left orbit into the left frontal lobe [47]. Two cases have recently been described of intraocular involvement of NK/T-cell lymphoma, having spread from its nasal- or paranasal site of primary disease [44, 46].

Hypocalcemia and Hypomagnesemia

Low levels of serum calcium and magnesium have been reported in patients with CTCL [48]. In a retrospective review of 80 mycosis fungoides patients evaluated at the M.D. Anderson Cancer Center prior to 2000, the authors found that hypomagnesemia was present in 22.2% of patients with early stage disease (stages I), 38.5% of those with intermediate stage disease (stages II), and 67.5% of those with advanced stage disease (stages III and IV) [48]. Hypocalcemia was found in 8.3% of early stage mycosis fungoides patients, 54.5% of those with intermediate stage disease, and 61% of those with advanced stage disease.

The etiology for these electrolyte disturbances is unclear. One possible explanation for the hypocalcemia is its relation to preexisting magnesium depletion. The release of parathyroid hormone is inhibited under conditions of hypomagnesemia, and this can result in secondary hypocalcemia [49]. Through its role in impairing immune function, magnesium deficiency may play a role in progression of mycosis fungoides [48]. Rats fed a magnesium-deficient diet that subsequently develop hypomagnesemia have been shown to develop T-cell lymphomas [50, 51].

Second Malignancies

CTCL patients are at risk for second malignancies, including malignant melanoma and second lymphomas [52–54]. Pielop et al. reported six cases of malignant melanoma among a database of 250 CTCL patients over a 3-year period [54]. In four of the melanoma cases, the melanoma was diagnosed prior to or concurrent with the diagnosis of CTCL. In the other two patients, dysplastic nevi were noted at the time of the CTCL diagnosis. The prevalence of malignant melanoma in the CTCL population under study was 2.4%, significantly higher than the 0.2% prevalence of melanoma in the general population [54]. Supporting data on the incidence of malignant melanoma in the CTCL population comes from a retrospective review of 285 cases of CTCL in London, England, in which six cases of melanoma were identified [52]. Of those six, four were diagnosed with melanoma after being diagnosed with CTCL, and two were diagnosed with melanoma prior to the CTCL diagnosis. While malignant melanoma was identified in 2.1% of the 285 cases of CTCL being studied, the crude rate of melanoma in the general population in England, London, in 1998 was 8.8/100,000 in men and 11.4/100,000 in women [52].

Huang and collaborators performed a retrospective study of two cohorts to assess the risks for developing second cancers in patients with mycosis fungoides or Sézary syndrome [53]. The first cohort consisted of the nine population-based U.S. cancer registries that make up the Surveillance, Epidemiology, and End Results Program (SEER-9); the second cohort consisted of the Stanford University referral center cohort of cutaneous lymphoma patients. The SEER-9 cohort included patients diagnosed between 1984 and 2001, and the Stanford cohort included those diagnosed between 1973 and 2001. Among the 1,798 CTCL patients that comprised the SEER-9 cohort, there were 197 second cancers diagnosed (standardized incidence ratio [SIR] of 1.32; 95% confidence interval [CI], 1.15–1.52). Patients with CTCL were at significantly increased risk for Hodgkin lymphoma (SIR = 17.14; 95% CI, 6.25–37.26), non-Hodgkin lymphoma

(SIR = 5.08; 95% CI, 3.34–7.38), melanoma (SIR = 2.6; 95% CI, 1.25–4.79), and urinary cancer (SIR = 1.74; 95% CI, 1.08–2.66). Among the 429 patients identified in the Stanford cohort, there were 37 second malignancies diagnosed (SIR = 1.04; 95% CI, 0.76–1.44). The Stanford University CTCL patients were at significantly increased risk for Hodgkin lymphoma (SIR = 27.27; 95% CI, 5.35–77.54) and cancer of the biliary system (SIR = 11.76; 95% CI, 1.51–42.02).

Management Issues Associated with Therapy

In the following section, we will review the unique management issues that exist for a variety of treatments used in T-cell lymphomas. The four FDA-approved drugs for CTCL—denileukin diftitox, bexarotene, vorinostat, and romidepsin—are each associated with distinctive side effect profiles, and these will be reviewed first. The unique features of pralatrexate, the first and only agent approved for peripheral T-cell lymphoma, will then be examined. Finally, we will review some investigational agents which have been demonstrated to have activity in T-cell lymphomas.

Denileukin Diftitox

Denileukin diftitox (DAB389IL; Ontak®) is a genetically engineered fusion protein that combines parts of the diphtheria toxin with the interleukin-2 (IL-2) receptor-binding domain. Denileukin diftitox has been shown to have activity in lymphoid malignancies. In 1999 the drug was granted approval by the FDA for the treatment of CTCL characterized by expression of the CD25 component of the IL-2 receptor.

Denileukin diftitox has been associated with a variety of acute infusion-related reactions. These include cutaneous reactions such as pruritis or flushing and systemic reactions such as dyspnea, chest pain or tightness, and back pain. Infusion-related symptoms typically occurred during or within 24 h of the infusion of the drug. Dyspnea occurred in 20% of patients in the pivotal phase III trial, back pain in 17%, hypotension in 17%, chest pain or tightness in 13%, pruritis in 13%, and flushing occurred in 13% of patients [55]. These reactions typically resolve after temporarily disrupting the infusion or after administration of antihistamines and/or corticosteroids [55]. Fever, chills, myalgias, arthralgias, headache, diarrhea, anorexia, and asthenia are also commonly associated with treatment with denileukin diftitox. Flu-like symptoms may be managed with antipyretics, antiemetics, and/or antidiarrheal agents. Vascular leak syndrome (VLS) occurs in up to 27% of patients receiving the drug [56]. VLS is characterized by edema, hypoalbuminemia (≤2.8 g/dL), and/or hypotension occurring within the first 14 days following treatment [55]. Steroid premedication prior to administration of denileukin diftitox with agents such as prednisone or dexamethasone can significantly reduce the risk of VLS [56].

Denileukin diftitox has been associated with visual changes in small numbers of patients [57, 58]. Dang et al. reported that two of 38 patients who received denileukin diftitox for relapsed/refractory B-cell non-Hodgkin lymphoma experienced visual changes felt to be associated with the drug [57]. The first patient experienced transient decreased visual acuity after receiving two cycles; however, the second patient experienced permanent loss of visual acuity after eight cycles. The exact mechanism is unclear. However, a potential link between altered T-cell immunity and autoimmune retinitis may exist as demonstrated in animal models [59].

Bexarotene

Bexarotene (Targretin®) is an oral synthetic retinoid that is selective for the retinoid X receptor (RXR). In 1999, bexarotene became the only retinoid to gain FDA approval for use in CTCL. Bexarotene leads to dose-dependent adverse effects including hypertriglyceridemia (82%), hypercholesterolemia (30%), central hypothyroidism (29%), and leukopenia (11%) [60].

Successful management of hypertriglyceridemia can be achieved through the use of lipid lowering agents, and there is evidence that response rates of bexarotene are higher when triglycerides are managed appropriately [61]. Fenofibrate has been shown to be effective as a triglyceride-lowering agent, either alone or in combination with a statin such as atorvastatin [61]. Patients should also be counseled on the adoption of a low-fat diet. Because of a paradoxical association with increased bexarotene levels, Gemfibrozil should not be used for the treatment of bexarotene-induced hypertriglyceridemia. In addition, Gemfibrozil has been associated with increased triglyceride levels and increased risk for pancreatitis [61]. Prescribing a lower starting dose of bexarotene (75–150 mg), monitoring weekly fasting triglyceride levels, and starting lipid-lowering agents 1 week prior to beginning therapy with bexarotene has been recommended as a useful therapeutic strategy [62].

Central hypothyroidism occurs in an estimated 29% of those receiving oral bexarotene therapy for CTCL [60]. Bexarotene has been shown to suppress thyrotropin secretion which results in reversible central hypothyroidism manifest by low thyroid stimulating hormone (TSH) and low T_4 levels [63]. TSH levels will remain low while the patient is taking bexarotene due to the drug's suppression of thyrotropin [61]. In view of its effect on thyroid hormonal axis, checking TSH and T_4 levels prior to beginning therapy with bexarotene followed by frequent monitoring of only free T_4 levels once bexarotene has been initiated would be recommended. Thyroid hormone supplementation should be administered and can improve T_4 levels as well as symptoms of cold intolerance and fatigue [61, 63].

Histone Deacetylase Inhibitors

Vorinostat (Zolinza®; Merck, Whitehouse Station, NJ) is an oral histone deacetylase (HDAC) inhibitor which was FDA approved for the treatment of relapsed or refractory CTCL in October 2006. In the pivotal phase IIB multicenter registration trial, the most common adverse events associated with the drug were gastrointestinal or constitutional symptoms, hematologic abnormalities (thrombocytopenia [21.6%]; anemia [12.2%]), or taste disturbances [64]. While most drug-related adverse events were grade 2 or lower, the grade 3 or higher adverse events included fatigue (5%), thromboembolic events (5%), thrombocytopenia (5%), and nausea (4%) [64]. Because of the risk for thromboembolic events, vorinostat should be used with caution in patients with a history of deep venous thrombosis or pulmonary embolism. Preclinical studies have raised concerns about the possibility of QTc prolongation as a class effect of the HDAC inhibitors. Electrocardiogram changes, including ST-T wave changes and QTc prolongation, were observed in the pivotal vorinostat trial; however, these electrocardiogram findings were clinically insignificant [64].

Romidepsin (Istotax®, Gloucester Pharmaceuticals, Cambridge, MA) is a novel HDAC inhibitor that, in early studies, has been shown to have activity in refractory CTCL and peripheral T-cell lymphoma [65–67]. Romidepsin was granted FDA approval for use in CTCL in November 2009. In a phase II multi-institutional trial of romidepsin, the drug was initially administered as a 4 h infusion at 18 mg/m² on days 1 and 5 of a 21-day cycle [66]. This schedule was altered, by amendment to the trial, to a more tolerable dosing schedule of 14 mg/m² on days 1, 8, and 15 of a 28-day cycle. In a total of 71 patients, the most common non-hematologic adverse events included nausea (52%), fatigue (41%), vomiting (20%), and anorexia (21%). The most common hematological adverse events included thrombocytopenia (37%), anemia (37%), neutropenia (37%), and lymphopenia (21%). Grade 1 hyperuricemia occurred in 11% of patients, and grade 4 hyperuricemia occurred in 4%. Other electrolyte abnormalities (any grade) that were seen included hypocalcemia in 42%, hypomagnesemia in 15%, and hypophosphatemia in 8%.

The evaluation of potential cardiac adverse effects was also systematically evaluated in the recently published phase II trial of romidepsin [66, 68]. In the 71 patients in the trial, 20 patients had cardiac events [66]. These included QTc prolongation in 16 patients, atrial fibrillation in three, supraventricular and ventricular ectopy in three, sinus bradycardia in two, and junctional rhythm in one patient. Piekarz and colleagues noted that eight of the 16 patients who experienced QTc prolongation were noted to have had preexisting abnormal QTc intervals of greater than 450 ms. In addition, there may be some effect on the QTc interval of antiemetics and concomitant medications which may be metabolized through CYP3A4 [66, 69]. The authors caution the use of drugs which prolong the QTc interval or inhibit the CYP3A4 enzyme concurrent with the use of romidepsin. In addition, electrolyte replacement and routine monitoring of serum potassium and magnesium levels is recommended [66, 68].

Pralatrexate

Pralatrexate (Folotyn®; Allos Therapeutics, Inc., Westminster, CO), structurally similar to methotrexate, is a drug in the 10-deazaaminopterin class of folate analogs. It has recently been shown to have activity in chemotherapy-refractory T-cell lymphomas [70, 71], and it gained FDA approval in September 2009 for use in relapsed or refractory peripheral T-cell lymphoma. The major toxicities of pralatrexate were dose-dependent and consisted of stomatitis and myelosuppression (grade 3 or 4 leukopenia, lymphopenia, and thrombocytopenia) [71]. Vitamin supplementation with folic acid (5 mg orally beginning 3 days prior to initiation of therapy) and vitamin B12 (1,000 μg orally daily or 100 μg intramuscularly every 8–9 weeks) reduces the risk of both stomatitis and myelosuppression [71].

Other Agents

Gemcitabine (Gemzar®; Eli Lilly and Company, Indianapolis, IN) is a nucleoside analog that inhibits DNA synthesis. It has activity in a wide variety of solid tumors as well as in hematologic malignancies [72]. Gemcitabine has been studied in relapsed or refractory peripheral T-cell lymphoma and CTCL [73–76]. The most common adverse effects of this drug include myelosuppression, elevation of hepatic transaminases, hyperpigmentation [76]. There have been rare cases of hemolytic-uremic syndrome during therapy with gemcitabine [76].

Horwitz et al. reported results from their phase I/IIA study evaluating the combination of pralatrexate and gemcitabine in patients with relapsed or refractory lymphoid malignancies [77]. Preliminary results revealed that when these drugs were used more frequently than once every 2 weeks, the grade 3 and 4 hematologic toxicity rendered the regimen very poorly tolerated by the heavily pretreated patients in the study. Grade 3 or 4 neutropenia and thrombocytopenia were experienced by 9 of 20 patients (45%), and grade 3 or 4 anemia was experienced by 8 of 20 patients (40%).

Pentostatin, an adenosine deaminase inhibitor that is selectively toxic to lymphocytes, has been shown to have activity in T-cell malignancies [78–81]. The major adverse effects of pentostatin include hematologic toxicity (including lymphopenia), renal insufficiency, nausea, and conjunctivitis [82]. Pentostatin-associated lymphopenia is likely due to selective depletion of CD26+ T-lymphocytes as demonstrated by Dang et al. [79]. CD26+ is a marker of activated T-lymphocytes, and their depletion—and subsequent suppression of the immune system—may explain the increased susceptibility to opportunistic infections in patients receiving pentostatin [79]. Cardiac toxicity has also been observed after pentostatin use. In patients with predisposing conditions—such as coronary artery disease, congestive heart failure, and hypertension—an association with angina, myocardial infarction, arrhythmias, and heart failure has been identified [83]. The risk of nephrotoxicity is dose-dependent, and renal toxicity is more likely to occur at doses higher than 4 mg/m^2/week [81, 84, 85]. Because of the risk for renal and cardiac toxicity, one should consider optimizing medical management of any preexisting cardiac disease, avoiding fluid overload or dehydration, and reducing the dose of pentostatin in those with impaired renal function [83].

Alemtuzumab (Campath®; Genzyme Corporation, Cambridge, MA/Berlex Oncology, Wayne, NJ) is a monoclonal antibody which targets CD52, an antigen expressed on most B and T lymphocytes. Approved for use in B-cell chronic lymphocytic lymphoma (CLL), alemtuzumab has also demonstrated activity in advanced CTCL and relapsed or refractory peripheral T-cell lymphoma [86, 87]. In clinical trials, patients have had a high risk of infectious complications, likely due to a combination of factors including underlying lymphoid malignancy, exposure to prior therapies, and possibly disease refractoriness [88]. Alemtuzumab, because of the prolonged depression of B and T lymphocytes, increases this risk for significant infectious complications, including reactivation of cytomegalovirus (CMV) and opportunistic infections. CMV reactivation may occur in 15–25% of patients who receive alemtuzumab [88]. It is recommended that patients receive prophylaxis for *Pneumocystis pneumonia* (PCP) and herpes virus infections, and these prophylactic anti-infective agents should be continued for at least 2 months after completing therapy [88].

In addition to the infectious complications resulting from immune suppression, alemtuzumab is associated with infusion-related toxicity and myelosuppression. Fever, rigors, rash, nausea and vomiting, and hypotension may occur with intravenous administration. Administration of premedications, such as acetaminophen and antihistamines, and administration of prophylactic steroids may reduce the risk of these infusion-related side effects [88, 89]. While the approved dosing of alemtuzumab is intravenous, subcutaneous administration has been shown to be feasible, effective, and associated with less risk of infusion-related toxicity in treatment of chronic lymphocytic leukemia [90]. Subcutaneous administration is associated with transient first-dose skin reactions (erythema and edema), and premedications can alleviate the risk of this reaction [90]. Patients may experience transient mild cytopenias including delayed neutropenia or, less commonly, thrombocytopenia [87].

Bortezomib (Velcade®; Millenium Pharmaceuticals, Cambridge, MA) is a proteasome inhibitor which is FDA-approved for use in multiple myeloma and in mantle cell lymphoma. A phase II trial in relapsed or refractory CTCL confirmed that bortezomib has activity in both in CTCL and in peripheral T-cell lymphoma with skin involvement [91]. In the small phase II trial, there was no grade 4 toxicity; however, grade 3 toxicities included neutropenia, thrombocytopenia, and peripheral neuropathy [91]. These toxicities are consistent with those experienced when using bortezomib in multiple myeloma and mantle cell lymphoma. Dose modifications are recommended (per package insert) in the event of neutropenia, thrombocytopenia, neuropathic pain, or peripheral neuropathy.

Pegylated liposomal doxorubicin (Doxil; Ortho Biotech Products LP, Bridgewater, NJ) is an anthracycline, doxorubicin, which has been formulated in such a way that allows for longer half-life, reduced toxicity, and improved efficacy [92, 93]. In addition to its activity in solid tumors, such as ovarian cancer, and multiple myeloma, this agent has been shown to have activity in CTCL [94, 95]. The dose-limiting toxicity of pegylated liposomal doxorubicin is mucositis, however, mucositis typically occurs at very high doses (70 mg/m^2) [93]. Palmar plantar erythroderma (PPE), also known as hand-foot syndrome, is a more commonly experienced side effect. The risk of PPE is reduced when the dose is lowered or when the frequency of administration of doses is decreased. The cardiac toxicity of pegylated liposomal doxorubicin is dose dependent, but there is some controversy about the cumulative dose limit. The risk of cardiac effects is less than that of traditional doxorubicin [93].

Zanolimumab (HuMax-CD4®; Genmab, Copenhagen, Denmark) is a humanized monoclonal antibody which targets CD4, found in the T-cell receptor complex, thus blocking receptor-mediated T-cell signaling. Through this action, the drug induces antibody-dependent cell-mediated toxicity of neoplastic CD4+ T-lymphocytes. Zanolimumab was shown to have dose-dependent activity in refractory CTCL [96]. Side effects of this antibody include low-grade infections, primarily of skin and upper respiratory tract, and eczematous dermatitis [96].

The chimeric monoclonal antibody, SGN-30, targets cells that express CD30. CD30 is expressed in several hematologic malignancies, including

ALCL, the Reed Sternberg cell of Hodgkin lymphoma, and lesions of mycosis fungoides. It is also expressed in lymphomatoid papulosis. Preliminary data from phase II studies have indicated that SGN-30 has activity in refractory CD30+ ALCL as well as other CD30+ lymphoproliferative disorders [97, 98]. In these preliminary reports, SGN-30 appears to be well tolerated.

Siplizumab (MEDI-507) is a humanized monoclonal antibody directed at the CD2 receptor on T- and NK-cells. Preliminary results from two phase I trials in CD2-positive T-cell lymphoproliferative disorders showed encouraging results [99, 100]. Because of an association with the development of EBV-associated lymphoproliferative diseases (LPD), these trials were stopped early [101]. In 29 patients who received siplizumab for their T-cell malignancy, four patients (13.7%) developed an EBV-associated LPD [101]. The incidence of EBV-associated LPD occurred more in those patients treated on a weekly schedule (3 out of 7 patients, or 43%) than in those treated biweekly (1 out of 22 patients, or 4.5%). The patients who developed EBV-associated LPD were found to have significantly greater T-cell and NK-cell depletion.

In addition to the FDA-approved HDAC inhibitors, vorinostat and romidepsin, there are other HDAC inhibitors under investigation for use in T-cell lymphomas. Panobinostat (LBH589), an HDAC inhibitor available in an oral and an intravenous formulation, is being evaluated in a phase I dose-escalation study in patients with solid tumors and non-Hodgkin's lymphoma, and the oral HDAC inhibitor induced responses in the cohort of CTCL patients ($n=10$) [102]. Two patients achieved a complete response, four achieved a partial response, and one achieved stable disease. The maximum tolerated dose and schedule was found to be 20 mg orally on days 1, 3, and 5, weekly. In this small sample size of patients, the most common side effects were nausea, anorexia, fatigue, diarrhea, and transient neutropenia and thrombocytopenia; one patient experienced atrial fibrillation [102]. A phase II trial of panobinostat in refractory CTCL is currently ongoing and preliminary results confirm similar adverse events but also identified a small incidence of QTc prolongation [103]. Of 4,542 electrocardiograms, four were noted to have a prolongation of more than 60 ms from baseline, and two were found to have QTc intervals of more than 480 ms [103]. As with vorinostat and romidepsin, it is not clear that these QTc interval prolongations are clinically relevant [104].

Lenalidomide (Revlimid®; Celgene, Summit, NJ) is an immunomodulatory drug which is FDA-approved for the treatment of multiple myeloma and myelodysplastic syndrome. It is currently under investigation in CTCL [105] and in T-cell lymphomas other than CTCL [106]. In the CTCL phase II study, four of the nine evaluable patients experienced grade 1 fatigue, three experienced grade 2 lower extremity edema, and one patient each experienced grade 1 gastrointestinal symptoms and grade 2 anemia [105]. Hematologic toxicity was the primary toxicity reported in the recent phase II trial using lenalidomide in other T-cell lymphomas. Out of 23 evaluable patients, grade 4 thrombocytopenia occurred in 33% and grade 3 neutropenia occurred in almost 21% [106]. Febrile neutropenia and pain were each reported in 16.7% of the 23 patients.

An inhibitor of purine nucleoside phosphorylase (PNP), forodesine leads to intracellular accumulation of deoxyguanosine triphosphate resulting in apoptosis. Oral forodesine has shown activity in refractory CTCL, and the optimal dose has been determined to be 80 mg/m^2 daily [107]. Of 56 patients treated on the phase I/II dose escalation trial, grade 3 or higher adverse which occurred in two patients each included diarrhea, rash, cellulitis, and acute renal failure [108]. Occurring in one patient each were grade 3 vertigo, edema, and pneumonia. Lymphopenia (grade 3 or higher) occurred in 71% of patients, and there was one episode each of neutropenia (grade 1) and anemia (grade 3) [108]. For nine patients who received forodesine for more than 12 months, the most common adverse events were nausea ($n=4$), fatigue ($n=2$), peripheral edema ($n=2$), dyspnea ($n=2$), and urinary casts ($n=2$) [107]. None of the nine patients experienced hematologic or infection-related adverse events due to forodesine.

References

1. Coiffier B, Brousse N, Peuchmaur M, et al. Peripheral T-cell lymphomas have a worse prognosis than B-cell lymphomas: a prospective study of 361 immunophenotyped patients treated with the LNH-84 regimen. The GELA (Groupe d'Etude des Lymphomes Agressives). Ann Oncol. 1990; 1:45–50.
2. Gisselbrecht C, Gaulard P, Lepage E, et al. Prognostic significance of T-cell phenotype in aggressive non-Hodgkin's lymphomas. Blood. 1998;92:76–82.
3. Melnyk A, Rodriguez A, Pugh WC, Cabannillas F. Evaluation of the revised European-American lymphoma classification confirms the clinical relevance of immunophenotype in 560 cases of aggressive non-Hodgkin's lymphoma. Blood. 1997;89: 4514–20.
4. Rudiger T, Weisenburger DD, Anderson JR, et al. Peripheral T-cell lymphoma (excluding anaplastic large-cell lymphoma): results from the non-Hodgkin's lymphoma classification project. Ann Oncol. 2002;13:140–9.
5. Chang CS, Wang CH, Su IJ, Chen YC, Shen MC. Hematophagic histiocytosis: a clinicopathologic analysis of 23 cases with special reference to the association with peripheral T-cell lymphoma. J Formos Med Assoc. 1994;93:421–8.
6. Falini B, Pileri S, De Solas I, et al. Peripheral T-cell lymphoma associated with hemophagocytic syndrome. Blood. 1990;75:434–44.
7. Saragoni A, Falini B, Medri L, et al. [Peripheral T-cell lymphoma associated with hemophagocytic syndrome: a recently identified entity. Clinicopathologic and immunohistochemical study of 2 cases]. Pathologica. 1990;82:359–69.
8. Imashuku S. Clinical features and treatment strategies of Epstein-Barr virus-associated hemophagocytic lymphohistiocytosis. Crit Rev Oncol Hematol. 2002;44:259–72.
9. Janka GE, Schneider EM. Modern management of children with haemophagocytic lymphohistiocytosis. Br J Haematol. 2004;124:4–14.
10. Han AR, Lee HR, Park BB, et al, Lymphoma-associated hemophagocytic syndrome: clinical features and treatment outcome. Ann Hematol. 2007; 86:493–498.
11. Tong H, Ren Y, Liu H, et al. Clinical characteristics of T-cell lymphoma associated with hemophagocytic syndrome: comparison of T-cell lymphoma with and without hemophagocytic syndrome. Leuk Lymphoma. 2008;49:81–7.
12. Tong H, Ren Y, Qian W, et al. Clinicopathological study on peripheral T-cell non-Hodgkin lymphoma with bone marrow involvement: a retrospective analysis from China. Int J Hematol. 2009;90(3):303–10.
13. Axelrod PI, Lorber B, Vonderheid EC. Infections complicating mycosis fungoides and Sezary syndrome. JAMA. 1992;267:1354–8.
14. Tokura Y, Heald PW, Yan SL, Edelson RL. Stimulation of cutaneous T-cell lymphoma cells with superantigenic staphylococcal toxins. J Invest Dermatol. 1992;98:33–7.
15. Tokura Y, Yagi H, Ohshima A, et al. Cutaneous colonization with staphylococci influences the disease activity of Sezary syndrome: a potential role for bacterial superantigens. Br J Dermatol. 1995;133:6–12.
16. Nguyen V, Huggins RH, Lertsburapa T, et al. Cutaneous T-cell lymphoma and Staphylococcus aureus colonization. J Am Acad Dermatol. 2008;59:949–52.
17. Talpur R, Bassett R, Duvic M. Prevalence and treatment of Staphylococcus aureus colonization in patients with mycosis fungoides and Sezary syndrome. Br J Dermatol. 2008;159:105–12.
18. Negro-Vilar A, Dziewanowska Z, Groves ES, Stevens V, Zhang JK, Prince M, et al. Efficacy and safety of denileukin diftitox (Dd) in a phase III, double-blind, placebo-controlled study of CD25+ patients with cutaneous T-cell lymphoma (CTCL). J Clin Oncol. 2007;18S:8026.
19. Cairo MS, Bishop M. Tumour lysis syndrome: new therapeutic strategies and classification. Br J Haematol. 2004;127:3–11.
20. Fer MF, Bottino GC, Sherwin SA, et al. Atypical tumor lysis syndrome in a patient with T cell lymphoma treated with recombinant leukocyte interferon. Am J Med. 1984;77:953–6.
21. Hirata Y, Yokote T, Kobayashi K, et al. Syndrome of inappropriate antidiuretic hormone associated with chemotherapy-induced tumor lysis in a patient with peripheral T-cell lymphoma unspecified. Leuk Lymphoma. 2009;50:1226–9.
22. Hsu HH, Huang CC. Acute spontaneous tumor lysis in anaplastic large T-cell lymphoma presenting with hyperuricemic acute renal failure. Int J Hematol. 2004;79:48–51.
23. Kaneki T, Hachiya T, Hayano T, et al. [Tumor lysis syndrome after treatment for mediastinal non-Hodgkin's lymphoma]. Nihon Kyobu Shikkan Gakkai Zasshi. 1997;35:414–9.
24. Lerza R, Botta M, Barsotti B, et al. Dexamethazone-induced acute tumor lysis syndrome in a T-cell malignant lymphoma. Leuk Lymphoma. 2002; 43:1129–32.
25. Tiley C, Grimwade D, Findlay M, et al. Tumour lysis following hydrocortisone prior to a blood product transfusion in T-cell acute lymphoblastic leukaemia. Leuk Lymphoma. 1992;8:143–6.
26. Wester JP, Breumelhof R, Geers AB, Meuwissen OJ. [Acute tumor lysis syndrome due to mono-therapy with a corticosteroid in a patient with non-Hodgkin lymphoma]. Ned Tijdschr Geneeskd. 1997;141:1621–3.
27. Fritsch-Stork RD, Leguit RJ, Derksen RH. Rapidly fatal HTLV-1-associated T-cell leukemia/lymphoma in a patient with SLE. Nat Rev Rheumatol. 2009;5:283–7.
28. Bouaziz J-D, Cordel N, Hickman G, Fieschi C, Ortonne N, Bagot M. Cutaneous tumor lysis

syndrome in a patient with HTLV-1 adult T-cell lymphoma/leukemia. Blood. 2009;114:4320–1.
29. Kopterides P, Lignos M, Mavrou I, Armaganidis A. Steroid-induced tumor lysis syndrome in a patient with mycosis fungoides treated for presumed Pneumocystis carinii pneumonia. Am J Hematol. 2005;80:309.
30. Paul T, Challa S, Tandon A, Panigrahi M, Purohit A. Primary central nervous system lymphomas: Indian experience, and review of literature. Indian J Cancer. 2008;45:112–8.
31. Salzburg J, Burkhardt B, Zimmermann M, et al. Prevalence, clinical pattern, and outcome of CNS involvement in childhood and adolescent non-Hodgkin's lymphoma differ by non-Hodgkin's lymphoma subtype: a Berlin-Frankfurt-Munster Group Report. J Clin Oncol. 2007;25:3915–22.
32. Kadan-Lottick NS, Skluzacek MC, Gurney JG. Decreasing incidence rates of primary central nervous system lymphoma. Cancer. 2002;95:193–202.
33. Colen CB, Rayes M, Kupsky WJ, Guthikonda M. Synchronous meningioma and anaplastic large cell lymphoma. Neuropathology. 2010;30(3):260–6.
34. Dungerwalla M, Osuji N, Waldman AD, et al. Isolated central nervous system involvement in adult T-cell lymphoma/leukaemia. Br J Haematol. 2005;130:511–5.
35. Kawamura T, Inamura T, Ikezaki K, Miyazono M, Ishihara S, Fukui M. Primary Ki-1 lymphoma in the central nervous system. J Clin Neurosci. 2001;8:574–7.
36. Omori N, Narai H, Tanaka T, et al. Epstein-Barr virus-associated T/NK cell-type central nervous system lymphoma which manifested as a post-transplantation lymphoproliferative disorder in a renal transplant recipient. J Neurooncol. 2008;87:189–91.
37. Shenkier TN, Blay JY, O'Neill BP, et al. Primary CNS lymphoma of T-cell origin: a descriptive analysis from the international primary CNS lymphoma collaborative group. J Clin Oncol. 2005;23:2233–9.
38. Levin N, Soffer D, Grissaru S, Aizikovich N, Gomori JM, Siegal T. Primary T-cell CNS lymphoma presenting with leptomeningeal spread and neurolymphomatosis. J Neurooncol. 2008;90:77–83.
39. Marsh Jr WL, Stevenson DR, Long Jr HJ. Primary leptomeningeal presentation of T cell lymphoma. Report of a patient and review of the literature. Cancer. 1983;51:1125–31.
40. Dulai MS, Park CY, Howell WD, et al. CNS T-cell lymphoma: an under-recognized entity? Acta Neuropathol. 2008;115:345–56.
41. Chua SL, Seymour JF, Prince HM. Deafness from eighth cranial nerve involvement in a patient with large cell transformation of mycosis fungoides. Eur J Haematol. 2000;64:340–3.
42. Stein M, Farrar N, Jones GW, et al. Central neurologic involvement in mycosis fungoides: ten cases, actuarial risk assessment, and predictive factors. Cancer J. 2006;12:55–62.
43. Vu BA, Duvic M. Central nervous system involvement in patients with mycosis fungoides and cutaneous large-cell transformation. J Am Acad Dermatol. 2008;59:S16–22.
44. Cimino L, Chan CC, Shen D, et al. Ocular involvement in nasal natural killer T-cell lymphoma. Int Ophthalmol. 2009;29:275–9.
45. Hon C, Kwok AKH, Shek TWH, Au WY. Unusual locations of involvement by malignancies: Case 4. Bilateral hypopyon heralding CNS relapse of cutaneous natural killer cell lymphoma. J Clin Oncol. 2003;21:3373–4.
46. Lee EJ, Kim TW, Heo JW, Yu HG, Chung H. Natural killer/T-cell lymphoma of nasal type with intraocular involvement: case report. Eur J Ophthalmol. 2010;20(1):215–7.
47. Luther N, Greenfield JP, Chadburn A, Schwartz TH. Intracranial nasal natural killer/T-cell lymphoma: immunopathologically-confirmed case and review of literature. J Neurooncol. 2005;75:185–8.
48. Morgan M, Maloney D, Duvic M. Hypomagnesemia and hypocalcemia in mycosis fungoides: a retrospective case series. Leuk Lymphoma. 2002;43:1297–302.
49. Cooper MS, Gittoes NJ. Diagnosis and management of hypocalcaemia. BMJ. 2008;336:1298–302.
50. Averdunk R, Bippus PH, Gunther T, Merker HJ. Development and properties of malignant lymphoma induced by magnesium deficiency in rats. J Cancer Res Clin Oncol. 1982;104:63–73.
51. Hass GM, Galt RM, Laing GH, Coogan PS, Maganini RO, Friese JA. Induction of a rat T cell lymphoma-leukemia by magnesium deficiency—a study of fetal defense against maternal neoplasia. Magnesium. 1989;8:45–55.
52. Evans AV, Scarisbrick JJ, Child FJ, Acland KM, Whittaker SJ, Russell-Jones R. Cutaneous malignant melanoma in association with mycosis fungoides. J Am Acad Dermatol. 2004;50:701–5.
53. Huang KP, Weinstock MA, Clarke CA, McMillan A, Hoppe RT, Kim YH. second lymphomas and other malignant neoplasms in patients with mycosis fungoides and Sezary syndrome: evidence from population-based and clinical cohorts. Arch Dermatol. 2007;143:45–50.
54. Pielop JA, Brownell I, Duvic M. Mycosis fungoides associated with malignant melanoma and dysplastic nevus syndrome. Int J Dermatol. 2003;42:116–22.
55. Olsen E, Duvic M, Frankel A, et al. Pivotal phase III trial of two dose levels of denileukin diftitox for the treatment of cutaneous T-cell lymphoma. J Clin Oncol. 2001;19:376–88.
56. Foss FM, Bacha P, Osann KE, Demierre MF, Bell T, Kuzel T. Biological correlates of acute hypersensitivity events with DAB(389)IL-2 (denileukin diftitox, ONTAK) in cutaneous T-cell lymphoma: decreased frequency and severity with steroid premedication. Clin Lymphoma. 2001;1:298–302.
57. Dang NH, Fayad L, McLaughlin P, et al. Phase II trial of the combination of denileukin diftitox and rituximab for relapsed/refractory B-cell non-Hodgkin lymphoma. Br J Haematol. 2007;138:502–5.

58. Ruddle JB, Harper CA, Honemann D, Seymour JF, Prince HM. A denileukin diftitox (Ontak) associated retinopathy? Br J Ophthalmol. 2006;90:1070–1.
59. Takeuchi M, Keino H, Kezuka T, Usui M, Taguchi O. Immune responses to retinal self-antigens in CD25(+)CD4(+) regulatory T-cell-depleted mice. Invest Ophthalmol Vis Sci. 2004;45:1879–86.
60. Duvic M, Hymes K, Heald P, et al. Bexarotene is effective and safe for treatment of refractory advanced-stage cutaneous T-cell lymphoma: multinational phase II–III trial results. J Clin Oncol. 2001;19:2456–71.
61. Talpur R, Ward S, Apisarnthanarax N, Breuer-Mcham J, Duvic M. Optimizing bexarotene therapy for cutaneous T-cell lymphoma. J Am Acad Dermatol. 2002;47:672–84.
62. Zhang C, Duvic M. Treatment of cutaneous T-cell lymphoma with retinoids. Dermatol Ther. 2006; 19:264–71.
63. Sherman SI, Gopal J, Haugen BR, et al. Central hypothyroidism associated with retinoid X receptor-selective ligands. N Engl J Med. 1999;340:1075–9.
64. Olsen EA, Kim YH, Kuzel TM, et al. Phase IIb multicenter trial of vorinostat in patients with persistent, progressive, or treatment refractory cutaneous T-cell lymphoma. J Clin Oncol. 2007;25:3109–15.
65. Kim Y, Reddy S, Kim EJ, et al. Romidepsin (depsipeptide) induces clinically significant responses in treatment-refractory CTCL: an international, multicenter study. Blood. 2007;110:123a.
66. Piekarz RL, Frye R, Turner M, et al. Phase II multi-institutional trial of the histone deacetylase inhibitor romidepsin as monotherapy for patients with cutaneous T-cell lymphoma. J Clin Oncol. 2009; 27:5410–7.
67. Piekarz RL, Robey R, Sandor V, et al. Inhibitor of histone deacetylation, depsipeptide (FR901228), in the treatment of peripheral and cutaneous T-cell lymphoma: a case report. Blood. 2001;98:2865–8.
68. Piekarz RL, Frye AR, Wright JJ, et al. Cardiac studies in patients treated with depsipeptide, FK228, in a phase II trial for T-cell lymphoma. Clin Cancer Res. 2006;12:3762–73.
69. Cabell C, Bates S, Piekarz R, et al. Systematic assessment of potential cardiac effects of the novel histone deacetylase (HDAC) inhibitor romidepsin [abstract]. J Clin Oncol. 2009;27:e19533.
70. O'Connor OA, Hamlin PA, Portlock C, et al. Pralatrexate, a novel class of antifol with high affinity for the reduced folate carrier-type 1, produces marked complete and durable remissions in a diversity of chemotherapy refractory cases of T-cell lymphoma. Br J Haematol. 2007;139:425–8.
71. O'Connor OA, Horwitz S, Hamlin P, et al. Phase II-I-II study of two different doses and schedules of pralatrexate, a high-affinity substrate for the reduced folate carrier, in patients with relapsed or refractory lymphoma reveals marked activity in T-cell malignancies. J Clin Oncol. 2009;27:4357–64.
72. Nabhan C, Krett N, Gandhi V, Rosen S. Gemcitabine in hematologic malignancies. Curr Opin Oncol. 2001;13:514–21.
73. Sallah S, Wan JY, Nguyen NP. Treatment of refractory T-cell malignancies using gemcitabine. Br J Haematol. 2001;113:185–7.
74. Zinzani PL, Baliva G, Magagnoli M, et al. Gemcitabine treatment in pretreated cutaneous T-cell lymphoma: experience in 44 patients. J Clin Oncol. 2000;18:2603–6.
75. Zinzani PL, Magagnoli M, Bendandi M, et al. Therapy with gemcitabine in pretreated peripheral T-cell lymphoma patients. Ann Oncol. 1998;9: 1351–3.
76. Duvic M, Talpur R, Wen S, Kurzrock R, David CL, Apisarnthanarax N. Phase II evaluation of gemcitabine monotherapy for cutaneous T-cell lymphoma. Clin Lymphoma Myeloma. 2006;7:51–8.
77. Horwitz SM, Vose JM, Advani R, et al. A phase 1/2A open-label study of pralatrexate and gemcitabine in patients with relapsed or refractory lymphoproliferative malignancies [ASH annual meeting abstracts]. Blood. 2008;112:1570.
78. Cummings FJ, Kim K, Neiman RS, et al. Phase II trial of pentostatin in refractory lymphomas and cutaneous T-cell disease. J Clin Oncol. 1991; 9:565–71.
79. Dang NH, Hagemeister FB, Duvic M, et al. Pentostatin in T-non-Hodgkin's lymphomas: efficacy and effect on CD26+ T lymphocytes. Oncol Rep. 2003;10:1513–8.
80. Greiner D, Olsen EA, Petroni G. Pentostatin (2′-deoxycoformycin) in the treatment of cutaneous T-cell lymphoma. J Am Acad Dermatol. 1997; 36:950–5.
81. Grever MR, Bisaccia E, Scarborough DA, Metz EN, Neidhart JA. An investigation of 2′-deoxycoformycin in the treatment of cutaneous T-cell lymphoma. Blood. 1983;61:279–82.
82. Foss FM. Activity of pentostatin (Nipent) in cutaneous T-cell lymphoma: single-agent and combination studies. Semin Oncol. 2000;27:58–63.
83. Grem JL, King SA, Chun HG, Grever MR. Cardiac complications observed in elderly patients following 2′-deoxycoformycin therapy. Am J Hematol. 1991;38:245–7.
84. Kintzel PE. Anticancer drug-induced kidney disorders. Drug Saf. 2001;24:19–38.
85. Major PP, Agarwal RP, Kufe DW. Clinical pharmacology of deoxycoformycin. Blood. 1981;58:91–6.
86. Enblad G, Hagberg H, Erlanson M, et al. A pilot study of alemtuzumab (anti-CD52 monoclonal antibody) therapy for patients with relapsed or chemotherapy-refractory peripheral T-cell lymphomas. Blood. 2004;103:2920–4.
87. Lundin J, Hagberg H, Repp R, et al. Phase 2 study of alemtuzumab (anti-CD52 monoclonal antibody) in patients with advanced mycosis fungoides/Sezary syndrome. Blood. 2003;101:4267–72.

88. Dearden CE. Alemtuzumab in lymphoproliferate disorders. Rev Clin Exp Hematol. 2002;6:435–48; discussion 49–50.
89. Dearden CE, Matutes E. Alemtuzumab in T-cell lymphoproliferative disorders. Best Pract Res Clin Haematol. 2006;19:795–810.
90. Osterborg A, Foa R, Bezares RF, et al. Management guidelines for the use of alemtuzumab in chronic lymphocytic leukemia. Leukemia. 2009;23:1980–8.
91. Zinzani PL, Musuraca G, Tani M, et al. Phase II trial of proteasome inhibitor bortezomib in patients with relapsed or refractory cutaneous T-cell lymphoma. J Clin Oncol. 2007;25:4293–7.
92. Gabizon AA. Selective tumor localization and improved therapeutic index of anthracyclines encapsulated in long-circulating liposomes. Cancer Res. 1992;52:891–6.
93. Gabizon AA. Pegylated liposomal doxorubicin: metamorphosis of an old drug into a new form of chemotherapy. Cancer Invest. 2001;19:424–36.
94. Wollina U, Dummer R, Brockmeyer NH, et al. Multicenter study of pegylated liposomal doxorubicin in patients with cutaneous T-cell lymphoma. Cancer. 2003;98:993–1001.
95. Wollina U, Graefe T, Kaatz M. Pegylated doxorubicin for primary cutaneous T cell lymphoma: a report on ten patients with follow-up. Ann N Y Acad Sci. 2001;941:214–6.
96. Kim YH, Duvic M, Obitz E, et al. Clinical efficacy of zanolimumab (HuMax-CD4): two phase 2 studies in refractory cutaneous T-cell lymphoma. Blood. 2007;109:4655–62.
97. Forero-Torres A, Bernstein SH, Gopal A, et al. SGN-30 (Anti-CD30 mAb) has a single-agent response rate of 21% in patients with refractory or recurrent systemic anaplastic large cell lymphoma (ALCL) [ASH annual meeting abstracts]. Blood. 2006;108:2718.
98. Duvic M, Kim Y, Reddy S, et al. Phase II preliminary results of SGN-30 (anti-CD30 mAb) in patients with cd30+ lymphoproliferative disorders [ASH annual meeting abstracts]. Blood. 2006;108:2733.
99. Casale DA, Bartlett NL, Hurd DD, et al. A phase I open label dose escalation study to evaluate MEDI-507 in patients with CD2-positive T-cell lymphoma/leukemia [ASH annual meeting abstracts]. Blood. 2006;108:2727.
100. O'Mahony D, Morris JC, Stetler-Stevenson M, Matthews H, Brown MR, Fleisher T, et al. Phase I trial of siplizumab in CD2-positive lymphoproliferative disorders. Blood. 2005;106:3353a.
101. O'Mahony D, Morris JC, Stetler-Stevenson M, et al. EBV-related lymphoproliferative disease complicating therapy with the anti-CD2 monoclonal antibody, siplizumab, in patients with T-cell malignancies. Clin Cancer Res. 2009;15:2514–22.
102. Ellis L, Pan Y, Smyth GK, et al. Histone deacetylase inhibitor panobinostat induces clinical responses with associated alterations in gene expression profiles in cutaneous T-cell lymphoma. Clin Cancer Res. 2008;14:4500–10.
103. Duvic M, Becker JC, Dalle S, et al. Phase II trial of oral panobinostat (LBH589) in patients with refractory cutaneous T-cell lymphoma (CTCL) [ASH annual meeting abstracts]. Blood. 2008;112:1005.
104. Zhang L, Lebwohl D, Masson E, Laird G, Cooper MR, Prince HM. Clinically relevant QTc prolongation is not associated with current dose schedules of LBH589 (panobinostat). J Clin Oncol. 2008;26: 332–3; discussion 3–4.
105. Querfeld C, Kuzel TM, Guitart J, Rosen ST. Preliminary results of a phase II study of CC-5013 (Lenalidomide, Revlimid(R)) in patients with cutaneous T-cell lymphoma [ASH annual meeting abstracts]. Blood. 2005;106:3351.
106. Dueck GS, Chua N, Prasad A, et al. Activity of lenalidomide in a phase II trial for T-cell lymphoma: report on the first 24 cases [abstract]. J Clin Oncol. 2009;27:8524.
107. Duvic M, Forero-Torres A, Foss F, Olsen E, Pinter-Brown L, Kim Y. Long-term treatment of CTCL with the oral PNP inhibitor, forodesine [abstract]. J Clin Oncol. 2009;27:8552.
108. Duvic M, Forero-Torres A, Foss F, Olsen E, Kim Y. Response to oral forodesine in refractory cutaneous T-cell lymphoma: interim results of a phase I/II study [abstract]. Blood. 2007;110:122.

Index

F. Foss (ed.), *T-Cell Lymphomas*, Contemporary Hematology,
DOI 10.1007/978-1-62703-170-7, © Springer Science+Business Media New York 2013

MIX
Papier aus verantwortungsvollen Quellen
Paper from responsible sources
FSC® C105338

If you have any concerns about our products,
you can contact us on
ProductSafety@springernature.com

In case Publisher is established outside the EU,
the EU authorized representative is:
Springer Nature Customer Service Center GmbH
Europaplatz 3, 69115 Heidelberg, Germany

Printed by Libri Plureos GmbH
in Hamburg, Germany